Handbuch der experimentellen Pharmakologie

Vol. 41 Heffter-Heubner New Series

Handbook of Experimental Pharmacology

Hypolipidemic Agents

Contributors

W. L. Bencze · Mary E. Dempsey · S. Eisenberg
J. M. Felts · I. D. Frantz · R. Hess · D. Kritchevsky
R. I. Levy · T. A. Miettinen · L. L. Rudel
H. S. Sodhi · W. Stäubli · T. Zemplényi

Editor

David Kritchevsky

With 81 Figures

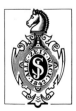

Springer-Verlag Berlin Heidelberg New York 1975

David Kritchevsky, Ph. D., The Wistar Institute of Anatomy and Biology, 36th Street at Spruce, Philadelphia PA 19104/USA

ISBN 3-540-07361-2 Springer-Verlag Berlin Heidelberg New York
ISBN 0-387-07361-2 Springer-Verlag New York Heidelberg Berlin

Library of Congress Cataloging in Publication Data. Main entry under title: Pharmacology of hypolipidemic agents. Handbuch der experimentellen Pharmakologie. New series; v. 41) Bibliography: p. Includes index. 1. Hyperlipoproteinemia. 2. Anticholesteremic agents. 3. Cholesterol metabolism. I. Kritchevsky, David, 1920- II. Series. QP905.H3 vol. 40, 1975 [RC632.H88] 615'.1'08s [616.3'99] 75-28022

© by Springer-Verlag Berlin · Heidelberg 1975.
Printed in Germany.

Type setting, printing, and binding: Brühlsche Universitätsdruckerei, Gießen

Preface

The major cause of death in the Western world is some form of vascular disease; and principal among these forms is atherosclerotic heart disease (ASHD). Although much is known about the etiology and treatment of ASHD, there is, as yet, no specific means of prognosis of an impending coronary episode. There are, however, several indications of susceptibility to coronary disease, generally known as risk factors, the foremost of which is hyperlipidemia. Hyperlipidemia is more commonly designated as hypercholesteremia or triglyceridemia, depending upon which moiety is elevated, but since lipids are transported in the blood as members of a lipoprotein complex, the most descriptive general term would be hyperlipoproteinemia.

This volume represents an effort to elucidate the origins and metabolic behavior of lipoproteins and their components, to describe aspects of the morphology, biochemistry and experimental induction of ASHD, and to describe modalities of treatment. The contributions to this book include descriptions of cholesterol synthesis and metabolism, as well as the metabolism of bile acids, the principal products of cholesterol metabolism. There are also chapters on the mechanisms of hyperlipidemia and on lipoprotein metabolism. The induction of experimental atherosclerosis and the aortic structural changes caused by this disease are discussed. Treatment of ASHD is described both in terms of these pharmaceutical preparations that lower levels of circulating lipids and in terms of the effect of drugs upon the metabolism of the aortic tissue, where effects relating to both induction and treatment of the disease are mediated. The rationale for such treatment is also discussed.

The field of atherosclerosis research is rapidly developing and major advances in diagnosis and treatment are anticipated. It is hoped that this book will serve as a basis for a greater understanding of current research and suggest fruitful directions for the future.

I would like to express my gratitude to Miss JANE T. KOLIMAGA for her skillful assistance in the preparation of the indices.

Philadelphia, PA, Summer 1975   DAVID KRITCHEVSKY

Table of Contents

CHAPTER 3

Bile Acid Metabolism. T. A. MIETTINEN. With 3 Figures

CHAPTER 4

Mechanisms of Hyperlipidemia. J. M. FELTS and L. L. RUDEL. With 3 Figures

CHAPTER 5

Lipoproteins and Lipoprotein Metabolism. S. EISENBERG and R. I. LEVY.
With 6 Figures

CHAPTER 6

Animal Models for Atherosclerosis Research. D. KRITCHEVSKY

CHAPTER 7

Lipoprotein Formation in the Liver Cell (Ultrastructural and Functional Aspects Relevant to Hypolipidemic Action). W. STÄUBLI and R. HESS. With 17 Figures

CHAPTER 8

Vascular Metabolism, Vascular Enzymes, and the Effect of Drugs. T. ZEMPLÉNYI. With 13 Figures

CHAPTER 9

Hypolipidemic Agents. W. L. BENCZE

CHAPTER 10

The Rationale for Hypolipemic Therapy. I. D. FRANTZ

List of Contributors

W. L. BENCZE, Ph. D., Research Laboratories of the Pharmaceutical Department of CIBA-GEIGY Limited, Basle/Switzerland

MARY E. DEMPSEY, Ph. D., Department of Biochemistry, University of Minnesota, Minneapolis, MN/USA

S. EISENBERG, M. D., Lipid Research Laboratory, Hadassah Medical School, Jerusalem/Israel

J. M. FELTS, Ph. D., Lipid Research Laboratory 151 G, Veterans Administration Hospital, San Francisco, CA/USA

I. D. FRANTZ, M. D., Department of Medicine, Medical School, Mayo-Memorial Building, University of Minnesota, Minneapolis, MN/USA

R. HESS, M. D., Research Laboratory of the Pharmaceutical Department of CIBA-GEIGY Limited, Basle/Switzerland

D. KRITCHEVSKY, Ph. D., The Wistar Institute of Anatomy and Biology, Philadelphia, PA/USA

R. I. LEVY, M. D., Section of Lipoproteins, Molecular Disease Branch, National Heart and Lung Institute, National Institutes of Health, Bethesda, MD/USA

T. A. MIETTINEN, M. D., Second Department of Medicine, University of Helsinki, Helsinki/Finland

L. L. RUDEL, Ph. D., Arterisclerosis Research Center, Bowman Gray School of Medicine of Wake Forest University, Winston-Salem, NC/USA

H. S. SODHI, M. D., Ph. D., Dept. of Medicine, University of Saskatchewan, Sakskatoon, Sask./Canada

W. STÄUBLI, Ph. D., Research Laboratory of the Pharmaceutical Department of CIBA-GEIGY Limited, Basle/Switzerland

T. ZEMPLENY, M. D., Department of Medicine, University of Southern California, School of Medicine, Cardiology Section, Los Angeles, CA/USA

CHAPTER 1

Cholesterol Biosynthesis in vitro

MARY E. DEMPSEY

With 27 Figures

The purpose of this chapter is to describe biochemical techniques (primarily those developed in this laboratory) for studying effects of hypolipidemic agents on cholesterol biosynthesis *in vitro*. Some current findings obtained by use of these techniques are included in the discussion of each procedure. The information presented here is not intended to be a comprehensive literature survey; it is meant to suggest approaches to an investigator desiring to study the mode of action of a potential hypolipidemic agent.

During development of a potential hypolipidemic agent it is essential to acquire as much information as possible on the site(s) and mechanism(s) of action of the new agent by studies *in vivo* and *in vitro*. Hypolipidemic agents having as one of their principal functions an inhibition of specific enzymic steps in cholesterol biosynthesis are readily characterized by experiments *in vitro*. In this regard, it is often desirable to demonstrate that a new agent does *not* act by blocking enzymic steps in the later stages of cholesterol biosyntheis (Fig. 1), i.e., agents acting specifically (at nanomolar or lower levels) in this manner are in general highly toxic *in vivo*, but useful tools for demonstrating pathways and intermediates in cholesterol synthesis and for preparation of biosynthetic intermediates (e. g. DEMPSEY 1965, 1967, 1968).

I. Cell-Free Homogenates

Applications. Homogenates prepared from rat liver are used for studies on the overall synthesis of cholesterol, i.e. the conversion of early precursors (acetate, mevalonate) through all the intermediate enzymic steps. If a potential hypolipidemic agent does not interfere with the overall conversion of labeled precursors to cholesterol by a liver homogenate, it is usually assumed that the site of action of the agent is not in this synthetic pathway. However, at elevated levels (e.g. greater than millimolar) a variety of compounds will interfere with cholesterol synthesis *in vitro* by blocking more than one enzymic step in a nonspecific manner, e.g. by detergent effects, chelation, etc. It is therefore important to ascertain the minimum level of an agent required for inhibition of cholesterol synthesis from early precursors and to determine, if possible, the site(s) of inhibition. Inhibitors acting at early stages (i.e. prior to squalene) in sterol synthesis cause a decrease in the level of nonsaponifiable compounds arising from acetate or mevalonate; those acting at later stages cause a change in the composition of the nonsaponifiable fraction. These inhibitors are usually found to block one enzymic step at low concentrations and additional steps when tested at higher concentrations.

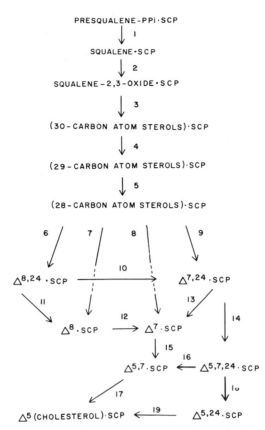

Fig. 1. An outline of pathways and intermediate compounds in the later stages of cholesterol biosynthesis; role of squalene and sterol carrier protein (SCP). Intermediates are shown as SCP complexes and positions of unsaturation are indicated by the delta (Δ) symbol. Adapted from DEMPSEY (1974)

If an agent at a low concentration blocks a specific step in cholesterol synthesis, the intermediate just prior to this step will accumulate. For example, agents acting on Δ^7-reductase (step 17, Fig. 1) cause the accumulation of $\Delta^{5,7}$-cholestadienol (7-dehydrocholesterol) (e.g. DVORNIK et al., 1963, 1964, 1966; RODNEY et al., 1965; those acting on Δ^{24}-reductase (step 19, Fig. 1) cause accumulation of $\Delta^{5,24}$-cholestadienol (demosterol) (e.g. BLOHM et al., 1970; RANNEY, 1967). Higher test concentrations of these agents cause accumulation of numerous intermediates and block early as well as later steps in cholesterol synthesis. As further illustration, studies *in vitro* with phenformin (DEMPSEY, 1967; 1968) and cholestane—3-β, 5α, 6β-triol and its analogs (DEMPSEY et al., 1970; WITIAK, et al., 1971a, 1971b; SCALLEN et al., 1971b) also indicate that more than one enzymic step in cholesterol synthesis was blocked, depending on the assay conditions employed.

Data presented in Fig. 2 are an indication of the type of results obtained with an inhibitor of cholesterol synthesis and a liver homogenate capable of converting acetate and mevalonate to cholesterol. In addition, Table 1 contains a selected list

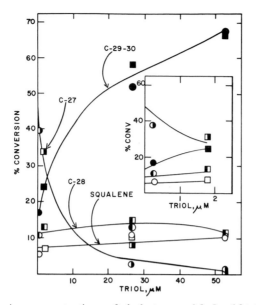

Fig. 2. Effects of varying concentrations of cholestane -3β, 5α, 6β-triol on the conversion of acetate and mevalonate to cholesterol by a liver homogenate; accumulation of 29—30-carbon atom sterols. Squares symbolize the conversions of mevalonate-2-^{14}C to products

(i.e. not comprehensive) of potential affectors of cholesterol synthesis recently studied using rat liver homogenates. For some purposes, it may be desirable to prepare homogenates from tissues other than liver by the technique described below. However the overall synthetic activity obtained with other tissues (e.g. brain (GROSSI-PAOLETTI, 1971) is usually lower than that of liver.

Preparation and Activity Assays. For preparation of a cell-free liver homogenate which will catalyze the conversion of acetate to cholesterol, it is essential to use a loose-fitting pestle during homogenization (BUCHER, 1953). Our procedure is as follows: female albino rats (150 to 200 g), fed *ad libitum*, are decapitated and exsanguinated. Livers are rapidly excised, trimmed of connective tissue, and chilled (4°, all the following manipulations are carried out at this temperature) in 0.1 M potassium phosphate buffer, pH 7.3. The livers are then minced and homogenized at moderate speed for 1.5 min in fresh buffer (2.5 ml per g liver) using a loose-fitting stainless steel pestle (1 mm clearance) and a thick-walled glass test tube. The total homogenate is centrifuged at 500 × g for 20 min and the sediment discarded. The supernatant is the cellfree homogenate. It is made fresh just prior to use. Many similar procedures are found in the literature; in our hands this is the most reliable.

A typical activity assay would contain the following constituents in addition to the agent to be tested: 0.1 M phosphate buffer (pH 7.35), 0.8 mM NADPH, NADP, and NAD, 5 mM ATP, and MgCl$_2$, sodium acetate or mevalonate (2 to 5 × 10^5 dpm; 2 to 4 mC/mmole), and 40 mg of cell-free homogenate (2 ml) in a final total incubation volume of 2.5 ml. Incubations are performed at 37° for 30 to 45 min in a Dubnoff shaker under air or oxygen. The enzymic reactions are terminated and saponifiable

Table 1. Selected list of recent studies employing liver homogenates to study factors affecting cholesterol synthesis *in vitro*[a]

Compound or factor tested	Substrate	Reference
Sex hormones, fatty acids	Mevalonate	CARROLL and PRITHAM (1966)
Bile salts	Lanosterol	MILLER and GAYLOR (1967)
Phenylalanine	Mevalonate	SHAH et al. (1968)
Vitamin E, Selenite, lipoic acid	Acetate and Mevalonate	ESKELSON and JACOBI (1969)
Phenformin and related biguanides	Cholest-5, 7-dienol, cholest-7-enol	DEMPSEY (1969 b)
Chlorophenoxyacetic acids	Acetate	WITIAK et al. (1969)
Cholestane derivatives	Acetate, mevalonate, cholest-7-enol	DEMPSEY et al (1970), WITIAK et al. (1971a), (1971b)
Ethanol	Acetate, mevalonate	ESKELSON et al. (1970a)
Fat soluble, vitamins	Acetate, mevalonate	ESKELSON et al. (1970b)
Plasma lipoproteins	Mevalonate	ONAJOBI and BOYD (1970)
Renal factors, kidney microsomes	Acetate, mevalonate	HAVEN and JACOBI (1971), THUY et al. (1973)
Steroid hormones	mevalonate	ONO and IMAI (1971)
3, 5-dihydroxy-3, 4, 4-trimethylvaleric acid	Mevalonate	HULCHER (1971)
Cyclic AMP	Acetate, squalene, lanosterol	BLOXHAM and AKHTAR (1971)
(—) Hydroxycitrate	Acetate	BARTH et al. (1972)
Liver factors	Acetate	GOODWIN and MARGOLIS (1973)

[a] This list does not include the numerous studies in which animals are fed a potential hypocholesterolemic agent and the effects of the agent *in vivo* examined by preparing homogenates of the livers of the animals to determine the possible occurrence of decreased synthesis rates (e. g. conversion of acetate or mevalonate to cholesterol; effects on HMG-CoA reductase activity).

compounds formed by addition of 2.5 ml of ethanol (95% v/v) and two KOH pellets. This mixture is allowed to stand at room temperature for at least one hour, followed by extraction of the nonsaponifiable fraction with petroleum ether (4×5 ml) and radioactivity measurement. Squalene, squalene epoxide, sterol intermediates (30-, 29-, 28-, and 27-carbon atom (including cholesterol) present in the nonsaponifiable fraction are separated and identified by their migration during silicic acid column chromatography relative to standard compounds according to the method of FRANTZ (1963). The latter technique is time consuming; however, it yields a wealth of information not obtainable with less sensitive methods (e.g. thin layer chromatography).

Typical levels of conversion of acetate and mevalonate to products by this method are given in Table 2. It should be noted that some investigators prefer to use tritiated water, labeled glucose, pyruvate, acetyl-CoA, or HMG-CoA (rather than labeled acetate or mevalonate) to measure cholesterol synthesis. With tritiated water, for example, there is no dilution of endogenous substrate levels (usually not accurately known in crude preparations) by addition of exogenous substrates and, therefore, rates of overall synthesis relative to the intact organ may be approached. This information is important in tissue culture and whole liver cell experiments; it is usually not essential for studies designed to determine the site of action of a hypolipidemic agent.

Table 2. Typical levels of conversion by a rat liver homogenate of acetate and mevalonate to products

Substrate	Nonsaponifiable[a] compounds	Cholesterol[b]
	%	%
Acetate-2-^{14}C	2.2	9.7
Mevalonate-2-^{14}C	94.0	37.3

[a] Expressed as percent of the total dpm in the incubation mixture.
[b] Expressed as percent of the total dpm in the nonsaponifiable extract of the incubatio mixture.

II. Microsomal and Soluble Enzymes; Squalene and Sterol Carrier Protein Applications

In addition to the cell-free homogenate preparations, just described, the 9000 to 10000 × *g* supernatant fraction or mixtures of the microsomal and soluble fractions are often employed as sources of enzyme systems catalyzing formation of cholesterol. These preparations are useful, for example, when it is desirable to exclude effects of a new drug on mitochondrial enzymes. In particular, once a new agent is shown to be effective in blocking overall sterol synthesis (e.g. by studies with cell-free homogenates), basic information on the site(s) and mechanism(s) of action of the agent can be obtained using purified or partially purified preparations of specific enzymes and proteins present in the microsomal and soluble fractions.

A. Enzymes in the Early Stages of Cholesterol Synthesis

Regarding the early stages of cholesterol synthesis, HMG (β-hydroxy-β-methyl glutaryl)-CoA reductase is an enzyme that should be examined during studies with a potential hypocholesterolemic agent. This enzyme is generally considered to be one important regulator of cholesterol synthesis. It is modified by several hypolipidemic agents in current clinical use (e.g. AVOY et al., 1965; WHITE, 1971, 1972; SHAFER et al., 1972). Recently, HMG-CoA reductase of yeast (which is more readily isolated in high activity yield than the liver enzyme) has been used to survey effects of a series of potential new hypolipidemic agents (BOOTS et al., 1973). It should be noted that effects observed with an enzyme from non-mammalian sources may not be predictive of findings with mammalian enzymes. In another regard, relatively little attention has been given to effects of potential hypolipidemic agents on other enzymes in the early stages of cholesterol synthesis; studies on these enzymes may be pertinent, especially in view of recent work indicating possible control of sterol synthesis by early enzymes in addition to HMG-CoA reductase (e.g. SUGIYAMA et al., 1972; CLINKENBEARD et al., 1973, 1975).

B. Enzymes in the Later Stages of Cholesterol Synthesis

Regarding the later stages of cholesterol synthesis, there are numerous recent examples of results obtained using microsomal enzyme preparations to study the effects of potential hypolipidemic agents. Several examples of these studies are listed in

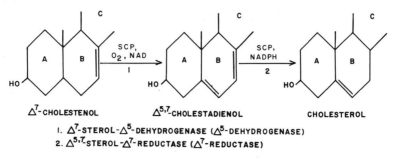

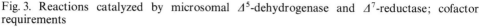

1. Δ^7-STEROL-Δ^5-DEHYDROGENASE (Δ^5-DEHYDROGENASE)
2. $\Delta^{5,7}$-STEROL-Δ^7-REDUCTASE (Δ^7-REDUCTASE)

Fig. 3. Reactions catalyzed by microsomal Δ^5-dehydrogenase and Δ^7-reductase; cofactor requirements

Table 1. GAYLOR (1972) has prepared an excellent review on the properties of micro-somal enzymes of sterol biosynthesis. His review also contains many useful descrip-tions of techniques for isolation and assay of a variety of these enzymes. A source of additional information is the volume edited by Clayton (1969). In our experience, two partially purified, well-characterized enzymes are easily isolated and assayed; they have been useful tools in studying effects of a variety of potential hypocholester-olemic agents. These enzymes are: Microsomal Δ^7-sterol Δ^5-dehydrogenase (steps 14 and 15, Fig. 1; or step 1, Fig. 3) and $\Delta^{5,7}$-sterol Δ^7-reductase (steps 17 and 18, Fig. 1; or step 2, Fig. 3). Similarly to other enzymes in later stages of cholesterol synthesis, these two enzymes require for full activity a protein present in the soluble fraction of homogenates (i.e. squalene and sterol carrier protein (SCP) (DEMPSEY et al., 1964, 1965, 1968; RITTER and DEMPSEY, 1970, 1971, 1973; SCALLEN et al., 1971a, 1972; DEMPSEY, 1974, 1975).

C. Characteristics of Δ^5-Dehydrogenase and Δ^7-Reductase; Role of Squalene and Sterol Carrier Protein (SCP)

Before describing typical studies with potential hypolipidemic agents and microso-mal Δ^5-dehydrogenase or Δ^7-reductase, it is pertinent to discuss some characteristics of these enzymes, the role of SCP in their functions, and the role of SCP in other reactions. The dehydrogenase (step 1, Fig. 3) has a rather broad pH optimum (Fig. 4); the optimum pH for the reductase (step 2, Fig. 5) is sharp (Fig. 5). The dehydrogenase requires for maximum activity (in addition to oxygen and SCP) a low level of pyridine nucleotide (e.g. NAD, Fig. 6). The reductase has a specific require-ment for NADPH (Fig. 7). The Km for pyridine nucleotides observed for these enzymes will vary with the experimental conditions chosen, i.e. SCP has a high affinity for pyridine nucleotides (RITTER and DEMPSEY, 1971; see also Fig. 7). In this regard, the apparent Km for the sterol substrates of these enzymes also varies with the experimental conditions, i.e. the enzymes have a high affinity for a preformed sterol·SCP complex (RITTER and DEMPSEY (1973) and see following paragraph). The mechanism of insertion of the Δ^5-bond by the dehydrogenase is not completely understood. It is known that other electron acceptors will not substitute for oxygen; our evidence suggests that cytochrome b_5 may participate in the reaction. Both the reductase and dehydrogenase have been purified >150-fold by detergent solubiliza-

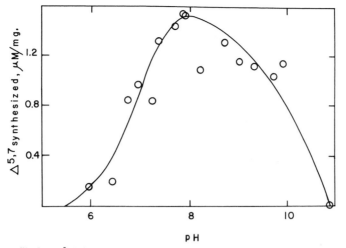

Fig. 4. pH profile for Δ^5-dehydrogenase

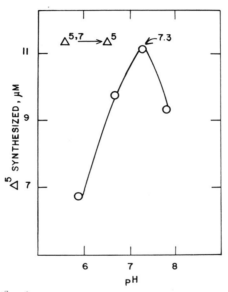

Fig. 5. pH profile for Δ^7-reductase

tion and salt fractionation (DEMPSEY, 1969b). The purified preparations, in particular, do not contain Δ^{24}-reductase activity (step 19, Fig. 1). Reduction of the Δ^7-bond (step 2, Fig. 3) is faster than insertion of the Δ^5-bond (step 1, Fig. 3); see also Fig. 8.

The requirement for the soluble or high-speed supernatant fraction for maximum activity of these enzymes is indicated by the data in Fig. 9 for the overall conversion of Δ^7-cholestenol to cholesterol and in Fig. 10 for the conversion of $\Delta^{5,7}$-cholestadienol (7-dehydrocholesterol) to cholesterol. Recently, the factor (now designated

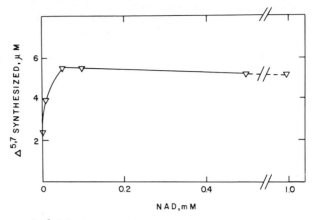

Fig. 6. Requirement of Δ^5-dehydrogenase for NAD

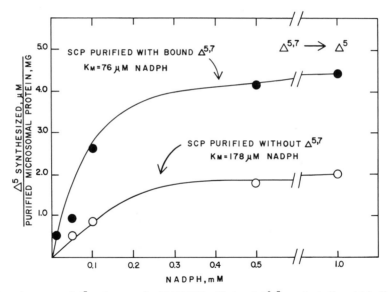

Fig. 7. Requirement of Δ^7-reductase for NADPH; effects of $\Delta^{5,\,7}$-cnolestadienol binding to SCP

SCP) present in the soluble fraction was shown to be an ubiquitous, heat-stable protein which binds sterols and other lipids and is essential for conversion of water insoluble precursors to cholesterol by microsomal enzymes (e.g. DEMPSEY, 1971; RITTER and DEMPSEY, 1970, 1971, 1973). SCALLEN et al. (1971a, 1972) have confirmed these observations, except for the heat stability property, ubiquitous occurrence in mammalian tissues, and molecular weight of the protomer form of SCP. The latter differences are readily accounted for by variations in assay conditions for SCP and methods used to determine molecular weight, e.g. ultracentrifugation (SCALLEN et al., 1972) versus gel filtration and SDS gel electrophoresis (RITTER and DEMPSEY, 1973; see also Figs. 11 and 12). In addition, SCP has a marked tendency to aggregate; it is

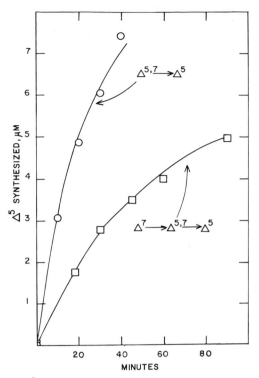

Fig. 8. Time course of the Δ^7-reductase reaction and the overall conversion of Δ^7-cholestenol to cholesterol by Δ^5-dehydrogenase and Δ^7-reductase

therefore possible to observe multiple molecular forms (cf. Fig. 26). Regarding this point, we consider the form of SCP which interacts with microsomal enzymes to be the high molecular weight sterol·SCP complex. Formation of this complex is facilitated by the presence of phospholipid (RITTER and DEMPSEY, 1973). SCP was first discovered in rat liver; more recently a structurally and functionally similar protein was purified from human liver (DEMPSEY et al., 1972; see also Fig. 13); from various mammalian tissues (McCoy et al., 1973; McCoy and DEMPSEY, 1973; see also Figs. 14 and 15); and from protozoa (CALIMBAS, 1972, 1973). The relative level of binding of the water soluble (acetate and mevalonate) and water insoluble precursors of cholesterol to SCP is indicated in Fig. 16.

The findings summarized above suggest the biological roles for SCP outlined in Fig. 17. SCP (the protomer-form, M.W. 16000) forms a noncovalent, high molecular weight (> 150000 daltons) complex with a water-insoluble precursor. This complex combines with a specific microsomal enzyme and the precursor·SCP is converted to its product, the following precursor·SCP, which then combines with the microsomal enzyme next in the sequence of cholesterol synthesis. Finally, cholesterol·SCP results (cf. also Fig. 1). Recent evidence further suggests that SCP may participate in the formation of lipoproteins and in the initial stages of metabolism of cholesterol to steroid hormones and bile acids. With regard to lipoprotein formation, the high density lipoprotein (HDL) fraction of plasma has been shown to contain SCP-like

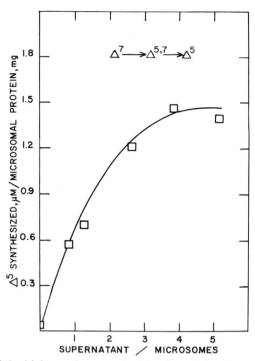

Fig. 9. Requirement of the high-speed supernatant fraction of liver homogenates for maximum cholesterol synthesis from Δ^7-cholesterol

activity (Fig. 18); this activity is associated predominantly with one of the HDL apo-peptides, apo-Gln-II (also designated apo-A-II) (DEMPSEY et al., 1972; see also Fig. 19). The possible structural similarity of apo-Gln-II (BREWER et al., 1972) and SCP is currently under investigation. With regard to the initial stages of steroid hormone synthesis, a cholesterol·liver-SCP complex is metabolized by adrenal mito-chondrial enzymes to pregnenolone (KAN et al., 1972; UNGAR et al., 1973; see also Fig. 20). Steroids formed from pregnenolone are progressively more water-soluble and not bound by SCP (cf. Fig. 21). In addition, KAN and UNGAR (1973) have isolated a heat-stable protein from adrenal tissue which is structurally similar to liver-SCP and functions with the adrenal mitochondrial enzymes catalyzing choles-terol side-chain cleavage yielding pregnenolone. With regard to bile acid formation, cholate and taurocholate are water-soluble and not bound by SCP (cf. Fig. 21). However, early products of cholesterol metabolism to bile acids (e.g. 7α-hydroxycho-lesterol; cf. also Fig. 22) are bound by SCP and the 12α-hydroxylase present in liver microsomes has a specific requirement for SCP (GRABOWSKI et al., 1973; see also Fig. 23).

D. Inhibition of the Later Stages of Cholesterol Synthesis

It is apparent from the characteristics of the microsomal enzymes and SCP, just described, that the mechanism by which an agent blocks a reaction in the later stages of cholesterol synthesis or in cholesterol metabolism may be quite complex. Some

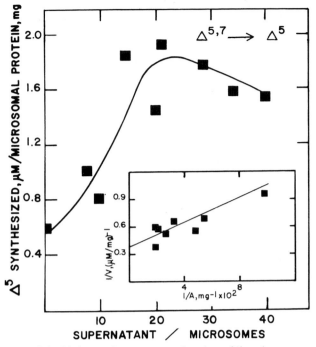

Fig. 10. Requirement of the high-speed supernatant fraction of liver homogenates for maximum activity of Δ^7-reductase

possibilities are: an agent could interact with SCP and prevent binding of a sterol; or an agent could change the conformation of a sterol·SCP complex to prevent interaction of the complex with a microsomal enzyme; or an agent ould block product formation by a sterol·SCP·microsomal enzyme complex. Furthermore, some agents, by acting at the level of SCP, could interfere with or accelerate the conversion of cholesterol to bile acids and steroid hormones. Another possibility is that the level of SCP or the cholesterol·SCP complex could regulate the early steps in cholesterol synthesis and these effects might then be modified by agents yet to be developed. Similar comments relate to the proposed role of SCP in lipoprotein formation. Clearly, there is need for new studies designed to obtain information in this area.

One approach to understanding the effects on a molecular level of potential hypolipidemic agents is to examine binding of an agent to both SCP and microsomal enzymes as well as the effects of this binding on the functions of SCP and the enzymes (DEMPSEY et al., 1972). For example, as shown in Fig. 21, cholestane-triol is bound by SCP at a level similar to that seen with cholesterol precursors (cf. Fig. 16). It also binds to microsomal enzymes. This compound blocks cholesterol synthesis at several steps in the later stages (cf. Figs. 2 and 24). Furthermore, the data given in Fig. 25 show that the triol and several of its analogs are capable of either stimulating or inhibiting cholesterol synthesis from a precursor (in this case $\Delta^{5,7}$-cholestadienol) depending on the levels of the precursor and SCP. These findings (Fig. 25) illustrate that some compounds (e.g. 3α-amino-5α, 6β-dihydroxy-cholestane) block cholesterol

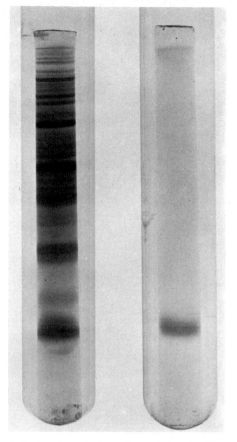

Fig. 11. Polyacrylamide gel electrophoresis in sodium dodecyl sulfate of the high-speed super-natant fraction of a liver homogenate (left) and purified SCP (right)

synthesis at the level of the microsomal enzyme, i.e. there was complete inhibition of effects observed when the substrate or SCP levels were varied. In addition, some compounds (e.g. 5α-amino-3β, 6β-dihydroxy-cholestane) interfere with the interaction of the sterol·SCP complex and the enzyme. Other compounds (e.g. 3,6-dioximino-5α-hydroxy-cholestane) favorably increase the interaction of the sterol·SCP complex with the enzyme.

III. Preparations and Activity Assays

Microsomal and Soluble Fractions of Homogenates. For preparation of the microsomal and soluble fractions, the cell-free supernatant of liver (described in the previous section of this chapter) is centrifuged for a further 15 min at $9000 \times g$. Many investigators use the supernatant of this centrifugation for studying cholesterol synthesis and its inhibition by various agents (cf. Table 1). The supernatant from the centrifugation at $9000 \times g$ is recentrifuged for 90 minutes at $105000 \times g$ and the floating fat

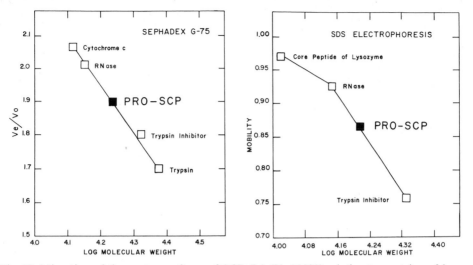

Fig. 12. Migration of the protomer form of SCP (M. W. 16000) relative to proteins of known molecular weight during gel filtration and electrophoresis

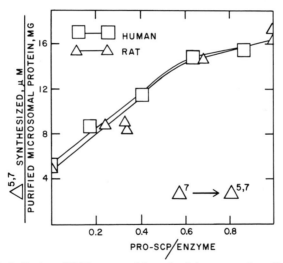

Fig. 13. Functional similarity of SCP prepared from both human and rat liver

layer is drawn off and either discarded or recentrifuged at $105000 \times g$ to obtain a higher yield of the soluble fraction for SCP preparation; see below. The supernatant is withdrawn from the microsomal pellet as two equal fractions: upper and lower. The lower fraction contains small particles of microsomes and in our experience may be used as source of soluble protein (SCP) plus microsomal enzymes (e.g. DEMPSEY, 1965, 1968, 1969b). The upper fraction (17 to 20 mg protein per ml) is used for purification of SCP; see below. The microsomal pellet is resuspended by homogenization, using a tight-fitting Teflon pestle and glass tube, in a volume of phosphate

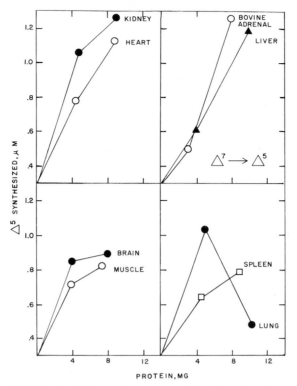

Fig. 14. Occurrence of SCP in the high-speed supernatant fraction of various mammalian tissues; determined by effects on the conversion of Δ^7-cholestenol to cholesterol

buffer equal to one-half the volume of the soluble fraction (upper plus lower fraction). The suspension is centrifuged for 60 minutes at $105000 \times g$. The supernatant fraction is decanted and the pellet resuspended in phosphate buffer by homogenization as just described. This suspension constitutes the washed microsomal fraction; it contains 10 to 15 mg protein per ml. The microsomal fraction may be used for incubations at this point or frozen for at least a week.

A. HMG-CoA Reductase

To prepare HMG-CoA reductase, we follow the procedure outlined above for isolation of washed microsomes—except the phosphate buffer also contains 0.1 mM EDTA and 1.0 mM DTT (dithiothreitol, also called Cleland's reagent). This preparation retains activity for several hours; it is not stored frozen.

B. Δ^5-Dehydrogenase and Δ^7-Reductase

To purify the Δ^7-sterol Δ^5-dehydrogenase and $\Delta^{5,7}$-sterol Δ^7-reductase a 10-ml aliquot of the washed microsomal fraction is thawed, then mixed with 32 mg sodium desoxycholate (special enzyme grade, Schwarz-Mann Laboratories) and centrifuged

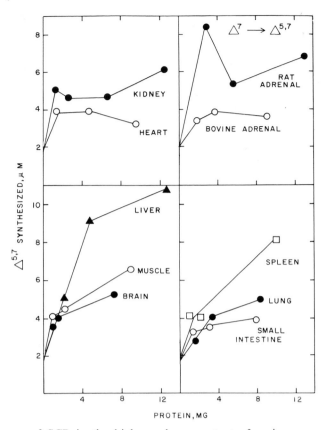

Fig. 15. Occurrence of SCP in the high-speed supernatant of various mammalian tissues; determined by effects on Δ^5-dehydrogenase

for 15 min at $270 \times g$. One gram $(NH_4)_2SO_4$ (special enzyme grade, Mann Research Laboratories) is added with stirring to 7 ml of the clear supernate and the $(NH_4)_2SO_4$ pellet is suspended by homogenization in 1.5 ml phosphate buffer, pH 7.3, and then applied to a column of Sephadex G-25, 2×13 cm, which has been equilibrated with the same buffer. The same buffer is used for elution. Approximately 10 ml of buffer are passed through the column at a rate of one ml per minute until the protein (light yellow color) begins to emerge from the column. This material is collected in one fraction (3 to 4 ml), containing 2 to 4 mg protein per ml. It is assayed immediately after preparation, i.e. not stored frozen.

C. Squalene and Sterol Carrier Protein (SCP)

We have developed two techniques for preparing purified SCP from the soluble fraction of homogenates; one involves heat treatment of the soluble fraction at high ionic strength (RITTER and DEMPSEY, 1970, 1971); the other avoids the heat step (McCoy et al., 1973; McCoy and DEMPSEY, 1975).

Cholesterol Precursor	% Bound
Acetate (C_2), Mevalonate (C_6)	4
Squalene (C_{30})	100
Lanosterol (C_{30})	85
Dihydrolanosterol (C_{30})	100
Δ^7-3-one (C_{30})	29
$\Delta^{8(14)}, \Delta^7$ (C_{29})	100
Δ^7, $HOCH_2$-Δ^7 (C_{28})	100
$\Delta^{8(14)}$ (C_{27})	90
$\Delta^{8,14}$ (C_{27})	50
$\Delta^{7,24}, \Delta^{5,7,24}, \Delta^{5,24}$ (C_{27})	94—97
Δ^7-3-one (C_{27})	86
$\Delta^7, \Delta^{5,7}$ (C_{27})	90—97
Cholesterol	95

Fig. 16. Relative level of binding of cholesterol precursors to SCP

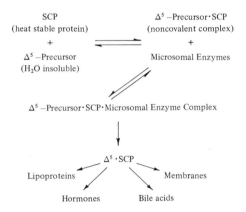

Fig. 17. Proposed biological roles of SCP

Preparation	Preincubation with Sterol	Enzymic Activation[a]
		-fold
Apo-SCP	−	1.0
	+	3.7
Apo-HDL (Rat) and	−	1.4
Apo-HDL$_3$ (Human)	+	3.6
BSA	−	1.1
	+	1.1
Serum (Rat and	−	0.6
Human)	+	1.3

[a] $\Delta^{5,7}$-sterol Δ^7-reductase and Δ^7-sterol Δ^5-dehydrogenase

Fig. 18. Similarity of function of plasma high density lipoprotein (HDL) and SCP

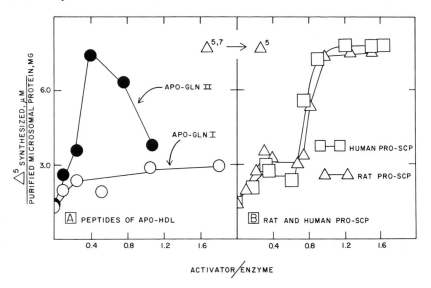

Fig. 19. Effects of purified human HDL apo-peptides and human and rat SCP on Δ^7-reductase activity

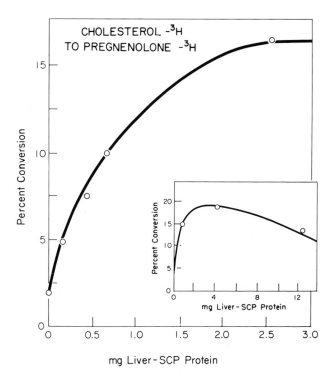

Fig. 20. Effects of liver SCP on the conversion of cholesterol to pregnenolone by adrenal mitochondrial enzymes

Compound	% Bound
Pregnenolone	27
Progesterone	16
Testosterone	4
Estradiol	3
Cholate	7
Taurocholate	7
Cholesteryl-acetate	36
Cholesteryl-palmitate	10
Cholesteryl-stearate	7
Cholesteryl-oleate	39
Δ^4-cholesten-3-one	<1
3-ketocholestane	<1
Cholestane	20
Cholestanol	30
3β, 5α-cholestanediol	50
3β, 5α 6β-cholestanetriol	94
Phenethylbiguanide	<1
AY-9944	4
Tetrahymanol	<1
$\Delta^{5,\,7,\,22}$-cholestatrienol	90
$\Delta^{5,\,7,\,22}$-cholestatrienyl-acetate	63

Fig. 21. Relative binding of various steroids and other compounds to SCP

D. Method 1

To purify SCP by heat treatment at high ionic strength, a 120 ml aliquot (2000 to 2500 mg protein) of the liver soluble fraction in 0.1 M phosphate buffer, pH 7.4, (see above), is increased in ionic strength by addition of 6 grams $(NH_4)_2SO_4$ (5%(w/v)). The pH of this mixture is readjusted to between 7.3 to 7.4 with 2N KOH. The mixture is then aliquoted equally into four 40 ml glass centrifuge tubes. The tubes are placed in a boiling water bath (500 ml) for 5 min. During this period, the contents of each tube are stirred with a glass rod and also flushed with oxygen-free nitrogen. The temperature of the contents of the tubes reaches 85° by the end of the 5-minute heating period. The tubes are cooled to 4°; the pH of the contents readjusted to 7.4; and coagulated protein removed by centrifugation ($10000 \times g$, 10 min). The resulting supernatant is concentrated at 4° to approximately 10 to 15 mls using an Amicon ultrafiltration cell (model 202) fitted with a PM-10 filter. The driving force for filtration is oxygen-free nitrogen at 20 lbs/in². The concentrate is then applied to a set of Sephadex G-75 columns (1.5×90 cm, down and 2.5×10 cm, up). Elution is at 4° with 0.1 M phosphate buffer, pH 7.4. Fractions (5 ml) are collected at the rate of 20 ml per hour. The protomer form of SCP elutes with 300 to 350 ml of buffer (cf. Fig. 26). Total protein as pro-SCP is 14 to 18 mg.

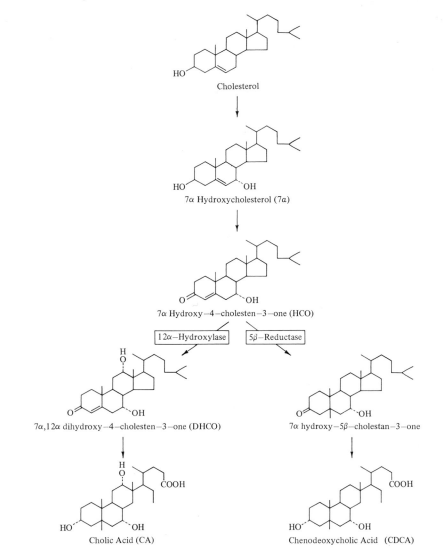

Fig. 22. Pathways of conversion of cholesterol to bile acids

E. Method 2

To purify SCP without heat treatment, a 40 ml aliquot of the liver soluble fraction is concentrated by the ultrafiltration procedure (see above) to 10 to 15 mls. The concentrate is applied and eluted using the Sephadex G-75 column system just described in Method 1. Pro-SCP prepared by this method elutes similarly to that prepared by heating at high ionic strength (Method 1; cf. Fig. 26). Total protein as pro-SCP is about 50 mg. Recently, homogeneous pro-SCP was prepared by an additional step involving passage over an ion-exchange resin column (McCoy, et al., 1975).

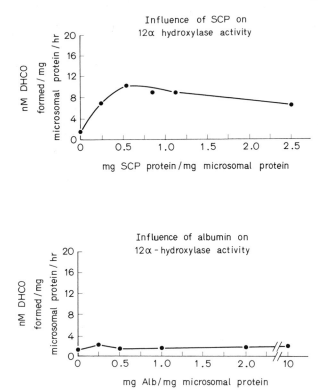

Fig. 23. Specific requirement by microsomal 12α-hydroxylase for SCP

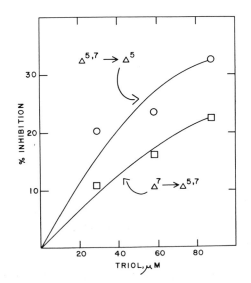

Fig. 24. Inhibition of Δ^5-dehydrogenase and Δ^7-reductase by cholestane- 3β, 5α 6β-triol

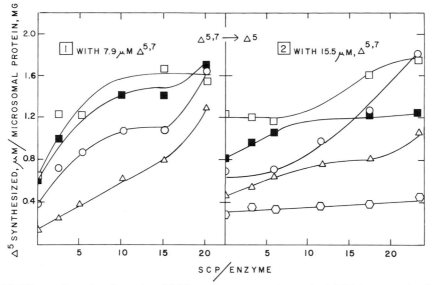

Fig. 25. Effects of varying the ratio of SCP to enzyme protein on the inhibition or activation of Δ^7-reductase by cholestane derivatives $\bigcirc — \bigcirc$, no inhibitor or activator; $\square — \square$, effect of 3,6-dioximino-5α-hydroxycholestane; $\triangle — \triangle$, effect of 5α-amino-3β, 6β-dihydroxy-cholestane; $\blacksquare — \blacksquare$ effect of 5α-cholestane-3β, 5α, 6β-triol; $\diamondsuit — \diamondsuit$ effect of 3α-amino-5α, 6β-dihydroxy-cholestane

Pro-SCP prepared by either of these methods may be stored at 4° for 48 hours or frozen in dry ice-ethanol for 2 weks. It is possible to reactivate older preparations with 5 mM reduced glutathione. Pro-SCP preparations may be concentrated by the ultrafiltration procedure, described above. Both methods of purification produce SCP having the same functional activity with microsomal enzymes and the same specific activity (based on the Δ^5-dehydrogenase assay; see bleow); however, the total SCP protein yield is greater with the method that does not include the heat step (Method 2). Both preparations of pro-SCP migrate as single bands with identical mobilities during polyacrylamide gel electrophoresis at pH 9.0 (McCoy and Dempsey, 1975).

The estimated degree of purification of pro-SCP depends on the method used for assay of SCP functional activity; using the Δ^5-dehydrogenase assay described below the estimated purification is greater than 20-fold (McCoy and Dempsey, 1975). Conversion of pro-SCP to the oligomer and subsequent assay by the Δ^5-dehydrogenase method results in an estimated purification of 720-fold (Ritter and Dempsey, 1973). The possible occurence of minor structural differences in the preparations of pro-SCP purified by the methods given here is currently being studied. It should be noted again that by both purification methods SCP activity is detected in column fractions in addition to that seen in the pro-SCP area (16000 daltons) of the chromatogram (cf. Fig. 26). In particular, SCP activity is found in the void volume of the Sephadex G-75 column. SCP present in the void volume is the oligomer form (> 150000 daltons) containing bound lipid and considered to be the active form of SCP with microsomal enzymes (Ritter and Dempsey, 1973); see also Fig. 17 and previous discussion under

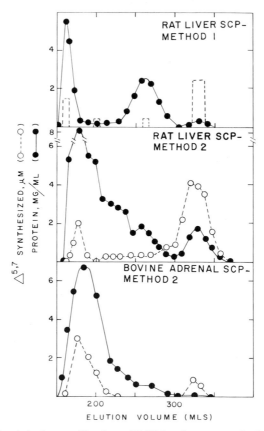

Fig. 26. Results obtained during purification of SCP by the two methods described in the text

Applications). The protomer form of SCP does not contain bound sterols; it is converted to the oligomer during lipid binding, as already discussed (RITTER and DEMPSEY, 1970, 1971, 1973). In this regard, when SCP is prepared from the soluble fraction of bovine adrenal glands, the majority of SCP is in the oligomer form (cf. Fig. 26).

F. Assay of HMG-CoA Reductase

For assay of microsomal HMG-CoA reductase activity, we follow the method described in detail by GOLDFARB and PITOT (1971). This is a thin layer chromatographic technique involving use of double isotopic labels to quantitate the amount of mevalonate formed from HMG-CoA. We also synthesize labeled HMG-CoA according to the procedure developed by these authors (GOLDFARB and PITOT, 1971).

G. Assay of Δ^5-Dehydrogenase

General conditions for assay of Δ^7-sterol Δ^5-dehydrogenase (step 1, Fig. 3) by a spectrophotometric method are as follows: Total incubation volume, 1 to 2 ml; 0.1 M phosphate, pH 7.4, 1 mM NAD, 120 mμM AY-9944 (Ayerst Laboratories);

60 µM Δ^7-cholestenol; and 1 to 1.5 ml of either the 9000 × g supernatant fraction of a liver homogenate; or a mixture of the upper soluble fraction and the washed microsomal fraction; or a mixture of the upper soluble fraction and the purified microsomal fraction; or a mixture of purified SCP and the washed or purified microsomal fraction. It is important for maximum or near maximum activity that the protein ratio of the soluble fraction (unpurified SCP) to microsomal enzyme be at least 15 (cf. Fig. 9) and that of purified SCP to enzyme between 0.5 and 1.0. The Δ^7-reductase inhibitor, AY-9944, is used to block conversion to cholesterol of $\Delta^{5,7}$-cholestadienol formed by action of Δ^5-dehydrogenase (DVORNIK et al., 1963). The substrate Δ^7-cholestenol, is dissolved in propylene glycol (34 µg per 0.2 ml).

Incubations are performed for 30 to 60 min at 37° in a Dubnoff shaker under air or oxygen. The reaction is stopped by addition of an equal volume of ethanol (95% v/v) and two KOH pellets. This mixture may be extracted immediately or stored overnight at −20°. The product, $\Delta^{5,7}$-cholestadienol, is extracted into spectral grade cyclohexane using a volume of cyclohexane equal to twice the total original incubation volume, i.e. for a 1.5 ml incubation mixture, the volume of cyclohexane would be 3 ml. Extraction is facilitated by subjecting each reaction tube to the mixing action of a Vortex mixer for one minute, followed by centrifugation at 2000 rpm for three minutes. The absorbance of the cyclohexane layer is read at 281.5 nm; each sample is scanned form 260 to 310 nm against its own cyclohexane blank at a spectrophotometer setting of 0 to 0.1 absorbance full scale. The cyclohexane blank for each incubation mixture is an extract of an identical incubation mixture, prepared without the substrate, Δ^7-cholestenol. The level of $\Delta^{5,7}$-cholestadienol synthesized from Δ^7-cholestenol is estimated by the following formula, using the absorptivity value of $\Delta^{5,7}$-cholestadienol at 281.5 mm (0.0102 μM^{-1} cm^{-1}): µM $\Delta^{5,7}$-cholestadienol synthesized

$$= \frac{\text{Absorbance (from difference spectrum)} \times 2}{0.0102}$$

The reference method for this spectrophotometric assay is the more time consuming epiperoxide derivative technique (DEMPSEY et al., 1964; DEMPSEY, 1965, 1969 b). The latter method depends on the conversion of labeled $\Delta^{5,7}$cholestadienol by photo-oxidation to its 5α, 8α-epiperoxide. As indicated by the data presented in Fig. 27, the two methods compare favorably (BISSET, 1971). We, therefore, utilize the rapid spectrophotometric assay described here for studies with potential hypolipidemic agents and for assay of SCP activity in chromatographic fractions (cf. Fig. 26).

H. Assay of Δ^7-Reductase

We commonly assay $\Delta^{5,7}$-sterol Δ^7-reductase (step 2, Fig. 3) by a specific, sensitive, isotope derivative technique for cholesterol, i.e. passage of the product of this reaction, cholesterol, through the dibromide derivative. General conditions for this assay are as follows: Total incubation volume 1 to 2 ml; 0.1 M phosphate buffer, pH 7.4; 0.8 mM NADPH; 5 mM reduced glutathione, 25 µM $\Delta^{5,7}$-cholestadienol-4-^{14}C (5 × 10^3 dpm); and 1 to 1.5 ml of the cell fractions or purified proteins, as given for the Δ^5-dehydrogenase assay (see above). Labeled $\Delta^{5,7}$-cholestadienol is dissolved in

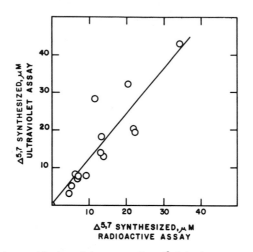

Fig. 27. Comparison of the rapid ultraviolet assay for Δ^5-dehydrogenase with the radioactive derivative method

propylene glycol (15 µg per 0.1 ml); it is prepared by the method of SCHROEPFER and FRANTZ (1961) and purified by column chromatography using silicic acid impregnated with silver nitrate (CARLSON, 1973). Incubations are performed in 20 ml beakers for 30 to 60 minutes at 37° in a Dubnoff shaker under nitrogen. The reaction is stopped by addition of an equal volume of ethanol (95% v/v). Sterols are extracted four times; each time with a volume of petroleum ether equal to four times the total original volume of the incubation mixture, i.e. for a one-ml incubation mixture the volume of petroleum ether (b.p. 30 to 60°) used for each extraction would be four ml. Extractions are performed in a 25×150 mm test tube using a Vortex mixer and disposable capillary pipet. The extract is filtered through shark skin paper (Schleicher and Schuell), dried under nitrogen, and dissolved in 10 ml of benzene. An aliquot (0.5 ml) is evaporated to dryness in a glass counting vial, dissolved in 10 ml of scintillation fluid (2,5-diphenyloxazole, 0.3% (v/v) in toluene), and assayed for radioactivity in a scintillation counter. To the remaining benzene solution (9.5 ml) containing the labeled sterols, a known weight (120 to 150 mg) of unlabeled cholesterol is added. The benzene is evaporated under nitrogen and the residual sterols are dissolved in 3 ml of anhydrous diethyl ether. The ether solution is cooled in an ice bath and bromine is added dropwise until a dark yellow color persists. After 1 hr in the ice bath, 1.5 ml of cooled glacial acetic acid is added with stirring. The precipitated cholesterol dibromide is collected on a sintered-glass funnel, washed until colorless with cooled glacial acetic acid, and dissolved in 5 ml of diethyl ether. Zinc dust (100 mg) is added and the suspension is stirred frequently with a Vortex mixer during 30 min. The zinc bromide is dissolved by addition of water (1 to 2 ml) and the suspension is stirred with the Vortex mixer until the ether and water layers separate completely. The ether layer is removed and washed with 1 ml of 0.7 N HCl, twice with 1 ml of water, and with 1 ml of 2 N NaOH. After evaporation of the ether, cholesterol (50 to 60 mg) is crystallized from aqueous acetone, dried, weighed, and assayed for radioactivity. The percentage of labeled $\Delta^{5,7}$-cholestadienol converted to cholesterol by Δ^7-reductase activity is calculated as follows:

Percentage conversion of $\Delta^{5,7}$-cholestadienol to cholesterol

$$= \left[\frac{\text{cpm cholesterol final)}}{\text{cpm sterol mixture}}\right]\left[\frac{\text{mg cholesterol (initial)}}{\text{mg cholesterol (final)}}\right] \times 100$$

   This percentage value is then multiplied by the original level of $\Delta^{5,7}$-cholesta-dienol-4-^{14}C present in the incubation mixture to give the µM cholesterol-4-^{14}C synthesized.
   The isotopic method, just described, for Δ^7-reductase may also be used for assay of conversion of Δ^7-cholestenol to cholesterol (steps 1 and 2, Fig. 3). For the latter assay, labeled Δ^7-cholestenol would be needed (DEMPSEY, 1969b) and incubations performed under oxygen. The rate of Δ^7-reductase is faster than the Δ^5-dehydrogen-ase and in the presence of excess NADPH there is no accumulation of $\Delta^{5,7}$-cholesta-dienol (DEMPSEY et al., 1964). It is also possible to use the spectrophotometric assay (as described for Δ^5-dehydrogenase activity) to measure Δ^7-reductase activity (Kan-dutsch, 1962). For this purpose, the substrate would be unlabeled $\Delta^{5,7}$-cholestadien-ol, and incubation mixtures would include excess NADPH. The incubation should be performed under nitrogen to avoid nonenzymic formation of the epiperoxide derivative of $\Delta^{5,7}$-cholestadienol, which if formed would result in falsely high conver-sion levels. For our studies with potential hypolipidemic agents, we have found the sensitivity and specificity of the isotopic method to be advantageous.

I. Linearity of Enzymic Assays; Optimum Substrate Levels

It is essential that an investigator determines the linearity with time and enzyme level, as well as the optimum substrate and SCP levels, for the reactions described here before studies with potential inhibitors of cholesterol synthesis are initiated. For example, it is possible that sources of animal tissues different than those described here will cause variations in observed reaction rates and the assay conditions will need to be modified. Similar comments apply to the use of cell-free homogenates for study of overall cholesterol synthesis; see the first section of this chapter.

J. Binding of Compounds to SCP and Microsomal Enzymes

Binding of labeled compounds to SCP (cf. Figs. 16 and 21) are performed by heat tratment (100°, 1 min) of the soluble fraction of liver homogenates (prepared as outlined above); removal of coagulated protein by centrifugation; incubation (37°, 15 min) of the supernatant fraction with a known level of the labeled compound; followed by $(NH_4)_2SO_4$ precipitation (40 to 80% saturation); and finally gel filtra-tion (Sephadex G-25) (RITTER and DEMPSEY, 1971, 1973).
Alternatively, pro-SCP, prepared by either Method 1 or 2, is incubated with the labeled compound under study and the SCP·compound complex (oligomer) is iso-lated by gel filtration (cf. Fig. 26).

Binding is expressed as the percentage of the total radioactivity applied to the gel column which emerges with the SCP complex (oligomer form). In order to obtain comparable data, binding studies are carried out at the same level of soluble protein (SCP) and compound to be tested. Ideally, the levels of protein and test compound should be varied in order to obtain binding constants. Studies of this type are in progress. We are also currently exploring the use of density gradient centrifugation to obtain more information on the molecular events occurring during binding by SCP (CARLSON et al., 1973). To measure the binding of compounds to microsomal enzymes, the protein bound species is separated from unbound compound by gel filtration (Sephadex G-25), as just described.

References

AVOY, D. R., SWYRD, E. A., GOULD, R. G.: Effects of α-p-Chloropenoxyisobutyryl Ethyl Ester (CPIB) With and Without Androsterone on Cholesterol Biosynthesis in Rat Liver. J. Lipid Res. **6**, 369—376 (1965).

BARTH, C., HACKENSCHMIDT, J., ULMANN, H., DECKER, K.: Inhibition of Cholesterol Synthesis by (—)-Hydroxycitrate in Perfused Rat Liver. Evidence for an Extramitochondrial Mevalonate Synthesis from Acetyl Coenzyme A. FEBS Letters **22**, 343—346 (1972).

BISSET, K. J.: Characteristics of an Enzyme System Catalyzing Formation of the Δ^5-Bond of Cholesterol. Master's Thesis. Minneapolis-University of Minnesota (1971).

BLOHM, T. R., STEVENS, V. L., KARUJA, T., ALIG, H. N.: Effects of Clomiphene cis and trans Isomers on Sterol Metabolism in the Rat. Biochem. Pharmacol. **19**, 2231—2241 (1970).

BLOXHAM, D. P., AKHTAR, M.: Studies on the Control of Cholesterol Biosynthesis: The Adenosine 3':5'-Cyclic Monophosphate—Dependent Accumulation of a Steroid Carboxylic Acid. Biochem. J. **123**, 275—278 (1971).

BOOTS, M. R., BOOTS, S. G., NOBLE, C. M., GUYER, K. E.: Hypocholesterolemic Agents II: Inhibition of β-Hydroxy-β-Methylglutaryl Coenzyme A Reductase by Arylalkyl Hydrogen Succinates and Glutarates. J. pharm. Sci. **62**, 953—957 (1973).

BREWER, H. B., JR., LUX, S. E., RONAN, R., JOHN, K. M.: Amino Acid Sequence of Human Apolp-Gen-II (apo A-II), an Apolipoprotein Isolated from the High-Density lipoprotein complex. Proc. nat. Acad. Sci. (Wash.) **69**, 1304—1308 (1972).

BUCHER, N. L. R.: The Formation of Radioactive Cholesterol and Fatty Acids from C^{14}-labeled Acetate by Rat Liver Homogenates. J. Amer. chem. Soc. **75**, 498 (1953).

CALIMBAS, T.: Requirement for a Carrier Protein in Sterol Conversions by a Protozoan. Fed. Proc. **31**, 430 (1972).

CALIMBAS, T.: Characteristics of a Protozoan Enzyme System Catalyzing Conversion of Cholesterol to $\Delta^{5,7,22}$-Cholestatrienol. Fed. Proc. **32**, 519 (1973).

CARLSON, J. P.: In Preparation (1975).

CARLSON, J. P., McCOY, K. E., DEMPSEY, M. E.: "Squalene and Sterol Carrier Protein: Model for Lipoprotein Structure and Function; Role in Control of Cholesterol Synthesis. Circulation **48**, IV—246 (1973).

CARROLL, J. J., PRITHAM, G. H.: Effects of Sex Hormones and of Potassium Salts of Fatty Acids on the Biosynthesis *In Vitro* of Cholesterol from $(2^{-14}$ C) Mevalonic Acid. Biochim. biophys. Acta (Amst.) **115**, 320—328 (1966).

CLAYTON, R. B.: Steroids and Terpenoids, Vol. 15 of Methods in Enzymology. New York: Academic 1969.

CLINKENBEARD, K. D., SUGIYAMA, T., MOSS, J., REED, W. D., LANE, M. D.: Molecular and Catalytic Properties of Cytosolic Acetoacetyl Coenzyme A Thiolase from Avian Liver. J. biol. Chem. **248**, 2275—2284 (1973).

CLINKENBEARD, K. D., REED, W. D., MOONEY, R. A., LANE, M. D.: Intracellular Localization of the 3-Hydroxy-3-methyl Coenzyme A Cycle Enzymes in Liver. J. biol. Chem. **250**, 3108—3116 (1975).

DEMPSEY, M. E., SEATON, J. D., SCHROEPFER, G. J., TROCKMAN, R. W.: The Intermediary Role of $\Delta^{5,7}$-Cholestadien-3β-ol in Cholesterol Biosynthesis. J. biol. Chem. **239**, 1381—1387 (1964).

DEMPSEY, M. E.: Pathways of Enzymic Synthesis and Conversion to Cholesterol of $\Delta^{5,7,24}$-Cholestatrien-3β-ol and Other Naturally Occurring Sterols. J. biol. Chem. **240**, 4176—4188 (1965).

DEMPSEY, M. E.: Pathways of Enzymic Cholesterol Synthesis Delineated by Use of Drugs. Progr. Biochem. Pharm. **2**, 21—29 (1967).

DEMPSEY, M. E.: Inhibition of Lipid Biosynthesis. Ann. N. Y. Acad. Sci. **148**, 631—646 (1968).

DEMPSEY, M. E.: The Effect of Hypoglycemic Agents on Cholesterol Biosynthesis. in Drugs Affecting Lipid Metabolism, pp. 511—520. New York: Plenum 1969a.

DEMPSEY, M. E.: Δ^7-Sterol Δ^5-Dehydrogenase and $\Delta^{5,7}$-Sterol Δ^7-Reductase of Rat Liver. Methods Enzymol. **15**, 501—514 (1969b).

DEMPSEY, M. E., RITTER, M. C., WITIAK, D. T., PARKER, R. A.: Effects of Cholestane -3β, 5α, 6β Triol and its Analogues on Cholesterol Biosynthesis *in Vitro*, in Atherosclerosis: Proceedings 2nd International Symposium, pp. 290—295. Berlin-Heidelberg-New York: Springer 1970.

DEMPSEY, M. E.: Cholesterol Biosynthesis in Liver Tissue, in Chemistry of Brain Development, pp. 31—39, New York: Plenum 1971.

DEMPSEY, M. E., RITTER, M. C., LUX, S. E.: Functions of a Specific Plasma Apo-Lipoprotein in Cholesterol Biosynthesis. Fed. Proc. **31**, 430 (1972).

DEMPSEY, M. E.: Regulation of Steroid Biosynthesis. Ann. Rev. Biochem. **43**, 967—990 (1974).

DEMPSEY, M. E.: Squalene and Sterol Carrier Protein in Sub-Unit Enzymes: Biochemistry and Function. New York: Dekker (in press) (1975).

DVORNIK, D., KRAML, M., DUBUC, J., GIVNER, M., GAUDRY, R.: A Novel Mode of Inhibition of Cholesterol Biosynthesis. J. Amer. chem. Soc. 3309—3310 (1963).

DVORNIK, D., KRAML, M., BAGLI, J. F.: Endogenous Formation of $\Delta^{5,7,24}$-Cholestatrien-3β-ol. J. Amer. chem. Soc. **86**, 2739—2740 (1964).

DVORNIK, D., KRAML, M., BAGLI, J. F.: Agents Affecting Lipid Metabolism. XVIII A 7-dehydrocholesterol Δ^7-Reductase Inhibitor (AY-9944) as Tool in Studies of Δ^7-Sterol Metabolism. Biochemistry **5**, 1060—1064 (1966).

ESKELSON, C. D., JACOBI, H. P.: Some Effects of Vitamin E, Selenite and Lipoic Acid on *in Vitro* Cholesterol Biosynthesis, Physiol. Chem. Phys. **1**, 487—494 (1969).

ESKELSON, C. D., CAZEE, C., TOWNE, J. C., WALSKE, B. R.: Cholesterolgensis *in Vitro* from Ethanol. Biochem. Pharmacol. **19**, 1419—1427 (1970a).

ESKELSON, C. D., JACOBI, H., CAZEE, C. R.: Some Effects of the Fat Soluble Vitamins on *in Vitro* Cholesterolgenesis. Physiol. Chem. Phys. **2**, 135—150 (1970b).

FRANTZ, I. D., JR.: Chromatography of Unesterified Sterols on Silicic Acid Super-Cell. J. Lipid Res. **4**, 176—178 (1963).

GAYLOR, J. L.: Microsomal Enzymes of Sterol Biosynthesis. Advan. Lipid Res. **10**, 89—141 (1972).

GOLDFARB, S., PITOT, H. C.: Improved Assay of 3-Hydroxy-3-Methylglutaryl Coenzyme A Reductase. J. Lipid Res. **12**, 512—515 (1971).

GOODWIN, C. D., MARGOLIS, S.: Specific Activation of *in Vitro* Cholesterol Biosynthesis by Preincubation of Rat Liver Homogenates J. biol. Chem. **248**, 7610—7613 (1973).

GRABOWSKI, G. A., DEMPSEY, M. E., HANSON, R. F.: Role of the Squalene and Sterol Carrier Protein (SCP) in Bile Acid Synthesis. Fed. Proc. **32**, 520 (1973).

GROSSI-PAOLETTI, E.: Biosynthesis of Sterols in Developing Brain, in Chemistry of Brain Development, pp. 41—51. New York: Plenum 1971.

HAVEN, G. T., JACOBI, H. P.: Effects of Renal Factors on *in Vitro* Hepatic Cholesterol Synthesis in the Rat. Lipids **6**, 751—757 (1971).

HULCHER, F. H.: Inhibition of Hepatic Cholesterol Biosynthesis by 3,5-Dihydroxy-3,4,4-Trimethylvaleric Acid & its Site of Action. Arch. Biochem. Biophys. **146**, 422—427 (1971).

KAN, K. W., RITTER, M. C., UNGAR, F., DEMPSEY, M. E.: The Role of a Carrier Protein in Cholesterol and Steroid Hormone Synthesis by Adrenal Enzymes. Biochem. Biophys. Res. Commun. **48**, 423—429 (1972).

KAN, K. W., UNGAR, F.: Characterization of an Adrenal Activator for Cholesterol Side Chain Cleavage. J. biol. Chem. **248**, 2868—2875 (1973).

KANDUTSCH, A. A.: Enzymatic Reduction of the Δ^7 Bond of 7-Dehydrocholesterol. J. biol. Chem. **237**, 358—362 (1962).

MILLER, W. L., GAYLOR, J. L.: Apparent Non-Specific Effect of Bile Salts on the Terminal reactions of Cholesterol Biosynthesis by Rat Liver. Biochem. Biophys. Acta **137**, 400—402 (1967).

ONOJOBI, F. D., BOYD, G. S.: Accumulation of Squalene During Hepatic Cholesterol Synthesis *in Virtro*, Role of a Plasma Apolipoprotein. Europ. J. Biochem. **13**, 203—222 (1970).

ONO, T., IMAI, Y.: Effects of Steroid Hormines on Synthesis of Cholesterol. J. Biochem. **70**, 45—54 (1971).

McCOY, K. E., DEMPSEY, M. E.: In Preparation (1975).

McCOY, K. E., KOEHLER, D. F., CARLSON, J. P.: Purification, Lipid Binding and Tissue Distribution of Squalene and Sterol Carrier Protein (SCP). Fed. Proc. **32**, 519 (1973).

RANNEY, R. E.: The Effects of Azasterols on Sterol Metabolism. Prog. Biochem. Pharm. **2**, 50—55 (1967).

RITTER, M. C., DEMPSEY, M. E.: Purification and Characterization of a Naturally Occuring Activator of Cholesterol Biosynthesis from $\Delta^{5,7}$-Cholestadienol and Other Precursors. Biochem. Biophys. Res. Commun. **38**, 921—929 (1970).

RITTER, M. C., DEMPSEY, M. E.: Specificity and Role in Cholesterol Biosynthesis of a Squalene and Sterol Carrier Protein. J. biol. Chem. **246**, 1536—1547 (1971).

RITTER, M. C., DEMPSEY, M. E.: Squalene and Sterol Carrier Protein: Structural Properties, Lipid-Binding, and Function in Cholesterol Biosynthesis. Proc. nat. Acad. Sci. (Wash.) **70**, 265—269 (1973).

RODNEY, G., BLACK, N. L., BIRD, O. D.: The Common Mode of Action of Three New Classes of Inhibitors of Cholesterol Biosynthesis. Biochem. Pharmacol. **14**, 445—456 (1965).

SCALLEN, T. J., SCHUSTER, M. W., DHAR, A. K.: Evidence for a Noncatalytic Carrier Protein in Cholesterol Biosynthesis. J. biol. Chem. **246**, 224—230 (1971a).

SCALLEN, T. J., DHAR, A. K., LOUGHRAN, E. D.: Isolation and Characterization of C-4 Methyl Intermediates in Cholesterol Biosynthesis After Treatment of Rat Liver *In Vitro* With Cholestan -3β, 5α, 6β-Triol. J. biol. Chem. **246**, 3168—3174 (1971b).

SCALLEN, T. J., SRIKANTAIAH, M. V., SKRALANT, H. B., HANSBURY, E.: Characterization of Native Sterol Carrier Protein. FEBS Letters **25**, 227—233 (1972).

SCHROEPFER, G. J., JR., FRANTZ, I. D., JR.: Conversion of Δ^7-Cholesterol-4-^{14}C and 7-Dehydrocholesterol-4-^{14}C to Cholesterol. J. biol. Chem. **236**, 3137—3140 (1961).

SHAH, S. N., PETERSON, N. A., McKEAN, C. M.: Inhibition of *In Vitro* Sterol Biosynthesis by Phenylalanine. Biochim. biophys. Acta (Amst.) **164**, 604—606 (1968).

SHEFER, S., HAUSER, S., LAPAR, V., MOSBACH, E. H.: HMG CoA Reductase of Intestinal Mucosa and Liver of the Rat. J. Lipid Res. **13**, 402—412 (1972).

SUGIYAMA, T., CLINKENBEARD, K., MOSS, J., LANE, M. D.: Multiple Cytosolic Forms of Hepatic β-Hydroxy-β Methyglutaryl CoA Synthase: Possible Regulatory Role in Cholesterol Synthesis. Biochem. Biophys. Res. Commun. **48**, 255—261 (1972).

THUY, L. P., HAVEN, G. T., JACOBI, H. P., RUEGAMER, W. R.: Study of an Inhibitor of Hepatic Cholesterol Synthesis Found in Kidney Microsomes. Res. Commun. Chem. Path. Pharm. **5**, 5—18 (173).

UNGAR, F., KAN, K. W., McCOY, K. E.: Activator and Inhibitor Factors in Cholesterol Side-Chain Cleavage. Ann N. Y. Acad. Sci. **212**, 276—288 (1973).

WHITE, L. W.: Regulation of Hepatic Cholesterol Biosynthesis by Clofibrate Administration. J. Pharm. exp. Ther. **178**, 361—370 (1971).

WHITE, L. W.: Feedback Regulation of Cholesterol Biosynthesis. Circulation Res. **31**, 899—907 (1972).

WITIAK, D. T., HACKNEY, R. E., WHITEHOUSE, M. W.: Inhibition of Cholesterolgenesis *in Vitro* by Chlorophenoxyacetic Acids. Effect of α-Methyl Groups. J. Med. Chem. **12**, 697—699 (1969).

WITIAK, D. T., PARKER, R. A., BRANN, D. R., DEMPSEY, M. E., RITTER, M. C., CONNOR, W. E., BRAHMANKAR, D. M.: Biological Evaluation *In Vivo* and *In Vitro* of Selected 5α-Cholestane-3β, 5α, 6β-Triol Analogs as Hypocholesterolemic Agents. J. med. Chem. **14**, 216—222 (1971a).

WITIAK, D. T., PARKER, R. A., DEMPSEY, M E., RITTER, M. C.: Inhibitors & Stimulators of Cholesterolgenesis Enzymes. A Structure Activity Study *in Vitro* of Amino and Selected N-Containing Analogs of 5α-Cholestane-3β, 5α, 6β-Triol. J. med. Chem. **14**, 684—693 (1971b).

CHAPTER 2

Cholesterol Metabolism in Man

H. S. SODHI

With 12 Figures

I. Introduction

Cholesterol is an important structural component of all cellular and intracellular membranes as well as of plasma lipoproteins. The cholesterol present in plasma is only a small fraction of the total present in the body but is, in many respects, the most important fraction. Patients with hypercholesterolemia have a greater risk of developing atherosclerosis of the coronary arteries. Conversely, reduction in plasma cholesterol may reduce the risk of death from myocardial infarction. Elevation of plasma cholesterol is assumed to increase the rate of deposition of cholesterol in tissues, including the arterial intima: the site of atherosclerotic lesions. The pathological effects of total circulating cholesterol may be significantly modified by the differences in the spectra of plasma lipoproteins. Attempts to decrease plasma cholesterol by diet or drugs are based on the hope that reduction in the rate of deposition of cholesterol may retard the development of lesions and also the risk of myocardial infarction.

A number of hypocholesterolemic agents have been developed, and many more are under active investigation. Studies on these agents have included their effects on absorption, synthesis, and excretion of cholesterol from the body. Changes in the total exchangeable pools have also been studied. Changes in the body pools of cholesterol are not necessarily associated with parallel and equal changes in plasma concentrations of cholesterol. Alteration in the rates of absorption, synthesis, or catabolism are not necessarily reflected by parallel changes in the plasma cholesterol. Furthermore, there is no evidence to indicate that alterations in the sizes of exchangeable pools parallel the changes in the cholesterol deposited in the atheromatous lesions. Although considerable data on many parameters of cholesterol metabolism are available, their exact relationships to the homeostatic mechanisms controlling the levels of plasma cholesterol are not fully understood. Since the cholesterol in plasma is transported by macromolecules in association with other lipids and proteins, it is essential to elucidate their metabolism in order to understand homeostatic control of plasma cholesterol.

Factors influencing deposition and mobilization of cholesterol from tissue pools are also not fully known. Plasma cholesterol concentration and the spectra of lipoproteins are two such factors. The existence of others is suggested by the development of xanthomata in diseases associated with normal concentrations of plasma cholesterol; e.g., cerbrotendinous xanthomatosis.

Many aspects of cholesterol metabolism have been intensively investigated in experimental animals during the last few decades. However, due to species' differences, the animal data cannot be indiscriminately extrapolated to man. The available methods for investigating cholesterol metabolism in man are so difficult and time consuming that only a small number of reliable studies have been done. Considerable information has, however, been collected by pioneering work of a small number of clinical investigators. However, there are still large areas which are either poorly understood or not understood at all. The need for simpler methods is obvious.

The phenomenon of exchange of free cholesterol between plasma and tissues has led not only to the definition of some concepts but also to considerable confusion in their use. Synthesis of cholesterol occurs in almost all tissues, but there is a lack of precise information concerning absolute contributions to plasma and total cholesterol pools. Endogenous synthesis and absorption of dietary cholesterol are two obvious sources for total body pools; but, as mentioned earlier, they do not necessarily have a direct and parallel effect on plasma cholesterol. Cholesterol concentration in plasma is determined by its rates of entry and exit into and out of that compartment. More is known about the sources and mechanisms of cholesterol entering plasma than about its modes of exit.

Several excellent recent reviews on different aspects of cholesterol metabolism are available (Danielsson, 1963; Goodman, 1965; Chevallier, 1967; Treadwell and Vahouny, 1968; Nestel, 1970a; Dietschy and Wilson, 1970). Enzymatic pathways for synthesis of cholesterol and bile acids—the major catabolic products—are discussed elsewhere in this volume. The emphasis in this chapter will be on the current understanding of homeostatic mechanisms controlling the concentration of plasma cholesterol in man and the relationship between plasma and tissue cholesterol pools. Finally a new concept of cholesterol metabolism in man is offered which, if accepted, will significantly influence our approach to the study and development of future hypocholesterolemic agents.

II. Distribution of Cholesterol in the Body

In an average male there is approximately 140 g of total cholesterol. Brain and nervous tissues contain a little less than 40 g, and of the remainder only about 5% is present in the plasma compartment (Cook, 1958; Maurizi et al., 1968). Traces can be detected in cerebrospinal fluid (Tourtellotte et al., 1959) and in urine (Kayser and Balat, 1952). Urinary concentration of cholesterol bears no relationship to the concentration in plasma (Vela and Acevedo, 1969).

Different samples of the same tissue in man show some variation in the content of cholesterol. The coefficients of variation were 4% for muscle, 10% for dura mater, and approximately 18% for skin and adipose tissue (Crouse et al., 1972). Although esterified cholesterol can be detected in almost all tissues, most of the cholesterol present in the body is unesterified. Esterified cholesterol present in plasma or in adrenal glands, however, may constitute more than 70% of the total (Boyd, 1942; Adams and Baxter, 1949). Liver contains about 20 to 25% in the esterified form (Ralli et al., 1941; Man et al., 1945). Cholesterol feeding can increase liver cholesterol many-fold in experimental animals, but its effects in man are not known. Liver cholesterol esters increased threefold in 12 hrs and tenfold in 7 days in rats given only 90 mg of cholesterol per day. The increase in liver free cholesterol, on the other hand, was seen only during the first few days (1.4-fold), and the values had returned to the starting levels by 7 days (KLEIN and MARTIN, 1959). Cholesterol feeding in rats has also been shown to be associated with a marked increase in adipose tissue cholesterol (ANGEL and FARKAS, 1970). In rabbits, on the other hand, cholesterol feeding did not appear to cause any increase in adipose tissue cholesterol (HO and TAYLOR, 1971).

Studies in man have been few and inconclusive (KHAN et al., 1963; NIEMINEN, 1965; MAURIZI et al., 1968; CROUSE et al., 1972). Earlier studies of KHAN et al. (1963) and of NIEMINEN (1965) did not suggest any systematic increase with age in the cholesterol content of tissues. Studies of INSULL et al. (1968) noted increases in adipose tissue and muscle, and MAURIZI et al. (1968) noted similar age-related increases in muscle cholesterol. CROUSE et al. (1972) examined subjects who had died suddenly and unexpectedly, in contrast to previous studies where tissues were examined from subjects dying of chronic debilitating diseases. Of the various tissues examined, connective tissue demonstrated the greatest increase in cholesterol content with age. Changes in the cholesterol content of muscle, adipose tissue, and skin were relatively minor. Most of the increase in the tissue cholesterol was noted in the esterified fraction, in accord with the observations in experimental animals.

Increases in the cholesterol pools have also been shown to occur when human volunteers were given large quantities of cholesterol in their diet (QUINTÃO et al., 1971 b).

III. Functions of Cholesterol

Unesterified cholesterol constitutes an important structural element of tissue or plasma lipoproteins. A considerable variety in membrane lipid composition is observed both in kind and relative abundance. The tissue content of cholesterol in eight autopsies on Masai subjects showed a striking similarity to the cholesterol content of similar tissues in dog, rat, and rabbit (HO and TAYLOR, 1968; HO et al., 1971). It was therefore suggested that histologically-similar tissues from the same organ from different species of mammals also have similar content of structural cholesterol. Cholesterol in mammalian cell membranes can be replaced by plant sterols such as campesterol and β-sitosterol. Their incorporation, however, is not as efficient as that of cholesterol (EDWARDS and GREEN, 1972).

Small amounts of esterified cholesterol present in tissues are generally assumed to represent a storage form of cholesterol. Esterification protects against auto-oxidation and enhances chemical stability. Of the various subcellular fractions of the liver cell, the microsomes, the mitochondria, and the nucleii contain 3 to 6% of their cholesterol as esters; whereas 25 to 75% of the cholesterol in the cell sap is esterified. The free cholesterol present in microsomes, mitochondria, and nucleii is assumed to be structural in function; whereas cholesterol in the cell sap may represent either a storage form or contamination from plasma (RICE et al., 1953; SCHOTZ et al., 1953; SPIRO and McKIBBIN, 1956).

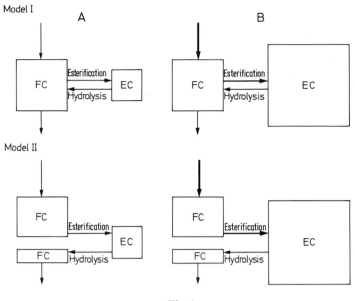

Fig. 1

The relationship of tissue free and esterified cholesterol may be represented by one of the two models shown in Fig. 1. In both models, entry and exit occur only into and form the free cholesterol pool(s). Free cholesterol entering in excess of the tissue requirement is converted into cholesterol esters. Thus an increase in the rate of entry or a decrease in the rate of exit from these pools is reflected more by changes in the size of cholesterol ester pools than by those of free cholesterol. Model 1 is exampli- fied by adrenal cortex, where cholesterol esters provide a ready source of free choles- terol for acute needs that may arise. Model 2 suggests that esterification of structural free cholesterol is an obligatory step in the turnover of tissue lipoproteins.

The role of cholesterol esters in plasma lipoproteins is more uncertain. A struc- tural role for cholesterol esters in plasma lipoproteins was suggested by VANDEN- HEUVEL (1962). He suggested that cholesterol esters were "generally wedge-shaped molecules and make appropriate components in lipid films with small radii of curva- ture. It is possible that cholesterol ester molecules serve to provide a stable, curved lipoprotein surface by means of their wedge shape together with the organized interactions of the ester groups with the protein chain. The free space at the end of the cholesterol molecule can easily accommodate the crooked ends of unsaturated fatty acids. The high proportion of polyunsaturated fatty acids in plasma cholesterol esters may therefore serve the geometric function of providing suitable structural wedges for lipoprotein construction."

However, most of the cholesterol in lipoproteins newly synthesized by the liver (as is in the case of tissues) may be unesterified (GLOMSET, 1968, 1970); and, as suggested by Model 2 in Fig. 1, esterification represents turnover of plasma lipoproteins. It is unlikely that cholesterol esters are primarily involved in the net transport of either cholesterol or of fatty acids. However, it is possible that under certain special conditions—such as during myelination—plasma cholesterol esters may be taken up by tissues for their use.

Cholesterol is the precursor of bile acids (BLOCH et al., 1943; BERGSTROM, 1952), which are necessary for the absorption of lipids from the intestinal lumen (ROTHS-CHILD, 1914; SIPERSTEIN et al., 1952a).

Cholesterol is the major precursor of all steroid hormones—including adrenal glucocorticoids, mineralocorticoids, androgens, and estrogens—testicular and ovarian hormones, and steroid hormones synthesized by placenta (ZAFFARONI et al., 1951; HECHTER et al., 1953; WERBIN et al., 1957).

Cholesterol is also the precursor for Vitamin D_3 in the body (BILLS, 1935; GLOVER et al., 1952).

IV. Synthesis of Cholesterol

Credit for the elucidation of the pathway for cholesterol synthesis (Fig. 2) goes to BLOCH, LYNEN, CORNFORTH, and POPJAK—among many others. Details can be found in excellent reviews published recently by BLOCH (1965), KRITCHEVSKY (1967), and FRANTZ and SCHROEPFER (1967). BLOCH et al. (1946) were the first to demonstrate the incorporation of labelled acetate into cholesterol by rat liver slices. Subsequently SRERE et al. (1950) and POPJAK and BEECKMANS (1950) showed that extrahepatic tissues can also actively incorporate acetate into sterols. These studies were confirmed in many laboratories (DIETSCHY and SIPERSTEIN, 1967; DIETSCHY and WILSON, 1968), and it is now apparent that every animal tissue is capable of at least some degree of cholesterol synthesis.

BUCHER and McGARRAHAN (1956) demonstrated that microsomes and the supernatant fractions of liver homogenates from rats were required for the conversion of acetate to cholesterol. The reduction of β-hydroxy-β-methyl glutarate (HMG) to mevalonate can occur both in microsomes and in the supernatant (BUCHER et al., 1960). Ninety percent of mevalonate synthesis occurs in the microsomes and 10% in the supernatant (KNAUSS et al., 1959; SIPERSTEIN and FAGAN, 1966). When microsomes were further subfractionated into ribosomes, endoplasmic reticulum, and the soluble interior, the HMG-CoA reductase activity was present exclusively in the endoplasmic reticulum or in the microsomal membrane (SIPERSTEIN and FAGEN, 1966). Subsequent reactions leading to cholesterol synthesis also take place in the microsomal fraction (CHESTERTON, 1966).

Every carbon in the cholesterol molecule may be derived from acetate (RITTEN-BERG and BLOCH, 1944, 1945; LITTLE and BLOCH, 1950; CORNFORTH et al., 1953, 1957). The first step is the activation of acetate by combination with coenzyme-A to give a high energy thiol-ester linkage. This reaction is catalyzed by an acetate-activating enzyme, which is widely distributed in animal tissues (JONES et al., 1953; HELE, 1954). Two molecules of acetyl-CoA are catalyzed to acetoacetyl-CoA by β-ketothiolase, and acetoacetyl-CoA serves as an intermediate for synthesis of fatty acids, ketone bodies, and cholesterol (LYNEN, 1955). Acetoacetyl-CoA condenses with another molecule of acetyl-CoA to form β-hydroxy-β-methylglutaryl-CoA (HMG-CoA) which can be converted either to ketone bodies or to cholesterol (LYNEN, 1959; CALDWELL and DRUMMOND, 1963). The conversion of HMG-CoA to mevalonic acid by HMG-CoA reductase is the irreversible step in cholesterol biosynthesis, and all reactions subsequent to it are almost specific for sterol synthesis. Ubiquinone is the only other compound known to be formed from mevalonate, but quantitatively it is of minor significance. Mevalonate is converted by a number of enzymatic steps, including the formation of farnesyl pyrophosphate to squalene: the last in a series of open-chain hydrocarbons. Squalene is converted to lanosterol by cyclization, and the latter is converted into cholesterol by either of the two independent pathways shown in Fig. 2. One pathway includes the conversion of lanosterol to desmosterol via the unsaturated side-chain series; and the other, conversion of lanosterol to Δ-7-cholestanol (lathosterol) via the saturated side-chain series.

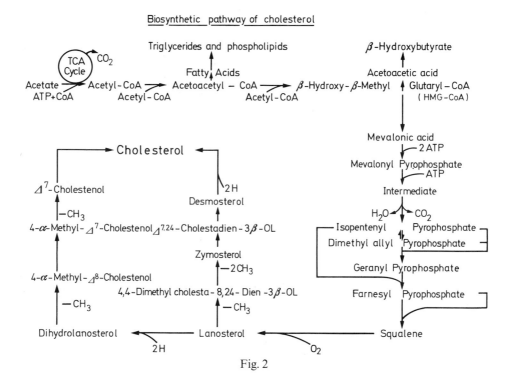

Fig. 2

A. Synthesis of Cholesterol in Various Tissues of the Body

Although all tissues are capable of synthesizing cholesterol from acetate (SRERE, et al., 1950; POPJAK and BEECKMANS, 1950), the rates differ markedly from one tissue to another (DIETSCHY and SIPERSTEIN, 1967; DIETSCHY and WILSON, 1968). In experimental studies on rats and monkeys, the highest rates of cholesterol synthesis per unit weight of tissue were noted in liver and ileum. In both species acetate incorporation into digitonin precipitable sterols was in excess of 100 nMoles/g for liver and ileum. For skin and most other viscera, it was between 5 and 15 nMoles/g of tissue. The lowest rates of synthesis were seen in muscle and mature central nervous system. The differences in the total amounts of cholesterol synthesized by various tissues from acetate became even more striking when organ weights were taken into consideration (DIETSCHY and WILSON, 1968). Of the total cholesterol synthesized in a squirrel monkey, more than 80% was produced in the liver. Both cell types in the liver—parenchymal and Kupffer cells — are capable of synthesis (CHEVALLIER, 1967). Since the vast bulk of liver is made up of parenchymal cells, the amount of cholesterol synthesized in the Kupffer cells is quantitatively unimportant.

There are many pathways open to newly-synthesized hepatic cholesterol: (1) incorporation into lipoproteins of membranes (cellular and subcellular) or of plasma, (2) secretion into bile either as such or as bile acids, (3) storage as cholesterol esters. DIETSCHY (1969) suggested that some of the newly-synthesized cholesterol may be converted to bile acids. However, preliminary studies of BRICKER (1971) showed that most of it was retained in the rat liver presumably as a structural component of tissue lipoproteins. About 10% appeared in the medium in three hours of liver perfusion. Contrary to the suggestion by DIETSCHY (1969), biliary excretion of newly-synthesized cholesterol was less than 0.5% of the total.

Data are not available to demonstrate that liver is as important an organ in cholesterol synthesis in man as it is in other experimental animals; however, this is generally assumed to be the case. Studies of human biopsy specimens showed that hepatic synthesis of cholesterol was more active than that of other tissues (DIETSCHY and WILSON, 1970).

The gastrointestinal tract is the next most important organ for endogenous synthesis of cholesterol (DIETSCHY and SIPERSTEIN, 1965; DIETSCHY and WILSON, 1968). The contribution of the G.I. tract amounted to about 10% of the total synthesis. The synthetic activity of the ileum was the maximum. The synthesis was lowest in the part of the duodenum just distal to the entry of the common bile duct, and it remained more or less constant in the middle portion of the small bowel. The synthesis increased in the proximal ileum and reached its maximum in the terminal ileum. Similar patterns were seen in the rat and the monkey. The same appeared to be the case in man. In the material obtained by suction biopsy from 29 normal subjects, the cholesterol synthesis was lowest in stomach and rectum, higher in the proximal duodenum than in the distal duodenum and the jejunum, and highest in the distal ileum (DIETSCHY and GAMEL, 1971).

It was reported by DIETSCHY and SIPERSTEIN (1965) that synthesis of cholesterol in the intestinal tract occurred only in the cells lining the crypts, with little, if any, activity in those lining the villi. In their *in vitro* studies they observed that mature epithelial cells of villi contributed less than 1% of digitonin precipitable sterols found in the whole wall preparation. Their preparations oxidized acetate-2-^{14}C to carbon dioxide, suggesting that their preparations were viable. Contrary to these observations, SODHI(1967) reported that intestinal villi were at least as active in cholesterol synthesis as intestinal crypts. In accord with this report, MAK and TRIER (1972) showed that radioactive mevalonic acid was incorporated into digitonin precipitable sterols in the absorptive cells of villi of rat ileum. They observed little conversion of radioactive mevalonate to digitonin precipitable sterols in the cells of intestinal crypts. Extensive *in vivo* and *in vitro* investigations in rats and guinea pigs carried out in the laboratories of GOULD and of SODHI (unpublished observations) clearly demonstrated that the synthesis of cholesterol in the cells of villi was at least as active as in the cells of crypts. Some of those results are shown in Tables 1 and 2.

Table 1. Cholesterol synthesis in rat intestinal fractions determined *in vivo*

Cholesterol (dpm per mg. protein)

Time (min)	Villi	Crypts	Muscle	Ratio: Villi/Crypts
10	286	476	35	0.60
20	324	427	30	0.76
40	550	597	68	0.92

A. Acetate-1-^{14}C (50 μC/100 g of body weight) was injected into the jugular vein, and one rat was killed at each interval. Intestinal villi from the distal portion of the ileum were scraped from crypts and muscle cells, and the ratio of radioactive cholesterol to tissue protein was determined

Cholesterol (dpm per mg. cholesterol)

Time (min)	Villi	Crypts	Ratio:	Percent of non-saponifiable fraction activity present as digitonin precipitable sterols	
				Villi	Crypts
7	11380	12360	0.92	14	18
11.5	9240	8390	1.10	20	24
10	2610	1710	1.53	43	39
10	3930	3750	1.05	15	11
8.5	12090	15920	0.76	31	30
20	4230	1520	2.78	58	50

B. Acetate-2-^{3}H (200 μC) was injected intraperitoneally, and one rat was killed at each interval. Intestinal villi from the duodenum above the entrance to the common bile duct were scraped from crypts and muscle cells, and the radioactivity in non-saponifiable fraction and in cholesterol was determined

Of the total cholesterol synthesized in the small intestine about one-half was absorbed into the intestinal lymph, and the remainder was discharged into the lumen (WILSON and REINKE, 1968). The radioautographic studies of MAK and TRIER (1972) suggested that recently-synthesized cholesterol tended to concentrate near the brush border of the intestinal cells. It is therefore possible that the experimental procedures employed by WILSON and REINKE (1968) might have removed some of the brush border and the newly-synthesized cholesterol from the intestinal mucosa into the intestinal lumen. SODHI et al. (unpublished data) found a significant fraction of the newly-synthesized cholesterol in the washings of rat intestine one hour after the injection of radioactive mevalonate. The radioactivity in the washings remained more or less the same up to 16 hrs. However, a fraction of the endogenous choles-terol would be expected through exfoliation of mature cells into the lumen. DIET-SCHY and WILSON (1970) have indicated that in man the contributions of endogenous cholesterol in the intestinal lumen from the mucosa were minor compared to those from bile.

Skin is the third most important organ. Calculated on the basis of the whole organ synthetic activity in a squirrel monkey, skin contributed about 5% of the total digitonin precipitable sterols, of which cholesterol constituted only 20% (DIETSCHY

Table 2. Cholesterol synthesis in Guinea pig intestinal fractions determined *in vitro*

Tissue Fraction	Radioactivity incorporated into non-saponifiable compounds (dpm/mg protein)	Radioactivity incorporated into digitonin precipitable sterols (dpm/mg protein)	Cholesterol synthesized (mμmoles/g. tissue/hr.)
	Mean $\pm$ SEM	Mean $\pm$ SEM	Mean $\pm$ SEM
Villi	1421 $\pm$ 124[a] (7)[b]	884 $\pm$ 90[a] (5)[b]	39.84 $\pm$ 4.08[a] (5)[b]
Crypts	612 $\pm$ 54 (7)	406 $\pm$ 90 (5)	18.30 $\pm$ 1.82 (5)
Muscle	111 $\pm$ 20[a] (7)	85 $\pm$ 15[a] (5)	3.85 $\pm$ 0.67[a] (5)
Intestinal Wall (incubated without scraping)	576 $\pm$ 40 (5)	371 $\pm$ 20 (5)	16.71 $\pm$ 0.90 (5)

Intestinal villi, crypts, and muscle cells were scraped from the distal ileum and incubated separately in 3.5 ml of Krebs-Ringer bicarbonate buffer, pH 7.2, containing 100 mg% glucose and 10 μmoles (1 μC) of acetate-2-^{14}C for 60 min at 37° under O_2/CO_2 (95%/5%). mμmoles cholesterol synthesized/g tissue/hr. was calculated as

$$\frac{(\text{dpm in digitonin precipitable sterols/mg. protein}) \times 150}{2.22 \times 10^3 \times 0.1 \times 15}$$

[a] $p < 0.002$ (difference with crypts).
[b] Number of samples examined.

and WILSON, 1968). SRERE et al. (1950) were the first to demonstrate that skin fragments incorporated acetate into sterols. The production of squalene from acetate occurred anaerobically, whereas its subsequent conversion to digitonin precipitable sterols occurred only in the presence of oxygen (GAYLOR, 1961, 1963). The conversion of squalene to sterols in the slices of epidermis was rapid, while the process was considerably slower in dermal slices (GAYLOR, 1963).

Differences in the rate of cholesterol synthesis have also been seen between the zones of the adrenal cortex. Although local production in the adrenal glands is insignificant when compared to the needs of cholesterol for steroid hormone production, synthesis was substantially greater in zona reticularis than in zona fasciculata. Most of the cholesterol necessary for synthesis of steroid hormones by the adrenal glands is derived from plasma free cholesterol (BORKOWSKI et al., 1972a, b).

Differences in the rates of cholesterol synthesis have also been observed between the cortex and medulla of the kidneys; however, the significance of the difference is not apparent (RASKIN and SIPERSTEIN, 1971; SODHI and KUDCHODKAR, unpublished observations).

Synthesis of cholesterol in adipose tissue was recently suggested by the studies of NESTEL et al. (1969) and of MIETTINEN (1971). Based on their studies in man, they concluded that increases in adiposity were related to increases in endogenous synthesis of cholesterol, suggesting that the site of the latter was adipose tissue. Studies on rats by ANGEL and FARKAS (1971) showed that adipose tissue was capable of active synthesis of cholesterol, especially when glucose was used as the precursor. However, studies of SCHREIBMAN (1974) indicate that synthesis of cholesterol in adipose tissue of man is insignificant, and it could not account for the observations of NESTEL et al. (1969) and of MIETTINEN (1971) in obesity.

It is noteworthy that in most of the above studies the end-point was digitonin precipitable sterols rather than the cholesterol itself. It has long been known that the significant incorporation of radioactive acetate into sterols other than cholesterol occurred in many tissues. The fraction incorporated into other sterols varies with different tissues. Of the total digitonin precipitable sterols synthesized in the liver, intestines, and the skin of a monkey, the fractions constituted by cholesterol were 94%, 82%, and 18% respectively (DIETSCHY and WILSON, 1968).

It is also worth emphasizing that acetate is not the only precursor from which tissues may synthesize cholesterol. Radioactive water, glucose, mevalonate, and leucine may also be used for this purpose. Results obtained with different precursors were strikingly different from each other. For example, if glucose-U-^{14}C is used, 70 to 85% of the radioactive cholesterol is recovered outside the (mouse) liver (JANSEN et al., 1972) in contradistinction to the results obtained with acetate. In other studies, the fetal brain has been shown to utilize glucose preferentially for cholesterol synthesis during myelination (PLOTZ et al., 1968). Similarly, the effects of cholesterol feeding were also very different when tested by different precursors of endogenous cholesterol. Cholesterol feeding almost eliminated liver cholesterol synthesis from glucose-U-^{14}C, but it reduced the extrahepatic synthesis by about 40% of the normal values (JANSEN et al., 1970). The incorporation of leucine into cholesterol by muscle was 200 times greater than that of acetate and 25 times greater than that of mevalonate (MIETTINEN and PENTTILA, 1968, 1971). Although leucine and acetate are both converted to HMG-CoA during sterol synthesis, the incorporation of leucine into cholesterol was inhibited by cholesterol feeding to a much smaller degree than the incorporation of acetate.

Radioactive water has been considered to be the best precursor for studies on synthesis of cholesterol. It mixes readily with the total body water, and significant changes in the latter rarely occur. GOULD et al. (1959) compared the results obtained with radioactive acetate and radioactive water. In the limited experimental conditions of those studies, the results were generally comparable.

Most data on relative rates of cholesterol synthesis were obtained from *in vitro* experiments, and it has been demonstrated that they do not always agree with the results of *in vivo* studies (KABARA, 1973). The results obtained from these studies should therefore not be extrapolated to man without some reservations.

B. Control of Endogenous Synthesis of Cholesterol

TAYLOR and GOULD (1950), GOULD et al. (1953), and subsequently many others (TOMKINS et al., 1953; LANGDON and BLOCH, 1953; FRANTZ et al., 1954) demonstrated that when animals were fed a high-cholesterol diet the ability of liver slices from such animals to synthesize cholesterol from acetate-^{14}C was markedly inhibited. As little as 0.1% cholesterol in the diet of the rat caused a 50% inhibition of cholesterol synthesis, and 0.5% cholesterol in the diet caused about 95% inhibition (SIPERSTEIN and GUEST, 1960). Similar negative feedback inhibition by dietary cholesterol has now been demonstrated in a large number of species, including birds (SAKAKIDA et al., 1963), rodents (SIPERSTEIN and GUEST, 1960), dogs (GOULD et al.,

1953), and primates (Cox et al., 1954). In fact, feedback control of cholesterol synthesis has been shown in all members of the animal kingdom that are capable of synthesizing cholesterol (SIPERSTEIN, 1965).

The results of studies on man, however, have been equivocal. The first studies on human liver slices suggested that the feedback system did not play an important role in compensating for variations in intake (DAVIS et al., 1958). Subsequent studies on human liver biopsy specimens indicated that dietary cholesterol in amounts of 3 to 4 g per day suppressed synthesis of cholesterol almost completely (BHATTATHIRY and SIPERSTEIN, 1963). From their isotopic balance studies, TAYLOR et al. (1960) and WILSON and LINDSEY (1965) came to the conclusion that negative feedback inhibition in man was insignificant. GRUNDY et al. (1969) suggested that in man the extent of feedback control by cholesterol could not be adequately evaluated through balance type studies. They argued that once the steady state had been attained the increment in absorption was balanced by an increment in the fecal excretion, thereby masking any decrease by inhibition of synthesis. They tested for the presence of negative feedback inhibition after giving large amounts of plant sterols to reduce the absorption of cholesterol. They noted continuous increase in the fecal excretion of endogenous steroids for as long as 112 days. The authors felt that this prolonged effect could not be explained on the basis of mobilization of tissue cholesterol. They concluded therefore that it must represent an increase in endogenous synthesis. Our observations (KUDCHODKAR et al., 1971a, 1973b) are also in support of this conclusion. Feeding plant sterols caused a significant increase in the specific activity slope of plasma cholesterol, and the changes were reversed when the treatment was stopped.

Most subjects in North America habitually consume moderate amounts of cholesterol. The hepatic synthesis therefore might have been partially inhibited even during the control periods. Assuming that the demonstration of feedback inhibition would be easier if hepatic synthesis were not inhibited during the control period, we investigated three subjects who ate less than 300 mg of cholesterol a day. Each subject was given two injections of a mixture of acetate-1-^{14}C and mevalonate-2-^{3}H, once before and once after the high-cholesterol diet, and the relative amounts of the two isotopes incorporated into plasma cholesterol were determined. From the ratios of the incorporation of acetate and mevalonate, the percentage inhibition of endogenous synthesis of cholesterol was calculated by the methods published by us previously (SODHI et al., 1971a). The results indicated that high-cholesterol diets for 4 to 6 weeks caused 14 to 30% inhibition of hepatic synthesis of cholesterol (SODHI and KUDCHODKAR, unpublished observations). Elegant studies of QUINTÃO et al. (1971b) recently demonstrated that increased absorption of cholesterol is compensated by a decrease in endogenous synthesis in some subjects and not in others.

Studies of GOULD and POPJAK (1957) and of BUCHER et al. (1959) indicated that the inhibition of cholesterol synthesis by dietary cholesterol occurred at a step between acetate and mevalonate. Specific biochemical localization was worked out by SIPERSTEIN and his associates (SIPERSTEIN and GUEST, 1960; SIPERSTEIN and FAGAN, 1964; SIPERSTEIN and FAGAN, 1966). They demonstrated that the dietary cholesterol caused a marked inhibition of synthesis of mevalonate but had no detectable effect on the synthesis of β-hydroxy-β-methyl glutarate. This was supported subsequently by the observation that cholesterol feeding specifically inhibited the direct conversion of β-hydroxy-β-methyl glutarate to mevalonate in cell-free systems (LINN, 1967; KANDUTSCH and SAUCIER, 1969; SHAPIRO and RODWELL, 1969). This is also the first unique and irreversible reaction in the biochemical pathway for synthesis of cholesterol. It was shown that over 90% of mevalonate production occurred in the microsomes, and it was the microsomal enzyme which was under the feedback control. The small amount of mevalonate synthesis that occurred in the supernatant of hepatic cells was relatively unaffected by short-term cholesterol feeding (SIPERSTEIN and FAGAN, 1966).

High levels of cholesterol in plasma in the form of very low density lipoproteins do not appear to cause inhibition of hepatic cholesterol synthesis (MARSH and DRABKIN, 1958; DUBACH et al., 1961; SAKAKIDA et al., 1963). Chylomicra, on the other hand, when infused in systemic circulation caused a prompt feedback inhibition in the liver (SAKAKIDA et al., 1963; WEIS and DIETSCHY, 1969). Conversely, lymph duct cannulation stimulated synthesis (SWELL et al., 1957; WEIS and DIETSCHY, 1969). It is therefore likely that the exogenous cholesterol absorbed from the intestine—but not the endogenous cholesterol present in plasma—is responsible for the activation of the cholesterol feedback system (WEIS and DIETSCHY, 1969; SIPERSTEIN, 1970).

It has also been suggested, from time to time, that bile acids may represent the feedback inhibitor that controls the synthesis of cholesterol in the liver. The role of bile acids was investigated recently by WEIS and DIETSCHY (1969). They demonstrated that both biliary diversion and biliary obstruction increased the rate of hepatic synthesis, though only one of them decreased the hepatic content of bile acids. Restoration of hepatic circulation of bile acids in animals with biliary diversion failed to prevent the rise in synthetic activity seen after this operation. This suggested that bile acids play no direct inhibitory role in the regulation of cholesterol synthesis by the liver. Increase in synthetic activity in animals with biliary diversion was prevented by infusions of approximately 7 mg of cholesterol per day in the form of chylomicra (WEIS and DIETSCHY, 1969). Most of the (reported) in vivo effects of bile acids on hepatic synthesis can therefore be explained on the basis of their action on intestinal absorption of cholesterol and on its rate of delivery into the circulation. Due to non-specific inhibition of homogenates by bile acids, their effects on in vitro systems cannot be seriously considered as evidence of their physiological role (POPE et al., 1966; DIETSCHY, 1968).

Cholesterol feeding (SIPERSTEIN and GUEST, 1960) and fasting (BUCHER et al., 1960) decreased HMG reductase in liver. Addition of HMG in vitro produced a dose-dependent decrease in the rate of cholesterol synthesis. This effect was specific for cholesterol synthesis, since HMG did not have any effect on the rate of oxidation of 1-^{14}C-acetate. The site of inhibition appeared to be the enzymatic step mediated by HMG-CoA reductase. HMG when injected into intact animals also inhibited cholesterol synthesis (BEG and LUPIEN, 1972).

In rat the inhibitory effect of a high-cholesterol diet was more marked in liver than in any other organ (GOULD et al., 1953; DIETSCHY and SIPERSTEIN, 1967). The effect could be seen as early as 12 hrs and was complete within 48 hrs (DIETSCHY and SIPERSTEIN, 1967; DIETSCHY and WILSON, 1968). Whereas cholesterol synthesis in the liver was suppressed more than a hundredfold, the suppression in the intestines was only 20 to 50% (DIETSCHY and SIPERSTEIN, 1967; DIETSCHY and WILSON, 1968). In a recent study on guinea pigs it was shown that cholesterol feeding caused 93% inhibition in the liver, 78% in the lungs, 79% in the intestines, 95% in the spleen, 81% in the lymph nodes, 72% in the adrenal glands, and 30% in the brain. Accumulation of cholesterol was present in all tissues studied. Except in brain and liver, inhibition of cholesterol synthesis was proportional to the tissue cholesterol accumulation (SWANN and SIPERSTEIN, 1972).

According to SIPERSTEIN (1970), all submammalian vertebrates possess a cholesterol-sensitive feedback system in their intestines. The mammals (according to SIPERSTEIN) have lost this response and retain, instead, mechanisms which are sensitive only to bile acids. Cholesterol synthesis in the intestines was enhanced when bile was diverted from the lumen, and the activity was inhibited when bile was infused into the lumen of these animals (DIETSCHY and SIPERSTEIN, 1965; DIETSCHY, 1968). The inhibition was not seen when bile acids were removed from the infusate, and the effect was completely reproduced by the intralumenal infusion of taurocholate: the normal bile acid of the rat. Similarly, cholestyramine, which binds the bile acids in the intestinal lumen, increased the intestinal synthesis (CAYEN, 1969). It was also shown by DIETSCHY (1968) that cholesterol synthesis from acetate—but not from mevalonate—was inhibited by bile acids. The biochemical site of the control is therefore, in all probability, located at the same reaction site that governs cholesterol synthesis in the liver.

CAYEN (1969) showed that addition of cholesterol reversed the increase in intestinal synthesis caused by feeding cholestyramine to rats. This suggested that cholesterol may also act as an inhibitor of intestinal synthesis. The bile acids in this case might serve simply to facilitate the entry of cholesterol into the mucosal cell.

C. Diurnal Variation

The available evidence from studies in rats indicates that there is a circadian rhythm in biosynthesis of cholesterol both in liver (KANDUTSCH and SAUCIER, 1969; BACK et al., 1969) and in intestines (EDWARDS et al., 1972). Sterol synthetic activity in ileum and jejunum exhibited a similar circadian rhythm (EDWARDS et al., 1972). Cholesterol synthesis gradually increased through the day, reaching a maximum between 8 p.m. and midnight, and decreased again to a minimum at approximately 8 a.m. (HAMPRECHT et al., 1969; SHAPIRO and RODWELL, 1969). The evidence available at present is not conclusive, though it suggests that the circadian rhythm is, to a degree, independent of food intake, although the major increase in activity appears to be in response to eating (EDWARDS et al., 1972).

In the fasting rat the highest level of HMG-CoA reductase activity is only a small fraction of that produced after ingestion of a normal diet. Fasting for three days caused a lowering of the rate of synthesis but did not abolish the circadian rhythm (HICKMAN et al., 1972). It could be abolished, however, by inhibitors of protein synthesis such as puromycin or cycloheximide, indicating a probable requirement for new enzymic protein synthesis in the process (BACK et al., 1969; KANDUTSCH and SAUCIER, 1969). Recently HICKMAN et al. (1972) found that adrenalectomy abolished the circadian rhythm and caused the cholesterol synthesis to remain at a uniformly high level. The authors suggested that corticosterone may play an essential role in the daily rhythm of cholesterogenesis.

Tomkins and Chaikoff (1952) found that fasting for as little as 24 hrs resulted in a pronounced reduction in the capacity of liver slices to incorporate acetate into cholesterol. This effect has been confirmed in experimental animals, both *in vitro* (Migicovsky and Wood, 1955; Dietschy and Siperstein, 1967) and *in vivo* (Lupien and Migicovsky, 1964; Jansen et al., 1966). Chronic undernutrition also resulted in a similar decrease (Tomkins and Chaikoff, 1952). Refeeding of any source of calories, fat, carbohydrate, or protein promptly restored cholesterogenesis to normal (Tomkins and Chaikoff, 1952; Jansen et al., 1966). Very little information is available on the effect of caloric restriction on cholesterol synthesis in man. Miettinen (1968 a) observed that starvation and weight reduction caused inhibition in man. Preliminary studies in man from our laboratories (Kudchodkar et al., 1973 d) are in accord with this observation. The enzymatic site of the regulation of cholesterol synthesis in fasting has been shown to be the same as that during cholesterol feeding; i.e., the reduction of β-hydroxy-β-methylglutaryl-CoA to mevalonate (Bucher et al., 1959, 1960; Linn, 1967). Fasting has also been shown to cause some depression of cholesterol synthesis in intestines. This effect, however, is minor compared to that observed in liver (Dietschy and Siperstein, 1967; Cayen, 1969).

The relationship of thyroid function to hepatic cholesterol synthesis is not absolutely clear. Some reports suggest depression of synthesis in hypothyroidism (Karp and Stetten, 1949; Byers et al., 1952), while others suggest increased synthesis in hypothyroidism (Frantz et al., 1954). The general body of evidence, however, favours the view that cholesterogenesis is decreased in hypothyroid animals and that thyroxin replacement causes a stimulation of synthesis (Fletcher and Myant, 1958, 1960). The changes in cholesterol synthesis with alterations in thyroid status are minor compared to those seen with cholesterol feeding. The incorporation of acetate-^{14}C into plasma cholesterol of man was decreased in hypothyroidism (Lipsky et al., 1955; Gould et al., 1955). Fletcher and Myant (1958), on the other hand, studied the incorporation of mevalonate into cholesterol and noted no significant effect of the thyroid state. They concluded, therefore, that thyroxin exerted its effect at a point prior to the synthesis of mevalonate. It has now been demonstrated that triiodothyronine when given to hypothyroid rats increased the HMG-CoA reductase. It was therefore suggested that thyroid hormones caused an increase in cholesterogenesis through a specific stimulation of the synthesis of this enzyme (Gries et al., 1962; Guder et al., 1968).

Recent studies of Nestel et al. (1969) and of Miettinen (1971) demonstrated a positive correlation between cholesterol synthesis and excess body weight in their subjects. They suggested that the additional synthesis might have occurred in adipose tissue.

Studies done in our laboratories (Sodhi and Kudchodkar, 1971 b, 1973 b) corroborated the above relationship, but the correlation between cholesterol synthesis and excess body weight was not nearly as good as that between cholesterol synthesis and the degree of hypertriglyceridemia. Most of the hypertriglyceridemic subjects had elevations of pre-β-lipoproteins, as judged from lipoprotein bands after agarose electrophoresis (Noble, 1968), and they had either type II b or type IV hyperlipoproteinemia (Beaumont et al., 1970). Cholesterol synthesis was measured by three independent methods: 1) cholesterol balance techniques developed at the Rockefeller University (Miettinen et al., 1965; Grundy et al., 1965), 2) kinetics of plasma cholesterol as reported by GOODMAN and NOBLE (1968), and 3) the relative incorporation of acetate and mevalonate into plasma cholesterol (MIETTINEN, 1970; SODHI et al., 1971a). Each of these methods demonstrated that cholesterol synthesis was much greater in hypercholesterolemic patients who had hypertriglyceridemia than in those who had normal plasma triglycerides. The correlation between the two parameters was excellent ($r > 0.91$). Since the group of patients who had hypertriglyceridemia were also heavier than those with only hypercholesterolemia, it could be argued that the primary relationship of endogenous synthesis of cholesterol was with body weight and that its relationship with hypertriglyceridemia was secondary. However, this did not appear to be so. When the effect of triglyceride concentrations on cholesterol synthesis was excluded from the correlation by appropriate statistical analysis, the relative body weight failed to have a significant correlation with cholesterol synthesis in our subjects. In contrast, the correlation between plasma triglycerides and cholesterol synthesis remained excellent whether or not the effect of body weight was excluded. This was true for all subjects. Furthermore, obese subjects in our studies failed to show a significant correlation between relative body weight and plasma triglycerides.

Our analysis of data published by GOODMAN and NOBLE (1968) and GRUNDY and AHRENS (1969) also tended to support our hypothesis. In the hyperlipemic subjects studied by GOODMAN and NOBLE, the plasma triglyceride concentrations had an excellent correlation ($r = 0.87$) with the production rate of cholesterol. Three of the eleven subjects reported by GRUNDY and AHRENS had type V hyperlipoproteinemia with triglyceride levels significantly above those of the other eight. Cholesterol synthesis was much greater in these three subjects, and the correlation between cholesterol synthesis and plasma triglycerides in the remaining eight was also excellent ($r = 0.75$). The correlations between cholesterol synthesis and relative body weight, in both of these studies, were either modest or insignificant.

Although studies on rat adipose tissue have shown that it can synthesize appreciable amounts of cholesterol (ANGEL and FARKAS, 1971), our results suggested that the increased cholesterol synthesis associated with hypertriglyceridemia can be explained by increased synthetic activity of the liver. The radioactive cholesterol appearing in plasma a few hours after the injection of radioactive precursors comes predominantly from the liver and not from other tissues. The kinetic data on the turnover of cholesterol synthesis in Pool A are also in accord with this suggestion (SODHI and KUDCHODKAR, 1973b). Thus, two of the three methods used in those studies indicated that liver may well be the most important site for increased endogenous synthesis of cholesterol. We have therefore suggested that hypertriglyceridemia is one of the major determinants of the rates of cholesterol synthesis in man Sodhi and KUDCHODKAR, 1971b, 1973b).

D. Methods to Study Synthesis of Cholesterol in Man

Reliable techniques for determining absolute values of cholesterol synthesis in man were developed by AHRENS and his associates (HELLMAN et al., 1957; MIETTINEN et al., 1965; GRUNDY et al., 1965). The proposed balance methods are based on the assumption that losses of endogenous cholesterol and its metabolites occur predominantly in the feces. Studies done in Connor's laboratories indicate that about 80 mg of cholesterol are lost daily from the skin surface (BHATTACHARYYA et al., 1972). At present, it is not known how much of this is derived from exchangeable pools and how much from local synthesis in epidermal cells. About 50 mg of cholesterol is converted into steroid hormones which are lost in the urine per day (BORKOWSKI et al., 1972 a, b).

On a cholesterol-free diet, the amounts of cholesterol and its metabolites lost in the feces are assumed to represent the net synthesis of cholesterol in the body. However, as indicated above, this method would underestimate daily synthesis by more than 100 mg a day.

Absolute values of cholesterol synthesis can be derived in subjects on cholesterol-free diets by the methods of HELLMAN et al. (1957) and of GOODMAN and NOBLE (1968). The isotopic balance method introduced by HELLMAN et al. (1957) involves the use of plasma cholesterol specific activity for the estimation of fecal neutral and acidic steroids. The specific activity values of cholesterol in different pools and those of bile acids reach equilibrium in 3 to 6 weeks after an intravenous injection of radioactive cholesterol. During this isotopic steady state, the synthesis of cholesterol (synthesis = fecal neutral + acidic steroids) can be calculated from the total radioactivity in the fecal neutral and acidic steroids and the specific activity of plasma cholesterol 24 to 48 hrs before the fecal collection period. Recently KUDCHODKAR et al. (1972 c) have suggested the use of plasma cholesterol specific activity 56 hrs before the midpoint in time of the fecal collections for the estimation of fecal bile acids.

In GOODMAN and NOBLE's method, data on plasma cholesterol specific activity are analyzed assuming a two-pool model for exchangeable cholesterol. WILSON's work in baboons (1970) suggested that the entry and exit of cholesterol occurred only in the first, or rapidly-exchangeable, pool and not in the second, or slowly-exchangeable, pool. However, significant synthesis and losses of cholesterol from the skin, which forms a part of the slowly-exchangeable pool, have been alluded to. Despite this, the values of cholesterol turnover obtained in baboons by this method were similar to those obtained by another independent method (WILSON, 1970).

Reports from the Rockefeller University (GRUNDY and AHRENS, 1969) and from our laboratories (SODHI and KUDCHODKAR, 1973 d) indicated that in man the values obtained by cholesterol balance techniques were 8 to 15% lower than the values obtained from the analysis of plasma cholesterol specific activity slopes. Since the production rates given by a two-pool model are somewhat higher than those given by a three-pool model, the difference in the values obtained by the two methods may be significantly reduced if a three-pool model rather than a two-pool model is assumed for calculations (GOODMAN et al., 1972).

Absolute values for synthesis cannot be obtained by either of the above methods when the subjects ingest cholesterol-containing foods. However, if the amounts of cholesterol absorbed are known, the net synthesis can be calculated. The amounts absorbed can be estimated by the method of GRUNDY and AHRENS (1966). Other methods for calculating absorption are given in a subsequent section.

The chemical balance method introduced by MIETTINEN et al. (1965) and GRUNDY et al. (1965), on the other hand, can give absolute values for synthesis whether the subjects eat cholesterol-containing or cholesterol-free diets.

Two simpler methods have been proposed to determine the relative rates of cholesterol synthesis in man. The first is based on the observations that only a small fraction of the acetate pool enters the pathway for cholesterol synthesis and that the site of its control is between acetate and mevalonate. The method was developed independently by MIETTINEN (1970) and by SODHI et al. (1971a). It was assumed that the sizes of precursor pools of acetate and mevalonate were not significantly different in the conditions compared. The data obtained indicated that the results obtained by this method were comparable to the results obtained by cholesterol balance techniques (MIETTINEN, 1970; SODHI and KUDCHODKAR, unpublished observations).

The other method is based on the assumption that precursors of cholesterol leak out of the liver during cholesterol synthesis and their amounts in plasma are directly proportional to the rates of hepatic synthesis. The quantities of cholesterol precursors in plasma are determined by gas-liquid chromatography, and it was shown by MIETTINEN (1970) that the results obtained were compatible with what might have been expected under different experimental conditions.

V. Absorption of Dietary Cholesterol

Cholesterol in body pools is derived from endogenous synthesis and from absorption of exogenous cholesterol. It is not an essential constituent of the diet, since endogenous synthesis is adequate for the normal growth of mammals (BILLS, 1935). Cholesterol is relatively insoluble in water and is, perhaps, one of the largest molecules to be readily absorbed from the intestinal tract. A number of successive steps can be delineated in absorption of dietary cholesterol: 1) transfer from lipid to micellar phase, 2) transfer from micellar phase into the mucosal cells, 3) esterification and incorporation of the cholesterol into chylomicra and intestinal lipoproteins, and finally 4) transfer from the mucosal cells into the lymph.

Considerable amounts of endogenous cholesterol also appear in the intestinal lumen every day. The endogenous cholesterol is secreted into the bile and other gastrointestinal secretions. It is also present in the mucosal cells exfoliated into the lumen. Exogenous and endogenous cholesterol mix in the intestinal lumen, and it is generally assumed that the absorption of both is similar (SWELL et al., 1959a; BORGSTROM, 1960). The suggestion has been made, however, that endogenous cholesterol present in the bile may be secreted in a form which is more readily absorbed than that from the diet (DORÉE and GARDNER, 1909). On the other hand, endogenous cholesterol present in the exfoliated cells cannot be incorporated into the micelles without prior disintegration of the cells. In man the most important source of endogenous cholesterol entering the intestinal lumen is bile, and the quantities derived from intestinal secretions or exfoliation of the intestinal cells are of relatively minor importance (DIETSCHY and WILSON, 1970).

Most of the endogenous cholesterol entering the intestinal lumen is in the form of free sterol, since only traces of cholesterol esters are present in the bile. The proportions of free and esterified cholesterol in the diet are not known, but most of it (approximately 85 to 90% of the total) is unesterified. Cholesterol esters are hydrolyzed in the intestinal lumen by pancreatic cholesterol esterase. There is sufficient evidence to indicate that the cholesterol esters are not absorbed intact. Hydrolysis must occur before absorption of the cholesterol moiety (PETERSON et al., 1954; SWELL et al., 1955; VAHOUNY and TREADWELL, 1958).

The presence of bile acids appears to be essential for absorption of the cholesterol from the intestinal lumen (Rothschild, 1914; Siperstein et al., 1952a; Borja et al., 1964). When cholesterol was fed along with cholic, taurocholic, glycocholic, deoxycholic, lithocholic, and cholanic acids, cholic, taurocholic, and glycocholic acids increased the cholesterol content of the thoracic duct lymph; but deoxycholic, lithocholic, and cholanic acids did not (Swell et al., 1953; Vahouny et al., 1959). These results are consistent with the observation that trihydroxy bile acids stimulate pancreatic cholesterol esterase, while di- or monohydroxy bile acids do not (Müller, 1916; Hernandez and Chaikoff, 1957; Korzenovsky et al., 1960; Murthy and Ganguly, 1962). Conjugated bile acids form micellar solutions with the products of pancreatic lipolysis. Cholesterol esters are hydrolyzed to free cholesterol and free fatty acids. Triglycerides are hydrolyzed to free fatty acids and monoglycerides (Treadwell and Vahouny, 1968).

The bile salts have two independent actions in relationship to the absorption of cholesterol:

1. They act as surface-active agents and thus help in the solubilization of cholesterol by forming micelles (Bashour and Bauman, 1937). Nonpolar hydrocarbon portions of the molecules aggregate in the micelles, and this core is surrounded by polar groups oriented towards the aqueous solvent. They possess the unique property of dissolving water-insoluble organic compounds within the hydrocarbon core (Hartley, 1936, 1955). Fatty acids and monoglycerides become oriented within the micelles with the polar group near the periphery and in contact with water molecules, thereby further stabilizing the micelles. It has been shown that the solubility of cholesterol in the bile salt micelles is low but can be significantly increased by the addition of monoglycerides or phospholipids (Fleisher and Brierly, 1961; Hofmann and Borgstrom, 1964).

2. The bile salts act as cofactors for cholesterol esterase systems in the intestines (Swell et al., 1953; Korzenovsky et al., 1960; Vahouny et al., 1965). The specific role of bile salts in relation to the enzymatic action of cholesterol esterase is uncertain. Murthy and Ganguly (1962) reported that taurocholate was effective in protecting the enzyme against pH inactivation. This was supported by the observations of Vahouny et al. (1964) that taurocholate protected pancreatic juice cholesterol esterase against proteolytic degradation by trypsin, chymotrypsin, or activated pancreatic juice.

It was generally assumed that micelles containing all lipids were passively transferred into the mucosa. However, studies on the time course of absorption of different lipids indicated that 95% or more of the triglycerides and their products were absorbed in 5 to 6 hrs, whereas only 25 to 40% of the cholesterol was absorbed in 24 hrs (Blomstrand and Ahrens, 1958; Borgstrom, 1960). Moreover, the peak absorption of triglycerides occurred approximately 3 hrs after their administration, but that of cholesterol occurred at 5 to 6 hrs after its administration (Borgstrom et al., 1958; Swell et al., 1959a). Most of the cholesterol and triglycerides are absorbed in the upper intestinal tract, and the absorption of bile acids is predominantly in the lower ileum. These data suggest that the intact micelles are not absorbed by the mucosal cells, but that they bring the various lipids in contact with the mucosal lining in a physical state most suited for their rapid absorption.

FAVARGER and METZGER (1952) suggested that prior to the entrance of cholesterol into the mucosal cells, the mucoprotein they secrete specifically binds cholesterol, which is then presumably transferred to lipoproteins of the cell membrane. This suggestion was supported by the observation that dietary sterol could not be extracted with ether unless the protein was first denatured (GLOVER and MORTON, 1958). Incubation of everted sacs of rat intestinal segments in cholesterol-free media allowed isolation of mucoprotein, which contained 64% protein, 11% carbohydrates, and 19% lipids (MAYER, 1963; SMITH and TREADWELL, 1958). When this mucoprotein was added to a cholesterol-containing medium, about 50% (by weight) of the cholesterol was complexed with the mucoprotein. However, when cholesterol-4-^{14}C mucoprotein complex was added to the incubation media, the cholesterol uptake by everted sacs was no greater than in controls containing no mucoprotein. This suggested that the mucoprotein was not involved in the direct transfer of cholesterol into the mucosal cells (MAYER, 1963).

Most of the experimental data indicate that bile salt micelle is necessary for the initial transfer of free cholesterol into the intestinal mucosa, although the mechanisms underlying this transfer are not completely known. After a short exposure of everted intestinal sac to mixed micelles of cholesterol-7α-^{3}H, bile salt-^{14}C, and monoglyceride, the absorbed radioactive cholesterol was present largely in the brush border fraction; whereas the bile salt was largely in the supernatant fraction of the epithelial cells (TREADWELL and VAHOUNY, 1968).

SIMMONDS et al. (1967) showed that fatty acids were important for solubilizing cholesterol in the bile acid micelles and for absorption in the jejunum of man. They perfused a micellar solution of monoglyceride, cholesterol, and bile salt through an intraduodenal triple lumen tube. As the monoglyceride and fatty acids were absorbed, cholesterol precipitated out of the solution. They suggested that the presence of polar lipid might critically influence the extent of absorption of cholesterol. However, recent studies from Isselbacher's laboratories indicated that the cholesterol in the micellar phase was in equilibrium with the cholesterol in the intestinal sediment, and any absorption of cholesterol from the micellar phase was replenished by the cholesterol in the insoluble phase (MCINTYRE et al., 1971).

Studies of GANGULY et al. (1959) demonstrated that the content of intestinal cholesterol did not increase during the absorption of dietary cholesterol in the rat. They suggested, therefore, that lumenal cholesterol merely replaced the molecules absorbed from the intestinal mucosa. This was in accord with the previous observations of GLOVER and co-workers (1957, 1958, 1959) and is also in accord with the recent suggestion of EDWARDS and GREEN (1972). The latter postulated that absorption of cholesterol from the lumen occurred by a process of successive exchanges among the intracellular membranes (of organelles) and soluble lipoproteins. This hypothesis can explain the appearance in lymph of cholesterol synthesized in the intestinal mucosa (SODHI, 1972; SODHI et al., 1973b) but fails to account for the differences in the rates of absorption between dietary and intestinal cholesterol (SODHI et al., 1965, 1967b, 1970, and 1973b). The fractional rate of absorption of dietary cholesterol was up to three times greater than that of intestinal cholesterol synthesized in the mucosa (SODHI et al., 1973b). It appears that the transport of dietary cholesterol across the mucosal cell is facilitated by mechanisms which are not available to cholesterol synthesized in situ (SODHI et al., 1973b).

The rate of cholesterol uptake by the intestinal mucosa was much greater than the rate of its transfer out of the mucosa (BORGSTROM et al., 1958; BORGSTROM, 1968). When radioactive cholesterol was fed to rats, its uptake by the intestinal wall was so rapid that at the very first interval (one hour) at which it was examined the intestinal wall contained the maximum amounts of radioactivity. On the other hand, the rate of transport of the cholesterol out of the intestinal mucosa was such that the absorbed cholesterol had a half-life of about 12 hrs in the wall before it reached the intestinal lymph. In accord with these observations, feeding large amounts of cholesterol to rats was followed by a detectable increase in the content of intestinal cholesterol (BORGSTROM et al., 1958). BORGSTROM et al. (1958) suggested that when radioactive cholesterol was given intralumenally it mixed first with endogenous cholesterol in the lumen and again with the cholesterol in the intestinal mucosa. As early as 1965 and 1967, SODHI and his associates had, however, suggested that the mixing of dietary and endogenous cholesterol in the mucosal cells was not complete and that the cholesterol derived from the two sources could be considered to be in separate pools. They had shown that the fractional rate of transfer from the mucosa to the lymph was greater for exogenous cholesterol than that for cholesterol synthesized in the intestine. It was also noted that the ratios of free to esterified cholesterol specific activity of the two isotopes were different after the administration of mevalonate-2-^{3}H (to label the endogenous cholesterol) and cholesterol-4-^{14}C (to label the exogenous cholesterol). This hypothesis was supported recently by the observations of RUDEL et al. (1972). They demonstrated that esterification of exogenous cholesterol occurred preferentially during its absorption. Their studies also suggested that mechanisms exist within the intestinal mucosa to keep exogenous cholesterol in different pools from those for endogenous cholesterol. Subcellular fractionation of rat intestine four hours after intraperitoneal injection of acetate-1-^{14}C and gastric intubation of cholesterol-^{3}H showed that the relative values of specific activity for the two isotopes in free and esterified cholesterol were different in different fractions (SODHI et al., unpublished observations).

During the transfer of cholesterol from intestinal mucosa to lymph, a major fraction of the cholesterol is esterified with long-chain fatty acids. The enzyme catalyzing this reaction has properties similar to those of pancreatic juice cholesterol esterase (SWELL et al., 1950). There is no evidence that the esterification requires activated fatty acid, as is true for other esterifications of fatty acids (TREADWELL and VAHOUNY, 1968). Although most of the cholesterol absorbed is esterified, esterification does not appear to be an absolute necessity. Between 15 and 40% of the cholesterol in the intestinal lymph is present as free sterol. Epicholesterol, which is not esterified by cholesterol esterase, is absorbed into the lymph, although at about one-half the rate of that of cholesterol (HERNANDEZ et al., 1954). GALLO and TREADWELL (1963) reported that 85 to 95% of the total mucosal cholesterol esterase activity was in the supernatant fraction, as opposed to the mucosal brush border; and it was suggested that sterol esterification occurs after passage of sterols through the brush border. More than 90% of the cholesterol present in the brush border is unesterified, whereas in the remainder of the cell the unesterified cholesterol makes up only two-thirds of the total sterols (GALLO and TREADWELL, 1963). It appears that pancreatic juice cholesterol esterase is intimately involved in cholesterol absorption, and in some manner it also effects the activity of mucosal esterase (LOSSOW et al., 1964).

Mucosal activity and cholesterol absorption are diminished, but not completely eliminated, in the absence of pancreatic juice. Bile without pancreatic juice can increase the level of mucosal cholesterol esterase and the absorption of cholesterol (BORJA et al., 1964).

Cholesterol is incorporated into chylomicra and lipoproteins synthesized by the intestinal mucosa. Studies in rabbits (ZILVERSMIT et al., 1967; RUDEL et al., 1972) indicated that very low density lipoproteins synthesized in the intestines were more important than chylomicra in the transport of cholesterol. Dietary cholesterol was preferentially incorporated into very low density lipoproteins, and the fraction of the dietary cholesterol transported in the lymph increased with time after a single meal containing radioactive cholesterol. The fraction transported in chylomicra, on the other hand, decreased with time after feeding of radioactive cholesterol in a fatty meal (RUDEL et al., 1972). The administration to rats of small doses of puromycin—a known inhibitor of protein synthesis—caused an accumulation of lipids within the mucosal cells and impaired transport to the lymphatics (SEBESIN and ISSELBACHER, 1965). Similar results have also been obtained with acetoxycycloheximide, another inhibitor of protein synthesis (GLICKMAN et al., 1972). These data suggest that there is a need for protein synthesis during cholesterol absorption. The inhibition of protein synthesis was associated with an increase in the size and a decrease in the number of intestinal lymph chylomicra, as compared to normal controls (GLICKMAN et al., 1972). In the disorder characterized by deficiency or absence of plasma β-lipoproteins in humans, dietary lipids accumulate in the mucosal cells (ISSELBACHER et al., 1964; LEVY et al., 1966)—a situation mimicking that in rats given puromycin.

Studies of WILSON and REINKE (1968) indicated that there was little, if any, reabsorption of the cholesterol synthesized in the mucosa and secreted into the intestinal lumen. Possibly a fraction of the dietary cholesterol taken up by the intestinal mucosa is also returned to the lumen without ever reaching the lymph.

In order to investigate the possible lumen-mucosa-lumen cycle for dietary cholesterol, rats were given a mixture of cholesterol-1-2-^{3}H and β-sitosterol-4-^{14}C by gastric intubation. Three hours later the animals were anesthetized, and the small intestine was divided into four, and the large intestine into two, equal segments. The contents of the small intestine were collected, and the ^{3}H/^{14}C ratios were determined. Since the absorption of β-sitosterol-^{14}C is insignificant, the ratios in intestinal contents were expected to decrease as cholesterol-^{3}H was absorbed. In actual fact, however, the ratios increased (Fig. 3). The following appears to be a likely explanation: Radioactive cholesterol was taken up by the intestinal wall, a fraction of it was absorbed into the intestinal lymph, and the remainder was released back into the lumen. During the time cholesterol was going through the "lumen-mucosa-lumen cycle", at the same level of the intestinal tract the β-sitosterol had moved down along the length of the intestines.

Other rats with bile fistulae were also given cholesterol-^{3}H and β-sitosterol-^{14}C, and fecal samples were collected over a period of a few days. The animals were infused with normal bile through a catheter placed in the duodenum. The ratios of the two isotopes in the various fecal specimens remained constant in 5 out of 6 rats. This suggested that the time taken for the lumen-mucosa-lumen cycle was so short that its effects were obscured by the daily timing of fecal collections (Table 3).

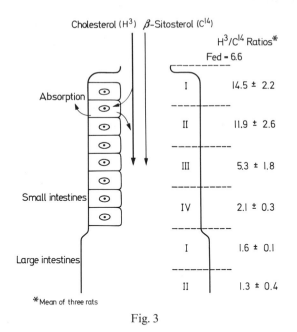

Fig. 3

The absorption of exogenous cholesterol occurs in the villi—most of it in the cells lining the distal halves of the villi (WILSON, 1962). Cells of the villi also synthesize cholesterol actively (SODHI, 1967; MAK and TRIER, 1972). Since these are also the earliest to be exfoliated, the losses of both endogenous and exogenous cholesterol from the mucosa may be through this process. This would also explain the lack of reabsorbability of (exogenous and endogenous) cholesterol. The results of BORG-STROM's (1968) experiments in rats are in accord with the concept that the fraction of dietary cholesterol which is discharged back into the lumen is not readily absorbed. He fed radioactive cholesterol to rats and noted that the maximum radioactivity in the intestinal wall was present at one hour: the earliest at which this determination was made. Thereafter, the radioactivity in the intestinal wall declined, although there was still considerable radioactive cholesterol in the lumen.

After administration of tracer and larger doses of cholesterol-4-^{14}C, the specific activity of the cholesterol fraction in the thoracic duct lymph increased and then decreased in parallel with the changes in its concentration (SWELL et al., 1950, 1959c, 1962).

Earlier studies had suggested that the absorption of dietary cholesterol occurred predominantly in the distal parts of the small intestine (BYERS et al., 1953), but studies by BORGSTROM (1960, 1968) indicated that the process took place over the entire length of the small intestine. It was demonstrated that the reversal of continuity of duodenal and ileal segments in rabbit did not result in any change in the total cholesterol absorption, indicating that all segments of the small intestine could absorb dietary cholesterol (GEBHARD and BUCHWALD, 1970). Since the duodenum and the upper jejunum are the first sections of intestine to come in contact with dietary cholesterol, most of the absorption takes place there (BORGSTROM, 1960, 1968).

Table 3. ^{3}H/^{14}C ratios in fecal neutral steroids at different times after duodenal intubation of cholesterol-^{3}H and β-sitosterol-^{14}C in rats with bile fistula

Without bile infusion					With bile infusion				
Rat. No.	Hours after feeding	^{3}H/^{14}C Ratio	Amount of the total ^{3}H (%)	^{14}C (%)	Rat. No.	Hours after feeding	^{3}H/^{14}C Ratio	Amount of the total ^{3}H (%)	^{14}C (%)
1	19	5.7	82.0	80.6	1	10	5.8	0.2	0.1
	23	5.2	8.6	9.3		12	4.0	9.1	11.8
	29	5.2	4.3	4.6		21	4.9	33.0	34.8
	42	5.2	5.0	5.4		29	5.6	13.0	12.0
	55	4.8	0.1	0.1		36	5.6	20.0	18.8
2	19	5.1	16.3	16.5		46	5.5	12.9	12.2
	23	5.1	25.0	25.0		51	5.6	1.6	1.4
	29	5.2	36.2	35.9		53	5.4	1.3	1.2
	42	5.2	17.4	17.1		60	5.6	2.9	2.7
	55	4.7	4.3	4.7		70	5.6	2.5	2.3
	73	5.2	0.6	0.6		74	5.7	0.3	0.3
3	19	5.0	37.8	38.0	2	23	3.9	65.3	68.4
	23	4.9	6.8	6.9		27	4.3	9.9	9.3
	29	5.1	14.1	13.6		48	4.6	14.4	12.9
	42	5.0	37.8	38.0		62	4.5	6.2	5.6
	55	5.0	1.7	1.7		73	4.7	1.8	1.6
	73	5.2	1.3	1.3		84	4.6	1.5	1.4
						95	4.7	0.4	0.3
						105	4.7	0.5	0.4
					3	38	2.2	1.0	1.8
						39	3.2	1.9	2.3
						43	3.3	10.7	12.5
						51	3.6	29.3	30.8
						63	4.1	44.1	42.6
						66	4.4	4.5	4.0
						71	4.8	2.0	1.7
						77	4.7	3.4	2.9

The rate of absorption seems to be largely determined by the chemical nature of the steroid. It was shown by BORGSTROM (1968) that a distinction between β-sitosterol and cholesterol was made during the process of their uptake, but once they were in the mucosal cells there was no difference in their subsequent transport into the intestinal lymph. This is supported by recent studies of EDWARDS and GREEN (1972). They demonstrated that plant sterols can exchange with the cholesterol in red blood cell membranes where cholesterol is a normal component. The rates of exchange suggested a marked preference for cholesterol over campesterol and for campesterol over sitosterol. Experimental studies in animals have also shown that the intestinal absorption of campesterol was better than that of sitosterol (KUKSIS and HUANG, 1962; SUBBIAH et al., 1970).

When radioactive cholesterol was given orally to rats with thoracic duct fistulae, its recovery from lymph in the hypercholesterolemic animals was twice that in controls during the first six hours. On the other hand, when rats without fistulae were used, the recovery of the administered radioactive cholesterol in plasma and liver at six hours was greater in the control than in the hypercholesterolemic rats (Iritani and Nogi, 1972). These data suggested that in the absence of the normal enterohepatic circulation of cholesterol and bile acids, observations on the amounts of cholesterol absorbed could not be extrapolated to normal animals. Furthermore, the course of absorption of dietary cholesterol in the rat is, in many respects, different from that in man. In the rat, the lymphatic transport can be increased fivefold when a high-cholesterol diet is given. The specific activity of the lymph cholesterol can also be increased to about 90% of that in the diet (Sylvén and Borgstrom, 1968). This does not appear to occur in man. The addition of cholesterol to dietary fat did not increase the lymphatic transport of cholesterol in subjects with thoracic duct fistulae (Borgstrom et al., 1970). The maximum specific activity of lymph cholesterol in man was 25% of that in the diet (Borgstrom et al., 1970).

Earlier investigations on cholesterol absorption in man suggested that 2 to 3 g of cholesterol could be absorbed in one day (Cook et al., 1956; Karvinen et al., 1957). Using more sophisticated techniques, however, Kaplan et al. (1963) and Wilson and Lindsey (1965) came to the conclusion that, regardless of the amount of dietary cholesterol, maximum absorption was generally at or below 300 mg per day. In contrast, studies by Borgstrom (1969) indicated that the capacity of man to absorb dietary cholesterol greatly exceeded the values suggested by Kaplan and his associates or by Wilson and Lindsey. He showed that absorption was directly proportional to the amounts ingested. Subsequent work (Quintão et al., 1971b; Connor and Lin, 1970; Kudchodkar et al., 1971b, 1973a) supported Borgstrom's findings. After comparing different methods for estimating absorption, Quintão et al. (1971a) concluded that the methods used by Kaplan et al. and by Wilson and Lindsey were not as satisfactory as those used by others, including ourselves. Our studies were designed to determine absorption of cholesterol in subjects eating ordinary North American diets. Cholesterol intake varied from 400 to 1200 mg per day, and the fat calories accounted for 20 to 50%. The range of the absorption percentage was narrow ($37 \pm 5\%$) and was not influenced by types of hyperlipoproteinemia (Kudchodkar et al., 1971b, 1973a).

On direct observation of thoracic duct lymph of man, Borgstrom et al. (1970) noted that the addition of cholesterol to the diet did not increase the concentration or the amount of cholesterol in the lymph. In order to explain the discrepancies between this report and his previous observations, as well as those of others, he suggested that the amounts of endogenous cholesterol secreted into the intestinal tract were almost sufficient to saturate the absorptive capacity in man. Any addition of cholesterol to the diet would only compete with and decrease the absorption of endogenous cholesterol. Based on this hypothesis, he postulated that the fraction of dietary cholesterol absorbed will decrease as the total intake increases, since the total absorption from endogenous and dietary sources remains constant. Our results (Kudchodkar et al., 1973a) failed to support this hypothesis, showing instead that the amounts of cholesterol (dietary plus endogenous) absorbed had a direct linear relationship to the amounts available, at least within the limits studied. Recent reports of Quintão et al. (1971b) have also indicated that as much as 1 gram of cholesterol can be absorbed from the diet. In most earlier studies, the presence of endogenous cholesterol secreted into the intestinal lumen and its effects on absorption of dietary cholesterol have been more or less completely ignored. BORGSTROM's reminder of their importance is timely.

A. Control Mechanisms Regulating Absorption of Cholesterol from the Intestinal Lumen

Cholesterol is not absorbed as efficiently as other fats. The absorption of triglycerides and phospholipids is almost quantitative, but the percent absorption of cholesterol is only half that of other dietary fats. The rate of uptake of cholesterol by mucosal cells is comparable to that of monoglycerides and fatty acids. It is not transferred out of the cell at anything like the rate for hydrolytic products of triglycerides. The actual rate of cholesterol absorption is determined by two independent factors: 1) the rate of transfer out of the cell to the lymph, and 2) the half-life of the mucosal cell containing the dietary cholesterol before it is exfoliated. The retention in the intestinal cell might be unique for cholesterol, since labelled triglycerides given to rats were absorbed so rapidly that only minor amounts of the radioactivity were found at any one time in any of the different parts of the intestinal tract. On the other hand, dietary cholesterol caused an appreciable increase in the cholesterol content of the intestinal wall and has a half-life of about 12 hrs before it appears in the lymph.

Among the factors which influence the amounts of cholesterol absorbed from the intestinal lumen, fats are perhaps the most important. There is good evidence that the absorption of exogenous cholesterol is facilitated by the dietary fats (COOK, 1936; KIM and IVY, 1952; PIHL, 1955). Crystalline cholesterol given in a fat-free diet is poorly absorbed (WILSON, 1962). The same cholesterol when dissolved in oil is well absorbed (STEINER et al., 1962; WELLS and BRONTE-STEWART, 1963). Since moderate amounts of endogenous fats become available in the intestinal lumen, considerable cholesterol absorption can occur on a fat-free diet. Fats, dietary or endogenous, provide the long-chain fatty acids needed to esterify cholesterol in the intestinal mucosa before its absorption. There is some degree of specificity with respect to utilization of these fatty acids for esterification. Cholesterol ester formation shows a marked specificity for oleic acid, relative to palmitic, stearic, and linoleic acids (KARMEN et al., 1963). The presence of fats also helps in the absorption of dietary cholesterol in another way. The hydrolytic products of triglycerides provide monoglycerides and free fatty acids, which are necessary to stabilize the micelles formed by bile salts. The hydrolytic products of fat also stimulate the flow of bile, which further aids in the absorption of cholesterol (BORGSTROM and LAURELL, 1953; FALOR et al., 1964). The greater the chain length of the fatty acids, the greater was the absorption of cholesterol. Dietary glycerides increased the lymphatic transport of cholesterol only when they had a chain length longer than C-6 (SYLVÉN and BORGSTROM, 1969). Once absorbed into the mucosa, cholesterol absorption into the lymph was independent of the chain length of dietary fatty acids (SYLVÉN and BORGSTROM, 1969).

When increasing amounts of cholesterol were fed in a constant amount of triolein to rats, the percentage absorbed decreased only gradually, and the total amounts absorbed increased rapidly (BORGSTROM, 1968). As indicated previously, the amounts absorbed by man can also be increased by dietary increment (BORGSTROM, 1969; QUINTÃO et al., 1971 b; KUDCHODKAR et al., 1971 b, 1973 a).

The amounts of protein and carbohydrates in the normal North American diet do not appear to affect cholesterol absorption significantly except insofar as they replace the dietary fats. Pectin, cellulose, and roughage in the diet have only negligible effects on the absorption of cholesterol, but they appear to bind bile acids and decrease their absorption from the intestinal tract (KRITCHEVSKY et al., 1973; BALMER and ZILVERSMIT, 1973).

The mechanisms controlling the absorption of endogenous cholesterol synthesized in the intestinal mucosa are not well elucidated. WILSON and REINKE (1968) showed that bile is required for the transfer of intestinal cholesterol from the wall to lymph. Feeding rats with medium- or short-chain triglycerides (C-12 to C-2) did not influence absorption of endogenous cholesterol (SYLVÉN and BORGSTROM, 1969).

Endogenous dilution of absorbed cholesterol in the intestinal mucosa differs for free and esterified fractions. The ratio of free to esterified cholesterol is generally higher for lymph total cholesterol than for newly-absorbed, labelled cholesterol. This finding appears to be related to the size of the exogenous dose, since it was apparent after a test dose of 3.3 mg of cholesterol-^{14}C but not after a test dose of 40 to 50 mg. The transfer of nonesterified cholesterol from the intestinal wall to the lymph is also not inhibited as strikingly by bile duct cannulation in rat as that of the esterified fraction, suggesting that the mechanism of the transfer for the two molecular forms may be different (SWELL et al., 1958, 1959 b).

B. Methods to Study Absorption of Dietary Cholesterol

The specific activity values of cholesterol in different pools and those of bile acids reach equilibrium in 3 to 6 weeks after an intravenous injection of radioactive cholesterol. During this isotopic steady state, the fecal neutral metabolites of endogenous (synthesized plus absorbed) cholesterol can be calculated from the total radioactivity in the fecal neutral steroids, and the specific activity of plasma cholesterol (HELLMAN et al., 1957). Cholesterol intake and the total fecal neutral steroids (unabsorbed dietary plus endogenous) are determined by gas-liquid chromatography. Unabsorbed dietary cholesterol alone can be derived from the values of total fecal neutral steroids and the steroids derived from endogenous cholesterol (GRUNDY and AHRENS, 1966, 1969).

BORGSTROM (1969) proposed that the difference between an orally-administered dose of radioactive cholesterol and its recovery in the feces gives the fraction absorbed. He assumed that it takes up to eight days for complete excretion of unabsorbed dietary cholesterol in the feces and that during this period biliary secretion of absorbed radioactive cholesterol is insignificant.

A simpler method was proposed by SODHI et al. (1971 b). Unknown to the authors, a similar approach had previously been taken by ARNESJO et al. (1969) to calculate absorption of cholesterol over different parts of the intestinal tract. A mixture of cholesterol-1-2-^{3}H and β-sitosterol-4-^{14}C in a known ratio is given orally with carmine red as a marker. The fecal sample containing most of the dietary (unabsorbed) sterols and the red color is tested for the ratio of the two isotopes. From the difference in the ratios of the isotopes administered and recovered, the fraction absorbed is calculated. A comparison of the values obtained by this method

Table 4. Comparison of the ratio method for calculating absorption of dietary cholesterol with the actual absorption determined[a] in rats

Rat number	Cholesterol fed (mg.)	Percent absorption		Difference (2)–(1)	Cholesterol absorbed (mg.) ratio method
		Actually determined[a] (1)	Ratio method (2)		
1	0.0	83.8	79.6	− 4.2	0
2	0.0	85.2	77.9	− 7.3	0
3	1.0	75.2	77.2	+ 2.0	0.77
4	1.0	80.0	91.8	+11.8	0.92
5	1.0	88.6	92.9	+ 4.3	0.93
6	1.6	82.7	71.5	−11.2	1.14
7	1.6	75.1	73.9	− 1.2	1.18
8	2.0	65.1	79.1	+14.0	1.58
9	2.0	53.6	62.0	+ 8.4	1.24
10	2.0	75.2	82.0	+ 6.8	1.64
11	2.7	70.9	78.4	+ 7.5	2.11
12	2.7	70.5	71.1	+ 0.6	1.92
13	4.0	42.0	48.0	+ 6.0	1.92
14	4.0	32.5	34.0	+ 1.5	1.36
15	4.0	33.4	43.1	+ 9.7	1.72
16	5.1	37.1	35.5	− 1.6	1.82
17	5.1	36.2	40.3	+ 3.6	2.05
18	6.0	30.8	40.0	+ 9.2	2.40
19	6.0	37.2	35.4	− 1.8	2.12
		$r = 0.95$	Mean ± SD	+ 3 ± 7	

[a] Percentage of the administered radioactivity in the carcass after removal of the contents from the gastrointestinal tract.

with actual absorption determined in rats (Table 4) and its comparison with BORG-STROM's method in man (Table 5) indicated that the method is satisfactory.

Another method was recently proposed by ZILVERSMIT (1972): The ratio of the two isotopes in plasma cholesterol is determined 24 hrs after the administration of radioactive cholesterol labelled with one isotope given orally and labelled by another isotope given by intravenous injection.

VI. Catabolism of Cholesterol and Its Losses from the Body Pools

Body cholesterol is derived from absorption and from endogenous synthesis. The most important organ involved in its catabolism is the liver, and the major catabolic products are bile acids. Cholesterol is lost primarily in the feces either as bile acids or as cholesterol.

Cholic and chenodeoxycholic are the two primary bile acids made from choles-terol in the liver. They are conjugated either with glycine or taurine (to form glyco-cholic, glycochenodeoxycholic, taurocholic, and taurochenodeoxycholic acids) and secreted in the bile and into the intestinal tract (BERGSTROM and DANIELSSON, 1968;

Table 5. Comparison of the ratio method with Borgstrom's method for calculating absorption of dietary cholesterol in man

Subject number	Percent absorption		Difference (2)–(1)
	Borgstrom's method (1)	Ratio method (2)	
1	49.2	55.0	+5.8
2	49.0	50.0	+1.0
3	54.5	53.8	−0.7
4	42.7	43.3	+0.6
5	62.1	65.9	+3.8
6	66.4	62.8	−3.6
7	47.0	54.3	+7.3
8	40.3	43.3	+3.0
9	58.0	58.0	0.0
10	70.5	68.5	−2.0
11	47.3	48.6	+1.3
12	59.7	61.9	+2.2
13	50.0	52.0	+2.0
14	63.7	71.0	+7.3
15	64.8	62.8	−2.0
16	55.4	55.8	+0.4
17	50.0	54.9	+4.9
18	50.0	50.0	0.0
19	54.5	67.7	+13.2
20	61.4	65.9	+4.5

$r = 0.89$ Mean ± SD $+2 \pm 4$

DANIELSSON, 1969). They are reabsorbed from the intestines; the reabsorption in the duodenum, jejunum, and colon is passive and quantitatively much less important than their active absorption in the ileum (LACK and WEINER, 1961; DIETSCHY et al., 1966). Secondary bile acids are produced by the action of intestinal microorganisms on the primary acids. Deoxycholic acid is derived from cholic acid; and lithocholic from chenodeoxycholic acid. Lithocholic acid differs from the other three in that it is poorly absorbed from the intestinal tract (NORMAN and SJOVALL, 1958; HELLSTRÖM and SJOVALL, 1961; SMALL et al., 1972). Intestinal microorganisms also produce small quantities of other ("tertiary", etc.) bile acids. Since the absorption of secondary and tertiary bile acids is different from that of primary bile acids, the activity of intestinal microflora can, in theory, influence the reabsorption of the latter. This influence, however, could not be important since most of the absorption occurs in the small intestine, and microorganisms are generally present only in the large intestine.

The conversion of cholesterol to bile acids involves oxidation of the sidechain and carboxylation of the ring (BERGSTROM and DANIELSSON, 1968; STAPLE, 1969). When cholesterol-4-^{14}C was administered intravenously to rats, 80 to 90% of the isotope was excreted in 15 days; and 90% of the excreted isotope was present in the bile acids (SIPERSTEIN et al., 1952b). Conversion of cholesterol to bile acids up to a level of 75 to 90% has also been reported in man by SIPERSTEIN and MURRAY (1955) and in rabbits by HELLSTRÖM (1965). It was reported that 0.5 to 1 gram of cholesterol is transformed into bile acids per day in young subjects on normal diets (LINDSTEDT, 1957; DANIELSSON et al., 1963). It was suggested that bile acids were the most important pathway for elimination of cholesterol from the body (SIPERSTEIN et al., 1952 b; BERGSTROM, 1952). Recent studies, however, indicate that losses of endogenous cholesterol as neutral steroids may be 1 to 2 times greater than the fecal losses of acidic steroids (GRUNDY and AHRENS, 1969, 1970; CONNOR et al., 1969; MIETTINEN, 1971; SODHI and KUDCHODKAR, 1973c).

SWELL et al. (1968) suggested that a specific macromolecular complex consisting of bile acids, cholesterol, lecithin, and water was made in the liver cells before its excretion into the biliary tract. Fractionation of biliary constituents, however, failed to confirm its existence (SCHERSTÉN et al., 1971). Recent studies in dogs suggested that conjugated bile acids are actively secreted by hepatocytes, and their surface activity in the cannulicular lumen is responsible for extraction of lecithin from cell membranes lining the biliary cannuliculi. A major fraction of biliary cholesterol is coupled to the biliary secretion of lecithin, although a small amount of cholesterol is assumed to be secreted independently of biliary lecithin (WHEELER and KING, 1972). Similar studies in five subjects (SCHERSTÉN et al., 1971) had shown that in two the rates of biliary excretion of bile acids and cholesterol had a linear relationship. In two others, the rates of biliary excretion of cholesterol were independent of bile acids. The total data from all five subjects, however, suggested a more or less linear relationship between the excretion of cholesterol and bile acids. In contrast to the findings in dogs, the ratio of cholesterol to lecithin was not constant in man. It appeared to decrease as biliary excretion of bile acids rose. Based on such data, it was suggested that biliary lecithin is derived from cell membranes due to the surface-active effects of bile acids; and the biliary cholesterol could either be extracted from cell membranes or transferred from the hepatic cells (SCHERSTÉN et al., 1971). An increase in biliary cholesterol associated with mobilization of tissue cholesterol (SODHI and KUDCHODKAR, 1971 a, GRUNDY et al., 1972; SODHI et al., 1973 a) would suggest that at least some of the biliary cholesterol is dependent directly on the amounts of cholesterol brought to the liver for catabolism (SODHI and KUDCHODKAR, 1973 a). Since both phospholipids and cholesterol are constituents of the lipoprotein structure, a relationship between the biliary excretion of free cholesterol and lecithin may well be expected whether they are derived from the lipoproteins of cell membranes or those of plasma.

The two primary bile acids are derived from a pool of cholesterol which is in equilibrium with plasma and biliary cholesterol (ROSENFELD and HELLMAN, 1959; LINDSTEDT and AHRENS, 1961; OGURA et al., 1971). There is some evidence, however, to suggest that at least some of the biliary cholesterol may be derived from a pool different from which biliary bile acids are formed. STAPLE and GURIN (1954) showed that in bile the specific activity of cholic acid was greater than that of cholesterol after injection of radioactive cholesterol. Other investigators observed that the bile acids became labelled more rapidly than cholesterol in the bile after injection of deuterated ethanol in rats. The relative abundance of deuterated molecules was highest in the first sample, but later the relative distribution of mono-, di-, and tri-deuterated molecules was similar to that found for cholesterol. Labelled bile acids continued to be excreted after the disappearance of the deuterated ethanol (CRONHOLM et al., 1972). The results of studies on rat liver perfusion by BRICKER (1971) are also in accord with this hypothesis. A similar situation appears to exist in man. Hypocholesterolemic agents, such as clofibrate and nicotinic acid, when given to man produce a mobilization of tissue cholesterol; it is transported to the liver and excreted into the bile (SODHI and KUDCHODKAR, 1971a; GRUNDY et al., 1972; SODHI et al., 1973a). The mobilized cholesterol does not appear to be secreted in the same proportion of neutral to acidic steroids as the cholesterol metabolized before treatment. The mobilized cholesterol appears in the feces predominantly as neutral steroids. QUINTÃO et al. (1971b) fed large amounts of cholesterol to volunteers. When the steady state was reached and a larger amount of cholesterol was excreted from the endogenous pools to balance the amounts from absorption, more of it was excreted as neutral steroids than as fecal bile acids. Data reported by DENBESTEN et al. (1973) are in accord with this observation.

Unabsorbed cholesterol in the intestinal lumen is also acted upon by microorganisms and converted into a number of neutral steroids (ROSENFELD et al., 1954; SNOG-KJER et al., 1956). Quantitatively the most important fecal neutral steroid in man is coprostanol. The formation of coprostanol from cholesterol has also been shown to occur *in vitro* using suspensions of feces (SNOG-KJER et al., 1956; COLEMAN and BAUMAN, 1957a). Coprostanol is absent in the feces of rats treated with antibiotics (COLEMAN and BAUMAN, 1957b) and in the feces of germ-free rats (DANIELSSON and GUSTAFSON, 1959). Coprostanone is another derivative which is commonly found in the feces of man (ANCHEL and SCHOENHEIMER, 1938; Rosenfeld et al., 1963), but generally its amounts are considerably less than those of fecal coprostanol.

In addition to cholesterol, a normal diet contains a number of plant sterols; e.g., β-sitosterol and campesterol. The intestinal mucosa can detect differences in the structure of these sterols and does not absorb plant sterols as efficiently as cholesterol (GOULD, 1955; SWELL et al., 1959b; BORGSTROM, 1968; SALEN et al., 1970). The intestinal microflora, however, do not appear to discriminate between these sterols, and they degrade all dietary sterols to the same degree—and by identical pathways (COLEMAN et al., 1956). GRUNDY et al. (1968) showed that after oral feeding of radioactive cholesterol and radioactive β-sitosterol, the proportions of radioactivity in fecal stanone and stanol derivatives of the two sterols were identical. This was confirmed by KUDCHODKAR et al. (1972a). They determined the amounts of stanone and stanol derivatives and those of their precursors in the feces by gas-liquid chromatography. The ratios of the products to their precursors were identical for cholesterol and β-sitosterol.

GRUNDY et al. (1968) presented evidence to indicate significant losses of dietary sterols despite the careful and meticulous methodology employed for their fecal recoveries. They postulated that the losses were due to degradation of the sterol nucleus and not to other possible causes of incomplete recovery of the sterols. The losses were noted in a number of subjects, and they differed from subject to subject. BORGSTROM (1969) studied 20 subjects, and CONNOR et al. (1969) studied 6 subjects, and there was only one case in each of the two studies where the recovery of dietary β-sitosterol was not quantitative. KUDCHODKAR et al. (1972a) and KOTTKE and SUBBIAH (1972) also failed to find evidence for losses of dietary β-sitosterol. In studies from this laboratory (KUDCHODKAR et al., 1972a), the percent recovery of β-sitosterol was $94 \pm 5\%$, indicating the absence of any significant degradation of dietary sterols in subjects examined by cholesterol balance techniques. These observations are in accord with the results of *in vitro* studies of WOOD and HATOFF (1970). They demonstrated complete recovery of radioactivity when radioactive cholesterol was incubated with fecal homogenates. The differences between the subjects examined by GRUNDY et al. (1968) and by us may be related to the differences in their diets. Subjects studied by AHRENS and his associates at the Rockefeller University were given liquid formula diets, whereas our subjects (and those of KOTTKE'S) were given solid food diets. It was shown by DENBESTEN et al. (1970) that losses of dietary β-sitosterol observed on liquid formula diets disappeared when cellulose was added to the diet or when the liquid formula was substituted with a solid diet of the same composition.

The concept of degradation assumes destruction of the steroid nucleus, resulting in fragments which are lost in the methods of extraction of fecal neutral steroids. In the absence of knowledge of the degradative products of cholesterol, it may be better to view its losses as an open question. However, it appears to be uncommon in subjects given solid food diets.

The total amount of cholesterol catabolised by the liver is equal to the sum of daily *fecal* excretion of bile acids ($\simeq 0.3$ g) and daily *biliary* secretion of cholesterol ($\simeq 1.0$ g).

A. Factors Influencing Catabolism of Endogenous Cholesterol

In man, increasing the dietary intake of cholesterol is associated with increased absorption, which in turn leads to an increase in fecal excretion of neutral steroids; the fecal excretion of bile acids does not increase (QUINTÃO et al., 1971b). The response of experimental animals to increased dietary cholesterol appears to be different from that of man. Animals respond by increasing the fecal excretion of bile acids rather than that of cholesterol. This has been shown in rats (WILSON, 1962; BEHER et al., 1970), dogs (ABELL et al., 1956), and monkeys (LOFLAND et al., 1972). Dietary fats also influence the catabolism of cholesterol. Substituting unsaturated for saturated fats increased the fecal excretion of bile acids and cholesterol in some subjects (WOOD et al., 1966; SODHI et al., 1967a; MOORE et al., 1968; CONNOR et al., 1969; NESTEL et al., 1973) but not in others (AVIGAN and STEINBERG, 1965; SPRITZ et al., 1965; GRUNDY and AHRENS, 1970).

Fecal excretion of neutral steroids and bile acids in a rat with normal intestinal microflora is twice that in a germ-free rat (WOSTMANN et al., 1966; KELLOGG and WOSTMANN, 1969). Bile acids in the intestinal lumen increase the turnover of mucosal cells suggesting therefore that the effect of microflora on bile acids may be responsible both for greater turnover of cells and for increases in fecal neutral steroids (KELLOGG, 1971).

Muscular activity has been shown to increase the rate of catabolism of cholesterol. After an injection of cholesterol labelled with ^{14}C in the side-chain and with ^{3}H in the ring, increased muscular activity was associated with increases both in the expired $^{14}CO_2$ and in the excretion of ^{3}H-labelled bile acids (MALINOW et al., 1970, 1972).

Subjects with hypertriglyceridemia appear to catabolise more cholesterol than those who have normal plasma triglycerides (KOTTKE, 1969; KUDCHODKAR and SODHI, 1972; SODHI and KUDCHODKAR, 1973c). The amount of endogenous cholesterol secreted into the intestinal tract was much greater in the former than in the latter group of subjects. The same was true not only for fecal neutral steroids—as might be expected from the above observation—but also for fecal bile acids. The ratios of fecal neutral to acidic steroids, however, were similar in both groups. The predominant bile acid in the former group was deoxycholic acid and in the latter, lithocholic acid (KUDCHODKAR and SODHI, 1971c; SODHI and KUDCHODKAR, 1973c). These observations suggested to us that synthesis of chenodeoxycholic acid does not increase to the same degree as that of cholic acid when the liver is confronted with increased amounts of cholesterol for catabolism.

B. Skin

The cholesterol content of skin (3 mg/g wet weight) is comparable to that of liver. Furthermore, the total skin weighs approximately three times as much as the liver (MASORO, 1968). Although the dermis constitutes 90% of the human skin, it is quantitatively less active in sterol metabolism than the epidermis, which forms only a few layers of epithelial cells (HSIA et al., 1970). BHATTACHARYYA et al. (1972) showed that sterols lost from the skin surface were the same for normal and hypercholesterolemic subjects. The mean 24-hour excretion of cholesterol in mg was 82.6 and 82.7. Cholesterol constituted 89% of the total sterol excretion through the skin surface in both groups. The authors suggested that at least some of the skin surface cholesterol is derived from plasma cholesterol. Since the skin surface sterols also contained plant sterols, which are not synthesized in the body, it was argued that net amounts of these plant sterols and cholesterol were transferred from plasma to the skin. The specific activity values of plasma and skin surface cholesterol suggested precursor-product relationship. However, in addition to net transfer some of this could have occurred from the exchange of plasma sterols, including plant sterols, with the cholesterol present in the cellular and intracellular membranes of skin cells, as has been shown to occur with red blood cell membranes (EDWARDS and GREEN, 1972). Since the epidermis is also the most active component of skin with regard to cholesterol biosynthesis (NICOLAIDES and ROTHMAN, 1955), a fraction of the cholesterol lost from the skin surface might also have been derived from local synthesis.

C. Adrenal Glands

Although only a small amount of endogenous cholesterol is catabolised in the adrenal glands, it is important in relationship to steroid hormones, which control the metabolism of most other body constituents. Cholesterol forms the main precursor for various steroid hormones synthesized by the adrenal glands and other steroid-producing organs (BLOCH, 1945; HECHTER et al., 1951; SABA et al., 1954).

In vitro studies suggest that the amount of cholesterol synthesized by the adrenal gland is much too low for its need (BORKOWSKI et al., 1972b). About 50 mg of free cholesterol in the adrenal glands are derived from plasma every day—which is about the daily production of steroid hormones (BORKOWSKI et al., 1972a, 1972b). A model of the cholesterol metabolism in the adrenal glands was recently suggested by BORKOWSKI et al. (1972a). They postulated two homogeneous intracellular compartments—one of free and the other of esterified cholesterol—exchanging with each other through esterification and hydrolysis. The turnover is dependent primarily on the inflow of cholesterol from plasma and to a small degree on local synthesis. The two zones of the adrenal cortex equilibrate differently with plasma cholesterol and synthesize different amounts of adrenal cholesterol. The free cholesterol in the adrenal glands turns over five to ten times per day, and it is a much smaller pool than that of cholesterol esters. It was suggested by FAWCETT et al. (1969) that structural cholesterol may also be a means of storing and making rapidly available a sufficient amount of free cholesterol for steroid synthesis in the adrenal glands. For reasons of structural stability, the concentration of free cholesterol in membranes must remain constant. The inflow of plasma cholesterol into the adrenal glands for synthesis of steroid hormones is continuous and autonomous and is not under control of ACTH (BORKOWSKI et al., 1972a). Hydrolysis of cholesterol esters in the adrenal glands, on the other hand, is under ACTH influence (SAYERS et al., 1944; SAYERS, 1950; DAVIS and GARREN, 1966). A fourth or fifth of the cholesterol ester compartment is turned over every day. ACTH stimulation and the reserve of esterified cholesterol in the adrenal glands constitute a biological mechanism to ensure a rapid supply of cholesterol under conditions of acute stress (BORKOWSKI et al., 1972a, 1972b).

The fatty acids esterifying the cholesterol in plasma are different from the fatty acids of adrenal cholesterol esters (DAILEY et al., 1960). It has been suggested that the adrenal cholesterol esters are synthesized within the glands rather than selectively accumulated from the plasma (LONGCOPE and WILLIAMS, 1963; MOORE and WILLIAMS, 1966). The concentration of adrenal cholesterol—particularly esterified cholesterol—appears to be higher in zona fasciculata than in zona reticularis (GRIFFITHS et al., 1963; BORKOWSKI et al., 1972a).

VII. Plasma Cholesterol

Cholesterol enters the plasma in association with macromolecules containing other lipids and proteins. Intestines and liver are known to produce these macromolecules; the mechanisms of contribution, if any, from other organs are not known.

In vitro studies on perfusion of intestinal segments demonstrated that not only chylomicra but all lipoproteins between the density of 1.006 and 1.21 g/ml (which are transported in intestinal lymph) are formed by the intestinal mucosa (WINDMÜLLER and LEVY, 1968; OCKNER et al., 1969a). The size of cholesterol-containing particles is generally larger in animals fed high-fat diets than when they are fed low-fat diets containing the same amount of cholesterol (ZILVERSMIT et al., 1967; OCKNER et al., 1969b). It was recently shown that very low density lipoproteins (VLDL) synthesized by the intestinal mucosa transport a greater percentage of exogenous cholesterol than that in chylomicra (RUDEL et al., 1972). On entering into circulation, the chylomicra and lipoproteins are enriched by serum proteins (LOSSOW et al., 1967). SODHI and GOULD (1970) showed that apo-HDL can readily transfer to VLDL and chylomicra under *in vitro* conditions, and this was corroborated by HAVEL et al. (1973) recently. They showed that high density lipoproteins contribute functionally-important apolipoproteins to chylomicra during alimentary lipemia in man (HAVEL et al., 1973).

NESTEL et al. (1963) reported that in functionally-hepatectomized dogs chylomicron triglyceride was cleared in extrahepatic peripheral tissue, whereas cholesterol esters remained in the blood. These observations were confirmed by REDGRAVE (1970) who showed in rat that chylomicra were rapidly divested of much of their triglycerides in peripheral tissues, and the cholesterol in the remnants remained in circulation. He characterized these cholesterol-rich remnants and demonstrated that their median particle size was considerably smaller than that of chylomicra. The flotation rates of remnants were also much less than those of chylomicra. Analyses of the remnant particles showed that their composition was different from that of chylomicra. The remnant composition was approximately 79% triglycerides, 4% unesterified cholesterol, 13% cholesterol esters, 3% phospholipids, and 1.5% protein. When injected intravenously into rats, the clearance of remnants was much faster than that of chylomicra. When chylomicra were injected intravenously, only 14% of the cholesterol esters was found in the liver one minute after the injection; whereas 40% of the injected cholesterol esters was found in the liver when remnants were injected. After intravenous injections into rats actively absorbing cholesterol, more than 80% of the chylomicron cholesterol—but only about 20% of their triglycerides—was seen in the liver (GOODMAN, 1962; REDGRAVE, 1970). Eighty to ninety percent of chylomicron cholesterol esters were removed from the plasma by the rat liver without prior hydrolysis. By one hour, 60% of the cholesterol esters removed by the liver were hydrolyzed; and by four hours, the percentage reached 85 to 95%. Twenty-four hours later only 20 to 28% of the labelled cholesterol was still present in the liver. The remainder had been transported out of the liver (QUARFORDT and GOODMAN, 1966). In contrast to the observations of GOODMAN (1962), LOSSOW et al. (1962) noted that cholesterol uptake by liver alone after an intravenous injection of chylomicra was only about 50%. The uptake by adipose tissue and muscle constituted about 20% of the total. Injection of heparin into rats accelerated the removal from circulation of labelled cholesterol in chylomicra (LOSSOW et al., 1963).

Although earlier studies had suggested that the removal of chylomicra was essentially by the reticuloendothelial cells of the liver (FRIEDMAN et al., 1956), recent studies have indicated that chylomicron cholesterol removed by KUPFFER cells constituted only a small fraction of the cholesterol taken up by the liver. The major amount was removed by the parenchymal cells (DiLUZIO and RIGGI, 1964; STEIN et al., 1969; NILSSON and ZILVERSMIT, 1971).

Fasting serum in man is free of chylomicra, and it therefore has been generally assumed that other lipoproteins synthesized by the intestine may also be absent from fasting samples of sera. Studies in rats, however, indicated that there was a continuous supply of VLDL from the intestinal mucosa to the circulation in a fasting animal, and the lipids for their synthesis were derived from bile (BAXTER, 1966; SHRIVASTAVA et al., 1967). Some differences in the composition of intestinal and hepatic VLDL have been documented (OCKNER et al., 1969a).

The total amount of cholesterol transported by chylomicra and intestinal lipoproteins is about 1.0 g/day. Most of it is either derived from bile ($\simeq 0.6$ g) or diet (0.3 g). Although more than 10% of endogenous cholesterol is synthesized in the gastrointestinal tract, it is not readily absorbed into intestinal lymph (SODHI et al., 1973b).

Three distinct classes of plasma lipoproteins are generally recognized to be synthesized by the liver and secreted into circulation: very low density lipoproteins (VLDL), low density lipoproteins (LDL), and high density lipoproteins (HDL).

Evidence is accumulating to suggest that plasma VLDL is catabolised to LDL, so that at least some of the latter may not be synthesized in the liver. Evidence for a structural and functional linkage between proteins of VLDL and LDL has recently been presented (BILHEIMER et al., 1972; GOTTO et al., 1972). Metabolic studies indicated that all the LDL present in plasma could be accounted for by the catabolism of VLDL (LANGER et al., 1972; BILHEIMER et al., 1972). Recent studies by WILSON and LEES (1972) have shown reciprocal changes in the concentrations of plasma VLDL and LDL in subjects treated with hypocholesterolemic agents. Since VLDL is rich in triglycerides and LDL is relatively rich in cholesterol, it may be assumed that during the catabolism of VLDL to LDL the losses of triglycerides are greater than those of cholesterol. It is conceivable that the triglycerides from VLDL are metabolized in the periphery in a fashion similar to that of chylomicra leaving their cholesterol-rich remnants (LDL) in the circulation. The half-life of VLDL proteins is between 6 and 12 hrs (GITLIN et al., 1958; GULBRANDSEN et al., 1972) and the corresponding half-life of LDL proteins is between 3 and 5 days (GITLIN et al., 1958; WALTON et al., 1963; LANGER et al., 1972). Calculations made from the cholesterol to protein ratios and the turnover of lipoprotein proteins suggest that significant fractions of VLDL cholesterol may be lost or catabolised during its conversion to LDL.

Until recently, designation of plasma lipoproteins was relatively simple. The three classes of lipoproteins isolated by ultracentrifugation (LDL, VLDL, and HDL) were considered synonymous with the three groups of lipoproteins fractionated by paper or agarose electrophoresis (β, pre-β, and α). Increasing interest in this area is bound to unravel complexities of lipoprotein structure and to generate newer concepts with regard to their function and classification.

Chylomicrons are generally absent from fasting plasma. A small fraction of plasma VLDL, however, may well be of intestinal origin reflecting the reabsorption of biliary lipids (OCKNER et al., 1969a). A lipoprotein (LpX) was described by SEIDEL et al., (1969) in patients with biliary obstruction. In similar patients QUARFORDT et al. (1972) described the presence of liquid crystals containing cholesterol, lecithin, and protein. The relationship between the two observations will be a subject for future investigations.

FREDRICKSON et al. (1967) described another "abnormal" lipoprotein in patients with relatively rare type III hyperlipoproteinemia. A lipoprotein of nearly the same composition is assumed to be an intermediate in the conversion of VLDL to LDL (LANGER, STROBER, and LEVY, 1972). However, the abnormal "floating β lipoprotein" of type III hyperlipoproteinemia has a density less than $1.006\,g/ml$, whereas the "intermediate" lipoprotein has a density between 1.006 and $1.019\,g/ml$. A sedimenting or sinking pre-β lipoprotein (as opposed to floating β lipoprotein) was first described by SODHI (1969) in a normal boy of 11 years, and subsequently the existence of such a lipoprotein was confirmed in a large group of subjects by RIDER et al. (1970). Another lipoprotein also having β mobility but the density of HDL was reported by SEEGERS et al. (1965).

Since exceptions to the old rule (that LDL, VLDL, and HDL are synonymous with β, pre-β, and α lipoproteins) are becoming increasingly evident, it will be desirable to designate lipoproteins by the nomenclature relevant to the method of its isolation or fractionation. When isolated only by ultracentrifugation the terminology of "VLDL", "LDL", and "HDL" should be applied and when examined only by electrophoresis the terminology of "β", "pre-β", and "α" should be used. However when both methods are used to characterize the lipoproteins it should be apparant from the designation using designations such as β-LDL, β-VLDL, pre-β-VLDL, pre-β-LDL, etc.

A new system of classification of plasma lipoproteins into three (A, B, and C) "families" based on three groups of apoproteins was recently proposed by ALAU-POVIC (1971; 1972). It appears desirable to restrict this terminology to the apoprotein groups (apoproteins A, B, and C) and to leave the clinical familiar designations of plasma lipoproteins as suggested earlier. Preliminary studies in our laboratories suggested the possibility of other "families" or subspecies. Plasma HDL_2, HDL_3, or LDL, previously considered to be homogeneous entities, yield a number of discrete lipoprotein species when subjected to isoelectric focussing (MACKENZIE et al., 1973; SUNDARAM et al., 1972; SODHI, 1974). Although the species are reproducible entities, the question of artefact has not been completely resolved. The ampholines used to fractionate the lipoproteins have been shown not to interact with lipoproteins, and the pooled fractions appear to have characteristics of original lipoproteins when tested by analytical ultracentrifugation and electrophoresis.

The cholesterol in plasma lipoproteins is present in two distinct chemical forms; namely, free or unesterified cholesterol and cholesterol esterified with long-chain fatty acids. Free cholesterol is believed to form a structural component of the lipoproteins, but the function of cholesterol esters in lipoproteins is not clear.

Of the total cholesterol in plasma, a major fraction is normally present in LDL, although the amount in VLDL may exceed that in LDL under abnormal conditions. About two-thirds of the total cholesterol present in plasma is esterified. Except for some rare exceptions (FREDRICKSON et al., 1967; NORUM and GJONE, 1967), it is generally believed that the ratio of plasma free to esterified cholesterol in man remains constant (BOYD and OLIVER, 1958; GOODMAN and NOBLE, 1970). However, preliminary observations from our laboratories suggested that the ratios of free to esterified cholesterol are different in subjects with hypercholesterolemia than in those with hypercholesterolemia and hypertriglyceridemia. The ratios of free to esterified cholesterol in the former were slightly—but significantly—greater than those in the latter (KUDCHODKAR and SODHI, 1973).

Free and esterified cholesterol are present in different ratios in different lipoproteins (LINDGREN et al., 1955; BRAGDON et al., 1956). The values shown in Table 6 represent circulating lipoproteins and do not necessarily represent their composition at the time of their synthesis or their release into plasma (GLOMSET, 1968, 1970). The composition of chylomicra and intestinal lipoproteins is well established. Of the total cholesterol present in the intestinal lymph, two-thirds to three-fourths is esterified; so that during the absorptive phase significant amounts of plasma cholesterol esters are of intestinal origin. It is possible that small amounts of plasma cholesterol esters, even during the postabsorptive phase, may also be of intestinal origin (OCKNER et al., 1969 a,b). The composition of lipoproteins synthesized by liver is not completely known. Studies on rat livers indicated that VLDL synthesized in the liver and secreted into the medium devoid of lipoproteins contained both esterified and free cholesterol (ROHEIM et al., 1963; SWELL and LAW, 1971). The situation in man, however, is not similar to that in rat. The composition of cholesterol esters in all plasma lipoproteins in man is similar (GOODMAN and SHIRATORI, 1964; NESTEL et al., 1965), suggesting that they may have originated from the same source; whereas in rats the composition of cholesterol esters in VLDL differs from the composition of cholesterol esters in other lipoproteins (SUGANO and PORTMAN, 1964; GIDEZ et al., 1965). In man, there is a marked difference between the composition of liver cholesterol esters and that of plasma cholesterol esters, making it unlikely that all liver cholesterol esters constitute the precursor pools of plasma cholesterol esters (SWELL et al., 1960; NESTEL and COUZENS, 1966). On the other hand, the composition of cholesterol esters in plasma VLDL of rats is similar to the composition of cholesterol esters in the liver (ROHEIM et al., 1963; SWELL and LAW, 1971). Recent evidence from Glomset's laboratories (GLOMSET, 1962; GLOMSET et al., 1962) suggests that in man all cholesterol esters in postabsorptive plasma may well be derived from plasma free cholesterol. Data supporting this hypothesis were presented recently (KUDCHODKAR and SODHI, 1973; BARTER, 1974).

VIII. Relationship of Cholesterol in Plasma and Tissue Pools

The relationship of cholesterol in plasma and tissue pools can be viewed under three separate categories.

1. Isotopic exchange. Except for the incidental exchange of one (radioactive) molecule for another (non-radioactive) molecule, the isotopic exchange has no direct relevance to the net turnover of cholesterol.

2. The transfer of net amounts of cholesterol from tissues to plasma. Most tissues synthesize cholesterol, and others acquire additional cholesterol; e.g., the spleen accumulates about 40 mg of cholesterol per day from entrapment and destruction of red blood cells. To prevent any progressive accumulation with time, mechanisms must therefore exist either for degradation of cholesterol in situ or for its transfer out of the tissues. Liver and intestine can transport cholesterol out in chylomicra and lipoproteins. Tissues such as skin and intestinal mucosa can lose cholesterol through exfoliation. Organs such as the adrenal glands convert cholesterol into other compounds and release them into circulation. Most other tissues are neither known to produce lipoproteins nor to convert cholesterol to other compounds. Although unknown at the present, it is necessary to postulate mechanisms by which net amounts of cholesterol are transported out. GLOMSET, in 1968, postulated one such mechanism. He suggested that LCAT present in the extracellular fluid reacts with HDL present in the interstitial fluid and esterifies the free cholesterol, thereby decreasing its free/esterified cholesterol ratio. During subsequent equilibrations, unesterified cholesterol from cell membranes is transferred to the plasma lipoproteins, which on re-entering into the vascular compartment release the excess cholesterol in the liver. This hypothesis implies that when in contact with each other, the distribution of unesterified cholesterol between different lipoproteins occurs as in two phases, each having a different partial coefficient of solubility. Only unesterified cholesterol above the minimum requirements for structural integrity of lipoproteins could participate in such an equilibrium. When plasma lipoproteins relatively poor in free cholesterol

(and relatively rich in cholesterol esters) are incubated with erythrocytes, there is a transfer of free cholesterol from RBC to plasma (MURPHY, 1962). Conversely, if the activity of LCAT is absent or below normal, the increased ratio of free to esterified cholesterol in plasma is associated with a transfer of cholesterol from plasma to RBC (NORUM and GJONE, 1967). Several liver diseases associated with LCAT deficiency are associated with an increase in RBC unesterified cholesterol. In general, there is a good correlation with LCAT activity and RBC cholesterol (NORUM and GJONE, 1967; SIMON, 1971). With improvement in the hepatic dysfunction, LCAT activity increases; and, correspondingly, the cholesterol content of RBC decreases (SIMON, 1971).

Other mechanisms for transport of tissue cholesterol into plasma may also be postulated. It was shown by AVIGAN (1959) that the amounts of cholesterol and other sterols in plasma low density lipoproteins can be increased by incubation with cholesterol dispersed on an inert surface. It was shown by SODHI and KALANT (1963c) that LDL + VLDL from nephrotic rats had a greater cholesterol to protein ratio than in those from normal rats. These observations suggest the possibility that circulating lipoproteins, particularly LDL and VLDL, may be enriched by cholesterol without the necessity of LCAT.

It has long been known that tissue deposits of cholesterol—e.g., xanthomata—can be reduced by long-term administration of hypocholesterolemic agents. Recent studies by SODHI et al. (1969, 1973a) showed that in most subjects acute reduction in plasma cholesterol was associated with prompt mobilization of tissue cholesterol. A number of other studies on hypocholesterolemic agents have shown that fecal losses of endogenous cholesterol may exceed the losses from plasma (WOOD et al., 1966; MIETTINEN, 1968a, b, c; HORLICK et al., 1971; GRUNDY et al., 1972; KUDCHODKAR et al., 1973e). In the absence of any increase in endogenous synthesis, these data implied that some of the fecal cholesterol was derived from tissues. It was not possible, however, to determine whether the tissue cholesterol came from Pool A or B. When the treatment is associated with an increase in endogenous synthesis, mobilization of tissue cholesterol cannot be assessed until methods become available for determination of synthesis during the nonsteady state conditions. Following studies, however, suggest that immediately after the administration of hypocholesterolemic agents, acute mobilization of cholesterol from Pool B commonly occurs (SODHI et al., 1969, 1973a).

Subjects were given intravenous injections of radioactive cholesterol, and four to six weeks were allowed for the specific activity of cholesterol in various pools to equilibrate and for the decline in plasma cholesterol specific activity to become exponential. The subjects were then put on cholesterol balance studies. After 12 to 15 days of control studies, they were given one of the three hypocholesterolemic agents (clofibrate, nicotinic acid, plant sterols). Nine of the eleven subjects showed prompt increases in the specific activity of plasma cholesterol soon after the start of treatment. Since no new source of radioactive cholesterol was introduced into the system, the only way in which the specific activity of plasma cholesterol could increase above its previous values was by an influx of higher specific activity cholesterol from pools other than plasma. Although it has generally been believed that the specific activity of exchangeable pools of cholesterol is the same as that of plasma cholesterol, this is only true of rapidly-exchangeable pools or Pool A. After pulse labelling of plasma

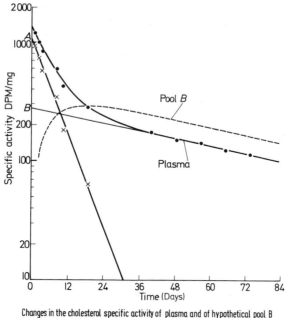

Changes in the cholesterol specific activity of plasma and of hypothetical pool B after an intravenous injection of labelled cholesterol.

Fig. 4

cholesterol, the specific activity of cholesterol in tissue pools belonging to Pool B would be greater than that of plasma cholesterol, as indicated by the precursor-product relationships (Fig. 4). This was validated by studies on rats (SODHI, 1967), rabbits (AVIGAN et al., 1962), baboons (WILSON, 1970), and man (MOUTAFIS and MYANT, 1969; SAMUEL et al., 1972). It therefore follows that contributions from the rapidly-exchangeable pool, or Pool A, are unlikely to cause appreciable changes in plasma cholesterol specific activity. Significant changes in plasma cholesterol specific activity must be due to the entry of cholesterol from the slowly-exchangeable pool, or Pool B. Mobilization of cholesterol from Pool A, however, is not excluded by these data.

Cholesterol from Pool B may enter plasma either through exchange or by mobilization. It was shown by us (SODHI et al., 1971a) that the rates of exchange of cholesterol between tissue pools and plasma were not affected by administration of clofibrate in man. It was, moreover, unlikely that drugs as different from each other as clofibrate, nicotinic acid, and plant sterols should have the same direct effect on the rates of exchange of cholesterol between plasma and tissues. Acute peaks in the specific activity of plasma cholesterol lasting only two to three days, by definition, could not be attributed to an exchange with *the slowly-exchangeable pool*. Therefore, mobilization is the only apparent explanation for the entry of higher specific activity cholesterol from Pool B. This hypothesis is supported by an earlier observation of SODHI et al. (1967a). They observed a dramatic increase in biliary cholesterol within a few hours after substitution of polyunsaturated for saturated fats in the diet. Furthermore, GRUNDY et al. (1972) and HORNING et al. (1972) reported increases in biliary cholesterol after the administration of clofibrate. Our recent studies have also shown that the increases in plasma cholesterol specific activity and the increases in the amounts of endogenous cholesterol secreted into the intestinal tract had a significant correlation, suggesting that both were dependent on mobilization of tissue cholesterol (Sodhi et al., 1969; 1973a).

3. The transfer of net amounts of cholesterol from plasma to tissues. Under physiological conditions, there is no net transfer of cholesterol from plasma to tissues (except in cases such as that of the adrenal glands where the synthesis is not sufficient for its needs). However, an abnormal increase in plasma cholesterol over a long period of time often leads to an increase in tissue cholesterol, manifested as deposits in tendons and the arterial intima (Taylor et al., 1962; Smith, 1965). The mechanisms by which plasma cholesterol is deposited into tissues are not entirely clear. It has been suggested that arterial elastin may interact with plasma VLDL or LDL, resulting in the transfer of the lipid to the elastin (Kramsch and Hollander, 1973). Evidence has also been presented that cholesterol may be deposited in tissues along with other lipid and protein moieties of lipoproteins (Watts, 1963; Kao and Wissler, 1965). The connective tissue components have been shown to precipitate plasma lipoproteins (Walton and Williamson, 1968). Since tissue deposits of cholesterol are particularly rich in cholesterol esters (Smith et al., 1967; Crouse et al., 1972), it is suggested that cholesterol may be esterified within the tissues (Mukherjee et al., 1958; Abdulla et al., 1968).

It is also conceivable that the increase of cholesterol in the tissues is analogous to the increase in the RBC membranes seen in conditions associated with deficiencies of LCAT. Since a deficiency of LCAT leads to an increase in the ratio of free/esterified cholesterol in plasma (Norum and Gjone, 1967; Simon, 1971), it is possible that the increased amount of free cholesterol in plasma on equilibration with tissues is accompanied by a transfer of some of the cholesterol to tissues. Since HDL is the preferred substrate for the action of LCAT (Glomset, 1968), the tissue deposits of cholesterol in Tangier's disease (Fredrickson, 1964) may also be explained by the above hypothesis. Although the tissue cholesterol deposits in Tangier's disease are those of cholesterol esters rather than of free cholesterol, it is to be expected that excess cholesterol will be esterified in the tissues (Fig. 1). Undoubtedly, there are additional factors, as illustrated by the following. Patients with cerebrotendinous xanthomatosis have normal cholesterol concentrations in plasma, but they develop tendon xanthomata rich in cholesterol. These patients also have elevations of plasma and tissue cholestanol (Menkes et al., 1968; Salen, 1971), but the relative proportion of stanol to cholesterol is so small that it is unlikely that the increase in plasma cholestanol is directly responsible for the deposition of cholesterol in the tissues. Substitution of cholesterol by cholestanol in plasma or tissue lipoproteins may interfere with the integrity of their structure, resulting in deposition of the lipid. The rates of isotopic exchange of cholesterol between patients' plasma lipoproteins and normal RBC, however, were normal (Sodhi, unpublished observations).

Patients fed large amounts of cholesterol also deposit excess cholesterol in tissues without significantly increasing the plasma concentration of cholesterol (Quintão et al., 1971b). Although most of the dietary cholesterol is normally taken up by liver in rats (Goodman, 1962), it is conceivable that when abnormal amounts are ingested and absorbed some cholesterol is deposited in extrahepatic tissues in man.

Ho and TAYLOR (1971) investigated the rate of increase in tissue cholesterol content in rabbits maintained on a diet which produced a moderate hypercholesterolemia. Tissues or organs in rabbits could be grouped into four categories according to their response to dietary-induced hypercholesterolemia. Aorta, liver, spleen, and skin showed an exponential increase in tissue cholesterol with time. Adrenal glands, kidney, small intestine, and lung showed a linear arithmetical increase. A random increase was seen in the third group constituted by testes and heart. No significant increase in tissue content of cholesterol was seen in muscle, fat, pancreas, or brain.

The deposition of excess cholesterol is determined to some degree by the species. In rats, liver receives the bulk of extra cholesterol (MORIN et al., 1962; BEHER et al., 1970); whereas in rabbits a lot of extrahepatic tissues also accumulate cholesterol (HO and TAYLOR, 1971).

IX. Homeostasis of Plasma Cholesterol

Cholesterol concentration in an apparently healthy population varies generally between 150 and 350 mg per 100 ml of plasma. The values are distributed in an almost "normal" curve with some skewing towards higher values. The average value reported in adults between the ages of 30 and 60 in most western societies is about 230 mg% (KANNEL, 1971). The so-called "normal" values are determined more by the frequency distribution than by the physiological considerations. Insofar as atherogenesis is concerned, there is no known concentration of serum cholesterol which is below the threshold for any risk. All other factors being equal, the higher values of total plasma cholesterol, even in the "normal" range, are associated with greater risk of atherosclerosis (KEYS et al., 1950; STAMLER, 1960). The relationship of plasma cholesterol concentration to coronary atherosclerosis is stronger the earlier in life the measurements are made (KANNEL, 1971). In most western countries the concentrations of plasma cholesterol increase with age (KEYS et al., 1950; KANNEL et al., 1964), and it has therefore been suggested that the values accepted as normal should be greater in older than in younger people (FREDRICKSON et al., 1967).

An increase in plasma cholesterol, however, is not a universal phenomenon. The Masai of Africa have plasma levels of 135 ± 33 mg per 100 ml, and no significant changes occur after the age of 15 (Ho et al., 1971). The Yemenite Jews in Israel also fail to show the age-related increase in their plasma cholesterol (BRUNNER et al., 1959). It would therefore appear that an increase in the levels of plasma cholesterol in older people is due mostly to environmental factors. It has also been shown that concentrations of cholesterol are highest in the spring and lowest in the autumn (FYFE et al., 1968). The genetic factors are also important, both in physiological states and in pathological conditions. Men belonging to blood group A have higher mean values of plasma cholesterol than those belonging to group 0 or B (ALLAN and DAWSON, 1968; OLIVER et al., 1969).

Although considerable information on cholesterol metabolism in man has become available, the mechanisms controlling its plasma concentrations are still not well understood. Changes in its absorption, synthesis, and catabolism have often been studied with a view to elucidate these mechanisms. Fecal excretion of neutral and acidic derivatives of endogenous cholesterol has also been examined to study the mechanisms responsible for the hypocholesterolemic action of drugs. However, it is not clear as to how changes in the above parameters bring about changes in the concentration of plasma cholesterol.

From a theoretical standpoint, the changes in the absorption, synthesis, and excretion of cholesterol bear more directly on the total amounts of cholesterol in the body than on plasma cholesterol concentrations. *The changes in plasma cholesterol are related primarily to the rates of entry of cholesterol and of lipoproteins with which cholesterol is associated and their exit from that compartment.* In order for changes in the absorption, synthesis, and catabolism of cholesterol to explain changes in concentration of plasma cholesterol, their effects on the entry and clearance of various lipoproteins in plasma must be known.

The entry of cholesterol into plasma from liver and intestines occurs in the form of chylomicra and lipoproteins. Other organs are not known to synthesize lipoproteins; therefore, mechanisms of contribution, if any, from other organs are not known. Biliary, dietary, and intestinal cholesterol is incorporated into chylomicra and intestinal lipoproteins and delivered to plasma through the lymph. The rates of its entry into and clearance from plasma are such that even during the absorption of a meal containing cholesterol, any increase in plasma levels is only minor (BOYD, 1935; SPERRY, 1936) except perhaps in patients with types I and V hyperlipoproteinemia. *The effects of dietary cholesterol on the levels of cholesterol in a fasting specimen, therefore, are dependent on its re-entry into circulation after having once been cleared.*

In experimental animals, most of the chylomicron cholesterol is removed by the liver (GOODMAN, 1962; NESTEL et al., 1963), although under certain conditions significant fractions may be removed by extrahepatic tissues (LOSSOW et al., 1963). Cholesterol removed by the liver can be incorporated into lipoproteins and secreted into plasma. It can also be excreted into the bile as such or after its conversion to bile acids, or it can be converted to cholesterol esters and stored in the liver. The cholesterol synthesized in the liver makes up by far the most important fraction of endogenous cholesterol, and this too has the same pathways open to it as those to the dietary and intestinal cholesterol in the liver. However, preliminary data from our laboratories (SODHI and AVIGAN, unpublished observations) and the work of BRICKER (1971) suggest that the biliary secretion of newly-synthesized cholesterol is only minor compared to its transfer into plasma.

The incorporation of cholesterol into hepatic lipoproteins and its secretion into plasma is the only important pathway by which exogenous or endogenous cholesterol can influence the plasma concentrations of cholesterol in a fasting specimen. This can be mediated, among others, through the following mechanisms.

1. Through changes in the concentration of the "substrate" in the liver: Changes in both the absorption and hepatic synthesis can increase or decrease the hepatic concentration of cholesterol, which in turn may influence its incorporation into plasma lipoproteins. Similarly, changes in the rates of catabolism of cholesterol will also lead to changes in the amounts of cholesterol in the liver and thus in its incorporation into lipoproteins. However, this does not appear to be a likely mechanism by which changes in the absorption, synthesis, or catabolism influence the plasma levels of cholesterol. Experimental studies in rats have shown that a signifi-

cant increase in the content of hepatic cholesterol did not lead to an increase in plasma concentration (WILSON, 1962; MORIN et al., 1962; BEHER et al., 1970).

2. Almost all of the exogenous (within the range of normal intake) and endogenous cholesterol in the liver is first incorporated into lipoproteins, and they may influence the levels of plasma cholesterol through this mechanism. This appears to us to be a likely possibility (SODHI and KUDCHODKAR, 1973a).

Although alterations in the absorption, synthesis, and excretion of cholesterol will cause changes in the total body pools of cholesterol, the latter does not produce parallel changes in plasma cholesterol. QUINTÃO et al. (1971b) fed large amounts of cholesterol to subjects, some of whom accumulated as much as 20 grams of cholesterol in the body pools. Plasma cholesterol concentrations rose in some, fell in others, and remained essentially unchanged in the remainder. NESTEL et al. (1969) and KUDCHODKAR et al. (1972b) have also observed that the turnover rates as well as the amounts of cholesterol in tissue pools had no relationship to the levels of plasma cholesterol.

Studies on insulin-deficient and control squirrel monkeys showed that plasma cholesterol concentrations were higher in the insulin-deficient than in the control animals. However, the amounts of cholesterol derived from absorption and endogenous synthesis were the same in the two groups. The amounts of cholesterol entering and leaving Pool A were also similar (LEHNER et al., 1972). Similarly, in squirrel monkeys fed cholesterol, hyporesponders and hyperresponders (with regard to the development of hypercholesterolemia) demonstrated essentially identical absorption and endogenous synthesis of cholesterol (LOFLAND et al., 1972).

Changes in endogenous synthesis of cholesterol are generally associated with corresponding changes in the synthesis of lipoproteins and their secretion into plasma. Therefore, if everything else remains equal, changes in endogenous synthesis may well be related to parallel changes in plasma cholesterol. However, changes in the synthesis of cholesterol and of lipoproteins are often associated with an alteration in the turnover rates of plasma lipoproteins; therefore, changes in synthesis are not always reflected in plasma cholesterol concentrations. The hepatic synthesis of cholesterol is increased in hyperthyroidism, but the cholesterol concentration in plasma is decreased. Conversely, in hypothyroidism cholesterol synthesis is decreased, but plasma levels are increased (GOULD, 1959; MIETTINEN, 1968c). In "chronic" experimental nephrosis of rats it was found that the hepatic synthesis of cholesterol was markedly decreased, while the concentration of plasma cholesterol remained elevated (SODHI and KALANT, 1963a, b). Furthermore, T-tube drainage of bile (DEPALMA et al., 1966), ileal exclusion (MOUTAFIS et al., 1968), cholestyramine (GRUNDY et al., 1971; NAZIR et al., 1972), and plant sterols (GRUNDY et al., 1969; KUDCHODKAR et al., 1971a, 1973b) all increase hepatic synthesis of cholesterol, although plasma levels may fall.

These data indicate that absorption and synthesis do not have as direct a relationship with plasma levels of cholesterol as the metabolism of plasma lipoproteins. It may be predicted that all conditions associated with increased synthesis and decreased plasma levels will show an increase in the net turnover of plasma lipoproteins, and vice versa. Similarly, the catabolism of cholesterol to bile acids and its biliary excretion are related to the metabolism of plasma lipoproteins, as suggested later; and therefore are not likely *to cause* changes in plasma cholesterol.

Turnover of Cholesterol in Exchangeable Pools

Unesterified cholesterol, phospholipids, and proteins of plasma lipoproteins are assumed to be structural in function. Plasma triglycerides and cholesterol esters on the other hand have been called "core" lipids, implying that they are not essential to the structural integrity of lipoproteins which transport them in plasma. In addition to mass transfers of proteins (HAVEL et al., 1973), triglycerides, and cholesterol esters between different classes of plasma lipoproteins (NICHOLS and SMITH, 1965), there are also isotopic exchanges of unesterified cholesterol (ECKLES et al., 1955; KRITCH-EVSKY et al., 1965), phospholipids (KUNKEL and BEARN, 1954; ZILVERSMIT, 1971; ILLINGWORTH and PORTMAN, 1972), and proteins (SODHI and GOULD, 1970; RUBEN-STEIN and RUBENSTEIN, 1972) between different lipoprotein molecules, although mass transfer of unesterified cholesterol from one lipoprotein to another has also been postulated (GLOMSET et al., 1970).

The isotopic exchange of unesterified cholesterol implies that one molecule of cholesterol in a lipoprotein is replaced by another molecule from another lipoprotein. This by definition precludes any net (or mass) transfers or changes in the content of free cholesterol in different lipoproteins. KRITCHEVSKY (1965, 1970) showed that the specific activity of α- and β-lipoproteins became equal three hours after the injection into a baboon of β-lipoproteins containing radioactive cholesterol. Equilibration of plasma free cholesterol specific activities between different lipoproteins without causing any changes in the content has also been shown to occur *in vitro* (SODHI and KALANT, 1963c; SHAPIRO et al., 1970), indicating that this equilibration is not mediated through the metabolic activity of liver or other organs. Isotopic exchange of unesterified cholesterol has also been shown between plasma and RBC (HAGERMAN and GOULD, 1951); and between plasma and other tissues, albeit at very different rates (ECKLES et al., 1955; SODHI, 1967). Equilibration is most rapid with liver and very slow with the nervous tissue (ECKLES et al., 1955; CHOBANIAN et al., 1962; AVIGAN et al., 1962; CHEVALLIER, 1967). The half-time of equilibration between plasma and liver is about one hour in man (GOULD et al., 1955), and the rate of equilibration between plasma and nervous tissue is so small that even after many weeks the specific activity of unesterified cholesterol in brain is only an insignificant fraction of that of plasma cholesterol (CHOBANIAN et al., 1962; CHEVALLIER, 1967). The half-time of equilibration between plasma and red blood cells is only a little longer than between plasma and liver. The cholesterol in spleen and lungs equilibrates with plasma more readily than the cholesterol in kidneys and intestines but much less readily than the cholesterol in red blood cells (CHOBANIAN et al., 1962; CHEVALLIER, 1967). The cholesterol in adipose tissue, muscle, and skin, etc., equilibrates more showly than most other organs (except nervous tissue). GURD (1960) postulated that the isotopic exchange of unesterified cholesterol between two lipoprotein molecules occurs as a result of their collisions with each other. However, all lipoproteins bear like electrical charges, which would tend to prevent them from coming in close contact with each other. VANDENHEUVEL has explained the same phenomenon as follows: "Local levels of thermal energy vary widely in biological structures such as membranes and lipoproteins, as postulated by Boltzmann's Law. Whenever this level of energy exceeds the relatively weak cohesional forces holding a molecule within a structure, the molecule may be ejected into the bathing medium. Molecules of the same type dispersed in the medium may enter the structure by the reverse process (VANDENHEUVEL, 1971). Hence, the lipoprotein not only maintains its compositional and structural integrity, but its units bathed in the same medium will exchange their constituent molecules, including cholesterol. The rate of exchange for a given molecule is dependent on the cohesional forces, its solubility (c.m. concentration) in the bathing medium, and the temperature" (VANDENHEUVEL, 1973).

When two lipoproteins, one labelled and the other unlabelled, were mixed in a test tube at equilibrium, the specific activity of unesterified cholesterol in both lipoproteins became identical. Similarly, when plasma labelled with radioactive cholesterol was mixed with unlabelled red blood cells in a test tube, the specific activity of free cholesterol at and after equilibration became identical for the two compartments (HAGERMAN and GOULD, 1951). Extrapolating the observations from closed systems such as these, it was generally believed that the specific activities of cholesterol in plasma and different tissue pools became equal on equilibration. However, unlike the in vitro systems, unlabelled cholesterol continues to enter into one compartment of the in vivo system; and, correspondingly, labelled as well as unlabelled cholesterol continues to leave the system. Since plasma cholesterol is a precursor of radioactive cholesterol in tissues, the specific activity of the latter becomes greater than that of plasma cholesterol and remains greater according to the precursor-product relationship. The differences between the specific activity values of tissue compartments and plasma cholesterol at and after equilibration depend on the rates of exchange and on relative sizes of the two compartments. The slower the rate of exchange and the larger the relative sizes of the product pool, the greater will be the difference (ZILVERSMIT, 1960). The relationship of specific activity of a hypothetical tissue pool (slowly-exchangeable or Pool B) to that of plasma cholesterol is shown in Fig. 4.

The rate of isotopic exchange of unesterified cholesterol between the liver and plasma is so rapid that in most metabolic studies changes in the specific activity of plasma and liver cholesterol are identical. Therefore, the unesterified cholesterol present in the two compartments has generally been considered to constitute a single metabolic pool. The validity of this concept is limited to the metabolic studies involving isotopes and where changes in the specific activity of unesterified cholesterol in liver and plasma are identical. Since the mechanisms controlling the content of cholesterol in the two compartments are more or less independent of each other, the isotopic exchange, by definition, cannot cause parallel and equal changes in both compartments. The concept of a single pool is also not valid when changes in the sizes of compartments are being considered. Similarly, changes in the rate of entry into or exit from one compartment do not necessarily imply that there will be related and parallel changes in entry or exit from the other compartment.

Isotopic exchange is not necessarily the only mechanism by which equilibration of specific activities of cholesterol in different tissues occurs, although it may be the most important. It is the only factor in equilibration between plasma and tissues which do not synthesize or catabolise cholesterol; e.g., mature red blood cells. Equilibration between free and esterified cholesterol in plasma, on the other hand, is brought about by mechanisms entirely different from the isotopic exchange, although the two have a precursor-product relationship. In other instances, specific activity equilibration between plasma and tissue cholesterol pools—e.g., intestines—

is brought about not by one but by many factors operating simultaneously. The rate of isotopic exchange of free cholesterol between plasma and intestines is so slow that for this alone to bring about equilibration would take many days (Sodhi, 1967; Connor et al., 1971). However, considerable amounts of cholesterol from the plasma-liver pool are secreted into the intestinal lumen and on reabsorption mix with cholesterol in the intestinal mucosa. Thus equilibration is generally complete by 24 hrs.

Depending on the rates of isotopic exchange between plasma and tissue cholesterol pools, the tissue cholesterol is designated either as readily-exchangeable or slowly-exchangeable. "Readily-exchangeable" tissue cholesterol is assumed to constitute a hypothetical "Pool A" and "slowly-exchangeable" tissue cholesterol, "Pool B" (Goodman and Noble, 1968). Nervous tissue and other cholesterol compartments which do not exchange have been designated as "Pool C" (Wilson, 1970). Cholesterol in RBC, liver, spleen, lungs, etc., appears to have rapid enough rates of exchange that it is considered to belong completely in Pool A. On the other hand, most of the cholesterol present in muscle, skin, and adipose tissue exchanges at much slower rates; and, traditionally, these organs have been considered to form parts of Pool B. Studies by Wilson (1970) in baboons, however, have indicated that, in addition to nervous tissue, large fractions of cholesterol in other tissues did not exchange, so that all of it should be considered to constitute Pool C. Of the total cholesterol present in tissues such as muscle, adipose tissue, and skin, significant fractions should also be considered to belong to Pool A by the same criteria as applied to the cholesterol in RBC, liver, spleen, and lungs (Wilson, 1970).

It is important to bear in mind that the concepts of Pool A and Pool B, based on the phenomenon of isotopic exchange, are entirely hypothetical; and they do not bear any relation to anatomical entities. From his experiments in baboons, Wilson (1970) suggested that portions of all pools (A, B, and C) may be found in many tissues.

When free cholesterol in the plasma compartment is pulse labelled, its rate of decay is given by a slope which (up to a period of about 12 weeks) can be broken into two exponentials. The second exponential begins 3 to 6 weeks after the injection (Fig. 4). If the specific activity of plasma cholesterol is followed for a longer period, a third exponential may become evident in the slope (Goodman et al., 1972). Two independent factors contribute to the slope of decline in plasma cholesterol specific activity: 1) isotopic exchange of free cholesterol between plasma and tissue pools, and 2) turnover of plasma free cholesterol.

Within minutes after its intravenous injection, radioactive cholesterol distributes itself in the plasma compartment, and the subsequent isotopic exchange between plasma and tissues may be viewed as a continuous process of dilution of the injected radioactivity in the total exchangeable cholesterol pool. This, by definition, precludes any net transfer or turnover. Turnover involves the entry of net amounts of unlabelled cholesterol and the exit of equal amounts of (labelled and unlabelled) cholesterol from exchangeable pools under steady-state conditions. The early curvilinear portion of the specific activity slope is determined more by the rates of exchange than the rates of turnover. The later exponential part of the slope is dependent more on the turnover than on the isotopic exchange. By that time the specific activities of cholesterol in different tissue pools have reached equilibrium with the specific activity of plasma cholesterol. Increased synthesis or increased absorption will be reflected by an increase in the slope; and, conversely, a decrease in synthesis or absorption will cause a decrease in the slope.

In earlier studies, the exponential part of the specific activity slope was assumed to reflect the turnover of the entire exchangeable pool (CHOBANIAN et al., 1962). The values obtained with this "one-pool" model were erroneously high. GOODMAN and NOBLE (1968) proposed a two-pool model for calculating various parameters of cholesterol metabolism from the specific activity slopes. The exponential part of the slope was assumed to reflect the turnover of only the second or slowly-exchangeable pool. If determinations of plasma cholesterol specific activity are made for longer periods of time when the third exponential becomes apparent, the last exponential, in this model, will reflect the turnover of the third or the slowest of the exchangeable pools. Based on a two-pool model, calculations by NESTEL et al. (1969) indicated that a subject with ideal body weight has a total of 60 grams of exchangeable cholesterol, one-third of which is in Pool A and the rest in Pool B. The production rate in such a man is about 1 gram a day, which includes about 300 mg from absorption and the remainder from endogenous synthesis. The values of production rate obtained by a three-pool model are approximately 10 percent lower than those obtained by a two-pool model.

It is worth noting that these values of cholesterol turnover derived from the data on plasma cholesterol specific activity refer to total cholesterol in exchangeable pools and not to plasma compartment alone. The turnover of plasma cholesterol is defined as the net amounts of cholesterol entering (and leaving) plasma per unit time. Most, if not all, of this occurs in the new lipoproteins or chylomicra synthesized by the liver and intestines. Although some information on the amounts and chemical state (free versus esterified) of cholesterol in intestinal lipoproteins, including chylomicra, is available, there is little information of this nature on hepatic lipoproteins.

Intestinal lipoproteins transport approximately one gram of cholesterol per day into blood (please see section on absorption). Cholesterol entering in hepatic lipoproteins cannot be estimated with any degree of confidence. There are mass transfers of unesterified cholesterol and of other lipids from one lipoprotein to another, and possibly from tissues to plasma lipoproteins. It is not certain if all or any fraction of plasma LDL is synthesized in the liver. Furthermore, the relationships between the turnover rates of different moieties in a given class of plasma lipoproteins have not yet been elucidated. If it is assumed that (1) newly synthesized hepatic lipoproteins contain only unesterified cholesterol (GLOMSET, 1968, 1970), (2) plasma LDL is derived only from plasma VLDL and none is synthesized in the liver (LANGER et al., 1972), and (3) fractional turnover of unesterified cholesterol in a lipoprotein is the same as that of the protein moiety, the approximate amounts of cholesterol entering circulation from the liver can be calculated from the unesterified cholesterol to protein ratios and the fractional turnover rates of the protein moieties of very low and high density lipoproteins. As a rough approximation, these assumptions suggest that about two grams of cholesterol enter plasma from the liver per day.

X. Plasma Cholesterol Esters

After pulse labelling of free cholesterol in plasma, the specific activity of plasma cholesterol esters begins to increase and it reaches peak values in about two days, at which time it is crossed by the declining specific activity slope of free cholesterol.

Thereafter, the specific activity slopes of plasma free and esterified cholesterol remain parallel, the specific activity of the latter remaining greater than that of free cholesterol, in accord with the precursor-product relationship. The incorporation of radioactive free cholesterol into cholesterol esters of HDL is greater than that in VLDL, and the incorporation is least in plasma LDL (Goodman, 1964; Nestel et al., 1965; Sodhi and Kudchodkar, 1973d).

The function of cholesterol esters in plasma lipoproteins and the mechanisms responsible for their turnover are not known. According to Glomset's hypothesis (1968, 1970), hepatic lipoproteins when newly-synthesized contain little, if any, esterified cholesterol, and he suggested (Glomset, 1962) that practically all cholesterol esters in fasting plasma are formed by the action of an enzyme called lecithin cholesterol acyltransferase (LCAT). This enzyme esterifies free cholesterol in the lipoproteins with the fatty acid in number 2 position of plasma lecithin. The fatty acid in number 2 position of lecithin is typically an unsaturated fatty acid. This may explain why most of the fatty acids in cholesterol esters are unsaturated. According to this hypothesis, newly-synthesized lipoproteins contain relatively large amounts of lecithin and unesterified cholesterol. According to Glomset, the composition of lipoproteins isolated from plasma reflect the effects of not only LCAT activity but also of equilibration of cholesterol between different plasma lipoproteins (Glomset, 1968, 1970).

When human or rat plasma was incubated at 37° C, the molar increase in plasma esterified cholesterol was identical to the molar decrement of free cholesterol and lecithin. The increase in cholesterol esters and the decrement in free cholesterol and the fatty acid in number 2 position of lecithin were parallel and equivalent. Lecithin was the only esterified lipid to decrease significantly in concentration during incubation of plasma. Incubation of labelled free fatty acids and plasma did not produce labelled cholesterol esters. When plasma was incubated with ^{14}C-tripalmitine, small amounts of cholesterol esters containing radioactive palmitate were formed. However, this transfer of radioactive fatty acids in triglycerides might either be direct or through lecithin, since labelled phospholipids were also formed (Shah et al., 1964).

Human plasma LCAT does not react with all plasma lipoproteins equally. After incubation of human plasma with cholesterol-4-^{14}C, the HDL cholesterol esters showed the highest specific activity. Furthermore, when human plasma was incubated with cholesterol-4-^{14}C, the specific activity of cholesterol esters within the subfractions of HDL was also different (Glomset et al., 1966). Similarly, after intravenous injection of radioactive free cholesterol, the specific activity of HDL cholesterol esters was greater than that of VLDL, which in turn had cholesterol esters of higher specific activity than those in plasma LDL (Goodman, 1964; Nestel et al., 1965; Sodhi and Kudchodkar, 1973d). When VLDL alone was incubated in vitro with LCAT, significant esterification of cholesterol did not occur. On the other hand, when plasma HDL was incubated with the same enzyme, considerable esterification of free cholesterol was observed (Akanuma and Glomset, 1968). After injection of radioactive mevalonate or acetate, the greatest fractional turnover rate of cholesterol esters was in HDL, then in VLDL, and then in LDL (Goodman, 1964; Nestel et al., 1965; Sodhi and Kudchodkar, 1973d). All cholesterol esters in a given lipoprotein, however, had the same turnover rate (Goodman, 1964; Wood et al., 1965; Nestel and Monger, 1967).

Table 6. Cholesterol composition of plasma lipoproteins

Class	Cholesterol[a] mg/100 ml plasma	Ratio[b] esterified/free
VLDL	21	1.01 ± 0.19
LDL	154	2.43 ± 0.21
HDL	58	4.08 ± 0.51

[a] Reference BLATON and PETERS, 1972.
[b] Reference ROSE, 1972.

Lecithin cholesterol acyltransferase also promotes nonenzymic transfer of cholesterol esters from HDL to VLDL and of triglycerides from VLDL to HDL. Much of the unesterified cholesterol in HDL that reacts with LCAT is probably derived from VLDL and LDL in the first instance, and much of the cholesterol esters formed in HDL is probably transferred to VLDL, which may ultimately become the major lipid component of LDL (GLOMSET, 1968). Glomset suggested that the esterification occurs in situ in plasma HDL, and then cholesterol esters formed by the action of LCAT are transferred en mass to plasma VLDL and LDL (GLOMSET, 1968). In accord with this suggestion, the cholesterol esters of human VLDL have been shown to be similar to those of human HDL (GOODMAN and SHIRATORI, 1964; NESTEL and COUZENS, 1966). In fact, the small difference in fatty acid composition which does exist (a higher percentage of monounsaturated fatty acid esters in VLDL than in HDL) may be caused by a disproportionate transfer of cholesterol esters from HDL to VLDL. It has also been suggested that "in exchange" for cholesterol esters there is a mass transfer of triglycerides from VLDL to LDL and HDL (REHNBORG and NICHOLS, 1964; NICHOLS and SMITH, 1965). However, even when the LCAT activity is inhibited, some of the cholesterol esters initially bound to LDL and HDL are transferred to VLDL; and there is a reciprocal transfer of triglycerides from VLDL to plasma HDL. Nichols' data (NICHOLS and SMITH, 1965) suggest that there is a reciprocal transfer of triglycerides from human VLDL and cholesterol esters from human HDL. NICHOLS et al. (1962) observed a strong positive statistical correlation between serum VLDL and HDL triglycerides in healthy males. NICHOLS and SMITH (1965) showed that incubation of human serum low in triglycerides resulted in a net increase in cholesterol esters in all three major lipoprotein classes and a small degree of transfer of triglycerides from VLDL to LDL and HDL. However, when serum rich in triglycerides was incubated, the increase in cholesterol esters produced by serum fatty acid transferase activity was seen only in VLDL which accepted some cholesterol esters initially bound to the LDL and HDL.

The physical transfer of cholesterol esters and of triglycerides between human serum lipoproteins appears to be the basic property of these macromolecules. Although LCAT facilitates this mass transfer, equilibration of cholesterol ester and triglyceride content of different lipoproteins can occur without the help of the enzyme.

MURPHY (1962) incubated erythrocytes in serum that had previously been incubated at 37° C for 24 hrs. He observed a transfer of unesterified cholesterol from erythrocytes to the serum, and he showed that the loss of erythrocyte cholesterol was

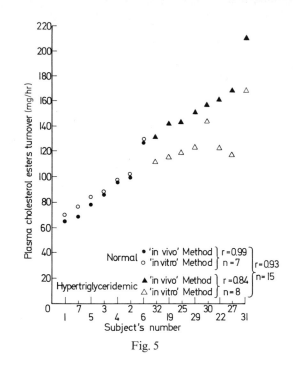

Fig. 5

related to the amount of esterified cholesterol formed in the serum during preincubation. He therefore concluded that the loss was due to a shift in the equilibration
between erythrocytes and lipoprotein unesterified cholesterol caused by the LCAT
reaction. Based on such findings, Glomset suggested that the unesterified cholesterol
and lecithin in different plasma lipoproteins reach an equilibrium distribution; so
that fresh samples of normal plasma contain lipoproteins that are at or near equilibrium insofar as the distribution of various lipids is concerned. According to him, the
enzyme LCAT preturbs this equilibrium by decreasing the concentration of unesterified cholesterol and lecithin in HDL and increasing the concentration of esterified
cholesterol. The increase in esterified cholesterol is perhaps responsible for the transfer of this lipid from HDL to VLDL and LDL, which in turn perhaps provokes the
transfer of triglycerides from VLDL to HDL (Glomset, 1970).

    Although the activity *in vitro* of lecithin: cholesterol acyltransferase is adequate
to explain the net turnover rates of plasma cholesterol esters, a direct comparison in
man of the turnover rates determined *in vivo* with the values derived from *in vitro*
studies had not been made until recently (Kudchodkar and Sodhi, 1973; Barter,
1974). We gave cholesterol-4-^{14}C intravenously to subjects with and without hypertriglyceridemia, and samples of blood were taken to determine the LCAT activity *in
vitro*. The results derived from *in vitro* studies were compared with *in vitro* esterification
of plasma free cholesterol. In normotriglyceridemic subjects the values obtained by the
two independent methods were in remarkable agreement with each other (Fig. 5). In
the hypertriglyceridemic subjects, however, the values derived from *in vitro* method
were consistently lower than the actual rates determined *in vivo* (Fig. 5). The reason
for this discrepancy is not known. Either the presence of hypertriglyceridemic

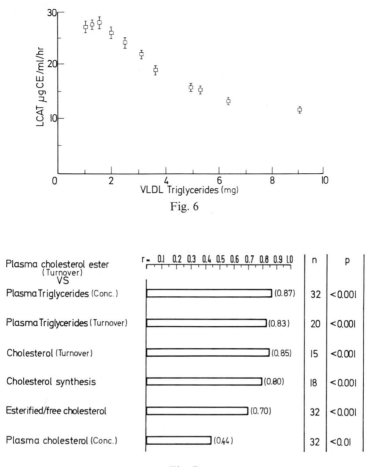

Fig. 6

Fig. 7

plasma inhibited the enzyme's activity *in vitro*; or the rapid turnover of VLDL, which acts as receptor for the product of the enzymatic activity (cholesterol esters), facilitated the reaction *in vivo*.

MARCEL and VEZINA (1973) showed that addition of VLDL or chylomicrons to the incubation medium increased the LCAT activity as determined by changes in the mass of plasma free cholesterol. Utilizing radioactive isotopes for *in vivo* labelling of plasma cholesterol, the investigations in our laboratories suggested that the increase in the *in vitro* activity of LCAT may be expected up to a concentration of 2 mg/ml of triglycerides (Fig.6). However, further increments in VLDL triglycerides caused a progressive decrease in esterification of free cholesterol (KUDCHODKAR and SODHI, 1973; SODHI, 1974; KUDCHODKAR, SUNDARAM, and SODHI, unpublished observations).

MONGER and NESTEL (1967) suggested that turnover rates of cholesterol esters in postabsorptive plasma were dependent on the concentration of plasma free cholesterol. Our studies, however, indicated that the correlation of the plasma cholesterol ester turnover (as determined *in vivo*) was much better with cholesterol synthesis than with its concentration in plasma (Fig. 7). Since an excellent correlation between cholesterol synthesis and hypertriglyceridemia has been shown by us, an excellent correlation between cholesterol ester turnover and plasma triglycerides was not unexpected (Fig. 7).

The concentrations of plasma triglycerides bear an excellent correlation ($r = 0.99$) with VLDL triglycerides (GOLDSTEIN et al., 1972), and the net turnover of plasma VLDL is directly proportional to the concentrations of plasma VLDL (except in severe hypertriglyceridemia) (REAVEN et al., 1965). These data therefore indicate that cholesterol synthesis, VLDL turnover, and turnover of plasma cholesterol esters are interrelated.

XI. Proposed Model for Cholesterol Metabolism in Man (Fig. 8)

In general, rates of cholesterol synthesis in any organ appear to parallel the activity in tissue turnover or in lipoprotein synthesis. All tissues have some degree of turnover, but only the liver and intestines synthesize plasma lipoproteins. Since the cholesterol synthetic activity from the latter two organs constitutes more than 90% of the total synthetic activity in animals, this suggests that lipoprotein synthesis is associated with greater cholesterol synthesis than the tissue turnover. This is further supported by marked changes in cholesterol synthesis associated with changes limited to hepatic synthesis of lipoproteins. Tissues that have a much greater turnover also appear to synthesize more cholesterol than those which have little turnover of their cellular membranes. Epidermal cells take about 27 days from their formation to their exfoliation on the skin surface (NICOLAIDES and KELLUM, 1965), and their turnover may be greater than that of cells in dermis. The synthesis of sterols in the latter is less than in the epidermis. The turnover appears to be minimum in mature nervous tissues and red blood cells; and they also synthesize little, if any, cholesterol. Incidentally, these tissues also contain little, if any, cholesterol esters, which may also be related somehow with cholesterol synthesis. In some tissues cholesterol esters serve as reservoirs of cholesterol needed by tissues for functions other than their turnover. Most cholesterol for the synthesis of steroid hormones by the adrenal glands is derived from plasma (BORKOWSKI et al., 1972a), the small amount of cholesterol synthesized by the gland may be related to its turnover. According to this view, synthesis of unesterified cholesterol is coupled to the formation of lipoproteins, be they for cellular membranes or for plasma.

Exogenous cholesterol can, however, replace endogenous cholesterol for synthesis of tissue or plasma lipoproteins. Recent studies demonstrated that after a high-cholesterol diet, the suppression of synthesis in various tissues of the guinea pig was proportional to the amounts of tissue cholesterol (SWANN and SIPERSTEIN, 1972). In rat, the synthesis is inhibited by exogenous cholesterol more in the liver than in any other organ (DIETSCHY and SIPERSTEIN, 1967). This may also be related to the fact that accumulation of cholesterol in liver is greater than in any other organ of the rat.

A corollary of this hypothesis is that abnormal deposition of cholesterol, such as seen after excessive intake, is not likely to occur due to excessive synthesis *in situ*.

The dietary and intestinal cholesterol removed by the liver enter into a pool concerned primarily with the synthesis of plasma lipoproteins. Hepatic cholesterol

Hypothesis

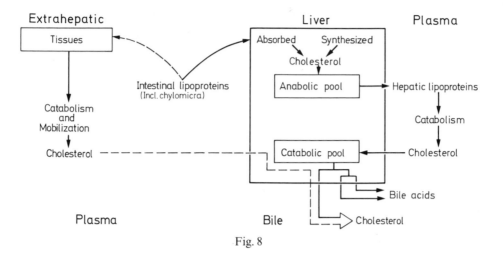

Fig. 8

for plasma lipoproteins also enters the same "anabolic" pool (Fig. 8). In addition to explaining the negative feedback inhibition, this suggests that the pathways for metabolism of absorbed (from normal intake) and synthesized cholesterol are similar.

We postulated that all dietary cholesterol removed by liver is first incorporated into plasma lipoproteins before being catabolised (SODHI and KUDCHODKAR, 1972a, b, 1973a). BHATTACHARYYA et al. (1971) noted that in normal subjects pool sizes and production rates calculated from changes in plasma cholesterol specific activity slopes were similar whether the radioactive cholesterol was given by intravenous injection or by oral feeding. This would not have been the case unless all the dietary cholesterol absorbed from the intestinal tract was first incorporated into plasma lipoproteins or at least into Pool A. ZILVERSMIT (1972) proposed a method for calculating absorption of dietary cholesterol based on the ratio of two isotopes in plasma after intravenous injection of one label and feeding of the other label. Validation of this method also implies that the absorbed dietary cholesterol was first incorporated quantitatively into plasma lipoproteins before it was catabolised. This is further supported by studies on β-sitosterol. The absorption of β-sitosterol calculated by the sterol balance method was the same as that calculated by isotopic kinetics of the sterol in plasma (SALEN et al., 1970). In a fashion somewhat similar to dietary cholesterol, particulate cholesterol injected intravenously is also removed primarily by the liver and is first quantitatively incorporated into plasma lipoproteins before it is catabolised and excreted into the bile (SODHI et al., 1969; NILSSON and ZILVERSMIT, 1972; SODHI and KUDCHODKAR, 1973d).

As is the case with absorbed cholesterol, newly-synthesized cholesterol in the liver is first incorporated into plasma lipoproteins before it is catabolised to bile acids. Although the specific activity of biliary cholesterol reaches its peak very rapidly after intravenous injection of radioactive precursors of cholesterol, the isotopic exchange may account for the appearance of at least some of the radioactivity in the bile. Quantitative information, which is not possible from such data, was provided by *in vitro* liver perfusion studies of BRICKER (1971). During the three hours after the addition of radioactive precursors to the perfusing medium, most of the newly-synthesized cholesterol either remained in the liver (presumably as a constituent of structural lipoproteins) or was released as lipoproteins into the circulating medium. Less than one-half of one percent was excreted into the bile during this period, indicating that newly-synthesized cholesterol is not directly excreted into bile.

Preliminary studies in our laboratories also support these observations. Rats were given radioactive mevalonate (I.V.), and the total radioactivity in hepatic and biliary cholesterol was determined. The loss of radioactive cholesterol between one and two hours from the liver was about 8% of the total injected radioactivity, whereas the total loss in biliary cholesterol and bile acids amounted to only 0.4%. This indicated that 95% of the newly-synthesized cholesterol lost from the liver was transported out into plasma (SODHI and AVIGAN, unpublished observations).

Most of the hepatic synthesis of cholesterol is coupled to the synthesis of plasma lipoproteins, especially that of very low density lipoproteins. The greater the synthesis of lipoproteins, the greater will be the synthesis of cholesterol. The fractional turnover rate of plasma VLDL protein is about ten times greater than that of LDL or HDL proteins (GITLIN et al., 1958). The net turnover of plasma lipoproteins is therefore greater when plasma VLDL is increased than when it is low or normal. This will hold true under most conditions, even if there is a moderate reduction in the clearance of VLDL or a moderate increase in the turnover of LDL or HDL. On this basis, it may be predicted that the turnover of lipoproteins will be greater in patients with types II b, IV, or V hyperlipoproteinemia than in normal subjects or in patients with type II a hyperlipoproteinemia.

Cholesterol absorption in patients with different types of hyperlipoproteinemia is not significantly different from that in normal subjects. Therefore, the synthesis of cholesterol in patients with types II b, IV, or V hyperlipoproteinemia is expected to be greater than in patients with type II a hyperlipoproteinemia or in normal subjects.

There does not appear to be any need for postulating homeostatic mechanisms specifically sensitive to the changes in the concentration of plasma cholesterol. Concentration of plasma cholesterol is determined by mechanisms primarily controlling the metabolism of plasma lipoproteins. The implication of this suggestion is that greater effort should be directed to the control of lipoproteins than on developing agents directly inhibiting cholesterol synthesis or absorption.

If it is assumed that most cholesterol in newly-synthesized lipoproteins is unesterified, as in tissue lipoproteins, the esterification of plasma cholesterol may only be a manifestation of lipoprotein metabolism in a manner similar to the one suggested by Fig. 1, Model II for turnover of tissue lipoproteins. The cholesterol entering the "anabolic pool" for synthesis of hepatic lipoproteins includes about 0.6 g of biliary and 0.3 g of dietary cholesterol absorbed from the intestinal tract. The absorbed cholesterol also includes cholesterol synthesized in the intestines. Hepatic synthesis of about 0.7 g also goes into the same pool. Thus there is close to 2 grams of cholesterol delivered by hepatic lipoproteins daily to plasma. Approximately the same amount of cholesterol in the plasma is esterified every day. As indicated previously, daily amounts of cholesterol catabolised by the liver in man are equal to daily *fecal* excretion of bile acids (0.3 g) and daily *biliary* excretion of cholesterol

(1.0 g). Thus this (1.3 g) amount is somewhat less than the cholesterol (2.0 g) incorporated daily into lipoproteins and esterified. Transfer of cholesterol between different pools in the body may conceivably account for the difference (KUDCHODKAR, unpublished observations).

Liver is the major organ concerned with the catabolism of cholesterol; therefore, the cholesterol released from the catabolism of plasma lipoproteins, whatever their sites, is transported back to the liver for conversion to bile acids and excretion into the bile. It is suggested that the cholesterol is brought back to the liver into a different ("catabolic") pool, and it is not reused for synthesis of new plasma lipoproteins. The greater the net turnover of plasma lipoproteins, the greater will be the amount of cholesterol brought to the catabolic pool in the liver. Relative to the amounts of cholesterol derived from the catabolism of plasma lipoproteins, the cholesterol derived from the turnover of tissue membranes is probably insignificant. Therefore the differences in hepatic synthesis and catabolism of cholesterol are related more to the net turnover of plasma lipoproteins than to the turnover of tissue membranes. On this assumption, it may be predicted that the fecal metabolites of endogenous cholesterol would be greater in types II b, IV, and V hyperlipoproteinemia than in types II a and in normal subjects.

Although the turnover of tissue membranes provides only insignificant amounts of cholesterol for catabolism, under certain conditions tissues may provide significant fractions of catabolised cholesterol; e.g., after the administration of hypocholesterolemic agents (SODHI et al., 1969, 1971 a, 1973 a; GRUNDY et al., 1972). Tissue cholesterol is promptly transported to the liver and is rapidly excreted into the bile without mixing completely with the pool of hepatic cholesterol from which bile acids are derived (SODHI et al., 1973 a). After feeding large amounts of cholesterol, tissue cholesterol also appears to be excreted as neutral steroids (QUINTÃO et al., 1971 b).

XII. Cholesterol Metabolism in Hyperlipoproteinemias

The available data are not sufficient for satisfactory analyses of cholesterol metabolism in all hyperlipoproteinemias; but when most reported data are pooled, some useful information can be derived. Comprehensive methods for reliable studies on cholesterol metabolism in man are so difficult and time consuming that only a small number of subjects have been examined. AHRENS, GRUNDY, and their associates at the Rockefeller University contributed the most to this area. The cholesterol balance method developed by them is perhaps the most satisfactory one available, and they have also published data on more subjects than any other group. Excellent studies on cholesterol balance have also been published by CONNOR, NESTEL, MIETTINEN, and MYANT—among others. Included in this report are the published and unpublished data from our own laboratories and that from most published reports (LEWIS and MYANT, 1967; Connor et al., 1969; GRUNDY and AHRENS, 1969, 1970; SALEN et al., 1970; QUINTAO et al., 1971 a, b; MIETTINEN, 1971; HORLICK et al., 1971; GRUNDY et al., 1971, 1972; NAZIR et al., 1972; SODHI and KUDCHODKAR, 1973 c; KUDCHODKAR et al., 1973 a, b, c, d, e).

Since the type of hyperlipoproteinemia was not recorded in most cases, we classified subjects on the basis of their plasma concentrations of cholesterol and triglycer-

Table 7. Cholesterol absorption in hyperlipoproteinemias

Type	Sex	Number of subjects	Cholesterol intake mg/day	Cholesterol absorption		
				mg/day	mg/day/kg	Percent
Normal	Male	8	627±212	252±101	3.5±1.5	40± 5
	Female	1	490	189	3.4	38
	Group	9	612±203	245± 97	3.5±1.4	39± 5
IIa	Male	6	516±144	163± 37	2.6±0.9	34± 9
	Female	7	550±207	233± 96	4.0±1.8	41± 9
	Group	13	534±174	201± 81	3.4±1.6	38± 9
IIb	Male	9	703±324	294±127	3.5±1.5	43±11
	Female	4	427±119	217± 35	4.6±1.3	49± 8
	Group	13	618±302	270±111	3.9±1.4	45±10
III	Male	1	679	251	3.6	37
IV	Male	3	578±175	210± 67	2.5±0.5	36± 2
	Female	1	586	248	4.6	42
	Group	4	580±143	220± 58	3.0±1.1	38± 3
V	Male	5	478±177	215± 92	3.1±1.5	44±10
	Female	1	682	334	10.6	48
	Group	6	512±179	234± 96	4.3±3.3	46±10
Mean			577	236		41

ides. The upper limits of normal were assumed to be 250 and 150 mg per 100 ml of plasma for cholesterol and triglycerides respectively. Type II a was defined as having elevations of only cholesterol, type II b of both cholesterol and triglycerides, and type IV of only triglycerides. In the absence of specific mention of types I, III, and V, hypertriglyceridemia was assumed to represent hyper-pre-β-lipoproteinemia; and hypercholesterolemia (without hypertriglyceridemia) was assumed to represent hyper-β-lipoproteinemia. The classification in this section of types I, III, and V hyperlipoproteinemia implies that they were mentioned specifically in the published reports. This arbitrary classification is not intended to represent discrete genetic conditions associated with elevations of different lipids (and presumably different lipoproteins). Goldstein et al. (1972) presented evidence recently to suggest that types II a, II b, or IV hyperlipoproteinemia classified according to Beaumont et al. (1970) cannot be considered specific entities. Considerations have therefore been given more to the presence or absence of hypertriglyceridemia and hypercholesterolemia.

The results of absorption studies in 32 men and 14 women are shown in Table 7. Reliable information on patients with type I hyperlipoproteinemia was not available. Subjects who were given abnormal diets containing extremely large amounts of cholesterol were also excluded for the purposes of this presentation. Dietary intake of cholesterol, shown in Table 7, was generally similar in all classes of subjects. The absolute amounts of cholesterol absorbed and the percentage absorbed are also given in the same table. The range of absorption was between 34 and 49%. Except in normals, the percentage absorption tended to be higher in females than in males, but the differences between them were not significant. The differences in the absorption

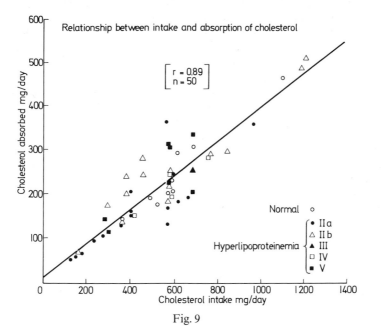

Fig. 9

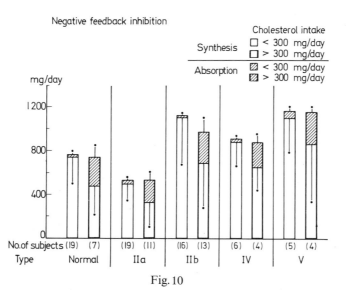

Fig. 10

between normal subjects and patients with different classes of hyperlipoproteinemias were also not statistically significant. Generally the number of subjects in various classes was not large enough to conclusively establish whether or not there are biologically significant differences between different hyperlipoproteinemias in the absorption of dietary cholesterol.

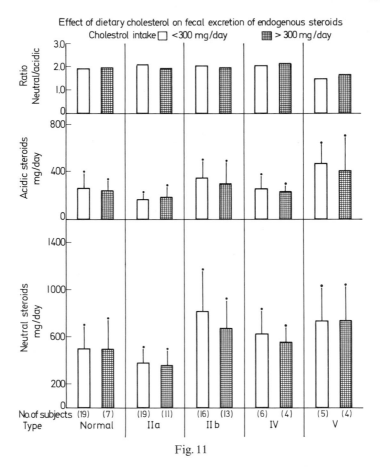

Fig. 11

We have presented evidence to suggest that the amounts of endogenous cholesterol secreted into the intestinal tract were greater in subjects with hypertriglyceridemia than in those with normal levels of plasma triglycerides (KUDCHODKAR and
SODHI, 1972; SODHI and KUDCHODKAR, 1973c). According to Borgstrom's hypothesis (BORGSTROM et al., 1970), therefore, patients with types IIb and IV hyperlipoproteinemia should have shown a smaller percentage absorption of dietary cholesterol
than those with type IIa hyperlipoproteinemia. However, the percentage absorption
in subjects with type IIb and type IV hyperlipoproteinemia was similar to that in
subjects with type IIa hyperlipoproteinemia.

The results shown in Fig. 9 also indicated that there was a positive correlation
between the amounts ingested and the amounts absorbed. There was more scatter in
the middle of the range than at the extremes, but this may have been due to the large
number of subjects in this range. In all subjects, the correlation between the amounts
absorbed and the amounts ingested was excellent ($r = 0.89$).

Endogenous synthesis was determined from the available data on cholesterol
balance. In order to determine the effects of absorbed cholesterol on synthesis,
subjects in each class were divided into two groups on the basis of cholesterol intake:

those with <300 mg/day and those with >300 mg/day (Fig. 10). In actual fact, most of the subjects in the first group consumed even less than 100 mg of cholesterol a day. Cholesterol synthesis was significantly greater in the low-cholesterol than in the high-cholesterol group in each class. The inhibition was approximately 36% in normal subjects and 34%, 40%, 24%, and 20% in types II a, II b, IV, and V hyperlipoproteinemia respectively. A moderate scatter of data and the small numbers in each group prevented conclusions about the validity of the differences in the degree of negative feedback inhibition of endogenous synthesis between the various classes. However, the data indicated clearly that endogenous synthesis was inhibited by dietary cholesterol in normal subjects as well as in patients with types II a, II b, IV, or V hyperlipoproteinemia. Results from these studies therefore do not support the suggestion that hepatic feedback inhibition may be defective in familial hypercholesterolemia (KHACHADURIAN, 1969), and they are in accord with the proposed model (SODHI and KUDCHODKAR, 1973 a).

When the amounts absorbed were added to the values for daily synthesis, the resultant values for daily turnover of cholesterol were remarkably similar for the two groups in each classification, suggesting that the absorbed cholesterol replaced the synthesized cholesterol. This observation gives considerable support to the thesis that absorbed and synthesized cholesterol enter the same metabolic pool in the liver.

The amounts of fecal metabolites of endogenous (synthesized plus absorbed) cholesterol were similar in the low- and high-cholesterol intake groups in each class (Fig. 11). Furthermore, the ratios of neutral to acidic steroids in the two grups were also the same in each class (Fig. 11), suggesting that the catabolic pathways for dietary and synthesized cholesterol were identical for all the groups. Since the data from only those subjects who consumed normal amounts of cholesterol were analyzed, it is conceivable that had the dietary cholesterol been grossly excessive and had the amounts of absorbed cholesterol exceeded the synthesis, catabolic pathways for dietary and endogenous cholesterol would have been different.

As predicted by the model, these data showed that cholesterol synthesis in type II a hyperlipoproteinemia was less than normal; and in types II b, IV, and V it was greater than normal. These conclusions were substantiated by the fecal excretion of metabolites of endogenous cholesterol in steady-state conditions. The excretion of neutral as well as acidic steroids in type II a hyperlipoproteinemia was less than normal. The total excretion of fecal metabolites of endogenous cholesterol in types II b, IV, and V hyperlipoproteinemia was greater than in normal subjects. The ratios of fecal neutral to acidic steroids in types II b and IV hyperlipoproteinemia, however, were the same as in normal subjects, indicating that the catabolic pathways for endogenous cholesterol in patients with types II b and IV hyperlipoproteinemia were similar to those in patients with type II a hyperlipoproteinemia and in normal subjects. This is in accord with our previous observations (SODHI and KUDCHODKAR, 1973b, c) and is contrary to the suggestion that hypercholesterolemia in type II hyperlipoproteinemia is due to a block in the catabolism of cholesterol to bile acids (MIETTINEN et al., 1967).

Cholesterol synthesis and its fecal excretion were somewhat higher in patients with type II b than in those with type IV hyperlipoproteinemia.

In an attempt to investigate the genetic defect in primary familial hypercholesterolemia, BROWN, DANA, and GOLDSTEIN (1974) examined the HMG-CoA reductase activity and synthesis of cholesterol in cultured fibroblasts. They found that the cells from homozygous patients had abnormally high HMG-CoA reductase activity; and unlike in normal cells, this was not inhibited by increasing concentrations of LDL in the medium. BROWN and GOLDSTEIN postulate (1974) that the primary genetic abnormality in familial hypercholesterolemia involves a deficiency in a cell surface receptor for LDL. They believe that the binding of LDL to this receptor regulates cholesterol metabolism by increasing LDL degradation and suppressing cholesterol synthesis in normal cells. Since cells from homozygotes failed to bind and degrade LDL, the HMG-CoA activity in them was not inhibited.

When these observations on skin fibroblasts cultured *in vitro* are extrapolated to intact man, the impression is created that the endogenous synthesis of cholesterol is above normal and the "negative feedback inhibition" is defective in patients with familial hypercholesterolemia. However, our analysis of the data pooled from various laboratories suggested that: 1) the cholesterol synthesis in such patients was certainly not greater than normal (in fact, it may well be below normal), and 2) they had normal "negative feedback inhibition". These discrepancies are unlikely to be entirely due to differences in the patients investigated, nor do they appear to be artefacts of the methods. They may, however, be due to the assumptions made. These discrepancies between the results obtained by BROWN and GOLDSTEIN from their *in vitro* system and the data obtained in *in vivo* studies disappear by substituting another set of at least equally plausible assumptions.

Synthesis of cholesterol (and the precursor of LDL) occurs predominantly in liver; and, although major sites for LDL catabolism are not known, it is possible that many extrahepatic tissues may be quite important. If the assumption that the metabolic activity investigated in cultured fibroblasts reflects the characteristics of *all* cells is replaced by the assumption that it reflects *only* the catabolism of LDL, the apparent discrepancies disappear. Observations of LANGER, STROBER, and LEVY (1972) are in accord with the suggestion that there may be a defect in catabolism of LDL in familial hypercholesterolemia. Even if in such patients the synthetic activity of fibroblasts (and tissues these cells represent) is abnormally high and is not subject to negative feedback control, the contributions from these extrahepatic tissues to total synthetic activity in man may still remain insignificantly small relative to the synthesis in liver. In fact, in steady-state conditions, a decrease in catabolism in LDL and thus of (released) cholesterol would not be expected to be associated with an increase in cholesterol synthesis. Furthermore, the control mechanisms in isolated cells are not necessarily the same as those in intact organism. There is no reason to believe that "medium" of *in vitro* systems represent the "plasma" in intact man, inasmuch as there is no reason to believe that metabolic characteristics of cultured fibroblasts will be the same as of liver cells in intact patients. The observations on cultured fibroblasts may still be extremely important to the genetic analysis of the basic abnormality in familial hypercholesterolemia.

In order to determine if there were any differences in the metabolism of cholesterol between males and females, data were analyzed for cholesterol synthesis and its catabolism (Fig. 12). To exclude the effects of differences in body weight, values were calculated on a per kg basis. Data were included from only those subjects who were on very low cholesterol intake, so that the effect of dietary cholesterol was also insignificant. Although there were no statistically significant differences in choles-

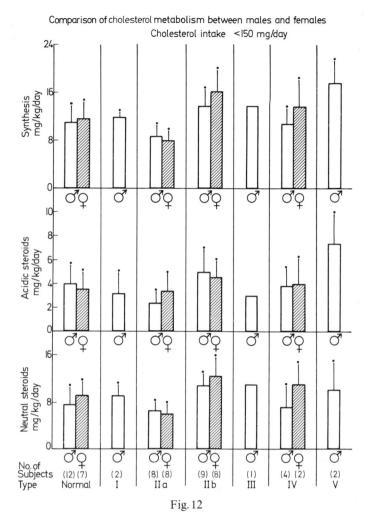

Fig. 12

terol synthesis between males and females, the values in females tended to be greater in all classes of patients except in those with type II a hyperlipoproteinemia. Correspondingly, the fecal excretion of neutral steroids tended to be greater in females in all classes of patients except in those with type I a hyperlipoproteinemia. Conversely, the fecal excretion of bile acids in type II a hyperlipoproteinemia was greater in females than in males. In normals and in patients with type II b hyperlipoproteinemia, the fecal excretion of bile acids was somewhat less in the females than in the males.

Acknowledgements

The invaluable assistance of my colleague Dr. B.J. KUDCHODKAR is gratefully acknowledged in the successful completion of this manuscript. Discussions with Doctors L. HORLICK and PETER WOOD were very useful in helping to clarify my thoughts and concepts. My thanks are also due to Ms. Kathy McCammon for preparing this manuscript.

Our work was supported by grants from the Medical Research Council of Canada and the Canadian and Saskatchewan Heart Foundations.

References

Abdulla, Y. H., Orton, C. C., Adams, C. M. M.: Cholesterol esterification by transacylation in human and experimental atheromatous lesions. J. Atheroscler. Res. **8**, 967—973 (1968).

Abell, L. L., Mosbach, E. H., Kendall, F. E.: Cholesterol metabolism in the dog. J. biol. Chem. **220**, 527—536 (1956).

Adams, E., Baxter, M.: Lipid fractions of human adrenals. Arch. Path. **48**, 13—26 (1949).

Akanuma, Y., Glomset, J. A.: In vitro incorporation of cholesterol ^{14}C into very low density lipoprotein cholesteryl esters. J. Lipid Res. **9**, 620—626 (1968).

Alaupovic, P.: Apolipoproteins and lipoproteins. Atherosclerosis **13**, 141—146 (1971).

Alaupovic, P.: Conceptual development of the classification systems of plasma lipoproteins. In: Peeters, H. (Ed.): Protides of the Biological fluids, pp. 9—19. Oxford-New York: Pergamon Press 1972.

Allan, T. M., Dawson, A. A.: ABO Blood groups and ischaemic heart disease in man. Brit. Heart J. **30**, 377—382 (1968).

Anchel, M., Schoenheimer, R.: Deuterium as an indicator in the study of intermediary metabolism. XV: Further studies in coprosterol formation. J. biol. Chem. **125**, 23—31 (1938).

Angel, A., Farkas, J.: Cholesterol storage in white adipose cells. Clin. Res. **18**, 690 (1970).

Angel, A., Farkas, J.: Cholesterol synthesis in white adipose tissue. Circulation **44**, II—1 (1971).

Armstrong, M. L., Connor, W. E., Warner, E. D.: Xanthomatosis in Rhesus Monkeys Fed a Hypercholesterolemic diet. Arch. Path. **84**, 227—237 (1967).

Arnesjö, B., Nilsson, A., Barrowman, J., Borgstrom, B.: Intestinal digestion and absorption of cholesterol and lecithin in humans. Scand. J. Gastroent. **4**, 653—665 (1969).

Ashworth, C. T., Riggi, S. J., Diluzio, N. R.: A morphologic study of the effect of reticuloendothelial stimulation upon hepatic removal of minute particles from the blood of rats. Exp. Mol. Path. Suppl. **1**, 86—103 (1963).

Avigan, J.: A method for incorporating cholesterol and other lipids into serum lipoproteins in vitro. J. biol. Chem. **234**, 787—790 (1959).

Avigan, J., Steinberg, D.: Sterol and bile acid excretion in man and the effects of dietary fat. J. clin. Invest. **44**, 1845—1856 (1965).

Avigan, J., Steinberg, D., Berman, M.: Distribution of labelled cholesterol in animal tissues. J. Lipid Res. **3**, 216—221 (1962).

Back, P., Hamprecht, B., Lynen, F.: Regulation of cholesterol biosynthesis in rat liver: diurnal changes of activity and influence of bile acids. Arch. Biochem. Biophys. **133**, 11—21 (1969).

Balmer, J., Zilversmit, D. B.: Cholesterol absorption and turnover in rats fed laboratory chow or semisynthetic diets. Fed. Proc. **1973**, 934.

Barter, P. J.: Origin of esterified cholesterol transported in the very low density lipoproteins of human plasma. J. Lipid Res. **15**, 11—19 (1974).

Bashour, J. T., Bauman, L.: The solubility of cholesterol in bile salt solutions. J. biol. Chem. **121**, 1—3 (1937).

Baxter, J. H.: Origin and characteristics of endogenous lipid in thoracic duct lymph in rat. J. Lipid Res. **7**, 158—165 (1966).

Beaumont, J. L., Carlson, L. A., Cooper, G. R., Fejfar, Z., Fredrickson, D. S., Strasser, T.: Classification of hyperlipidemias and hyperlipoproteinemias. Bull. Wld. Hlth Org. **43**, 891—915 (1970).

Beg, Z. H., Lupien, P. J.: In vitro and in vivo inhibition of hepatic cholesterol synthesis by 3-Hydroxy-3-methylglutaric acid. Biochim. biophys. Acta (Amst.) **260**, 439—448 (1972).

Beher, W. T., Casazza, K. K., Beher, M. E., Filus, A. M., Bertasius, J.: Effects of cholesterol on bile acid metabolism in the rat. Proc. Soc. exp. Biol. (N.Y.) **134**, 595—602 (1970).

Bergström, S.: The formation of bile acids from cholesterol in the rat. Fysiografiska, Sallskapets **22**, 1—5 (1952).

BERGSTRÖM,S., DANIELSSON, H.: Formation and metabolism of bile acids. In: CODE,C.F.: HEI-DEL, W. (Eds.): Handbook of Physiology, Vol. 5, pp. 2391—2407. Washington D.C.: Amer. Physiol. Soc. 1968.

BHATTACHARYYA,A., CONNOR, W.E., SPECTOR,A.A.: Excretion of sterols from the skin of normal and hypercholesterolemic humans. J. clin. Invest. **51**, 2060—2070 (1972).

BHATTACHARYYA,A., CONNOR, W.E., SPECTOR,A.A.: Serum cholesterol turnover in normal and type II hypercholesterolemic subjects. Circulation **44**, II-2 (1971).

BHATTATHIRY, E.P.M., SIPERSTEIN, M.D.: Feedback control of cholesterol synthesis in man. J. clin. Invest. **42**, 1613—1618 (1963).

BILHEIMER, D.W., EISENBERG,S., LEVY,R.I.: The metabolism of very low density lipoprotein proteins. I. Preliminary in vitro and in vivo observations. Biochim. biophys. Acta (Amst.) **260**, 212—221 (1972).

BILLS,C.E.: Physiology of sterols, including Vitamin D. Physiol. Rev.**15**, 1—97 (1935).

BLATON,V.H., PEETERS,H.: Integrated approach to plasma lipid and lipoprotein analysis. In: Nelson, G.J.(Ed.): Blood lipids and lipoproteins: Quantitation, Composition and Metabolism, pp. 275—313. New York: Wiley-Interscience 1972.

BLOCH, K.: The biological conversion of cholesterol to pregnanediol. J. biol. Chem. **157**, 661—666 (1945).

BLOCH, K.: The biological synthesis of cholesterol. Science **150**, 19—28 (1965).

BLOCH, K., BERG, B.N., RITTENBERG, D.: The biological conversion of cholesterol to cholic acid. J. biol. Chem.**149**, 511—517 (1943).

BLOCH, K., BOREK, E., RITTENBERG, D.: Synthesis of cholesterol in surviving liver. J. biol. Chem. **162**, 441—449 (1946).

BLOMSTRAND,R., AHRENS, E.H.,JR.: The absorption of fats studied in a patient with chyluria III cholesterol. J. biol. Chem. **233**, 327—330 (1958).

BORGSTRÖM,B.: Studies on intestinal cholesterol absorption in the human. J. clin. Invest. **39**, 809—815 (1960).

BORGSTRÖM, B.: Quantitative aspects of the intestinal absorption and metabolism of cholesterol and β-sitosterol in the rat. J. Lipid Res. **9**, 473—481 (1968).

BORGSTRÖM, B.: Quantification of cholesterol absorption in man by fecal analysis after the feeding of a single isotope labelled meal. J. Lipid Res. **10**, 331—337 (1969).

BORGSTRÖM, B., LAURELL,C.B.: Studies on lymph flow and lymph proteins during absorption of fat and saline in rats. Acta physiol. scand. **29**, 264—267 (1953).

BORGSTRÖM, B., LINDHE, B.A., WLODAWER, P.: Absorption and distribution of cholesterol -4-^{14}C in the rat. Proc. Soc. exp. Biol. (N.Y.) **99**, 365—368 (1958).

BORGSTRÖM, B., RADNER,S., WERNER, B.: Lymphatic transport of cholesterol in the human being. Effect of dietary cholesterol. Scand. J. clin. Lab. Invest. **26**, 227—235 (1970).

BORJA,C.R., VAHOUNY,G.V., TREADWELL,C.R.: Role of bile and pancreatic juice in cholesterol absorption and esterification. Amer. J. Physiol. **206**, 223—228 (1964).

BORKOWSKI,A., DELCROIX,C., LEVIN,S.: Metabolism of adrenal cholesterol in man I. In vivo studies. J. clin. Invest. **51**, 1664—1678 (1972a).

BORKOWSKI,A., DELCROIX,C., LEVIN,S.: Metabolism of adrenal cholesterol in man. II. In vitro studies including a comparison of adrenal cholesterol synthesis with the synthesis of glucocorticosteroid hormones. J. clin. Invest. **51**, 1679—1687 (1972b).

BOYD, E.M.: Diurnal variations in plasma lipids. J. biol. Chem. **110**, 61—70 (1935).

BOYD,E.M.: Species variation in normal plasma lipids estimated by oxidative micromethods. J. biol. Chem. **143**, 131—132 (1942).

BOYD,G.S., OLIVER,M.F.: The physiology of the circulating cholesterol and lipoproteins in Cholesterol. In: Cook, R. P. (Ed.): Chemistry, Biochemistry and Pathology, pp. 181—208. New York: Academic Press Inc. 1958.

BRAGDON,J.H., HAVEL,R.J., BOYLE,E.: Human serum lipoproteins. I. chemical composition of four fractions. J. Lab. clin. Med. **48**, 36—42 (1956).

BRICKER,L.A.: Effects of dietary cholesterol on sterol synthesis and release by the perfused rat liver. J. clin. Invest. **50**, 12a (1971).

BROWN,M.S., GOLDSTEIN,J.L.: Expression of the familial hypercholesterolemic gene in heterozygotes: Mechanism for a dominant disorder in man. Science **185**, 61—63 (1974).

Brown, M.S., Dana, S.E., Goldstein, J.L.: Regulation of 3-hydroxy-3-methylglutaryl coenzyme A reductase activity in cultured human fibroblasts. J. biol. Chem. **249**, 789—796 (1974).

Brunner, D., Manelis, G., Loebel, K.: Influence of age and race on lipid levels in Israel. Lancet **1959V**, 1071—1073.

Bucher, N.L.R., McGarrahan, K.: The biosynthesis of cholesterol from acetate-1-^{14}C by cellular fractions of rat liver. J. biol. Chem. **222**, 1—16 (1956).

Bucher, N.L.R., McGarrahan, K., Gould, E., Loud, A.V.: Liver from normal fasting, X-irridiated cholesterol-fed, triton, or Δ^4cholesten-3-l-treated rats. J. biol. Chem. **234**, 262—267 (1959).

Bucher, N.L.R., Overath, P., Lynen, F.: β-hydroxy-methylglutaryl Coenzyme A reductase cleavage and condensing enzymes in relation to cholesterol formation in rat liver. Biochim. biophys. Acta (Amst.) **40**, 491—501 (1960).

Byers, S.O., Rosenman, R.H., Friedman, M., Biggs, M.W.: Rate of cholesterol synthesis in hypo- and hyperthyroid rats. J. exp. Med. **96**, 513—516 (1952).

Byers, S.O., Friedman, M., Gunning, B.: Observations concerning the production and excretion of cholesterol in mammals. XI. The intestinal site of absorption and excretion of cholesterol. Amer. J. Physiol. **175**, 375—379 (1953).

Caldwell, I.C., Drummond, G.I.: Synthesis of acetoacetate by liver enzymes. J. biol. Chem. **238**, 64—68 (1963).

Cayen, M.N.: The effect of starvation and cholesterol feeding on the intestinal cholesterol synthesis in the rat. Biochim. biophys. Acta (Amst.) **187**, 546—554 (1969).

Chesterton, C.J.: The subcellular site of cholesterol synthesis in rat liver. Biochim. Biophys. Res. Commun. **25**, 205—209 (1966).

Chevallier, F.: Dynamics of cholesterol in rats, studied by the isotopic equilibrium method. Advanc. Lipid Res. **5**, 209—239 (1967).

Chobanian, A.V., Burrows, B.A., Hollander, W.: Body cholesterol metabolism in man. II. measurement of the body cholesterol miscible pool and turnover rate. J. clin. Invest. **41**, 1738—1744 (1962).

Clifton-Bligh, P., Miller, N.E., Nestel, P.J.: Cholesterol influx in very low density and efflux from low density lipoproteins. Circulation **46**, II-249 (1972).

Coleman, D.L., Baumann, C.A.: Intestinal sterols. IV. Δ^7-coprostanol. Arch. biochim. Biophys. (Amst.) **71**, 287—292 (1957a).

Coleman, D.L., Baumann, C.A.: Intestinal sterols. V. Reduction of sterols by intestinal microorganisms. Arch. biochim. Biophys. (Amst.) **72**, 219—225 (1957b).

Coleman, D.L., Wells, W.W., Baumann, C.A.: Intestinal sterols. II. Determination of coprostanol and certain related sterols. Arch. biochim. Biophys. (Amst.) **60**, 412—418 (1956).

Connor, W.E., Lin, D.: The intestinal absorption of dietary cholesterol in human being. Effect of dietary cholesterol. J. Lab. clin. Med. **76**, 870 (1970).

Connor, W.E., Bhattacharyya, A., Nestel, P.J.: The intestinal biosynthesis and exchange of cholesterol in intact animals. Circulation **44**, II—14 (1971).

Connor, W.E., Witiak, D.T., Stone, D.B., Armstrong, M.L.: Cholesterol balance and fecal neutral steroid and bile acid excretion in normal men, fed dietary fats of different fatty acid composition. J. clin. Invest. **48**, 1363—1375 (1969).

Cook, R.P.: Cholesterol feeding and fat metabolism. Biochem. J. **30**, 1630—1636 (1936).

Cook, R.P.: Distribution of sterols in organisms and in tissues. In: R.P. Cook (Ed.): Cholesterol, Chemistry, Biochemistry and Pathology, pp. 145—180. New York: Academic Press Inc. 1958.

Cook, R.P., Edwards, D.C., Riddell, C.: Cholesterol metabolism. 7. Cholesterol absorption and excretion in man. Biochem. J. **62**, 225—234 (1956).

Cornforth, J.W., Hunter, G.D., Popjak, G.: Studies of cholesterol biosynthesis. I. A new chemical degradation of cholesterol. Biochem. J. **54**, 590—597 (1953).

Cornforth, J.W., Gore, I.Y., Popjak, G.: Studies on the biosynthesis of cholesterol. Degradation of rings C and D. Biochem. J. **65**, 94—109 (1957).

Cox, G.E., Nelson, L.G., Wood, W.B., Taylor, C.B.: Effect of dietary cholesterol on cholesterol synthesis in monkey's tissue *in vitro*. Fed. Proc. **13**, 31 (1954).

Cronholm, T., Makino, I., Sjovall, J.: Steroid metabolism in rats given $[1-^2H_2]$ ethanol: Biosynthesis of bile acids and reduction of 3-keto-5-β Cholanic acid. Europ. J. Biochem. **24**, 507—519 (1972).

CROUSE, J. R., GRUNDY, S. M., AHRENS, E. H. JR.: Cholesterol distribution in the bulk tissues of man. Variation with age. J. clin. Invest. **51**, 1292—1296 (1972).

DAILEY, R. C., SWELL, L., FIELD, H. JR., TREADWELL, C. R.: Adrenal cholesterol ester fatty acid composition of different species. Proc. Soc. exp. Biol. (N.Y.) **105**, 4—6 (1960).

DANIELSSON, H.: Present status of research on catabolism and excretion of cholesterol. Advanc. Lipid Res. **1**, 335—385 (1963).

DANIELSSON, H.: In: SCHIFF, L., CAREY, J. B. JR. and DIETSCHY, J. M. (Eds.): Mechanisms of bile acid formation of bile salt metabolism, pp. 91—102. Springfield, Ill.: Charles C. Thomas Publ. 1969.

DANIELSSON, H., GUSTAFSSON, B.: On serum cholesterol levels and neutral fecal sterols in germ free rats. Bile acids and steroids 59. Arch. Biochem. **83**, 482—485 (1959).

DANIELSSON, H., ENEROTH, P., HELLSTRÖM, K., LINDSTEDT, S., SJÖVALL, J.: On the turnover and excretory products of cholic and chenodeoxycholic acid in man. J. biol. Chem. **238**, 2299—2304 (1963).

DAVIS, C. B. JR., COX, G. E., TAYLOR, C. B., CROSS, S. L.: Cholesterol synthesis in human liver. Surg. Forum **9**, 486—489 (1958).

DAVIS, W. W., GARREN, L. D.: Evidence for the stimulation by adenocortico-trophic hormone on the conversion of cholesterol esters to cholesterol in the adrenal in vivo. Biochem. Biophys. Res. Commun. **24**, 805—810 (1966).

DEPALMA, R. G., HUBAY, C. A., INSULL, W. JR.: The effect of T-tube drainage on cholesterol and bile acid metabolism in man. Surg. Gynec. Obstet. **123**, 269—273 (1966).

DENBESTEN, L., CONNOR, W. E., BELL, S.: The effect of dietary cholesterol on the composition of human bile. Surgery **73**, 266—273 (1973).

DENBESTEN, L., CONNOR, W. E., KENT, T. H., LIN, D.: Effect of cellulose in the diet on the recovery of dietary plant sterols from the feces. J. Lipid Res. **11**, 341—345 (1970).

DIETSCHY, J.: The role of bile salts in controlling the rate of intestinal cholesterogenesis. J. clin. Invest. **47**, 286—300 (1968).

DIETSCHY, J. M.: The role of the intestines in the control of cholesterol metabolism. Gastroenterology **57**, 461—464 (1969).

DIETSCHY, J. M., SIPERSTEIN, M. D.: Cholesterol synthesis by the gastrointestinal tract: Localization and mechanisms of control. J. clin. Invest. **44**, 1311—1327 (1965).

DIETSCHY, J. M., SIPERSTEIN, M. D.: Effect of cholesterol feeding and fasting on sterol synthesis in seventeen tissues of the rat. J. Lipid Res. **8**, 97—104 (1967).

DIETSCHY, J. M., WILSON, J. D.: Cholesterol synthesis in the squirrel monkey relative rates of synthesis in various tissues and mechanisms of control. J. clin. Invest. **47**, 166—174 (1968).

DIETSCHY, J. M., WILSON, J. D.: Regulation of cholesterol metabolism. Parts 1 to 3. New Engl. J. Med. **282**, 1128—1138; 1179—1183; 1241—1249 (1970).

DIETSCHY, J. M., GAMEL, W. G.: Cholesterol synthesis in the intestine of man. Regional differences and control mechanisms. J. clin. Invest. **50**, 872—880 (1971).

DIETSCHY, J. M., SALOMON, H. S., SIPERSTEIN, M. D.: Bile acid metabolism. I — Studies on the mechanisms of intestinal transport. J. clin. Invest. **45**, 832—846 (1966).

DILUZIO, N. R., RIGGI, S. J.: The development of a lipid emulsion for the measurement of reticuloendothelial function. J. Reticuloendothelial Soc. **1**, 136—149 (1964).

DORÉE, C., GARDNER, J. A.: The origin and destiny of cholesterol in the animal organism. Part III. The absorption of cholesterol from the food and its appearance in the blood. Proc. roy. Soc. (Biol.) **81**, 109—132 (1909).

DUBACH, U., RECANT, L., HATCH, E., KOCH, M. B.: Negative feedback mechanism of cholesterol synthesis in experimental nephrosis. Proc. Soc. exp. Biol. (N.Y.) **106**, 136—139 (1961).

ECKLES, N. E., TAYLOR, C. B., CAMPBELL, D. J., GOULD, R. G.: The origin of plasma cholesterol and the rates of equilibration of liver, plasma and erythrocyte cholesterol. J. Lab. clin. Med. **46**, 359—371 (1955).

EDWARDS, P. A., GREEN, C.: Incorporation of plant sterols into membranes and its relation to sterol absorption. F.E.B.S. Letters **20**, 97—99 (1972).

EDWARDS, P. A., MUROYA, H. H., GOULD, R. G.: In vivo demonstration of the circadian rhythm of cholesterol biosynthesis in the liver and intestine of the rat. J. Lipid Res. **13**, 396—401 (1972).

FALOR, W. H., KELLY, J. R., BOECKMAN, L. R.: Bilateral thoracic duct cannulation. Arch. Surg. **88**, 787—792 (1964).

FAVARGER, P., METZGER, E. F.: La resorption intestinale du deuteriocholesterol et sa re'partition dans l'organisme animal sous forme libre et esterifee. Helv. chim. Acta **35**, 1811—1819 (1952).

FAWCETT, D. W., LONG, J. A., JONES, A. L.: The ultra structure of endocrine glands. Recent Progr. Hormone Res. **25**, 315—380 (1969).

FLEISHER, S., BRIERLY, G.: Solubilization of cholesterol in phospholipid micelles in water. Biochem. Biophys. Res. Commun. **5**, 367—373 (1961).

FLETCHER, K., MYANT, N. B.: Influence of the thyroid on the synthesis of cholesterol by liver and skin in vitro. J. Physiol. **144**, 361—372 (1958).

FLECHTER, K., MYANT, N. B.: Effects of thyroxine on the synthesis of cholesterol and fatty acids by cell free fractions of rat liver. J. Physiol. **154**, 145—152 (1960).

FRANTZ, I. D., Jr., SCHROEPFER, G. J.: Sterol Biosynthesis. Ann. Rev. Biochem. **36**, 691—726 (1967).

FRANTZ, I. D., Jr., SCHNEIDER, H. S., HINKELMAN, B. T.: Supression of hepatic cholesterol synthesis in the rat by cholesterol feeding. J. Biol. Chem. **206**, 465—469 (1954).

FREDRICKSON, D. S.: Inheritance of high density lipoprotein deficiency (Tangier disease). J. Clin. Invest. **43**, 228—236 (1964).

FREDRICKSON, D. S., ALTROCCHI, P. H., AVIOLO, L. V., GOODMAN, D. S., GOODMAN, H. C.: Tangier disease: Combined clinical staff Conference at the National Institutes of Health. Ann. Intern. Med. **55**, 1016—1031 (1967).

FRIEDMAN, M. S., BYERS, S. O., ST. GEORGE, S.: Detection of dietary cholesterol-4-^{14}C in the hepatic reticuloendothelial cell of the rat. Am. J. Physiol. **184**, 141—144 (1956).

FYFE, T., DUNNIGAN, M. A., HAMILTON, E., RAE, R. J.: Seasonal variation in serum lipids, and incidence and mortality of Ischaemic heart disease. J. Atheroscler. Res. **8**, 591—596 (1968).

GALLO, L. L., TREADWELL, C. R.: Localization of cholesterol esterase and cholesterol in mucosal fractions of rat small intestine. Proc. Soc. Exp. Biol. Med. **114**, 69—72 (1963).

GANGULY, J., KRISHNAMURTHY, S., MAHADEVAN, S.: The transport of carotenoids, Vitamin A and cholesterol across the intestines of rats and chickens. Biochem. J. **71**, 756—762 (1959).

GAYLOR, J. L.: Biosynthesis of Skin sterols. III. Conversion of squalene to sterols by rat skin. J. Biol. Chem. **238**, 1643—1648 (1963).

GAYLOR, J. L.: Anaerobic conversion of acetate to squalene by rat skin. Proc. Soc. Exp. Biol. Med. **106**, 576—579 (1961).

GEBHARD, R. L., BUCHWALD, H.: Cholesterol absorption following reversal of the upper and lower halves of the small intestine. Surgery, **67**, 474—477 (1970).

GIDEZ, L. I., ROHEIM, P. S., EDER, H. A.: Effect of diet on the cholesterol ester composition of liver and plasma lipoproteins in the rat. J. Lipid Res. **6**, 377—382 (1965).

GILTIN, D., CORNWELL, D. G., NIKASATO, D., ONCLEY, J. L., HUGHES, W. L., Jr., JANEWAY, C. A.: Studies on metabolism of plasma proteins in nephrotic syndrome. II. Lipoproteins. J. Clin. Invest. **37**, 172—184 (1958).

GLICKMAN, R. M., KIRSCH, K., ISSELBACHER, K. J.: Fat absorption during inhibition of protein synthesis. Studies of lymph chylomicrons. J. Clin. Invest. **51**, 356—363 (1972).

GLOMSET, J. A.: The mechanism of the plasma cholesterol esterification reaction and plasma fatty acid transferase. Biochim. biophys. Acta (Amst.) **65**, 128—135 (1962).

GLOMSET, J. A.: Further studies of the mechanism of the plasma cholesterol esterification reaction. Biochim. biophys. Acta. (Amst.) **70**, 389—395 (1963).

GLOMSET, J. A.: The plasma lecithin: Cholesterol acyltransferase reaction. J. Lipid Res. **9**, 155—167 (1968).

GLOMSET, J. A.: Physiological role of Lecithin — Cholesterol Acyltransferase. Amer. J. Clin. Nutr. **23**, 1129—1136 (1970).

GLOMSET, J. A., PARKER, F., TJADEN, M., WILLIAMS, R. H.: The esterification in vitro of free cholesterol in human and rat plasma. Biochim. biophys. Acta (Amst.) **58**, 398—406 (1962).

GLOMSET, J. A., JANSSEN, F. T., KENNEDY, R., DOBBINS, J.: Role of plasma lecithin:cholesterol acyltransferase in the metabolism of high density lipoproteins. J. Lipid Res. **7**, 638—648 (1966).

GLOMSET, J. A., NORUM, K. R., KING, W.: Plasma lipoproteins in familial lecithin: cholesterol acyl-transferase deficiency: Lipid composition and reactivity in vitro. J. clin. Invest. **49**, 1827—1837 (1970).

GLOVER, J., GREEN, C.: The distribution and transport of sterols across the intestinal mucosa of the guinea pig. Biochem. J. **67**, 308—316 (1957).

GLOVER, J., MORTON, R. A.: The absorption and metabolism of sterols. Brit. med. Bull. **14**, 226—233 (1958).

GLOVER, J., STAINER, D. W.: Sterol metabolism. 4 — The absorption of 7-dehydrocholesterol in the rat. Biochem. J. **72**, 79—82 (1959).

GLOVER, M., GLOVER, J., MORTON, R. A.: Provitamin D_3 in tissues and the conversion of cholesterol to 7-dehydrocholesterol in vivo. Biochem. J. **51**, 1—9 (1952).

GLOVER, J., GREEN, C., STAINER, D. W.: Sterol metabolism. 5: The uptake of sterols by organelles of intestinal mucosa and the site of their esterification during absorption. Biochem. J. **72**, 82—87 (1959).

GOLDSTEIN, J. L., SCHROTT, H. G., HAZZARD, W. R., BIERMAN, E. L., MOTULSKY, A. G.: Combined hyperlipidemia: Genetic evidence for a distinct disorder. Circulation **46**, 11—17 (1972).

GOODMAN, D. S.: The metabolism of chylomicron cholesterol ester in the rat. J. clin. Invest. **41**, 1886—1896 (1962).

GOODMAN, D. S.: The in vivo turnover of individual cholesterol esters in human lipoproteins. J. clin. Invest. **43**, 2026—2038 (1964).

GOODMAN, D. S.: Cholesterol ester metabolism. Physiol. Rev. **45**, 747—839 (1965).

GOODMAN, D. S., SHIRATORI, T.: In vivo turnover of different cholesterol esters in rat liver and plasma. J. Lipid Res. **5**, 578—586 (1964).

GOODMAN, D. S., NOBLE, R. P.: Turnover of plasma cholesterol in man. J. clin. Invest. **47**, 231—241 (1968).

GOODMAN, D. S., NOBLE, R. P.: Cholesteryl ester turnover in human plasma lipoproteins during cholestyramine and clofibrate therapy. J. Lipid Res. **11**, 183—189 (1970).

GOODMAN, D. S., NOBLE, R. P., DELL, R. B.: Three pool model of long-term turnover of plasma cholesterol in man. Circulation **46**, II—249 (1972).

GOTTO, A. M., BROWN, W. V., LEVY, R. I., BIRNBAUMER, M., FREDRICKSON, D. S.: Evidence for the identity of the major apoprotein in low density and very low density lipoproteins in normal subjects and patients with familial hyperlipoproteinemia. J. clin. Invest. **51**, 1486—1494 (1972).

GOULD, R. G.: Symposium on sitosterol. IV. Absorbability of Beta sitosterol. Trans. N.Y. Acad. Sci. **18**, 129—134 (1955).

GOULD, R. G.: In: PINCUS, G. (Ed.): The relationship between thyroid hormones and cholesterol biosynthesis and turnover in hormones and atherosclerosis, pp. 76—82. New York: Academic Press Inc. 1959.

GOULD, R. G., POPJAK, G.: Biosynthesis of cholesterol in vivo and in vitro from DL-β-hydroxy-β-methyl-δ-[2-^{14}C] valerolactone. Biochem. J. **66**, 51p (1957).

GOULD, R. G., COOK, R. P.: The metabolism of cholesterol and other sterols in the animal organism. In: COOK, R. P. (Ed.): Cholesterol: Chemistry, Biochemistry and Pathology, pp. 237—307. New York: Academic Press. Inc. 1958.

GOULD, R. G., BELL, V. L., LILLY, E. H.: Stimulation of cholesterol biosyntheis from acetate in rat liver and adrenals by whole body X-irridiation. Amer. J. Physiol. **196**, 1231—1237 (1959).

GOULD, R. G., TAYLOR, C. B., HAGERMAN, J. S., WARNER, I., CAMPBELL, D. J.: Cholesterol metabolism: I. Effect of dietary cholesterol on the synthesis of cholesterol in dog tissue in vitro. J. biol. Chem. **201**, 519—528 (1953).

GOULD, R. C., LEROY, G. V., OKITA, G. T., KABARA, J. J., KEEGAN, P., BERGENSTAL, D. M.: Use of ^{14}C labelled acetate to study cholesterol metabolism in man. J. Lab. clin. Med. **46**, 374—384 (1955).

GRIES, F. A., MATSCHINSKY, F., WIELAND, O.: Induktion der Hydroxy-β-methylglutaryl reduktase durch Schilddrüsenhormone. Biochim. biophys. Acta (Amst.) **56**, 615—617 (1962).

GRIFFITHS, K., GRANT, J. K., SYMINGTON, T.: A biochemical investigation of the functional zonation of the adrenal cortex in man. J. clin. Endocr. **23**, 776—785 (1963).

GRUNDY, S. M., AHRENS, E. H. JR.: An evaluation of the relative merits of two methods for measuring the balance of sterols in man: Isotopic balance versus chromatographic analysis. J. clin. Invest. **45**, 1503—1515 (1966).

GRUNDY, S. M., AHRENS, E. H. JR.: Measurements of cholesterol turnover, synthesis and absorption in man, carried out by isotope kinetic and sterol balance methods. J. Lipid Res. **10**, 91—107 (1969).

GRUNDY, S. M., AHRENS, E. H. JR.: The effects of unsaturated dietary fats on absorption, excretion, synthesis and distribution of cholesterol in man. J. clin. Invest. **49**, 1135—1152 (1970).

GRUNDY, S. M., AHRENS, E. H. JR., MIETTINEN, T. A.: Quantitative isolation and gas-liquid chromatographic analysis of total fecal bile acids. J. Lipid Res. **6**, 397—410 (1965).

GRUNDY, S. M., AHRENS, E. H., JR., SALEN, G.: Dietary β-sitosterol as an internal standard to correct for cholesterol losses in sterol balance studies. J. Lipid Res. **9**, 374—387 (1968).

GRUNDY, S. M., AHRENS, E. H. JR., DAVIGNON, J.: The interaction of cholesterol absorption and cholesterol synthesis in man. J. Lipid Res. **10**, 304—315 (1969).

GRUNDY, S. M., AHRENS, E. H. JR., SALEN, G.: Interruption of the enterohepatic circulation of bile acids in man: comparative effects of cholestyramine and ileal exclusion on cholesterol metabolism. J. Lab. clin. Med. **78**, 94—121 (1971).

GRUNDY, S. M., AHRENS, E. H. JR., SALEN, G., SCHREIBMAN, P. H., NESTEL, P. J.: Mechanisms of action of clofibrate on cholesterol metabolism in patients with hyperlipidemia J. Lipid Res. **13**, 531—551 (1972).

GUDER, W., NOLTE, I., WIELAND, O.: The influence of thyroid hormones on β-methyl-glutaryl-Coenzyme A reductase of rat liver. Europ. J. Biochem. **4**, 273—278 (1968).

GULBRANDSEN, C., EVANS, V., NICHOLS, A., LEES, R. S.: Very low density lipoprotein metabolism in abetalipoproteinemia. J. clin. Invest. **51**, 40 a (1972).

GURD, F. R. N.: In: HANAHAN, D. J. (Ed.): Some naturally occuring lipoprotein systems in Lipide chemistry, p. 260. New York: Wiley 1960.

HAGERMAN, J. S., GOULD, R. G.: The in vitro interchange of cholesterol between plasma and red cells. Proc. Soc. exp. Biol. (N.Y.) **78**, 329—332 (1951).

HAMPRECHT, B., NUSSLER, C., LYNEN, F.: Rhythmic changes for hydroxymethylglutaryl Coenzyme A reductase activity in livers of fed and fasted rats. F.E.B.S. Letters **4**, 117—121 (1969).

HARTLEY, G. S.: Aqueous solutions of paraffin chain salts. A study in micelle formation. Actualites Sci. Ind. No 387 (1936).

HARTLEY, G. S.: Solutions of soap like substances. Progr. Chem. Fats. Lipids **3**, 19—55 (1955).

HAVEL, R. J., KANE, J. P., KASHYAP, M. L.: Interchange of apolipoproteins between chylomicrons and high density lipoproteins during alimentary lipemia in man. J. clin. Invest. **52**, 32—38 (1973).

HECHTER, O., ZAFFARONI, A., JACOBSEN, R. P., LEVY, H., JEANLOZ, R. W., SCHENKER, V., PINCUS, G.: The nature and the biogenesis of adrenal secretory product. Recent Progr. Hormone Res. **6**, 215—241 (1951).

HECHTER, O., SOLOMON, M. M., ZAFFARONI, A., PINCUS, G.: Transformation of cholesterol and acetate to adrenal cortical hormones. Arch. Biochem. **46**, 201—213 (1953).

HELE, P.: The acetate activating enzyme of beef heart. J. biol. Chem. **206**, 671—676 (1954).

HELLMAN, L., ROSENFELD, R. S., INSULL, W. JR., AHRENS, E. H. JR.: Intestinal excretion of cholesterol: A mechanism for regulation of plasma levels. J. clin. Invest. **36**, 898 a (1957).

HELLSTRÖM, K.: On the bile acids and neutral steroid excretion in man and rabbits following cholesterol feeding. Bile acids and steroids 150. Acta physiol. scand. **63**, 21—35 (1965).

HELLSTRÖM, K. SJÖVALL, J.: On the origin of lithocholic acid and ursodeoxycholic acids in man. Bile acids and steroids 106. Acta physiol. scand. **51**, 218—223 (1961).

HERNANDEZ, H. H., CHAIKOFF, I. L.: Purification and properties of pancreatic cholesterol esterase. J. biol. Chem. **228**, 447—457 (1957).

HERNANDEZ, H. H., CHAIKOFF, I. L., DAUBEN, W. G., ABRAHAM, S.: The absorption of ^{14}C labelled epicholesterol in the rat. J. biol. Chem. **206**, 757—765 (1954).

HICKMAN, P. E., HORTON, B. J., SABINE, J. R.: Effect of adrenalectomy on the diurnal variation of hepatic cholesterogenesis in the rat. J. Lipid Res. **13**, 17—22 (1972).

HO, K. J., TAYLOR, C. B.: Comparative studies on tissue cholesterol. Arch. Path. **86**, 585—596 (1968).

HO, K. J., TAYLOR, C. B.: Mode of cholesterol accumulation in various tissues of rabbits with moderate hypercholesteremia. Proc. Soc. exp. Biol. (N.Y.) **136**, 249—252 (1971).

HO, K. J., BISS, K., MIKKELSON, B., LEWIS, L. A., TAYLOR, C. B.: The Masai of East Africa: some unique biological characteristics. Arch. Path. **91**, 387—410 (1971).

HOFMANN, A. F., BORGSTRÖM, B.: The intraluminal phase of fat digestion in man. The lipid content of the micellar and oil phases of intestinal content obtained during fat digestion and absorption. J. clin. Invest. **43**, 247—257 (1964).

HORLICK, L., KUDCHODKAR, B.J., SODHI, H.S.: Mode of action of chlorophenoxyisobutyric acid on cholesterol metabolism in man. Circulation **43**, 299—309 (1971).

HORNING, M.G., HEBERT, R.M., ROTH, R.J., DAVIS, D.L., HORNNING, E.C., FISCHER, E.P., JORDAN, C.C., JR.: Effects of Ethyl-p-chlorophenoxyisobutyrate on biliary secretion of bile acids, cholesterol and phosphatidyl choline. Lipids **7**, 114—120 (1972).

HSIA, S.L., FULTON, J.E. JR., FULGHUM, D., BUCH, M.M.: Lipid synthesis from acetate -1-^{14}C by suction blister epidermis and other skin components. Proc. Soc. exp. Biol. (N.Y.) **135**, 285—291 (1970).

ILLINGWORTH, D.R., PORTMAN, O.W.: Exchange of phospholipids between low and high density lipoprotein of squirrel monkeys. J. Lipid Res. **13**, 220—227 (1972).

INSULL, W., HSI, B., YOSHIMURA, S.: Comparison of tissue cholesterols in Japanese and American men. J. Lab. clin. Med. **72**, 885 (1968).

IRITANI, N., NOGI, J.: Cholesterol absorption and lymphatic transport in rat. Atherosclerosis **15**, 231—239 (1972).

ISSELBACHER, K.J., SCHEIG, R., PLOTKIN, G.R., CAULFIELD, J.B.: Congenital β-lipoprotein deficiency: Heriditary disorder involving defect in absorption and transport of lipids. Medicine **43**, 347—361 (1964).

JANSEN, G.R., ZANETTI, M.E., HUTCHISON, C.F.: Studies in lipogenesis in vivo: fatty acid and cholesterol synthesis during starvation and re-feeding. Biochem. J. **101**, 811—818 (1966).

JANSEN, G.R., ZANETTI, M.E., HUTCHISON, C.F.: Synthesis of cholesterol from glucose-U-^{14}C in the liver and extrahepatic tissues of the mouse. Arch. Biochim. Biophys. **138**, 433—442 (1972).

JONES, M.E., BLACK, S., FLYNN, R.M., LIPMANN, F.: Acetyl-Coenzyme A synthesis through pyrophosphoryl split of ATD. Biochim. biophys. Acta (Amst.) **12**, 141—149 (1953).

KABARA, J.J.: Brain cholesterol: XVI. Incorporation of different precursors into baboon tissue sterol. Lipids **8**, 56—60 (1973).

KANDUTSCH, A.A., SAUCIER, S.E.: Prevention of cyclic and triton induced increases in hydroxymethyl glutaryl Coenzyme A reductase and sterol synthesis by puromycin. J. biol. Chem. **244**, 2299—2305 (1969).

KANNEL, H.S.: Normal limits for serum cholesterol. In: CASDORPH, H.R. (Ed.): Treatment of Hyperlipidemic States. Springfield, Ill: Charles C. Thomas 1971.

KANNEL, W.B., DAWBER, T.R., FRIEDMAN, C.D., GLENNON, W.E., MCNAMARA, P.M.: Risk factors in coronary artery disease: An evaluation of several serum lipids as predictors of coronary heart disease: The Framingham study. Ann. intern. Med. **61**, 888—899 (1964).

KAO, V.C.Y., WISSLER, R.W.: A study of immunohistochemical localization of serum lipoproteins and other plasma proteins in human atherosclerotic lesions. Exp. Mol. Path. **4**, 465—479 (1965).

KAPLAN, J.A., COX, G.C., TAYLOR, C.B.: Cholesterol metabolism in man: Studies on absorption. Arch. Path. **76**, 359—368 (1963).

KARMEN, A., WHYTE, H.M., GOODMAN, D.S.: Fatty acid esterification and chylomicron formation during fat absorption. 1. Triglycerides and cholesterol esters. J. Lipid Res. **4**, 312—321 (1963).

KARP, A., STETTEN, D. JR.: The effect of thyroid activity on certain anabolic processes studied with the aid of deuterium. J. biol. Chem. **179**, 819—830 (1949).

KARVINEN, E., LIN, T.M., IVY, A.C.: Capacity of human intestine to absorb exogenous cholesterol. J. appl. Physiol. **11**, 143—147 (1957).

KAYSER, F., BALAT, R.: Sur la presence et sur l'origine du cholesterol dans l'urine. Bull. Soc. chim. Biol. **34**, 806—812 (1952).

KELLOG, T.F.: Microbiological aspects of enterohepatic neutral sterol and bile acid metabolism. Fed. Proc. **30**, 1808—1814 (1971).

KELLOG, T.F., WOSTMANN, B.S.: Fecal neutral steroids and bile acids from germ free rats. J. Lipid Res. **10**, 495—503 (1969).

KEYS, A., MICHELSEN, O., MILLER, E.O., HAYES, E.R., TODD, R.L.: The concentration of cholesterol in the blood serum of normal man and its relation to age. J. clin. Invest. **29**, 1347—1353 (1950).

KHACHADURIAN, A.K.: Lack of inhibition of cholesterol synthesis of dietary cholesterol in cases of familial hypercholesterolemia. Lancet **1969 II**, 778—780.

KHAN, B., COX, G. E., ASDEL, K.: Cholesterol in human tissues. Arch. Path. **76**, 369—381 (1963).

KIM, K. S., IVY, A. C.: Factors influencing cholesterol absorption. Amer. J. Physiol. **17**, 302—318 (1952).

KLEIN, P. D., MARTIN, R. A.: Some transitory changes in cholesterol metabolism induced by dietary cholesterol. J. biol. Chem. **234**, 3129—3132 (1959).

KNAUSS, H. J., PORTER, J. W., WASSON, G.: The biosynthesis of mevalonic acid from 1-^{14}C acetate by a rat liver enzyme system. J. biol. Chem. **234**, 2835—2840 (1959).

KORZENOVSKY, M. WALTERS, C. P., HARVEY, O. A., DILLER, E. R.: Some factors which influence the catalytic activity of pancreatic cholesterol esterase. Proc. Soc. exp. Biol. (N.Y.) **105**, 303—305 (1960).

KOTTKE, B. A.: Differences in bile acid excretion. Primary hypercholesterolemia compared to combined hypercholesterolemia and hypertriglyceridemia. Circulation **40**, 13—20 (1969).

KOTTKE, B. A., SUBBIAH, M. T. R.: Sterol balance studies in patients on solid diets. Comparison of two nonabsorbable markers. J. Lab. clin. Med. **80**, 530—538 (1972).

KRAMSCH, D. M., HOLLANDER, W.: The interaction of serum and arterial lipoproteins with elastin of the arterial intima and its role in the lipid accumulation in atherosclerotic plaques. J. clin. Invest. **52**, 236—247 (1973).

KRITCHEVSKY, D.: In: SCHETTLER, G. (Ed.): Biochemistry of steroids in Lipids and Lipidoses, pp. 66—92. New York: Springer-Verlag Inc. 1967.

KRITCHEVSKY, D.: Cholesterol metabolism in the baboon. Trans. N.Y. Acad. Sc. **32**, 821—831 (1970).

KRITCHEVSKY, D., WERTHESSEN, N. T., SHAPIRO, I. L.: Studies on the biosynthesis of lipids in the baboon. Bisoynthesis and transport of cholesterol. Clin. chim. Acta **11**, 44—52 (1965).

KRITCHEVSKY, D., CASEY, R. P., TEPPER, S. A.: Isocaloric, isogravic diets in rats. II. Effects on cholesterol absorption and excretion. Nutrition Reports International **7**, 61—69 (1973).

KUDCHODKAR, B. J., HORLICK, L., SODHI, H. S.: Effects of nicotinic acid and plant sterols on cholesterol metabolism in man. Proceedings of fourth International Symposium on Drugs affecting lipid metabolism. Philadelphia, U.S.A. Sept. (1971 a).

KUDCHODKAR, B. J., HORLICK, L., SODHI, H. S.: Mechanism of action of nicotinic acid on cholesterol metabolism in man. To be published (1973 c).

KUDCHODKAR, B. J., SODHI, H. S.: Enterohepatic metabolism of cholesterol in types IIa and IIb hyperlipoproteinemia. Circulation **46**, II—267 (1972).

KUDCHODKAR, B. J., SODHI, H. S.: Turnover of cholesterol esters in hyperlipoproteinemias. Proc. Can. Fed. Biol. Soc. **16**, 93 (1973).

KUDCHODKAR, B. J., SODHI, H. S., HORLICK, L.: Absorption of dietary cholesterol in man. Circulation **44**, II-3 (1971 b).

KUDCHODKAR, B. J., SODHI, H. S., HORLICK, L.: Effects of clofibrate on the fecal excretion of individual bile acids in hyperlipemic subjects. Clin. Res. **19**, 4 (1971 c).

KUDCHODKAR, B. J., SODHI, H. S., HORLICK, L.: Lack of degradation of dietary and endogenous sterols in gastrointestinal tract of man. Metabolism **21**, 343—349 (1972 a).

KUDCHODKAR, B. J., SODHI, H. S., HORLICK, L.: Cholesterol pools and their turnover rates in types IIa and IIb hyperlipoproteinemia. Circulation **46**, II—250 (1972 b).

KUDCHODKAR, B. J., SODHI, H. S., HORLICK, L.: Comparison of isotopic and chromatographic methods for estimating fecal bile acids. Clin. chim. Acta. **41**, 47—54 (1972 c).

KUDCHODKAR, B. J., SODHI, H. S., HORLICK, L.: Absorption of dietary cholesterol in man. Metabolism **22**, 155—163 (1973 a).

KUDCHODKAR, B. J., SODHI, H. S., HORLICK, L.: Effect of positol on cholesterol metabolism in man. To be published (1973 b).

KUDCHODKAR, B. J., SODHI, H. S., HORLICK, L.: Effect of low calorie diet on cholesterol metabolism in man. To be published (1973 d).

KUDCHODKAR, B. J., SODHI, H. S., HORLICK, L.: Effects of clofibrate on cholesterol metabolism in man. To be published (1973 e).

KUKSIS, A., HUANG, T. C.: Differential absorption of plant sterols in the dog. Canad. J. Biochem. **40**, 1493—1504 (1962).

KUNKEL, H. G., BEARN, A. G.: Phospholipid studies of different serum lipoproteins employing ^{32}p. Proc. Soc. exp. Biol. (N.Y.) **86**, 887—891 (1954).

LACK, L., WEINER, I. M.: In vitro absorption of bile salts by small intestine of rats and guinea pigs. Amer. J. Physiol. **200**, 313—317 (1961).

LANGDON, R. G., BLOCH, K.: The effect of some dietary additions on the synthesis of cholesterol from acetate in vitro. J. biol. Chem. **202**, 77—81 (1953).

LANGER, T., LEVY, R. I.: The effect of nicotinic acid on the turnover of low density lipoproteins in Type II hyperlipoproteinemia. In: GEY, K. F., CARLSON, L. A. (Eds.): Metabolic effects of nicotinic acid and its derivatives, pp. 641—647. Bern: Hans Huber Publ. 1971.

LANGER, T., STROBER, W., LEVY, R. I.: The metabolism of low density lipoprotein in familial Type II hyperlipoproteinemia. J. clin. Invest. **51**, 1528—1536 (1972).

LEBLOND, C. P., STEVENS, C. E.: The constant renewal of the intestinal epithelium in the albino rat. Anat. Rec. **100**, 357—377 (1948).

LEHNER, N. D. M., CLARKSON, T. B., BELL, F. P., ST.CLAIR, R. W., LOFLAND, H. B.: Effects of insulin deficiency, hypothyroidism and hypertension of cholesterol metabolism in squirrel monkey. Expt. Mol. Path. **16**, 109—123 (1972).

LEVY, R. I., FREDRICKSON, D. S., LASTER, L.: Lipoproteins and lipid transport in abetalipoproteinemia. J. clin. Invest. **45**, 531 531—541 (1966).

LEWIS, B., MYANT, N. B.: Studies in the metabolism of cholesterol in subjects with normal plasma cholesterol levels and in patients with essential hypercholesterolemia. Clin. Sci. **32**. 201—213 (1967).

LINDGREN, F. T., NICHOLS, A. V.: Structure and function of human serum lipoproteins. In: PUTNAM, F. W. (Ed.): The plasma proteins, Vol. II, p. I—58. Biosynthesis, metabolism, alterations in disease. New York: Academic Press 1960.

LINDGREN, F. T., NICHOLS, A. V., FREEMAN, N. K.: Physical and chemical composition studies on the lipoproteins of fasting and heparinized sera. J. Phys. Chem. **59**, 930—938 (1955).

LINDSEY, C. A., JR., WILSON, J. D.: Evidence for a contribution by the intestinal wall to the serum cholesterol of the rat. J. Lipid Res. **6**, 173—181 (1965).

LINDSTEDT, S.: Turnover of cholic acid in man. Acta physiol. scand. **40**, 1—9 (1957).

LINDSTEDT, S., AHRENS, E. H. JR.: Conversion of cholesterol to bile acids in man. Proc. Soc. exp. Biol. (N.Y.) **108**, 286—288 (1961).

LINN, T. C.: The effect of cholesterol feeding and fasting upon β-hydroxy-β-methylglutaryl Coenzyme A reductase. J. biol. Chem. **242**, 990—993 (1967).

LIPSKY, S. R., BONDY, P. K., MAN, E. B., McGUIRE, J. S. JR.: The effects of triiodothyronine on the biosynthesis of plasma lipids from acetate-l-^{14}C in myxedematous subjects. J. clin. Invest. **34**, 950 a (1955).

LITTLE, H. N., BLOCH, K.: Studies on the utilization of acetic acid for the biological synthesis of cholesterol. J. biol. Chem. **183**, 33—46 (1950).

LOFLAND, H. B. JR., CLARKSON, T. B., ST.CLAIR, R. W., LEHNER, N. D. M.: Studies on the regulation of plasma cholesterol levels in squirrel monkeys of two genotypes. J. Lipid Res. **13**, 39—47 (1972).

LONGCOPE, C., WILLIAMS, R. H.: Cholesterol esterification by adrenal homogenates. Proc. Soc. exp. Biol. (N.Y.) **113**, 754—756 (1963).

LOSSOW, W. J., BROT, N., CHAIKOFF, I. L.: Disposition of the cholesterol moiety of a chylomicron containing lipoprotein fraction of chyle in the rat. J. Lipid Res. **3**, 207—215 (1962).

LOSSOW, W. J., NAIDOO, S. S., CHAIKOFF, I. L.: Effect of heparin on disappearances of the cholesterol moiety of an injected cholesterol ^{14}C labelled, very low density chyle lipoprotein fraction from the circulation of the rat. J. Lipid Res. **4**, 419—423 (1963).

LOSSOW, W. J., MIGLIONIM, R. H., BROT, N., CHAIKOFF, I. L.: Effect of total exclusion of the exocrine pancreas in the rat upon in vitro esterification of ^{14}C labelled cholesterol by the intestine and upon lymphatic absorption of ^{14}C cholesterol. J. Lipid Res. **5**, 198—202 (1964).

LOSSOW, W. J., LINDGREN, F. T., JENSEN, L. C.: Net uptake of rat serum protein by Sf 400 Lymph chylomicrons in vitro. Biochim. biophys. Acta. (Amst.) **144**, 670—677 (1967).

LUPIEN, P. J., MIGICOVSKY, B. B.: Effect of deutectomy on levels of blood and liver cholesterol and on the incorporation of acetate and mevalonate into liver cholesterol by the chick. Canad. J. Biochem. **42**, 179—185 (1964).

LYNEN, F.: Lipide metabolism. Ann. Rev. Biochem. **24**, 653—688 (1955).

LYNEN, F.: Biosynthesis. Terpenes sterols. Ciba Found. Symp. 1958 pp. 95—118 (1959).

MacKenzie, S. L., Sundaram, G. S., Sodhi, H. S.: Heterogeneity of human serum high density lipoprotein (HDL$_2$). Clin. chim. Acta **43**, 223—229 (1973).

Mak, K. M., Trier, J. S.: Radioautographic and chemical evidence for [5-^{3}H]-mevalonate incorporation into cholesterol by rat villous absorptive cells. Biochim. biophys. Acta (Amst.) **280**, 316—328 (1972).

Malinow, M. R., McLaughlin, P., Pierovich, I.: Muscular activity and degradation of cholesterol by the liver. Atherosclerosis **15**, 153—162 (1972).

Malinow, M. R., McLaughlin, P., Perley, A., Laestuen, L.: Effect of muscular activity on bile acid excretion in rats. J. appl. Physiol. **29**, 610—614 (1970).

Man, E. B., Kartin, B. L., Durlacher, S. H., Peters, J. E.: The lipids of serum and liver in patients with hepatic diseases. J. clin. Invest. **24**, 623—643 (1945).

Marcel, Y. L., Vezina, C.: Lecithin: cholesterol acyltransferase of human plasma — Role of chylomicrons, very low, and high density lipoproteins in the reaction. J. biol. Chem. **248**, 8254—8259 (1973).

Marsh, J. B., Drabkin, D. L.: Metabolic channeling in experimental nephrosis V. Lipid metabolism in the early stages of the disease. J. biol. Chem. **230**, 1083—1091 (1958).

Masoro, E. J.: Physiological chemistry of lipids in mammals, pp. 116—123. Philadelphia: W. B. Saunders Co. 1968.

Maurizi, C. P., Alvarez, C., Fischer, G. C., Taylor, C. B.: Human tissue cholesterol. Arch. Path. **86**, 644—646 (1968).

Mayer, R. M.: In vitro studies on cholesterol absorption (doctoral thesis). Washington D. C.: The George Washington University 1963.

McIntyre, N., Kirsch, K., Orr, J. C., Isselbacher, K. J.: Sterols in the small intestine of the rat, guinea pig and rabbit, J. Lipid **12**, 336—346 (1971).

Menkes, J. H., Schimshock, J. R., Swanson, P. D.: Cerebrotendinous xanthomatosis: The storage of cholestanol within the nervous system. Arch. Neurol. **19**, 47—53 (1968).

Miettinen, T. A.: Fecal steroid excretion during weight reduction in obese patients with hyperlipidemia. Clin. chim. Acta **19**, 341—344 (1968a).

Miettinen, T. A.: Effect of nicotinic acid on catabolism and synthesis of cholesterol in man. Clin. chim. Acta **20**, 43—51 (1968b).

Miettinen, T. A.: Mechanism of serum cholesterol reduction by thyroid hormones in hyperthyroidism. J. Lab. clin. Med. **71**, 537—547 (1968c).

Miettinen, T. A.: Detection of changes in human cholesterol metabolism. Ann. Clin. Res. **2**, 300—320 (1970).

Miettinen, T. A.: Cholesterol production in obesity. Circulation **44**, 842—850 (1971).

Miettinen, T. A., Penttila, I. M.: Leucine and mevalonate as precursors of serum cholesterol in man. Acta med. scand. **184**, 159—164 (1968).

Miettinen, T. A., Penttila, I. M.: Comparison of leucine with mevalonate and acetate as precursor of tissue and serum cholesterol in the rat. Ann. Med. Exp. Biol. Fenn. **49**, 20—28 (1971).

Miettinen, T. A., Ahrens, E. H. Jr., Grundy, S. M.: Quantitative isolation and gas liquid chromatographic analysis of total dietary and fecal neutral steroids. J. Lipid Res. **6**, 411—424 (1965).

Miettinen, T. A., Pelkonen, R., Nikkila, E. A., Heinonen, O.: Low excretion of fecal bile acids in a family with hypercholesterolemia. Acta med. scand. **182**, 645—650 (1967).

Migicovsky, B. B., Wood, J. D.: Effect of starvation on cholesterol biosynthesis in vitro. Canad. J. Biochem. **33**, 858—866 (1955).

Monger, E. A., Nestel, P. J.: Relationship between the concentration and the rate of esterification of free cholesterol by the plasma esterification system. Clin. chim. Acta **15**, 269—273 (1967).

Moore, J. H., Williams, D. L.: Studies on the cholesterol esters of the adrenal glands and other tissues of the rabbit. Biochim. biophys. Acta **125**, 352—366 (1966).

Moore, R. B., Anderson, J. T., Taylor, H. L., Keys, A., Frantz, I. D. Jr.: Effect of dietary fat on the fecal excretion of cholesterol and its degradation products in man. J. clin. Invest. **47**, 1517—1534 (1968).

Moore, R. B., Frantz, I. D., Buchwald, H.: Changes in cholesterol excretion after partial ileal bypass in hypercholesterolemic patients. Surgery **65**, 98—108 (1969).

MORIN, R.J., BERNICK, S., MEAD, J.F., ALFIN-SLATER, R.B.: The influence of exogenous cholesterol on hepatic lipid composition of the rat. J. Lipid Res. **3**, 432—438 (1962).
MOUTAFIS, C.D., MYANT, N.B.: The metabolism of cholesterol in two hypercholesterolemic patients treated with cholestyramine. Clin. Sci. **37**, 443—454 (1969).
MOUTAFIS, C.D., MYANT, N.B., TABAQEHALI, S.: The metabolism of cholesterol after resection or
   by-pass of the lower small intestine. Clin. Sci. **35**, 534—545 (1968).
MUELLER, J.H.: The mechanism of cholesterol absorption. J. biol. Chem. **27**, 463—480 (1916).
MUKHERJEE, S., KUNITAKE, G., ALFIN-SLATER, R.B.: The esterification of cholesterol with palmitic
   acid by rat liver homogenates. J. biol. Chem. **230**, 91—96 (1958).
MURPHY, J.R.: Erythrocyte metabolism. III. Relationship of energy metabolism and serum fac-
   tors to the osmotic fragility following incubation. J. Lab. clin. Med. **60**, 86—109 (1962).
MURTHY, S.K., GANGULY, J.: Studies on cholesterol esterases of the small intestine and pancreas
   of rats. Biochem. J. **83**, 460—469 (1962).
NAZIR, D.J., HORLICK, L., KUDCHODKAR, B.J., SODHI, H.S.: Mechanisms of action of cholestyr-
   amine in the treatment of hypercholesterolemia. Circulation **46**, 95—102 (1972).
NESTEL, P.J.: Cholesterol turnover in man. Advanc. Lipid Res. **8**, 1—39 (1970a).
NESTEL, P.J.: Turnover of plasma esterified cholesterol. Influence of dietary fat and carbohydrate
   and relation to plasma lipids and body weight. Clin. Sci. **38**, 593—600 (1970b).
NESTEL, P.J., COUZENS, E.A.: Turnover of individual cholesterol esters in human liver and
   plasma. J. clin. Invest. **45**, 1234—1240 (1966).
NESTEL, P.J., MONGER, E.A.: Turnover of plasma esterified cholesterol in normocholesterolemic
   and hypercholesterolemic subjects and its relation to body build. J. clin. Invest. **46**, 967—974
   (1967).
NESTEL, P.J., HAVEL, R.J., BEZMAN, A.: Metabolism of constituent lipids of dog chylomicrons. J.
   clin. Invest. **42**, 1313—1321 (1963).
NESTEL, P.J., COUZENS, E., HIRSCH, E.Z.: Comparison of turnover of individual cholesterol esters
   in subjects with low and high plasma cholesterol concentration. J. Lab. clin. Med. **66**, 582—
   595 (1965).
NESTEL, P.J., WHYTE, H.M., GOODMAN, D.S.: Distribution and turnover of cholesterol in humans. J. clin. Invest. **48**, 982—991 (1969).
NESTEL, P.J., HAVENSTEIN, N., WHYTE, H.M., SCOTT, T.J., COOK, L.J.: Lower plasma cholesterol
   after eating polyunsaturated ruminant fats. New Engl. J. Med. **288**, 379—382 (1973).
NICHOLS, A.V., SMITH, L.: Effect of very low density lipoproteins on lipid transfer in incubated
   serum. J. Lipid Res. **6**, 206—210 (1965).
NICHOLS, A.V., REHNBORG, C.S., LINDGREN, F.T., WILLS, R.D.: Effects of oil ingestion on lipo-
   protein fatty acids in man. J. Lipid Res. **3**, 320—326 (1962).
NICOLAIDES, N., ROTHMAN, S.: The site of sterol and squalene synthesis in the human skin. J.
   Invest. Dermatol. **24**, 125—129 (1955).
NICOLAIDES, N., KELLUM, R.E.: Skin lipids. I. sampling problems of the skin and its appendages.
   J. Amer. Oil chem. Soc. **42**, 685—690 (1965).
NIEMINEN, E.: Free and esterified cholesterol in human organs and tissues. Ann. Acad. Sci. Fenn.
   (Med.). **118**, 1—104 (1965).
NILSSON, A., ZILVERSMIT, D.B.: Distribution of chylomicron cholesteryl ester between parenchy-
   mal and Kupffer cells of rat liver. Biochim. biophys. Acta (Amst.) **248**, 137—142 (1971).
NILSSON, A., ZILVERSMIT, D.B.: Fate of intravenously injected particulate and lipoprotein choles-
   terol in the rat. J. Lipid Res. **13**, 32—38 (1972).
NOBLE, R.P.: Electrophoretic separation of plasma lipoproteins in agarose gel. J. Lipid Res. **9**,
   693—700 (1968).
NORMAN, A., SJOVALL, J.: On the transformation and enterohepatic circulation of cholic acid in
   the rat. Bile acids and steroids. 68. J. biol. Chem. **233**, 872—885 (1958).
NORUM, K.R., GJONE, E.: Familial plasma lecithin:cholesterol acyltransferase deficiency: Biochemical study of a new inborn error of metabolism. Scand. J. clin. Lab. Invest. **20**,
   231—243 (1967).
OCKNER, R.K., HUGHES, F.B., ISSELBACHER, K.J.: Very low density lipoproteins in intestinal
   lymph origin, composition, and role in lipid transport in the fasting state. J. clin. Invest. **48**,
   2079—2088 (1969a).

OCKNER, R. K., HUGHES, F. B., ISSELBACHER, K. J.: Very low density lipoproteins in intestinal lymph: role in triglyceride and cholesterol transport during fat absorption. J. clin. Invest. **48**, 2367—2373 (1969b).

OGURA, M., SHIGA, J., YAMASAKI, K.: Studies on the cholesterol pool as the precursor of bile acids in the rat. J. Biochem. **70**, 967—972 (1971).

OLIVER, M. F., GEIZEROVA, H., CUMMING, R. A., HEADY, J. A.: Serum cholesterol and ABO and Rhesus blood groups. Lancet **9**, 605—607 (1969).

PETERSON, D. W., SHNEOUR, E. A., PEEK, N. F.: Effects of dietary sterols and sterol esters on plasma and liver cholesterol in the chick. J. Nutr. **53**, 451—459 (1954).

PIHL, A.: The effect of dietary fat on the intestinal cholesterol absorption and on the cholesterol metabolism in the liver of rats. Acta physiol. scand. **34**, 197—205 (1955).

PLOTZ, E. J., KABARA, J. J., DAVIS, M. E.: Studies on the synthesis of cholesterol in the brain of the human fetus. Amer. J. Obstet. Gynec. **101**, 534—538 (1968).

POPE, J. L., PARKINSON, T. M., OLSON, J. A.: Action of bile salts on the metabolism and transport of water soluble nutrients by perfused rat jejunum in vitro. Biochim. biophys. Acta (Amst.) **130**, 218—232 (1966).

POPJAK, G., BEECKMANS, M. L.: Extrahepatic lipid synthesis. Biochem. J. **47**, 233—238 (1950).

QUARFORDT, S. H., GOODMAN, D. S.: Heterogeneity in the rate of plasma clearance of chylomicrons of different size. Biochim. biophys. Acta (Amst.) **116**, 382—385 (1966).

QUARFORDT, S. H., OLLSCHLAEGER, H., KRIGBAUM, W. R.: Liquid crystalline lipid in the plasma of humans with biliary obstruction. J. clin. Invest. **51**, 1979—1988 (1972).

QUINTAO, E., GRUNDY, S. M., AHRENS, E. H. JR.: An evaluation of four methods for measuring cholesterol absorption by the intestine in man. J. Lipid Res. **12**, 221—232 (1971a).

QUINTAO, E., GRUNDY, S. M., AHRENS, E. H., JR.: Effects of dietary cholesterol on the regulation of total body cholesterol in man. J. Lipid Res. **12**, 233—247 (1971b).

RALLI, E. P., RUBIN, S. H., RINSLER, S.: The liver lipids in normal human livers and in cases of cirrhosis and fatty infiltration of the liver. J. clin. Invest. **20**, 93—97 (1941).

RASKIN, P., SIPERSTEIN, M. D.: The metabolism of mevalonic acid by the kidney. Clin. Res. **19**, 484 (1971).

REAVEN, G. M., HILL, D. B., GROSS, R. C., FARQUHAR, J. W.: Kinetics of triglyceride turnover of very low density lipoproteins of human plasma. J. clin. Invest. **44**, 1826—1833 (1965).

REDGRAVE, T. G.: Formation of cholesteryl ester rich particulate lipid during metabolism of chylomicrons. J. clin. Invest. **49**, 465—471 (1970).

REHNBORG, C. S., NICHOLS, A. V.: The fate of cholesteryl esters in human serum incubated in vitro at 38°. Biochim. biophys. Acta (Amst.) **84**, 596—603 (1964).

RICE, L. I., SCHOTZ, M. C., ALFIN-SLATER, R. B., DEUEL, H. J. JR.: Changes in cholesterol distribution in liver cell fractions of rats fed cholesterol. J. biol. Chem. **201**, 867—871 (1953).

RIDER, A. K., LEVY, R. I., FREDRICKSON, D. S.: "Sinking" prebeta lipoprotein and the Lp antigen. Circulation **42**, III-10 (1970).

RITTENBERG, D., BLOCK, K.: The utilization of acetic acid for fatty acid synthesis. J. biol. Chem. **154**, 311—312 (1944).

RITTENBERG, D., BLOCH, K.: The utilization of acetic acid for the synthesis of fatty acids. J. biol. Chem. **160**, 417—424 (1945).

ROHEIM, P. S., HAFT, D. E., GIDEZ, L. I., WHITE, A., EDER, H. A.: Plasma lipoprotein metabolism in perfused rat livers. II. Transfer of free and esterified cholesterol into plasma. J. clin. Invest. **42**, 1277—1285 (1963).

ROSE, H. G.: Influence of plasma lipoprotein levels on lipoprotein cholesterol esterification in normal and hyperlipemic subjects. Circulation **46**, II—274 (1972).

ROSENFELD, R. S., HELLMAN, L.: The relation of plasma and biliary cholesterol to bile acid synthesis in man. J. clin. Invest. **38**, 1334—1338 (1959).

ROSENFELD, R. S., FUKUSHIMA, D. K., HELLMAN, L., GALLAGHER, T. F.: The transformation of cholesterol to coprostanol. J. biol. Chem. **211**, 301—311 (1954).

ROSENFELD, R. S., ZUMOFF, B., HELLMAN, L.: Metabolism of coprostanol-^{14}C and cholestanol-4-^{14}C in man. J. Lipid Res. **4**, 337—340 (1963).

ROTHSCHILD, M. A.: The relationship of the liver to the cholesterin metabolism. Proc. N.Y. Pathol. Soc. **14**, 229—238 (1914).

RUBENSTEIN, B., RUBINSTEIN, D.: Interrelationship between rat serum very low density and high
    density lipoproteins. J. Lipid Res. **13**, 317—324 (1972).
RUDEL, L. L., MORRIS, M. D., FELTS, J. M.: The transport of exogenous cholesterol in the rabbit. I.
    Role of cholesterol ester of lymph chylomicra and lymph very low density lipoproteins in
    absorption. J. clin. Invest. **51**, 2686—2692 (1972).
SABA, N., HECHTER, O., STONE, D.: Conversion of cholesterol to pregnenolone in bovine adrenal
    homogenates. J. Amer. chem. Soc. **76**, 3862—3864 (1954).
SAKAKIDA, H., SHEDIAC, C. C., SIPERSTEIN, M. D.: Effect of endogenous and exogenous cholesterol
    on the feedback control of cholesterol synthesis. J. clin. Invest. **42**, 1521—1528 (1963).
SALEN, G. S.: Cholesterol deposition in cerebrotendinous xanthomatosis. Ann. intern. Med. **75**,
    843—851 (1971).
SALEN, G., AHRENS, E. H. JR., GRUNDY, S. M.: Metabolism of β-sitosterol in man. J. clin. Invest.
    49, 952—967 (1970).
SAMUEL, P., PERL, W., HOLTZMAN, C., ROCHMAN, N. D., LIEBERMAN, S.: Long term kinetics of
    serum and xanthoma cholesterol radioactivity in patients with hypercholesterolemia. J. clin.
    Invest. **51**, 266—278 (1972).
SAYERS, G.: The adrenal cortex and homeostasis. Physiol. Rev. **30**, 241—320 (1950).
SAYERS, G., SAYERS, M. A., FRY, E. G., WHITE, A., LONG, E. N. H.: The effect of adrenotrophic hor-
    mone of the anterior pituitary on the cholesterol content of the adrenals. Yale J. Biol. Med.
    16, 361—392 (1944).
SCHERSTEN, T., NILSSON, S., CAHLIN, E., FILIPSON, M., BRODIN-PERSSON, A.: Relationship between
    the biliary excretion of bile acids and the excretion of water, lecithin and cholesterol in man.
    Europ. J. clin. Invest. **1**, 242—247 (1971).
SCHOTZ, M. C., RICE, L. I., ALFIN-SLATER, R. B.: Further studies on cholesterol in liver cell frac-
    tions of normal and cholesterol fed rats. J. biol. Chem. **204**, 19—26 (1953).
SCHREIBMAN, P. J.: Cholesterol metabolism in human adipose tissue. Bull. N.Y. Acad. Med. **50**,
    413, 1974.
SEBESIN, S. M., ISSELBACHER, K. J.: Protein synthesis inhibition: Mechanism for the production of
    impaired fat absorption. Science **147**, 1149—1150 (1965).
SEEGERS, W., HIRSCHHORN, K., BURNETT, L., ROBSON, E., HARRIS, H.: Double beta lipoprotein: A
    new genetic variant in man. Science **149**, 303—304 (1965).
SEIDEL, D., ALAUPOVIC, P., FURMAN, R. H.: A lipoprotein characterizing obstructive jaundice. I.
    Method for quantitative separation and identification of lipoproteins in jaundiced subjects. J.
    clin. Invest. **48**, 1211—1223 (1969).
SHAH, S. N., LOSSOW, W. J., CHAIKOFF, I. L.: The esterification of cholesterol in vitro by rat plasma.
    I. Relative participation of triglycerides and phospholipids. II. Effect of snake venom.
    Biochim. biophys. Acta (Amst.) **84**, 176—181 (1964).
SHAPIRO, D. J., RODWELL, V. W.: Diurnal variation and cholesterol regulation of hepatic HMG—
    CoA reductase activity. Biochem. Biophys. Res. Commun. **37**, 867—872 (1969).
SHAPIRO, I. L., DAVIDSON, L. M., KRITCHEVSKY, D.: Free cholesterol exchange in vitro: A compar-
    ison of endogenous and exogenous cholesterol. Proc. Soc. exp. Biol. (N.Y.) **133**, 993—996
    (1970).
SHORE, B., SHORE, V.: Heterogeneity in protein subunits of human serum high density lipopro-
    teins. Biochemistry **7**, 2773—2777 (1968).
SHORE, B., SHORE, V.: Isolation and characterization of polypeptides of human serum lipopro-
    teins. Biochemistry **8**, 4510—4516 (1969).
SHRIVASTAVA, B. K., REDGRAVE, T. G., SIMMONDS, W. J.: The source of endogenous lipid in the
    thoracic duct lymph of fasting rats. Quart. J. exp. Physiol. **52**, 305—312 (1967).
SIMMONDS, W. J., HOFMANN, A. F., THEODOR, E.: Absorption of cholesterol from micellar solution:
    Intestinal perfusion studies in man. J. clin. Invest. **46**, 874—890 (1967).
SIMON, J. B.: Red cell lipids in liver disease: Relationship to serum lipids and to lecithin-choles-
    terol acyltransferase. J. Lab. clin. Med. **77**, 891—900 (1971).
SIPERSTEIN, M. D.: Comparison of the feedback control of cholesterol metabolism in liver and
    hepatomas in developmental and metabolic control mechanism and neoplasia, pp. 427—451.
    Baltimore, Maryland: Williams and Wilkins 1965.
SIPERSTEIN, M. D.: Regulation of cholesterol biosynthesis in normal and malignant tissues. Cur-
    rent topics Cell Reg. **2**, 65—100 (1970).

SIPERSTEIN, M. D., MURRAY, A. W.: Cholesterol metabolism in man. J. clin. Invest. **34**, 1449—1453 (1955).

SIPERSTEIN, M. D., GUEST, M. H.: Studies on the site of the feedback control of cholesterol synthesis. J. clin. Invest. **39**, 642—652 (1960).

SIPERSTEIN, M. D., FAGAN, V. M.: Studies on the feedback regulation of cholesterol synthesis. Advanc. Enzyme Regul. **2**, 249—264 (1964).

SIPERSTEIN, M. D., FAGAN, V. M.: Feedback control of mevalonate synthesis by dietary cholesterol. J. biol. Chem. **241**, 602—609 (1966).

SIPERSTEIN, M. D., CHAIKOFF, I. L., REINHARDT, W. O.: ^{14}C cholesterol: V. obligatory function of bile in intestinal absorption of cholesterol. J. biol. Chem. **198**, 111—114 (1952a).

SIPERSTEIN, M. D., JAYKO, M. E., CHAIKOFF, I. L., DAUBEN, W. A.: Nature of the metabolic products of ^{14}C cholesterol excreted in bile and feces. Proc. Soc. exp. Biol. (N.Y.) **81**, 720—724 (1952b).

SMALL, D. M., DOWLING, R. H., REDINGER, R. N.: The enterohepatic circulation of bile salts. Arch. intern. Med. **130**, 552—573 (1972).

SMITH, A. L., TREADWELL, C. R.: Effect of bile acids and other factors on cholesterol uptake by inverted intestinal sacs. Amer. J. Physiol. **193**, 34—40 (1958).

SMITH, E. B.: The influence of age and atherosclerosis on the chemistry of aortic intima. I. The lipids. J. Atheroscler. Res. **5**, 241—248 (1965).

SMITH, E. B., EVANS, P. H., DOWNHAM, M. D.: Lipid in the aortic intima: The correlation of morphological and chemical characteristics. J. Atheroscler. Res. **7**, 171—186 (1967).

SNOG-KJAER, A., PRANGE, I., DAM, H.: Conversion of cholesterol into coprosterol by bacteria in vitro. J. gen. Microbiol. **14**, 256—260 (1956).

SODHI, H. S.: Disposition of dietary versus endogenous cholesterol: The fate of dietary lipids. In: G. COWGILL, L. W. KINSELL, (Eds.): Proceed. of the 1967 Deuel Conference on lipids, pp. 75—87. Washington, D.C.: U.S. Government Printing Office 1967.

SODHI, H. S.: New lipoprotein differing in charge and density from known plasma lipoproteins. Metabolism **18**, 852—859 (1969).

SODHI, H. S.: Relative rates of absorption into lymph of dietary and endogenous cholesterol from intestinal mucosa and their signficance. Circulation **46**, II—276 (1972).

SODHI, H. S.: Current concepts of cholesterol metabolism and their relationship to lecithin:cholesterol acyltransferase. Scand. J. clin. Lab. Invest. **33**, Suppl. 137, 161—163 (1974).

SODHI, H. S., KALANT, N.: Hyperlipemia of antiserum nephrosis. I. Rate of synthesis of plasma cholesterol. Metabolism **12**, 404—413 (1963a).

SODHI, H. S., KALANT, N.: Hyperlipemia of antiserum nephrosis. II. Turnover of plasma cholesterol. Metabolism **12**, 414—419 (1963b).

SODHI, H. S., KALANT, N.: Hyperlipemia of antiserum nephrosis. III. Plasma lipoproteins. Metabolism **12**, 420—427 (1963c).

SODHI, H. S., GOULD, R. G.: Interactions of apoHDL with HDL and with other lipoproteins. Atherosclerosis **12**, 439—450 (1970).

SODHI, H. S., KUDCHODKAR, B. J.: Is there a need for in vitro incorporation of radioactive cholesterol into plasma lipoproteins? Circulation **42**, III-24 (1970).

SODHI, H. S., KUDCHODKAR, B. J.: Acute effects of change in concentrations of plasma cholesterol on the fluxes of cholesterol from adipose and other normal tissues in man. Endocrinology **88**, A258 (1971a).

SODHI, H. S., KUDCHODKAR, B. J.: Relationship of hypertriglyceridemia and endogenous synthesis of cholesterol in man. Circulation **44**, II—57 (1971b).

SODHI, H. S., KUDCHODKAR, B. J.: Catabolism of plasma cholesterol in man; a new hypothesis. Clin. Res. **20**, 946 (1972a).

SODHI, H. S., KUDCHODKAR, B. J.: A new hypothesis correlating metabolism of cholesterol with the type of hyperlipoproteinemia in man. Clin. Res. **20**, 946 (1972b).

SODHI, H. S., KUDCHODKAR, B. J.: Hypothesis correlating metabolism of plasma and tissue cholesterol with that of plasma lipoproteins. Lancet **1973a I**, 513—519.

SODHI, H. S., KUDCHODKAR, B. J.: Synthesis of cholesterol in hypercholesterolemia and its relationship to plasma triglycerides. Metabolism **22**, 895—912 (1973b).

SODHI, H. S., KUDCHODKAR, B. J.: Catabolism of cholesterol in hypercholesterolemia and its relationship to plasma triglycerides. Clin. chim. Acta **46**, 161—171 (1973c).

SODHI, H. S., KUDCHODKAR, B. J.: Labelling plasma lipoproteins with radioactive cholesterol. J. Lab. clin. Med. **82**, 111—124 (1973 d).

SODHI, H. S., WOOD, P. D. S., SCHLIERF, G., KINSELL, L. W.: Plasma, bile and fecal sterols in relation to diet. Metabolism **16**, 334—343 (1967 a).

SODHI, H. S., BERGER, E. A., GOULD, R. G.: Evidence for two pools of cholesterol in small intestines. Fed. Proc. **26**, 471 (1967 b).

SODHI, H. S., HORLICK, L., KUDCHODKAR, B. J.: Evidence for net transfer of cholesterol from tissues into plasma. Clin. Res. **17**, 395 (1969).

SODHI, H. S., ORCHARD, R., AGNISH, N.: Pools of exogenous and endogenous cholesterol in the intestines of the rat. Clin. Res. **18**, 373 (1970).

SODHI, H. S., KUDCHODKAR, B. J., HORLICK, L.: Hypocholesterolemic agents and mobilization of tissue cholesterol in man. Atherosclerosis **17**, 1—19 (1973 a).

SODHI, H. S., BERGER, E. A., SWYRYD, E. A., GOULD, R. G.: Studies on the metabolism and fate of intestinal cholesterol. Circulation **32**, II-11 (1965).

SODHI, H. S., KUDCHODKAR, B. J., HORLICK, L., WEDER, C. H.: Effects of chlorophenoxyisobutyrate on the synthesis and metabolism of cholesterol in man. Metabolism **20**, 348—359 (1971 a).

SODHI, H. S., HORLICK, L., NAZIR, D. J., KUDCHODKAR, B. J.: A simple method for calculating absorption of dietary cholesterol in man. Proc. Soc. exp. Biol. (N.Y.) **137**, 277—279 (1971 b).

SODHI, H. S., ORCHARD, R. C., AGNISH, N. D., VARUGHESE, P. V., KUDCHODKAR, B. J.: Separate pools for endogenous and exogenous cholesterol in rat intestines. Atherosclerosis **17**, 197—210 (1973).

SODHI, H. S., SUNDARAM, G. S., MACKENZIE, S. L.: Isoelectric fractionation of plasma high density lipoproteins. Scand. J. clin. Lab. Invest. **33**, Suppl. 137, 71—72 (1974).

SPERRY, W. M.: The relationship between total and free cholesterol in human blood serum. J. biol. Chem. **114**, 125—133 (1936).

SPIRO, M. J., MCKIBBIN, J. M.: The lipides of rat liver cell fractions. J. biol. Chem. **219**, 643—651 (1956).

SPRITZ, N., AHRENS, E. H., GRUNDY, S. M.: Sterol balance in man as plasma cholesterol concentrations are altered by exchanges of dietary fats. J. clin. Invest. **44**, 1482—1493 (1965).

SRERE, P. A., CHAIKOFF, I. L., TREITMAN, S. S., BURSTEIN, L. S.: The extrahepatic synthesis of cholesterol. J. biol. Chem. **182**, 629—634 (1950).

STAMLER, J.: The problem of elevated blood cholesterol. Amer. J. Publ. Hlth **50**, 14—19 (1960).

STAPLE, E.: In: SCHIFF, L., CAREY, J. B. JR., DIETSCHY, J. M. (Eds.): Mechanism of cleavage of the cholestane side chain in bile acid formation/Bile salt metabolism, pp. 127—139. Springfield, Ill.: Charles C. Thomas 1969.

STAPLE, E., GURIN, S.: The incorporation of radioactive acetate into biliary cholesterol and cholic acid. Biochim. biophys. Acta **15**, 372—376 (1954).

STEIN, O., STEIN, Y., GOODMAN, D. S., FIDGE, N. H.: The metabolism of chylomicron cholesteryl ester in rat liver: A combined radioautographic electron microscopic and biochemical study. J. Cell Biol. **43**, 410—431 (1969).

STEINER, A., HOWARD, E. J., AKGUN, S.: Importance of dietary cholesterol in man. J. Amer. med. Ass. **181**, 186—190 (1962).

SUBBIAH, M. T. R., KOTTKE, B. A., CARLO, I. A.: Experimental studies in the spontaneous atherosclerosis-susceptible white carneau pigeon: nature of biliary and fecal neutral steroids. Mayo Clin. **45**, 729—737 (1970).

SUGANO, M., PORTMAN, O. W.: Fatty acid specificities and rates of cholesterol esterification in vivo and in vitro. Arch. Biochem. Biophys. **107**, 341—351 (1964).

SUNDARAM, G. S., SODHI, H. S., MACKENZIE, S. L.: Heterogeneity of human plasma high density lipoprotein. Proc. Soc. exp. Biol. (N.Y.) **141**, 842—845 (1972).

SWANN, A., SIPERSTEIN, M. D.: Distribution of cholesterol feedback control in the guinea pig. J. clin. Invest. **51**, 95 a (1972).

SWELL, L., LAW, M. D.: Release of lipoprotein cholesterol esters by the isolated perfused rat liver. Biochim. biophys. Acta (Amst.) **231**, 302—313 (1971).

SWELL, L., BYRON, J. E., TREADWELL, C. R.: Cholesterol esterases. IV. cholesterol esterase of rat intestinal mucosa. J. biol. Chem. **186**, 543—548 (1950).

SWELL, L., FIELD, H. JR., TREADWELL, C. R.: Role of bile salts in activity of cholesterol esterase. Proc. Soc. exp. Biol. (N.Y.) **84**, 417—420 (1953).

Swell, L., Boiler, T. A., Field, H. Jr., Treadwell, C. R.: Absorption of dietary cholesterol esters. Amer. J. Physiol. **180**, 129—132 (1955).

Swell, L., Trout, E. C., Jr., Field, H. Jr., Treadwell, C. R.: Regulation of liver cholesterol synthesis by lymph cholesterol. Science **125**, 1194—1195 (1957).

Swell, L., Trout, E. C. Jr., Hopper, J. R., Field, H. Jr., Treadwell, C. R.: Mechanism of cholesterol absorption. 1. Endogenous dilution and esterification of fed cholesterol 4^{14}C. J. biol. Chem. **232**, 1—8 (1958).

Swell, L., Trout, E. C. Jr., Hopper, J. R., Field, H. Jr., Treadwell, C. R.: The mechanism of cholesterol absorption. Ann. N.Y. Acad. Si. Sci. **72**, 813—825 (1959a).

Swell, L., Trout, E. C., Field, H. Jr., Treadwell, C. R.: Absorption of $H^3\beta$-sitosterol in the lymph fistula rat. Proc. Soc. exp. Biol. (N.Y.) **100**, 140—142 (1959b).

Swell, L., Trout, E. C. Jr., Field, H. Jr., Treadwell, C. R.: Labelling of intestinal and lymph cholesterol after administration of tracer doses of cholesterol-4-^{14}C Proc. Soc. exp. Biol. (N.Y.) **101**, 519—521 (1959c).

Swell, L., Field, H. Jr., Schools, P. E. Jr., Treadwell, C. R.: Fatty acid composition of tissue cholesterol esters in elderly humans with atherosclerosis. Proc. Soc. exp. Biol. (N.Y.) **103**, 651—655 (1960).

Swell, L., Stutzman, E., Law, M. D., Treadwell, C. R.: Intestinal metabolism of epicholesterol -4-^{14}C. Arch. Biochem. Biophys. **97**, 411—416 (1962).

Swell, L., Bell, C. C., Enteman, C.: Bile acids and lipid metabolism. III. Influence of bile acids on phospholipids in liver and bile of the isolated perfused dog liver. Biochim. biophys. Acta (Amst.) **164**, 278—284 (1968).

Sylvén, C., Borgstrom, B.: Absorption and lymphatic transport of cholesterol in the rat. J. Lipid Res. **9**, 596—601 (1968).

Sylvén, C., Borgstrom, B.: Intestinal absorption and lymphatic transport of cholesterol in the rat. Influence of the fatty acid chain length of the carrier triglycerides. J. Lipid Res. **10**, 351—355 (1969).

Taylor, C. B., Gould, R. G.: Effect of dietary cholesterol on rate of cholesterol synthesis in the intact animal measured by means of radioactive carbon. Circulation **2**, 467—468 (1950).

Taylor, C. B., Patton, D., Yogi, N., Cox, G. E.: Diet as source of serum cholesterol in man. Proc. Soc. exp. Biol. (N.Y.) **103**, 768—772 (1960).

Taylor, C. B., Cox, G. E., Manalo-Estrella, P.: Atherosclerosis in rhesus monkeys: II. Arterial lesions associated with hypercholesterolemia induced by dietary fat and cholesterol. Arch. Path. **74**, 16—34 (1962).

Tomkins, G. M., Chaikoff, I. L.: Cholesterol synthesis by liver. I. Influence of fasting and of diet. J. biol. Chem. **196**, 569—573 (1952).

Tomkins, G. M., Sheppard, H., Chaikoff, I. L.: Cholesterol synthesis by liver. III. Its regulation by ingested cholesterol. J. biol. Chem. **201**, 137—141 (1953).

Tourtellotte, W. W., Skrentry, B. A., Dejong, R. N.: A study of lipids in the cerebrospinal fluid. IV. The determination of free and total cholesterol. J. Lab. clin. Med. **54**, 197—206 (1959).

Treadwell, C. R., Vahouny, G. V.: Cholesterol Absorption. Handbook of Physiology: A critical, comprehensive presentation of physiological knowledge and concepts. Section 6. Alimentary canal, Vol. 3, pp. 1407—1438. Intestinal Absorption. Section editor: C.F. Code. Washington, D.C.: Amer. Physiol. Soc. 1968.

Vahouny, G. V., Treadwell, C. R.: Absorption of cholesterol esters in the lymph fistula rat. Amer. J. Physiol. **195**, 516—520 (1958).

Vahouny, G. V., Gregorian, H. M., Treadwell, C. R.: Comparative effects of bile acids on intestinal absorption of cholesterol. Proc. Soc. exp. Biol. (N.Y.) **101**, 538—540 (1959).

Vahouny, G. V., Weersing, S., Treadwell, C. R.: Taurocholate protection of cholesterol esterase against proteolytic inactivation. Biochim. Biophys. Res. Commun. **15**, 224—229 (1964).

Vahouny, G. V., Weersing, S., Treadwell, C. R.: Function of specific bile acids in cholesterol esterase activity in vitro. Biochim. biophys. Acta (Amst.) **98**, 607—616 (1965).

Vandenheuvel, F. A.: The origin, metabolism and structure of normal human serum lipoproteins. Canad. J. Biochem. Physiol. **40**, 1299—1326 (1962).

Vandenheuvel, F. A.: Structure of membranes and role of lipids therein. Advanc. Lipid Res. **9**, 161—248 (1971).

VANDENHEUVEL, F. A.: 1973 (Personal communication).

VELA, B. A., ACEVEDO, H. F.: Urinary cholesterol. I. Isolation and characterization of "free" cholesterol in normal and pregnant subjects. J. clin. Endocr. **29**, 1251—1258 (1969).

WALTON, K. W., WILLIAMSON, N.: Histological and immunofluorescent studies on the evolution of the human atheromatous plaque. J. Atheroscler. Res. **8**, 599—624 (1968).

WALTON, K. W., SCOTT, P. J., JONES, V. J., FLETCHER, R. F., WHITEHEAD, T.: Studies on low density lipoprotein turnover in relation to atromid therapy. J. Atheroscler. Res. **3**, 396—414 (1963).

WATTS, H. F.: In: JONES, R. J. (Ed.): Role of lipoproteins in the formation of atherosclerotic lesions in evolution of the atherosclerotic plaque, p. 117. Chicago: University of Chicago Press 1963.

WEIS, H. J., DIETSCHY, J. M.: Failure of bile acids to control hepatic cholesterogenesis: Evidence for endogenous cholesterol feedback. J. clin. Invest. **48**, 2398—2408 (1969).

WELLS, V. M., BRONTE-STEWART, B.: Egg yolk and serum cholesterol levels. Importance of dietary cholesterol intake. Brit. med. J. **1963 I**, 577—581. WERBIN, H., PLOTZ, J., LEROY, G. V., DAYIS, E. M.: Cholesterol — a precursor of estrone in vivo, J. Amer. chem. Soc. **79**, 1012—1013 (1957).

WHEELER, H. O., KING, K. K.: Biliary excretion of lecithin and cholesterol in the dog. J. clin. Invest. **51**, 1337—1350 (1972).

WILSON, D. E., LEES, R. S.: Metabolic relationships among the plasma lipoproteins. Reciprocal changes in the concentrations of very low and low density lipoproteins. J. clin. Invest. **51**, 1051—1057 (1972).

WILSON, J. D.: Influence of dietary cholesterol on excretion of cholesterol -4-^{14}C by the rat. Amer. J. Physiol. **202**, 1073—1076 (1962).

WILSON, J. D.: Biosynthetic origin of serum cholesterol in the squirrel monkey: Evidence for a contribution by the intestinal wall. J. clin. Invest. **47**, 175—187 (1968).

WILSON, J. D.: The measurement of the exchangeable pools of cholesterol in the baboon. J. clin. Invest. **49**, 655—665 (1970).

WILSON, J. D., LINDSEY, C. A. JR.: Studies on the influence of dietary cholesterol on cholesterol metabolism in the isotopic steady state in man. J. clin. Invest. **44**, 1805—1814 (1965).

WILSON, J. D., REINKE, R. T.: Transfer of locally synthesized cholesterol from intestinal wall to intestinal lymph. J. Lipid Res. **9**, 85—92 (1968).

WILSON, T. H.: Intestinal absorption. Philadelphia: Saunders 1962.

WINDMUELLER, H. G., LEVY, R. I.: Production of β-lipoprotein by intestine in the rat. J. biol. Chem. **243**, 4878—4884 (1968).

WOOD, P. D. S., HATOFF, D.: Incubation of human fecal homogenates with 4-^{14}C cholesterol. Lipids **5**, 702—706 (1970).

WOOD, P. D. S., GABRIEL, J., KINSELL, L.: Turnover of individual plasma cholesterol esters in humans on diets rich in different fats. Fed. Proc. **24**, 262 (1965).

WOOD, P. D. S., SHIODA, R., KINSELL, L. W.: Dietary regulation of cholesterol metabolism Lancet **1966 II**, 604—607.

WOSTMANN, B. S., WIECH, N. L., KUNG, E.: Catabolism and elimination of cholesterol in germ free rats. J. Lipid Res. **7**, 77—82 (1966).

ZAFFARONI, A., HECHTER, O., PINCUS, G.: Adrenal conversion of ^{14}C labelled cholesterol and acetate to adrenal cortical hormones. J. Amer. chem. Soc. **73**, 1390—1391 (1951).

ZILVERSMIT, D. B.: The design and analysis of isotope experiments. Amer. J. Med. **29**, 832—848 (1960).

ZILVERSMIT, D. B.: Exchange of phospholipid classes between liver, microsomes and plasma. Comparison of rat, rabbit and guinea pig. J. Lipid Res. **12**, 36—42 (1971).

ZILVERSMIT, D. B.: A single blood sample dual isotope method for the measurement of cholesterol absorption. Proc. Soc. exp. Biol. (N.Y.) **140**, 862—865 (1972).

ZILVERSMIT, D. B., COURTICE, F. C., FRASER, R.: Cholesterol transport in thoracic duct lymph of the rabbit. J. Atheroscler. Res. **7**, 319—329 (1967).

CHAPTER 3

Bile Acid Metabolism

T. A. MIETTINEN

With 3 Figures

I. Introduction

Bile acids which are formed from cholesterol in the liver via a series of reactions initiated by 7α-hydroxylation of cholesterol (DANIELSSON and EINARSSON, 1969) have several functions in the animal organism. Within the intestinal lumen the biliary bile acids facilitate formation of the micellar phase which appears to be obligatory for absorption of cholesterol and plays an essential role in the absorption of fat-soluble vitamins and hydrolysis products of triglycerides during fat digestion. Decrease of the intestinal bile acid concentration below a certain level (critical micellar concentration) prevents formation of the micellar phase, resulting in lipid malabsorption. Within the intestinal mucosa the bile acids seem to promote esterification of cholesterol and fatty acids and to inhibit cholesterol synthesis.

Bile acids form also a catabolic pathway for cholesterol metabolism. As a matter of fact, the cholesterol molecule can be removed from the body only as a bile acid or as cholesterol itself mainly via the intestinal route when biliary secretion and intestinal reabsorption of the two compounds, or of the one or the other, are the major factors determining the overall elimination of steroid nucleus into faeces. The secretion of bile and that of biliary cholesterol are partly dependent on bile acids. Changes in the biliary secretion or intestinal reabsorption of bile acids can markedly alter the metabolism not only of bile acids but also of cholesterol, being reflected ultimately in the blood cholesterol level and possibly also in tissue cholesterol, especially in that of the arterial wall. A relative defect in biliary secretion of bile acids results in formation of supersaturated bile for cholesterol, thus predisposing the development of cholesterol gallstones. In biliary obstruction an impaired biliary bile acid secretion is associated with fat malabsorption, accumulation of bile acids into the blood and tissues, enhanced urinary excretion of bile acids, and marked hypercholesterolaemia which in long-standing obstruction is associated with a decreased cholesterol and bile acid synthesis and an enhanced tissue deposition of cholesterol. But impaired catabolism of cholesterol via bile acids might lead to hypercholesterolaemia even without biliary obstruction; damage to hepatic parenchymal cells reduces bile acid and cholesterol synthesis, the blood cholesterol remaining normal or even subnormal; in familial hypercholesterolaemia the bile acid production is subnormal and may essentially contribute to defective removal of blood cholesterol in that disease. In contributing to the development of the hypercholesterolaemia, a condition believed to enhance formation of arterial atheromata, the impaired catabolism of cholesterol via bile acids may be a significant pathogenetic factor of atherosclerosis.

Therefore, increasing attention has recently been paid to the experimental and clinical conditions in which cholesterol catabolism to bile acids is enhanced. Promotion of endogenous cholesterol synthesis by obesity is associated with enhanced bile acid production. The latter can be induced also indirectly by inhibiting the reabsorption of bile acids (interruption of enterohepatic circulation), thereby enhancing their faecal output, e.g. with ion exchangers or by ileal exclusion. Under these conditions the conversion of cholesterol to bile acids is markedly augmented, resulting, despite increased cholesterol synthesis, in reduction of the blood cholesterol level and possibly also in enhanced flux of tissue cholesterol to the blood. As a rule of thumb it can be said that with some exceptions an increasing elimination of cholesterol as bile acids decreases serum cholesterol, while a diminishing production of bile acids is associated with an increase of the serum cholesterol level.

Many extensive papers and symposia on bile acids have been published in the past (BERGSTRÖM et al., 1960; DANIELSSON, 1963; HASLEWOOD, 1964) and more recently (BOYD and PERCY-ROBB, 1971; DANIELSSON, 1972; DANIELSSON and EINARSSON, 1969; DIETSCHY, 1972; DOWLING, 1972; ELLIOTT and HYDE, 1971; MIETTINEN, 1973; WEINER and LACK, 1968), dealing with different aspects of bile acid synthesis, metabolism and functions in experimental animals and in man. Therefore the present paper does not exhaustively handle the literature in this area but deals primarily with some clinical aspects of bile acid metabolism, especially the role of bile acids in cholesterol catabolism and in the development and treatment of hypercholesterolaemia.

II. Enterohepatic Circulation

Since bile acids are secreted by the liver into the bile, reabsorbed from the intestine and taken up from the portal blood and resecreted by the liver they are said to have an enterohepatic circulation. The amount of bile acids participating in this recirculation forms the bile acid pool. The two major primary bile acids, cholic acid and chenodeoxycholic acid taken up from the portal blood by hepatic parenchymal cells and mixed with a small amount of newly synthesized bile acids, and the main secondary bile acid, deoxycholic acid taken up by the hepatocytes from the portal blood, are excreted as glycine and taurine conjugates into the bile. These three bile acid conjugates form the bulk of biliary bile acids in man (SJÖVALL, 1960). Trace amounts of other primary bile acids, such as trihydroxy- (converted to cholic acid) and dihydroxy- (converted to chenodeoxy-cholic acid) coprostanic acids (CAREY, 1964; CAREY and HASLEWOOD, 1963; STAPLE and RABINOWITZ, 1962), and secondary bile acids, primarily lithocholic, are found in human bile. In some children with intrahepatic bile duct anomalies almost a half of the biliary bile acids consist of trihydroxy coprostanic acid (EYSSEN et al., 1972), which is one of the major bile acids in reptiles (HASLEWOOD, 1964). In addition to the taurine and glycine conjugates human bile contains sulfate and even ornitine derivatives (GORDON et al., 1963; PALMER, 1967; PALMER and BOLT, 1971). Only negligible amounts of the biliary bile acids are in the unconjugated form (PERIC-GOLIA and SOCIC, 1968; POLEY et al., 1964; SJÖVALL, 1960) in man and in most animal species. They may originate either from the liver or are released from their conjugates by bacterial action (NAIR et al., 1967).

It is interesting to note that in the dog a lack of taurine, which apparently develops readily in many species when bile salts are lost excessively, e.g. by biliary drainage or in connection of ileal dysfunction (ABAURRE et al., 1969; GARBUTT et al., 1969; HEATON et al., 1968; McLEOD and WIGGINS, 1968), leads to secretion of unconjugated bile acids into the bile (O'MAILLE and RICHARDS, 1967). Taurine given orally or parenterally usually normalizes the conjugation of bile acids with taurine and restores the high glycine/taurine ratio of bile acid conjugates found in conjunction with interrupted enterohepatic circulation of bile acids (BRUUSGAARD and HESS THAYSEN, 1970; GARBUTT et al., 1969; O'MAILLE and RICHARDS, 1967; SJÖVALL, 1959).

In the morning, after an overnight fast, the bile acid pool is concentrated into the gallbladder, from where it is secreted into the duodenum in connection with the meal by gallbladder contraction. Under these conditions the bile acid concentration of the intestinal contents usually exeeds 4 mmoles/l (BADLEY et al., 1969; BADLEY et al., 1970; VAN DEEST et al., 1968; McLEOD and WIGGINS, 1968; MIETTINEN and SIURALA, 1971a), an especially high concentration being found initially when concentrated gallbladder bile (bile acid concentration above 30 mM) enters the intestinal lumen. In the absence of the gallbladder, e.g. after cholecystectomy, bile salts apparently pass continuously into the intestine; under these conditions the fluctuation of the intestinal bile salt concentration should be less marked than normally (NAHRWOLD and GROSSMAN, 1970). Conjugated bile salts facilitate intestinal absorption of hydrolysis products of triglycerides, sterols and fat soluble vitamins by enhancing their micellar solubilization during fat digestion (cf. BORGSTRÖM, 1960; HOFMANN, 1966; HOFMANN and BORGSTRÖM, 1964; JOHNSTON, 1968; TREADWELL and VAHOUNY, 1968). Under normal conditions intestinal bile acids remain in the conjugated form during fat absorption and are transported downwards by the gut motility because their absorption, especially that of taurine derivatives, is negligible in the proximal small intestine (cf. DIETSCHY, 1968a; WEINER and LACK, 1968). Less polar bile acids, glycine conjugates of chenodeoxy- and deoxycholic acids and unconjugated bile acids (HISLOP et al., 1967), are reabsorbed to a small extent along the whole small intestine by passive diffusion. The terminal ileum reabsorbs bile acid conjugates effectively by an active transport mechanism even against the concentration gradient. Thus the bulk of bile acids entering the terminal ileum is reabsorbed and only traces, about 2 to 5%, escape during each cycle into the colon. Studies (HEPNER et al., 1972; NORMAN, 1970) performed after administration of double labeled conjugates [label(s) present in the steroid moiety and in glycine or taurine] have revealed that in man about 80% of bile acids is normally absorbed in the conjugated form and 20% as free acids. The site of formation of the latter is not known exactly. Though trace amounts of free bile acids are constantly found in the upper intestinal contents (MIETTINEN and SIURALA, 1971a; SJÖVALL, 1960) and though the proximal small intestine effectively absorbs unconjugated bile acids by diffusion (DIETSCHY, 1968a) it is improbable that normally any significant deconjugation would take place in the duodenum and jejunum; this can occur in the terminal ileum, where free bile acids are found in man (NORTHFIELD et al., 1970, 1972), or most likely in the colon. In gastrectomized patients (MIDTVEDT et al., 1970) or in subjects with ileal resection, blind loop or intestinal stasis syndrome (DONALDSON, 1965, HAMILTON et al., 1970; ROSENBERG et al., 1967; TABAQCHALI, 1970; TABAQCHALI and BOOTH, 1966), i.e. in cases with bacterial overgrowth in the proximal small intestine, bacterial deconjugation may become extensive. Unter these conditions the reabsorption of bile acids in unconjugated form is markedly enhanced in the upper intestine (HISLOP et al., 1967), less conjugates being passed to the terminal ileum; then reabsorption should be effective. However, because of the reduced transit time the overall reabsorption of bile acids may be normal or subnormal even in cases in which the terminal ileum is intact. Enhanced deconjugation by bacterial overgrowth can be detected quite sensitively and simply with the breath test (FROMM and HOFMANN, 1971; SHERR et al., 1971). In this procedure glycine-labeled bile acid conjugate is given orally. Glycine released from the conjugate by bacteria is partly converted to $^{14}CO_2$ and can be measured from the expired air; the greater the deconjugation, the greater the specific activity of expired CO_2 and the greater should be the absorption of bile acid in unconjugated form. Despite increased bacterial action the formation of secondary bile acids in the small intestine, first of all 7-dehydroxylation of cholic acid to deoxycholic acid, is not consistently enhanced, as indicated by the intestinal and serum bile acid pattern (ABAURRE et al., 1969; MIDTVEDT et al., 1970; SHIMADA et al., 1969; TABAQCHALI, 1970; TABAQCHALI and BOOTH, 1966; TABAQCHALI et al., 1968).

It is interesting to note that in colectomized patients with ileostoma, in whom the terminal ileum serves as a "reservoir" of intestinal contents and contains large amounts of different bacteria (GORBACH et al., 1967), bacterial transformation of bile acids is quite negligible (MIETTINEN and PELTOKALLIO, 1971; PERCY-ROBB et al., 1969a and b, 1971). Thus, deconjugation is rarely complete in these subjects and deoxycholic acid can be detected in the bile and ileostomal fluid in occasional cases only, unless a small rectal stump is present (MIETTINEN and PELTOKALLIO, 1971). Furthermore, colectomized patients lose quantitatively normal amounts of bile acids into the ileostomal fluid provided that the remaining terminal ileum is quite intact, suggesting that normally only negligible amounts of bile acids are absorbed by the colon, or that after colectomy the remaining gut adapts itself to conserve bile acids effectively.

It seems to be quite clear that of the two bacterial processes, deconjugation and transformation of hydroxyl groups of the steroid nucleus, the former takes place primarily and the latter almost exclusively in the colon under normal conditions (cf. DANIELSSON and EINARSSON, 1969). As a result of 7-dehydroxylation, deoxycholic and lithocholic acids are formed from cholic and chenodeoxycholic acids, respectively, lithocholic acid, as a poorly soluble compound, being reabsorbed only in trace amounts, while deoxycholic acid seems to be reabsorbed from the colon at a higher rate. Usually deconjugation precedes 7-dehydroxylation (NORMAN, 1970), though the latter and subsequent absorption can take place to a certain extent without preceding deconjugation (HEPNER et al., 1972). Though colonic absorption of bile acids is apparent its quantitative significance is unknown (DANIELSSON and EINARSSON, 1969; MEKHJIAN et al., 1968, 1972; SAMUEL et al., 1968; WEINER and LACK, 1968). Estimates in man range from 1 to 15% of the total daily absorption (HEPNER et al., 1972). In view of the quite normal faecal output of bile acids (340 mg as compared to 250 mg/day normally) in colectomized patients (MIETTINEN and PELTOKALLIO, 1971), even the former percentage sounds high because at an assumed total intestinal reabsorption of 20 g/day (calculated from GRUNDY and METZGER, 1972) the colonic contribution would be 200 mg/day.

The small amount of bile acids which is not absorbed by the terminal ileum and subsequently by the colon is quite completely deconjugated by colonic bacteria and excreted into faeces mainly after bacterial transformations affecting chiefly hydroxyl group at position 7 and to a lesser extent at positions 3 and 12. As a result of these processes faecal bile acids are composed of a mixture of about 20 different compounds, the bulk being formed by deoxycholic, lithocholic and isolithocholic acids (DANIELSSON et al., 1963; ENEROTH et al., 1966a and b; ROSENFELD and HELLMAN, 1962).

Reabsorption of both dihydroxy bile acids (deoxy- and chenodeoxycholic acids) in man appears to be similar to and perhaps even better than that of cholic acid (HEPNER et al., 1972). Thus the pattern of bile salts in the portal blood should resemble that in the small intestinal contents (SANDBERG et al., 1965) except that absorption of newly synthesized deoxycholic acid in the colon may increase its proportion in the portal blood mixture. Virtually all of the reabsorbed bile acids, i.e. 5 to 33 g/day (calculated from BRUNNER et al., 1972; GRUNDY and METZGER, 1972), are rapidly cleared by the liver so that the hepatic and consequently also the peripheral venous blood contain only small amounts of bile acids (SANDBERG et al., 1965), their concentration increasing minimally even during digestion or after intraduodenal bile acid infusion when the ileal reabsorption is markedly enhanced (BODE and FRANZ, 1972; KAPLOWITZ et al., 1972; SANDBERG et al., 1965). It has been calculated that normally about 98% of bile acids are transported by the portal blood back to the liver and 2% by the hepatic artery (SMALL et al., 1972). If the hepatic uptake of bile acids is decreased, as in biliary obstruction or parenchymal cell damage, or if the portal vein is occluded the proportion of bile acids released into the general circulation and the subsequent return to the liver via the hepatic artery may increase enormously. The same appears to apply to the intestinal bacterial overgrowth in which the intestinal absorption of free bile acids is increased. Because the latter are apparently bound to plasma albumin (BURKE et al., 1971; RUDMAN and KENDALL, 1957b) their hepatic clearance may be lower (BLUM and SPRITZ, 1966; O'MAILLE and RICHARDS, 1967) than that of conjugated bile acids and consequently the plasma concentration of free bile acids is increased in patients with intestinal bacterial overgrowth (LEWIS et al., 1969).

The liver resecretes rapidly the cleared, either free or conjugated bile acids into the bile in the conjugated form, thus completing the enterohepatic circulation. In some animal species, as in the rat, the secondary bile acids are rehydroxylated back to the primary bile acids before the biliary resecretion (DANIELSSON and EINARSSON, 1969). This type of "reconstruction" has not been detected in man (DANIELSSON and EINARSSON, 1969), though in vitro studies have suggested that 6α-hydroxylation takes place (TRÜLZSCH et al., 1972).

III. Different Parameters of Bile Acid Metabolism

The rate of cholesterol catabolism by way of bile acids (daily bile acid synthesis) is reflected directly in many parameters of bile acid metabolism. Thus, changes in daily bile acid synthesis may alter, for instance, the pool size, biliary secretion rate, intestinal concentration, intestinal reabsorption and faecal excretion of bile acids. On the other hand, a change in one or another of these parameters modifies the rate of bile acid production and may finally alter the cholesterol synthesis and the blood cholesterol level. Understanding of the interplay between the different parameters and their measurement would be important for complete understanding of bile acid metabolism.

A. Pool Size

The size of the bile acids pool can be measured in man by the isotope dilution technique described by Lindstedt (1957). In this procedure a labeled bile acid (either cholic or chenodeoxycholic acid, or both, labeled with different isotopes) is administered and the bile acid pool is sampled serially over 5 to 7 days by duodenal intubation. The semilogarithmic plot of the specific activity of the bile acids shows a straight line. Extrapolation of the line to zero time allows the pool size of the bile acid to be measured, while the slope of the line reveals the turnover (synthesis) and half-life of this bile acid. Since the kinetics of different major bile acids appear to differ (Danielsson et al., 1963; Meihoff and Kern, 1968), the kinetic parameters of the individual bile acids should be measured separately. However, a rough estimate can be obtained if the kinetic characteristics of one is determined, and those of the others are calculated from the relative proportions of the main bile acids (Lindstedt, 1957, 1970). The pool size of the total and individual bile acids varies greatly in different studies; the range of the total bile acid pool appears to be from 2 to 5 g (Austad et al., 1967; Danielsson et al., 1963; Hepner et al., 1972; Hofmann, 1963; Lindstedt, 1957, 1970; Vlahcevic et al., 1971b).

If after an overnight fast a tracer bile acid is given intravenously it is rapidly secreted into the bile and gallbladder, where in man under those conditions the effective bile acid pool is accumulated almost quantitatively (Abaurre et al., 1969; Heaton et al., 1968). Subsequent determination of the specific activity of the tracer bile acid in the duodenal aspirate reveals the size of the pool, which under normal conditions appears to be of the same magnitude as that obtained by the original Lindstedt's method. The intestinal bile salt concentration (Hofmann et al., 1970) and the intestinal bile salt pool (Miettinen, 1971b) during a fat meal also reflect roughly the size of the bile salt pool.

The pool size is known to be decreased in some clinical and experimental conditions, such as ileal dysfunction (Abaurre et al., 1969) and interruption of the enterohepatic circulation in general (Small et al., 1972), liver cirrhosis (Vlahcevic et al., 1971a, 1972a) and gallstone disease (Vlahcevic, 1970, 1972b) and in β-hyperlipoproteinaemia (Einarsson and Hellström, 1972; Wollenweber and Stiehl, 1972). In the latter state the size of the cholic acid pool, but not that of chenodeoxycholic acid, is reduced. Since in many occasions an altered cholesterol synthesis is associated with a comparable change in bile acid production (Dietschy and Wilson, 1970; Miettinen, 1971a, 1973) it is reasonable to assume that the conditions associated with enhanced or reduced cholesterol synthesis lead via promoted or depressed bile acid synthesis to expansion (interrupted enterohepatic circulation excluded) or decrease of the bile acid pool, respectively. Thus patients with pre-β-hyperlipoproteinaemia (Einarsson and Hellström, 1972) and obese subjects probably have a large bile acid pool while fasting (Small et al., 1972), hypothyroidism (HELLSTRÖM and LINDSTEDT, 1964) and hypercholesterolaemia (EINARSSON and HELLSTRÖM, 1972) may reduce the bile acid pool. It should be borne in mind, however, that patients with gallstones frequently are obese yet their bile acid pool is subnormal. Hyperglyceridaemic subjects with present or previous gallstones, on the other hand, may have an increased pool (EINARSSON and HELLSTRÖM, 1972). Oral administration of bile acids can markedly expand the bile acid pool (DANZINGER et al., 1972).

B. Biliary Secretion

Measurement of the daily biliary secretion of bile acids without interrupting the enterohepatic circulation appears to be a difficult task in man, though promising results have been presented recently by GRUNDY and METZGER (1972). These authors infused liquid formula diets with markers at a constant rate and estimated the hourly biliary bile acid secretion rates by marker dilution techniques. The average secretion ranged from 234 to 1440 mg/h, the values being significantly higher on a high fat than low fat diet. BRUNNER et al. (1972) have modified the method by giving the liquid formula by mouth and infusing the markers into the duodenum. As yet no information is available in man about the relationship between biliary secretion of bile acids and their synthesis, pool size, reabsorption and faecal excretion. In Indian women with gallstones, who usually have a small bile acid pool (VLAHCEVIC et al., 1970, 1972b), bile acid secretion is low but its faecal excretion somewhat enhanced, indicating that reabsorption is impaired (GRUNDY et al., 1972). Animal experiments (SMALL et al., 1972) and studies of biliary diversion (SCHERSTÉN et al., 1971; THUREBORN, 1962) indicate that interruption of the enterohepatic circulation by ileal exclusion or biliary diversion, i.e. reduction of ileal reabsorption of bile acids, reduces the biliary secretion of bile acids. This process is diminished by fasting and stimulated by eating, especially by overeating (GARDINER and SMALL, 1972; SARLES et al., 1970; SMALL et al., 1972; SOLOWAY et al., 1971).

C. Intestinal Concentration

It is quite clear that if the biliary bile acid secretion decreases, the bile salt concentration in the upper intestinal contents diminishes and, depending on the degree of this diminution, the critical micellar bile acid concentration may not be reached, resulting in impaired fat and especially sterol absorption. A slightly decreased secretion, as found in gallstone disease (GRUNDY et al., 1972), may have little influence on intestinal bile acids. As already mentioned, studies performed with a fat test meal have indicated that normally the intestinal bile acid concentration during fat digestion is maintained at or above 4 mM even after successive meals. Except biliary secretion, dilution of intestinal contents either by enhanced water secretion, e.g. in the Ellison-Zollinger syndrome, or impaired water absorption, e.g. in the malabsorption syndrome and diabetes, can reduce the intestinal bile salt concentration and may also impair the reabsorption and enterohepatic circulation of bile acids. A reduced intestinal volume probably increases the bile salt concentration and enhances reabsorption. Enhanced absorption of free bile acids in the upper intestine during bacterial overgrowth probably reduces the total bile salt level (TABAQCHALI, 1970) from what it should be without bacterial deconjugation. A low intestinal bile acid concentration due to decreased biliary secretion is found when the portal flux of bile acids to the liver is diminshed in ileal dysfunction (ileal resection, by-pass or inflammation, enhanced motility; cf. MIETTINEN, 1973), when bile acid synthesis is decreased owing to parenchymal cell damage (cirrhosis hepatis or hepatitis; BADLEY et al., 1970; MIETTINEN, and SIURALA, 1967, 1971 b; MODAI and THEODOR, 1970), or when the delivery of bile into the intestine is impaired by intra- and extrahepatic obstruction (VAN DEEST et al., 1968; MCLEOD and WIGGINS, 1968; MIETTINEN and SIURALA, 1971 b) or by gallbladder dysfunction (LOW-BEER et al., 1971; MIETTINEN and PERHEENTUPA, 1971; TURNBERG and GRAHAME, 1970).

D. Reabsorption

As already mentioned, bile acids are mostly absorbed in conjugated form in the terminal ileum by an active mechanism, a small amount being absorbed quite quickly by diffusion in the free form and from the colon. The quantitation of the reabsorption is difficult in man but it can be calculated as the difference between the daily biliary secretion rate and the daily faecal excretion (equals synthesis) or turnover (determined by the isotope dilution technique). Factors regulating reabsorption are poorly understood but it can be inferred that this process is reduced when the intestinal mucosa of the terminal ileum is damaged (atrophy or inflammation), absorptive surface is decreased (ileal exclusion), intestinal transit time is reduced, intestinal motility is too low to allow a proper mixing of the intestinal contents, intestinal contents become bulkier, bile acids are bound to any components of intestinal contents (e.g. ion exchangers, dietary fibres, bacteria), or the chemical structure of bile acids is altered by bacteria (precipitation of non-polar secondary bile acids, e.g. lithocholic acid). Under normal conditions the absorbed fraction of the total circulating bile acid pool is about 95%, though no exact measurements, with simultaneous determination of biliary secretion and faecal excretion, have been performed. It can be calculated from the data of GRUNDY et al. (1972) that in the Indians in whom the two determinations were performed the reabsorption was 96% in women with gallstones and 98% in men without gallstones. The reason for this decrease of reabsorption in patients with gallstones is not yet clear.

The capacity of the intestine to reabsorb bile acids is not known; biliary secretion data indicate that normally reabsorption ranges from 5 to 33 g/day (GRUNDY and METZGER, 1972). In view of these high figures it is interesting to note that a single 1 to 1.5 g oral dose of bile acids may sometimes overload reabsorption and result in diarrhoea. Owing to recirculation and limited reduction of endogenous production the actual absolute increase in the bile acid load to the small intestine and in reabsorption may markedly exceed the oral dose, however. Continuous oral administration of bile acids, used, e.g., in the medical treatment of gallstone disease (DANZINGER et al., 1972), finally exceeds the reabsorption capacity in every case provided the daily dose exceeds the endogenous synthesis. Under these conditions the reabsorption and the reduction of endogenous synthesis determine the magnitude of bile acid pool expansion. A marked increase in reabsorption may take place in the conditions in which endogenous bile acid production is primarily increased, as in obesity. Thus, one of the present author's obese patients excreted exceptionally high amounts, 1.5 g, into faeces without diarrhoea. At the 96% reabsorption level this would mean a 38 g daily load of bile acid to the small intestine, this figure being 70 g at the 98% reabsorption. Turnover data have indicated that some hyperglyceri-daemic patients would produce daily (and excrete into faeces) more than 2 g of bile acids (KOTTKE, 1969; EINARSSON and HELLSTRÖM, 1972; WOLLENWEBER and STIEHL, 1972), exposing the small intestine to a 45 to 100 g daily bile acid load at 96 to 98% reabsorption.

E. Number of Enterohepatic Circulations

Determination of the number of enterohepatic cycles can be performed only when the daily biliary secretion rate and the pool size are known. Then, the secretion rate divided by the pool size equals the number of cycles. No exact information is available regarding the number or alterations in the number of cycles. According to earlier experiments in man (BORGSTRÖM et al., 1963) the pool has been estimated to circulate three times per meal. Assuming that the mean secretion rate is 800 mg/h according to GRUNDY and METZGER (1972) and the mean pool size 3 g it can be calculated that the bile acid pool circulates six times daily, a figure which has been reported according to more recent experiments (BRUNNER et al., 1972; HEPNER et al., 1972). Since during fasting most of the bile salt pool is located in the gallbladder (ABAURRE et al., 1969), fasting can markedly reduce the number of daily circulations (SMALL et al., 1972) while frequent meals apparently increase it. Continuous biliary secretion of bile in cholecystectomized subjects may also increase the number of daily cycles. The latter may be reduced in subjects with sluggish gallbladder contraction.

F. Faecal Excretion

Daily loss of bile acids into faeces must be balanced by equal hepatic synthesis from cholesterol so as to keep the size of the bile acid pool constant. Thus, faecal bile acids reveal the daily synthesis of bile acids and catabolism of cholesterol by way of bile acids. The measurement can be performed either with chemical analyses (GRUNDY et al., 1965), turnover technique (LINDSTEDT, 1957) or isotope balance (GRUNDY and AHRENS, JR., 1966; MOORE et al., 1962; ROSENFELD and HELLMAN, 1962). At the 96% reabsorption and 800 mg/h (19.2 g/day) biliary secretion it can be calculated that about 750 mg of bile acids escapes daily into the stools. This figure is clearly higher than the value of 250 mg/day obtained by the direct chemical measurement (chemical balance) of faecal bile acids (MIETTINEN, 1973). The discrepancy between the two values is not known, but the fraction of reabsorption may be higher and/or the biliary secretion lower. The measurement of bile acid kinetics also indicates that, for unknown reasons, the isotopic turnover of bile acids is higher than that revealed by chemical analyses of faecal bile acids. In the isotopic balance method radioactive cholesterol is administered either orally or parenterally and after the isotopic steady state is reached the faecal bile acids can be quantitated by dividing the radioactivity in faecal acidic steroids by the specific activity of blood cholesterol. The half life of faecal bile acids can be obtained by measuring the daily faecal excretion of radioactivity after administration of labeled bile acids (LINDSTEDT and NORMAN, 1956;

MEIHOFF and KERN, JR., 1968; STANLEY and NEMCHAUSKY, 1967). Faecal bile acid excretion is markedly increased in the conditions in which ileal reabsorption of bile acids is decreased, as in ileal dysfunction, altered intestinal motility or trapping of bile acids by intestinal contents. It is owing to the enhanced drainage of serum cholesterol into the faeces as bile acids that a negative correlation can be found between the serum cholesterol level and the faecal bile acids under those conditions, indicating that the higher the faecal loss of bile acids the lower the serum cholesterol level (MIETTINEN, 1971 b). On the other hand, even under basal conditions a similar negative correlation can be detected in hypercholesterolaemic subjects, indicating that an impaired bile acid production can contribute to the development of hyper-cholesterolaemia (MIETTINEN, 1969, 1970 b, 1971 c, 1973 a and b). Studies in primates have also suggested that plasma cholesterol levels may rise solely as a result of a reduced excretion of bile acids (LOFLAND et al., 1972). A primarily enhanced bile acid synthesis occurring in obesity and in certain types of hyperglyceridaemia(s) can also increase the faecal bile salt excretion (MIETTINEN, 1971 a), while a diminished output is found if the biliary secretion is reduced in connection with impaired hepatic parenchymal cell function or biliary obstruction (MIETTINEN, 1972 a). Fasting and negative calorie balance (MIETTINEN, 1968 b, 1970 b, 1973; STANLEY, 1970) as well as hypercholesterolaemia (MIETTINEN, 1973) reduce faecal bile acid excretion.

G. Serum Bile Acids

Under normal conditions only a small amount of bile acids, 30 to 230 µg/100 ml, are present in serum (SANDBERG et al., 1965). In patients with disturbed liver function the removal of bile acids from the circulation is slow (BLUM and SPRITZ, 1966; THEODOR et al., 1968). Thus, markedly high plasma bile acid levels have been found in liver cirrhosis and other hepatobiliary disorders, especially in biliary obstruction (CAR-EY, JR., 1958; CRONHOLM et al., 1970; FROSCH and WAGENER, 1968 a and b; MAKINO et al., 1969; SJÖVALL and SJÖVALL, 1966; NEALE et al., 1971; ROOVERS et al., 1968; RUD-MAN and KENDALL, 1957 a; SANDBERG et al., 1965), indicating that because of defective uptake by parenchymal cells, of biliary obstruction and/or of portal-systemic shunts a sizeable portion of the enterohepatic bile acid pool is located in the systemic circulation and tissues. Under these conditions any increase of intestinal bile acid absorption may markedly raise the plasma level. As a matter of fact, serum bile acids can increase several fold postprandially (KAPLOWITZ et al., 1972), after intraduodenal taurocholate infusion (BODE and FRANZ, 1972), or after oral bile acid administration (CAREY, JR., 1958) in patients with impaired liver function while normally only a negligible change is recorded. The pattern of serum bile acids may be markedly altered in different hepatobiliary diseases (cf. CAREY, JR., 1973). In biliary occlusion the proportion of cholic acid increases conspicuously, a change found also in liver tissue (GREIM et al., 1972) and interpreted to be the result of a protective pathway favouring the production of cholic acid. The latter, in contrast to chenodeoxycholic and lithocholic acids (MIYAI et al., 1971; PALMER, 1972), has been shown to be relatively little toxic for the liver (BOYD et al., 1966). In severe forms of biliary obstruction the liver apparently starts to synthesize abnormal bile acids (MAKINO et al., 1971; MURPHY and BILLING, 1972). Under those conditions unsaturated mono-hydroxy bile acids can be found in the blood and comprise up to 35% of the serum bile acids (MURPHY et al., 1972a and b). Cholestyramine, which is known to reduce elevated serum bile acid levels (CAREY,JR. and WILLIAMS 1961; DATTA and SHERLOCK, 1963; VAN ITALLIE and HASHIM, 1963; LOTTSFELDT et al., 1963; NEALE et al., 1971; SJÖVALL and SJÖVALL, 1966), appears to decrease the serum concentration of these abnormal bile acids in patients with biliary cirrhosis (MURPHY et al., 1972b), indicating that these compounds have an enterohepatic circulation because they apparently are not formed by bacteria in the gastrointestinal tract. It is interesting to note that in cholestyramine treated rats the ligation of bile ducts increases the plasma bile acids only slightly (BOYD et al., 1966), suggesting that bile acid synthesis acutally is low in biliary obstruction. Patients with intrahepatic cholestasis respond by a marked reduction in plasma bile acids to phenobarbital treatment (EARNEST, 1972; STIEHL et al., 1972).

In liver cirrhosis chenodeoxycholic acid predominates in the bile acid pattern, the proportion of deoxycholic acid being characteristically low (cf. CAREY,JR., 1973; MIETTINEN, 1973). Under these conditions the formation of lithocholic acid from chenodeoxycholic acid can be increased and lithocholic acid has been associated with the development of liver damage (cf. PALMER, 1972). Lithocholic acid can be frequently found in high concentrations in the serum of cirrhotic patients (CAREY,JR. and WILLIAMS, 1965; CAREY,JR. et al., 1967).

H. Urinary Bile Acids

Urine contains normally only negligible amounts (usually less than 2 mg/day; MIETTINEN, 1973) of bile acids, partly because the renal clearance of these compounds is quite low (GREGG, 1968; GRUNDY et al., 1965; RUDMAN and KENDALL, 1957a). This applies only to unconjugated bile acids and to taurine and glycine conjugates; the renal clearance of sulfate conjugates is much higher and the mono-, di- and trisulfates of bile acids, which apparently form the bulk of urinary bile acids, have been recently detected in the urine of subjects with biliary obstruction (ADMIRAND et al., 1972; STIEHL, 1972). It is owing to the high renal clearance (about 100-fold as compared to non-sulfated derivatives) that the concentration of these derivatives is usually low in serum. Thus, because the sulfation of different bile acids may vary, the pattern of urinary bile acids may differ from that of the plasma especially in biliary obstruction; furthermore, under these conditions the plasma bile acid pool consists apparently of two compartments, a small sulfated pool with a fast turnover and a larger non-sulfated pool with a relatively slow turnover. Urinary bile acids cleared from the latter pool may originate directly from reabsorbed bile acids and to a lesser extent form bile acids regurgitating from bile canaliculi, while bile acids of the plasma sulfated pool apparently originate mostly from the liver. Sulfated unsaturated monohydroxy bile acids have been found in urine, too (BACK, 1972; MAKINO et al., 1971). Since in biliary obstruction the normal excretory pathway of bile acids into the bile is blocked, an excessive accumulation of poorly cleared taurine and glycine conjugates into the blood stream is partly prevented by the production of sulfate conjugates with a high renal clearance. The urine of patients with cholestasis is known to contain, in addition to the normal components cholic, deoxycholic, chenodeoxycholic and lithocholic acids, also ursodeoxycholic acid and various unsaturated monohydroxy bile acids (BACK, 1972; MAKINO et al., 1971), suggesting that

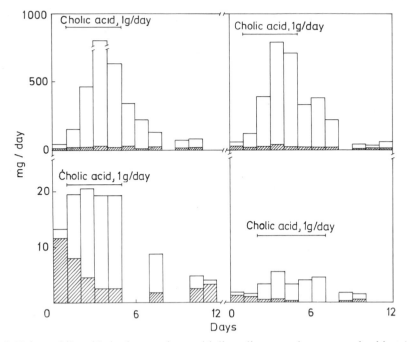

Fig. 1. Urinary bile acids in three patients with liver disease and one normal subject (right lower panel) prior to, during and after oral cholic acid 1 g/day. Chenodeoxycholic acid and lithocholic acid are indicated by shaded part of the columns. Interrupted column (left upper panel) amounted to 1427 mg/day

under those conditions the mithochondrial pathway described by MITROPOULOS and MYANT (1967) *in vitro* for lithocholic acid synthesis in the rat becomes activated for catabolism of cholesterol in man.

In biliary atrasia and in other severe forms of biliary obstruction bile acids are mostly eliminated via the urinary route (NORMAN et al., 1969; STIEHL, 1972) while in parenchymal liver diseases a relatively small fraction is excreted in the urine (ALSTRÖM and NORMAN, 1972; BLUM and SPRITZ, 1966; THEODOR et al., 1968; VLAHCEVIC et al., 1972a). Even in quite complete biliary occlusion the urinary output of bile acids appears to remain usually below 100 mg/day, a figure distinctly lower than normal bile acid production (250 mg/day), indicating that bile acid synthesis is inhibited by chronic biliary stasis (MIETTINEN, 1972a). One of the present author's patients with liver cirrhosis excreted, however, almost 250 mg of bile acids into the urine. In the rat, acute cholestasis is associated with a marked increase in urinary bile acids during the first day after bile duct ligation, followed by a gradual decrease during the subsequent days (BOYD et al., 1966), a finding also suggesting a decreased conversion of cholesterol to bile acids. Cholestyramine reduces rather effectively the urinary bile salt output in man and alters the pattern by almost eliminating the occurrence of deoxycholic acid so that cholic and chenodeoxycholic acids are predominant (MIETTINEN, 1973). This may be due to inhibition of intestinal bacterial action and of reabsorption of deoxycholic acid, but it may also be caused by enhanced release of newly synthesized bile acids into the blood stream from the liver.

It is interesting to note that phenobarbital, which effectively stimulates the microsomal drug metabolizing enzyme system in the liver (cf. MIETTINEN and LESKINEN, 1970), reduces plasma and urinary and increases faecal bile acids and normalizes the peripheral bile acid pool in patients with partial biliary obstruction (EARNEST, 1972). This suggests that the drug stimulates also the uptake and release of bile acids from the blood into the bile.

In connection with studies dealing with the diagnostic significance of urinary bile acids in hepatobiliary disorders it was found that oral administration of 1 g of cholic acid per day to normal human subjects may remove urinary chenodeoxycholic acid and lithocholic acid and result in a marked relative increase in the output of cholic and deoxycholic acids, though quantitatively this increase was quite small (Fig. 1). Thus, in man this extra load of cholic acid apparently can normally inhibit synthesis of chenodeoxycholic acid and slightly exceed the hepatic clearance of bile acids so that the blood bile acid pool tends to expand and the urinary excretion of bile acids to increase. In patients with hepatobiliary diseases the administration of cholic acid was frequently but not consistently associated with a marked increase in urinary cholic acid, sometimes also in deoxycholic acid, while chenodeoxycholic and lithocholic acids disappeared inconsistently. In occasional patients with liver disease most (up to 70%) of the administered bile acids appeared relatively rapidly in the urine, probably in sulfated form, the maximum value being almost 1.5 g/day (Fig. 1). It is not known whether the presumably increased hepatic sulfation of bile acids enhances also the biliary secretion of sulfated bile acids.

Daily Synthesis

Under normal conditions the faecal route is the major pathway of bile salt elimination, the output into the urine (DANIELSSON, 1963) and through the skin (SCHOENFIELD et al., 1967) being negligible. Thus, because bile acids are not degraded during intestinal transit (GRUNDY et al., 1965, 1968) the amount of faecal bile acids equals the synthesis and can be measured either by the chemical or isotopic balance or by the turnover of the isotope dilution technique. The values obtained by the latter method appear to be, for unkown reason(s), 2 to 3 times as high as those of the chemical balance (MIETTINEN, 1973). Since simultaneous measurements of bile acid synthesis have not been performed with the two methods in the same subjects it cannot be concluded whether the relative difference is the same from patient to patient and from one experimental and clinical condition to another or whether the difference is variable. According to the chemical method, daily bile acid synthesis is about 250 mg/day (about 4 mg/kg of body weight); according to the isotope dilution method the daily production of cholic acid ranges from 190 to 690 mg and that of chenodeoxycholic acid from 290 to 390 mg, the total synthesis being about 700 mg.

Though the isotope dilution technique has been used for the determination of bile acid kinetics in hepatitis and liver cirrhosis (BLUM and SPRITZ, 1966; THEODOR et al., 1968; VLAHCEVIC et al., 1971a, 1972a) it is not always valid in hepatobiliary diseases because an unknown portion of the bile acid pool may remain prehepatically in the general circulation and tissues, and the mixing of this pool with the biliary and intestinal pool may be incomplete. The determination of faecal and urinary bile acids by the chemical methods reveals accurately the bile acid synthesis under these conditions, especially because bile salts secreted through the skin appear to be quantitatively unimportant. In ileal dysfunction or in any other condition with markedly impaired bile acid reabsorption the isotope technique may be invalid because of rapid disappearance of radioactivity from the bile acid pool.

In man bile acid synthesis is markedly enhanced by interruption of the entero-hepatic circulation of bile acids, less markedly by excessive calorie intake and obesity, by hyperpre-β-lipoproteinaemia, and frequently by unsaturated fats (MIETTINEN, 1973). Absorbable hypolipidaemic drugs appear to have inconsistent effects though clofibrate frequently decreases (GRUNDY et al., 1972b) and phenobarbital (ERNEST, 1972) and DH-581 (MIETTINEN, 1972d) enhance bile acid production. Bile acid synthesis is reduced in hypercholesterolaemia, total fast and negative calorie balance, long-standing biliary obstruction and impaired parenchymal cell function (cf. MIETTINEN, 1973). A negative correlation exists frequently between blood cholesterol and bile acid synthesis, though e.g. obesity, imbalance of calorie intake and impaired hepatic parenchymal cell function are exceptions.

IV. Regulation of Cholesterol Catabolism via Bile Acids

In the light of current knowledge on factors influencing the catabolism of cholesterol by way of bile acid it seems apparent that 1) altered portal flow of bile acids 2) altered lymphatic flow of cholesterol, 3) altered endogenous synthesis of cholesterol, and 4) even an altered plasma lipoprotein concentration and/or composition can modify this process. In experimental animals the hepatic bile acid synthesis or at least the activity of the key enzyme, cholesterol 7α-hydroxylase, exhibits a marked diurnal variation (GIELEN et al., 1970; RENSON et al., 1969), the maximum being, as that of HMG-CoA dehydrogenase (HAMPRECHT et al., 1969), at midnight. It is not known whether a similar diurnal rhythm occurs in man and whether any of the afore-mentioned factors are basically responsible for this rhythm. Animal experiments have suggested that the hypophysis regulates the elimination of bile acids, especially that of chenodeoxycholic acid (BEHER et al., 1967, 1970), and that hypophysectomy abolishes the diurnal variation of cholesterol 7α-hydroxylase (cf. MAYER, 1972).

The studies by BERGSTRÖM and DANIELSSON (1958) demonstrated that in bile fistula rats the enhanced bile acid production could be suppressed by intestinal bile acid infusion. However, CRONHOLM and SJÖVALL (1967) studied portal bile acids in the rat and concluded that "the data obtained do not support the theory that the production of bile acids from cholesterol is regulated through a direct feedback inhibition by the bile acids returned to the liver via the portal blood". Some other studies (LEE et al., 1965; WEIS and DIETSCHY, 1969; WILSON et al., 1969) dealing with the effect of bile salt infusion on cholesterol catabolism and taurocholate synthesis have failed to disclose a feedback control of bile acid synthesis by bile acids. On the other hand, SHEFER et al., (1969, 1970) presented convincing data demonstrating that if bile salts in high enough amounts, but still ranging within physiological limits, are administered intraduodenally to rats with bile fistula bile acid synthesis is inhibited. They concluded that "previous attempts to demonstrate the feedback control have been unsuccesful because too little bile salt was infused".

It is not known exactly whether the primary action of bile acids is on cholesterol 7α-hydroxylase or HMG-CoA reductase enzyme steps, the activities of which are markedly stimulated by interrupted enterohepatic circulation of bile acids (cf. DAN-IELSSON et al., 1967; DIETSCHY and WILSON, 1970; SHEFER et al., 1970). In rats with bile fistula taurocholate infusion inhibits the conversion of both acetate and meva-lonate into cholesterol, indicating that both of the two enzymes are under a feedback control of bile acids (SHEFER et al., 1970). As a matter of fact, BEHER et al. (1960, 1962) have suggested that there is a double feedback mechanism; bile acid feeding inhibits the synthesis of bile acids followed by inhibition of cholesterol synthesis via accumulated liver cholesterol. In taurocholate-fed rats increase of liver cholesterol has been ascribed to an increased absorption of cholesterol, to a decreased conver-sion of cholesterol to bile acids (low 7α-hydroxylase activity and low endogenous bile acid production), or to a combination of these effects (MOSBACH, 1972). The temporal relationship between the activation and inhibition of 7α-hydroxylase and HMG-CoA reductase is not clear, though in bile fistula rats the activation of cholesterol synthesis appears to precede that of bile acid synthesis (MYANT and EDER, 1961).

Though it appears evident that in the rat the conversion of cholesterol to bile acids is at least partly regulated directly by the bile acids themselves, it would be important to know whether cholic acid feeding suppresses the synthesis of both cholic and chenodeoxycholic acids and whether the latter has a similar action on the synthesis of both primary bile acids. In man, oral administration of cholic acid inhibits bile acid synthesis (GRUNDY et al., 1966) and chenodeoxycholic acid feeding decreases production of cholic acid, even though the latter inhibition may not be complete (DANZINGER et al., 1972; THISTLE and SCHOENFIELD, 1971). The urinary bile salt pattern reveals (Fig. 1) that cholic acid feeding can normally be accompanied by a relatively rapid disappearance of chenodeoxycholic and lithocholic acids, while in patients with liver diseases this is not consistently the case. Deoxycholic acid in doses of 150 mg/day has been reported to suppress the synthesis of chenodeoxycholic acid but not that of cholic acid, a finding suggesting that the negative feedback mechanism is a separate one for each of the two primary bile salts (LOW-BEER et al., 1972). Decrease of deoxycholate in patients with cirrhosis and hypercholester-olaemia is associated with a relative increase of chenodeoxycholate (cf. CAREY, JR., 1973; EINARSSON and HELLSTRÖM, 1972; MIETTINEN, 1973), while in cholestyramine-treated subjects chenodeoxycholate is markedly decreased despite an almost com-plete absence of deoxycholate, the increased synthesis occurring mainly via the production of glycocholate (GARBUTT and KENNEY, 1972). In the rat taurocholate feeding effectively decreases (by 90%) the biliary secretion of taurochenodeox-ycholate plus muricholate and suppresses 7α-hydroxylase activity; the latter is only slightly inhibited by taurochenodeoxycholate feeding, the biliary secretion of cholic acid being reduced by 70% (MOSBACH, 1972).

It seems to be clear that a decreased portal bile acid flux enhances cholesterol synthesis, though in total fast the latter is suppressed despite an apparently low enterohepatic circulation of bile acids (cf. MIETTINEN, 1973). Absence of bile acids stimulates and their presence inhibits cholesterol synthesis in intestinal mucosal cells via an altered HMG-CoA reductase activity (DIETSCHY, 1968b; DIETSCHY and GA-MEL, 1971; SHEFER et al., 1972). The same appears to be true with the liver, even though it is difficult to differentiate between the effects of bile acids and cholesterol itself on the hepatic cholesterol synthesis *in vivo*. With a view to gallstone dissolution with chronic oral chenodeoxycholate treatment (DANZINGER et al., 1972; THISTLE and SCHOENFIELD, 1971) it would be important to know the effect of an excessive portal bile acid flux on cholesterol synthesis because bile acid-induced suppression of the conversion of cholesterol to bile acids may lead to accumulation of cholesterol into tissues and blood. In man cholic acid has been reported to inhibit cholesterol synthesis (GRUNDY et al., 1966). Taurocholate administered to rats on a low cholesterol diet (enhanced cholesterol synthesis) slightly reduced the cholesterol synthesis between acetate and mevalonate *in vivo*, while in human subjects on a "normal" cholesterol intake no consistent effects could be recorded (MIETTINEN, 1968a). In cholestyramine-treated patients, in whom the acetate-mevalonate test showed a markedly enhanced cholesterol synthesis (MIETTINEN, 1970b), the simultaneous administration of cholic acid (given 1 to 2 hrs before each cholestyramine dose so as to facilitate cholic acid absorption in the absence of resin) clearly reduced cholesterol synthesis (Table 1). The final value of the latter, however, was still about 50% above the initial level; together with an unaltered (or even slightly decreased) sterol balance value this indicates that cholesterol was accumulating within the body. Under this condition chenodeoxycholic acid production was not inhibited completely by oral cholic acid (Table 1).

In the rat feeding of cholic acid in the diet prevents the diurnal variation of the activity of HMG-CoA reductase, suggesting that cholesterol synthesis is inhibited (HAMPRECHT et al., 1971a). It has been suggested, however, that it is cholesterol, not bile acids, which regulates hepatic cholesterol synthesis (DIETSCHY and WILSON, 1970; WEIS and DIETSCHY, 1969). Accordingly, an interrupted enterohepatic circulation of bile acids would impair cholesterol absorption and reduce the return of cholesterol as chylomicrons and VLDL to the liver, thus resulting in enhanced hepatic cholesterol synthesis via the released feedback inhibition. The enhanced synthesis would then passively stimulate bile acid production. On the other hand, feeding of bile acids would promote cholesterol absorption and lymphatic flux of cholesterol back to the liver, cholesterol production being inhibited via the feedback mechanism and bile acid synthesis from newly synthesized cholesterol decreased. However, administration of cholic acid to lymph fistula rats with lacking lymphatic flux of cholesterol and increased HMG-CoA reductase activity caused a strong depression in the activity of HMG-CoA reductase especially when the diurnal activity of the enzyme was high (HAMPRECHT et al., 1971b). In addition, feeding cholic acid to rats results in a more rapid depression of hepatic cholesterogenesis than feeding cholesterol (BACK et al., 1969). Furthermore, in monkeys interruption of enterohepatic circulation of bile acids with ileal diversion (associated with high cholesterol production) did not interfere with cholesterol absorption. Yet, in contrast to intact animals, a high cholesterol diet had no effect on cholesterol synthesis (WILSON, 1972). Thus, a direct action of bile acids on cholesterol synthesis seems apparent from many studies.

The actual role of dietary cholesterol as precursor of bile acids is poorly understood. In the dog (ABELL et al., 1956) and rat (WILSON, 1964) cholesterol feeding enhances bile acid excretion, suggesting that increased amounts of absorbed cholesterol are eliminated as bile acids. However, 7α-hydroxylase is not activated (MOSBACH, 1972). In view of the possible heterogeneity of human subjects to eliminate cholesterol (MIETTINEN, 1972c) it is interesting to note that some individuals among squirrel monkeys are unable to compensate for increased cholesterol absorption by enhanced elimination of cholesterol as bile acids and develop a marked hypercholesterolaemia in response to cholesterol feeding while others are able to do so and

Table 1. Effect of cholestyramine and cholic acid on faecal steroids and cholesterol synthesis in man. Mean ± SE of four subjects

Treatment	Serum chol., mg%	Faecal steroids, mg/day		NS	Sterol balance, mg/day	$^{14}C/^{3}H \times 100$[1]
		Bile acids				
		Cheno	Total			
None	317 + 57	—	477 + 124	867 + 112	− 1229 + 144	11 + 1
Resin	264 + 37[a]	311 + 6	1631 + 155[a]	711 + 79	− 2227 + 102[a]	27 + 6[a]
Resin + Cha	289 + 34	252 + 29	2480 + 150[a]	624 + 74	− 989 + 128	16 + 2[a]

NS = neutral steroids; resin = cholestyramine 32 g/day for 10 days during each period; Cha = cholic acid 2 g/day for 10 days. [1]The ratio of $^{14}C/^{3}H \times 100$ in plasma cholesterol 8 hrs after i.v. injection of a mixture of ^{14}C-acetate-^{3}H-mevalonate.
[a] Statistically different ($P < 0.05$) from the none-treatment values. -Bile acid excretion significantly exeeded the administered dose of 2 g during cholic acid treatment, and neutral sterol and chenodeoxycholic acid (cheno; includes faecal derivatives of chenodeoxycholic acid) excretions were significantly decreased by cholic acid

remain quite normocholesterolaemic (LOFLAND, JR. et al., 1972). The enhancement of bile acid production appears to develop slowly over several weeks in the latter animals. It is generally accepted that cholesterol feeding has no consistent effect on bile acid synthesis in man (cf. MIETTINEN, 1972b). However, all these studies have been performed under special conditions and most of them are relatively short-term experiments. Bearing in mind the quite a long time needed for induction of enhanced bile acid production in monkeys and the possible heterogeneity of the human population, long-term experiments should be performed on a reasonable large number of human subjects under normal dietary and living habits so as to explore the ultimate effect of dietary cholesterol on bile acid synthesis.

It is not known exactly in which form dietary cholesterol is utilized for bile acid synthesis. Chylomicrons, the major vehicle in addition to very low density lipoproteins for the transport of dietary cholesterol to the liver, or their cholesterol-rich remnants are rapidly taken up by the liver (REDGRAVE, 1970); cholesterol may be stored in the liver, secreted as bile acids and cholesterol into the bile, or secreted as newly synthesized lipoproteins into the blood where it is mixed with endogenously synthesized cholesterol. Catabolism of these lipoproteins may solely generate cholesterol for bile acid synthesis (SODHI and KUDCHODKAR, 1973). Particulate cholesterol injected intravenously is also rapidly removed by the liver and is utilized for biliary cholesterol and bile acid secretion only after it has been released into the blood stream as lipoproteins (NILSSON and ZILVERSMIT, 1972).

Enhanced fluxes of both lymphatic cholesterol and portal bile acids to the liver seem apparent in obesity and in patients with type IV hyperlipoproteinaemia (MIETTINEN, 1973), yet the synthesis both of cholesterol and bile acids is increased. On the other hand, owing to disturbed absorption the flux of cholesterol to the liver may be markedly reduced (interrupted entero-lymphohepatic circulation of cholesterol) in patients with gluten enteropathy, or in those treated with neomycin or β-sitosterol, yet, despite enhanced cholesterol synthesis, bile acid production is usually not increased. It is interesting to note that, with exception of DH-581 (MIETTINEN, 1972d), absorbable hypocholesterolaemic drugs, e.g. nicotinic acid (MIETTINEN, 1968e, 1971d), thyroxine (MIETTINEN, 1968d, 1972b), clofibrate (GRUNDY et al., 1972b;

HORLICK et al., 1971; MITCHELL and MURCHISON, 1972) which apparently stimulate the flux of cholesterol from tissues to the liver, enhance elimination of cholesterol only as neutral steroids but not as bile acids (cf. MIETTINEN, 1970c, 1973c). Thus, different findings suggest that in man the enhanced flux of cholesterol from the gut and tissues to the liver is usually not, while that from primarily excessive endogenous synthesis (obesity, type IV hyperlipoproteinaemie) is, associated with an augmented catabolism of cholesterol by way of bile acids. On the other hand, the secondarily enhanced cholesterol synthesis in subjects with interrupted entero-lympho-hepatic circulation of cholesterol but intact enterohepatic circulation of bile acids has no consistent effect on bile acid production, while the high cholesterol synthesis in subjects with interrupted enterohepatic circulation of bile acids consistently increases bile acid production no matter whether cholesterol absorption is interrupted or not.

The association of bile acid production with types of hyperlipoproteinaemia and its severity will be discussed later on (cf. VII).

V. Dietary Factors Influencing Bile Acid Metabolism

A. Quantity of Diet

Dietary alterations, both from quantitative and qualitative points of view, can affect bile acid metabolism. Excessive amounts of calories as such enhance cholesterol synthesis, which then may lead to increased bile acid production (exceptions can occur, cf. MIETTINEN, 1973) before any marked gain in weight has yet taken place. Under these conditions, and mormally as well, the frequency of daily meals may affect bile acid elimination and synthesis; one daily meal is associated with few enterohepatic circulations of bile acids and may thus result in low faecal bile acid elimination; several daily meals, on the other hand, increase markedly the number of enterohepatic circulations of bile acids and can be expected to enhance faecal bile acid excretion and synthesis of bile acids as well.

During total fast or low-calorie diet the intestinal contents and nondigestable residue are reduced, allowing better reabsorption of bile acids, a factor which may, together with a reduced bile flow, diminished enterohepatic circulation of bile acids and reduced cholesterol synthesis, contribute to a low faecal bile acid excretion (MIETTINEN, 1968b and c, 1970b, 1973). Binding of intestinal bile acids with ion exchange resin under those conditions or making the intestinal contents more bulky with cellulose or mucillaneous substances increases faecal bile salt elimination (MIETTINEN, 1968b, 1973; STANLEY, 1970), indicating that even during a negative calorie balance and total fast the enterohepatic circulation of bile acids can be interrupted, resulting in enhanced bile acid synthesis. Animal experiments have shown that starvation reduces biliary bile salt secretion to one third and that this is associated with decreased pool size and number of enterohepatic circulations of bile acids (cf. SMALL et al., 1972).

B. Dietary Fibre

Large amounts of nondigestable residue in the intestinal contents may prevent reabsorption of bile acids either by trapping bile salts or favouring the transformation of primary bile acids by intestinal bacteria to less absorbable secondary products. Thus, rats eliminate more cholic acid on Purine Chow than on a purified sucrose diet, the addition of cellulose fibre to the latter greatly increasing the daily cholic acid output, while administration of sulfa reduces it again (PORTMAN, 1960; PORTMAN and MURPHY, 1958). Total faecal bile acid excretion is also markedly higher on rat chow than on low-residue fat-free diet (cf. GRUNDY et al., 1965). Secondary bile acids are known to be adsorbed to intestinal contents. Lithocholic acid and its major metabolites are partly adsorbed in cultures to the micro-organisms of intestinal contents from conventional rats (MIDVEDT and NORMAN, 1972) but lithocholic acid can also be adsorbed to residue of intestinal contents from germfree rats (GUSTAFSSON and NORMAN, 1968).

In man a high residue diet has been generally held to enhance bile acid and cholesterol elimination and subsequently reduce serum cholesterol. As a matter of fact, dietary supplement with pectin, but not with cellulose, has been reported to lower serum cholesterol (KEYS et al., 1961). A hydrophilic colloid (Metamucil) derived from the blond psyllium seed reduce serum cholesterol in man and increases faecal bile acid excretion in man (FORMAN et al., 1968) and rat (BEHER and CASAZZA, 1971). Cellulose, but not methyl cellulose, administered to human subjects enhances bile acid elimination to the same extent as Metamucil (STANLEY et al., 1972). In view of these findings our observation of quite normal daily quantities of bile acids in stools of vegetarians is somewhat surprising, even though the dietary analysis and high faecal plant sterol values suggested that consumption of vegetables and nondigestable fibrous material had been considerable (unpublished results). It is interesting to note that in vegetarians the formation of secondary bile acids and the faecal bile acid concentrations are greatly reduced as compared to subjects on a normal western mixed diet (ARIES et al., 1971). Western people, consuming the latter type of diet, pass relatively small amounts of faeces with high concentrations of secondary and total bile acids, whereas Indians and Ugandans, consuming largely a vegetarian type of diet with little animal matter (and probably low in calories), pass bulky stools with a low concentration and low daily output of total bile acids; bacterial transformation to secondary products is also low (HILL and ARIES, 1971).

C. Dietary Fat

The effects of dietary fats on bile acid metabolism have been rather extensively studied in man because of the well known cholesterol-lowering action of polyunsaturated fats. Though the results are variable, a review of the literature revealed that the majority of the studies demonstrate an increase in bile acid elimination by unsaturated fats (MIETTINEN, 1973). More recent sterol balance studies have shown that both neutral and acidic steroid excretion is increased by vegetable oils (GROEN, 1972, personal communication). Similar results have been obtained in monkey experiments in which the biliary secretion of bile acids was significantly increased by a corn oil diet as compared to that obtained during the olive oil period. The pool size was slightly expanded by corn oil supplementation and the number of enterohepatic circulations was increased (CAMPBELL et al., 1972).

D. Dietary Cholesterol

As already presented, dietary cholesterol enhances bile acid synthesis in some species but usually not in man. Our sterol balance studies in normolipidaemic healthy human subjects living at home under their normal dietary habits showed a positive correlation between the dietary cholesterol intake and the faecal bile acids, a finding which was mostly explainable by differences in body weight (unpublished results). Supplementation of their basic diet for four weeks with 1 g of cholesterol dissolved in olive oil had no consistent effect on the faecal bile acids; since the sterol balance data indicated that cholesterol synthesis was reduced, the finding suggests that a relatively large portion of the faecal bile acids originated now from the dietary cholesterol and that in relation to cholesterol synthesis the bile acid production was high. In another study (DAM et al., 1971a) 1 to 2 g/day of cholesterol in the form of eggs for 6 weeks increased the serum cholesterol by about 30% and, even though biliary cholesterol secretion is increased under those conditions (QUINTAO et al., 1971), the bile maintained cholesterol in solution, the ratio of total bile acids to cholesterol even increasing slightly as a sign of a relative increase in bile acid secretion.

E. Dietary Carbohydrates

It is generally known that a high carbohydrate diet enhances the hepatic fatty acid synthesis and induces a more or less permanent increase in the plasma triglyceride and VLDL concentrations. Since under these conditions the absolute turnover of VLDL is enhanced and since VLDL is believed to be converted to LDL (BILHEIMER et al., 1972, GITLIN et al., 1958) the formation and catabolism of LDL may be markedly increased. It can be speculated that this is also associated with an increased removal of cholesterol as cholesterol and bile acids. However, the biliary secretion rate of both cholesterol and bile acids is higher in man on a high-fat than a high-carbohydrate diet (GRUNDY and METZGER, 1972). Similar results have been obtained in monkeys. A no-fat diet was associated with a low biliary secretion of bile acids and cholesterol; this was caused by a reduced pool size because the number of enterohepatic circulations of bile acids remained unchanged (cf. SMALL et al., 1972). Furthermore, our sterol balance studies in patients in whom the serum triglyceride concentration was on an average 2.41 mmol/l on a high fat diet an 4.14 mmol/l on a high carbohydrate diet (equal cholesterol intake on both diets) revealed that cholesterol elimination as faecal neutral sterols was significantly (about 20%) higher on the former than on the latter diet, while bile acid excretion was unaffected (Table 2). This suggests that the high biliary secretion of bile acids is balanced by their effective reabsorption during the high-fat diet, preventing excessive bile salt loss into the stools. Cholestyramine resulted in a slightly greater faecal bile acid elimination on the low- than the high-fat diet, as if the high intestinal fatty acid concentration had been interfering with the cholestyramine action or the capacity of the liver to synthesize bile acids were great on a high carbohydrate diet.

F. Vitamins

Among the vitamins, ascorbic acid influences bile acid metabolism by stimulating transformation of cholesterol to bile acids in liver mitochondria from scorbutic guinea-pigs (GUCHHAIT et al., 1963). In agreement with these findings the extensive studies by GINTER's groups (cf. GINTER, 1970) have revealed that hypovitaminotic animals excrete subnormal amounts of labelled bile acids into stools after administration of labelled cholesterol, and the oxidation of intraperitoneally administered

Table 2. Serum lipids and faecal steroids during high fat and high carbohydrate diets in hyperlipidaemic patients

Diet	Serum lipids, mmol/l		Faecal steroids		
	Cholest.	Triglyc.	Acidic	Neutral	Total
Fat[a]	6.3 ± 0.4	2.41 ± 0.41	306 ± 45	877 ± 90	1183 ± 111
CHO[b]	5.9 ± 0.3	4.14 ± 0.66	323 ± 33	710 ± 71	1033 ± 88
Change	-0.4 ± 0.2	$+1.73 \pm 0.68*$	$+ 16 \pm 25$	$-167 \pm 59*$	$- 151 \pm 65*$

[a] Caloric composition: 60% fat, 20% protein and 20% carbohydrate (no sugar).
[b] Caloric composition: 70% carbohydrates (20% as sucrose, 80% as starch), 10% fat and 20% protein. Fat consisted of equal amounts of coconut oil and olive oil, cholesterol contents of both solid food diets being 150 mg/day. $n = 15$. Statistically significant changes are indicated by *

^{14}C-26-cholesterol to $^{14}CO_2$ increases significantly after injection of ascorbic acid to scorbutic guinea-pigs (GINTER et al., 1971, 1972). The authors suggested that the hypercholesterolaemia and increase of tissue cholesterol which occur in scorbutic guinea-pigs is due to the defective elimination of cholesterol as bile acids.

Pyridoxine-deficient rats produce greater than normal amounts of bile acids; under those conditions chenodeoxycholate predominates and the conjugation of bile acids with glycine is increased (AVERY, 1970). Large doses of nicotinic acid, used widely for the treatment of hyperlipidaemias appear to stimulate the oxidation of cholesterol to bile acids in the rat (KRITCHEVSKY et al., 1960; LENGSFELD and GEY, 1971) but apparently not in man. Thus, lowering of serum cholesterol by nicotinic acid in hyperlipidaemic patients is associated with a significant increase in the cholesterol elimination as faecal neutral sterols while bile acid excretion is inconsistently affected (MIETTINEN, 1968e, 1971d). Isotope studies have also indicated that nicotinic acid has no constant effect on turnover of either cholic or chenodeoxycholic acid in man (WOLLENWEBER et al., 1967). The few faecal bile acid determinations performed in patients with pernicious anaemia before and after vitamin B_{12} supplementation suggested that this vitamin has little if any effect on cholesterol elimination as bile acids in man (unpublished results).

VI. Effects of Hormones on Bile Acids

A. Pituitary Hormones

Growth hormone (GH)-deficient children have usually a marked hypercholesterolaemia (MERIMEE et al., 1972), and adult human subjects with type A behavioural pattern who also are hypercholesterolaemic have an impaired somatotropin response to arginin and insulin stimuli (FRIEDMAN and ROSENMAN, 1971). Patients with familial hypercholesterolaemia have an impaired cholesterol elimination especially in the form of bile acids; they also have frequently a short stature (MIETTINEN and ARO, 1972), which may be associated with abnormal cholesterol metabolism or abnormal GH action. These findings suggest that GH may have some bearing on cholesterol and bile acid metabolism in man. As a matter of fact, POLEY et al. (1972b) have shown that growth hormone-deficient patients have a very low intestinal bile salt concentration (at or even below the critical micellar concentration) during fat meal and that administration of human GH corrects this defect; in controls the GH effect was less pronounced. Though the correction of the intestinal bile salt deficiency could be due to enhanced intestinal reabsorption of bile salts, the absence of choler-rhoic diarrhoea in untreated pituitary dwarfs suggests that the hepatic effect of improved bile acid production and secretion by GH is more likely. How the GH effect on bile acids and cholesterol is related to the action of somatomedin is not known at present; GH treatment oversaturated the bile with cholesterol in the GH-deficient patients who showed a good growth acceleration, but had no effects in those with lacking growth acceleration (POLEY et al., 1972a).

According to our clinical experience serum cholesterol or triglycerides are not consistently changed by cryohypophysectomy in agromegalic subjects with an ade-quate thyroid and adrenal hormone substitution. Nor was there any gross abnormal-ity in faecal bile salt elimination under basal conditions or when bile acid production was enhanced by cholestyramine treatment prior to and after hypophysectomy. This appears to be in contrast to what has been found in experimental animals *in vivo* or on the enzyme level. In the rat hypophysectomy markedly inhibits or completely suppres-ses the diurnal variation in the activity of the key-enzyme, cholesterol-7α-hydroxylase, of bile acid synthesis; furthermore, cholestyramine, which normally markedly stimu-lates the activity of this enzyme, and cholic acid, which inhibits it, have no effects on the 7α-hydroxylation of cholesterol in hypophysectomized animals (MAYER, 1972; MAYER and VOGES, 1972). The *in vivo* experiments have revealed that hypophysec-tomized rats exhibit a prolonged half life and a greatly reduced excretion and syn-thesis of bile acids, the production of chenodeoxycholic acid being decreased to undetectable levels (BEHER et al., 1966, 1967, 1970). Despite the low elimination of cholesterol as bile acids the serum and tissue cholesterol of those animals are main-tained normal on a low cholesterol intake, while increase occurs more sensitively than normally on a high cholesterol diet, suggesting an impaired elimination of cholesterol. Hypophysectomized rats are, however, able to increase their bile acid synthesis in response to the high cholesterol diet and the interruption of entero-hepatic circulation of bile acids by cholestyramime or Metamucil, but to a lesser extent than the non-hypophysectomized controls (BEHER et al., 1967, 1970, 1971). Since in the latter experiments the hypophysectomized rats maintained or even increased their bile acid pool sizes despite the increased excretion of bile acids caused by cholestyramine and Metamucil it was concluded that these animals have no defect in their ability to convert cholesterol to bile acids but that elimination of bile acids from the pool is defective. Thyroidectomy as such had virtually no effect on sterol and bile acid secretion in the rat; administration of thyroid hormones to hypophysectomized rats increased the conversion of cholesterol to bile acids and the bile acid excretion, demonstrating the role of thyrotropin in maintaining a normal bile acid production (BEHER et al., 1964, 1966).

B. Sex Hormones

The serum cholesterol level of women in the child-bearing age is usually lower than that of men of comparative age. The basic reason for this is unknown, though the effective removal of plasma triglycerides (NIKKILÄ and KEKKI, 1971), and probably also VLDL as a whole, suggests that elimination of all plasma lipoproteins and also of cholesterol as such or as bile acids would take place more effectively in young

women. The serum cholesterol lowering effect of oestrogens is well known (KRITCH-
EVSKY, 1958).

In the rat the bile acid pool contains virtually no chenodeoxycholic acid during
the first weeks of life; this bile acid appears at about the age of one month and
comprises roughly 15% of the pool in females during the rest of life but almost
disappears again from the pool of male rats at the age of $1^{1}/_{2}$ months, a finding
related to the beginning androgen or estrogen action on the catabolism of cholesterol by way of bile acids (BEHER et al., 1971). A somewhat different sex difference of
the bile acid pattern has been found in bile of rats with a biliary fistula (YOUSEF et al.,
1972). Several animal studies have indicated that oestrogens might stimulate the
conversion of cholesterol to bile acids, while androgens either inhibit or have no
effect on this process (KRITCHEVSKY et al., 1961, 1963; MUKHERJEE and GUPTA,
1967). The faecal bile acid excretion, however, tends to be lower in women than in
men not only normally but also in obesity (high cholesterol production) and in
familial hypercholesterolaemia (low cholesterol production) (MIETTINEN, 1973). Furthermore, the relative catabolism of cholesterol by way of bile acids is significantly
lower in obese women than obese man. This type of difference is not seen between
Indian women with gallstones and men without gallstones though both groups are
overweight (GRUNDY et al., 1972a). Our experiments with cholestyramine in some
young females and male subjects have indicated that the increase of bile acid excretion is at least as great or even greater in women ($+33$ mg ± 4 mg/kg/day) than in
men ($+27$ mg ± 3 mg/kg/day) under comparable conditions.

Also in human infants cholic acid is the major component of the bile acids, the
proportion of chenodeoxycholate increasing markedly long before the beginning of
sexual maturation (BONGIOVANNI, 1965; ENCRANTZ and SJÖVALL, 1959; POLEY et
al., 1964). In adult human subjects chenodeoxycholate comprises about one third of
the total biliary bile acids, some sex differences being detected in the bile composition
(DAM et al., 1971b; SJÖVALL, 1960). More recent studies indicate that the amount of
chenodeoxycholate is higher in bile from female than male subjects (YOUSEF and
FISHER, 1972). Furthermore, the ratio of biliary bile acids to cholesterol appears to be
lower in women than in men (DAM et al., 1971b), and the biliary secretion rate of bile
acids also tends to be lower in women than in men without gallstones, the reverse
being true of the cholesterol secretion rate (GRUNDY et al., 1972a). If the woman
actually has a relative defect in catabolizing cholesterol as bile acids she will, e.g. in
obesity with cholesterol overproduction, more easily produce lithogenic bile (cf.
MIETTINEN, 1973) and develop gallstone disease, an ailment occurring more frequently in women than in men. In women with gallstones and/or lithogenic bile in
whom the bile salt pool is clearly subnormal (VLACHEVIC et al., 1972c), the cholesterol synthesis is increased and cholesterol is inadequately converted into bile acids
(GRUNDY et al., 1972a).

C. Thyroid Hormones

Of the hormones, thyroxine and its derivatives have the most drastic and consistent
effect on not only serum cholesterol but also triglycerides. Both of these components,
especially serum cholesterol, are markedly elevated in hypothyroidism and decreased in hyperthyroidism, parallel changes being seen in the plasma concentrations

of the LDL and VLDL fractions as an apparent consequence of altered removal of these lipoproteins from the circulation (NIKKILÄ and KEKKI, 1972; WALTON et al., 1965). Therefore, the effect of an enhanced and an impaired removal of lipoproteins (and of cholesterol) would be seen on cholesterol catabolism via bile acids in, respectively, hyper- and hypothyroidism even though this may be interfered with by changes in lipoprotein, cholesterol and bile acid synthesis, calorie balance, and intestinal contents and motility (cf. MIETTINEN, 1973).

Rat experiments indicate that thyroxine stimulates the biliary cholesterol and chenodeoxycholate secretions in bile fistula rats in which bile acid production may be maximal, but has negligible effect on the total bile acids (ERIKSSON, 1957; LIN et al., 1963; STRAND, 1962). In intact animals the thyroid hormones stimulate also the total bile acid production, the increase being mainly due to enhanced chenodeoxycholate synthesis; the pool size of the latter increases, too, while its half life remains unchanged (STRAND, 1963). These studies have shown that in the hypothyroid state the bile acid production is normal or slightly decreased, while cholesterol elimination as neutral sterols is sensitively reduced. It is interesting to note that a cholesterol feeding-induced increase of bile acid production is not seen in propylthiouracil-treated dogs (ABELL et al., 1956; MOSBACH and KENDALL, 1957) and that in the rat thyroidectomy does not interfere with bile acid production while in secondary hypothyroidism after hypophysectomy the bile acid metabolism is clearly disturbed, this disturbance being corrected with thyroid hormones (see VI A). The latter appear to stimulate the side chain oxidation of cholesterol before 12α-hydroxylation of the steroid nucleus takes place, thus allowing an enhanced production of chenodeoxycholate, especially because these hormones also inactivate 12α-hydroxylation, a process activated by the hypothyroid state (BERSEUS, 1965; BJÖRKHEM, 1967; MITROPOULOS et al., 1968).

It remains to be shown whether in the rat the enhanced removal of cholesterol in hyperthyroidism, primarily as cholesterol but also as bile acids, especially chenodeoxycholate, is secondary to an enhanced flux of cholesterol from an increased catabolism of plasma lipoproteins, or whether the thyroid hormones have a special action on hepatic cholesterol and bile acid metabolism. Relatively unaffected bile acid production, even during interrupted enterohepatic circulation of bile acids in hypothyroid rats, suggests that bile acid synthesis at least can proceed effectively even in the absence of thyroid hormones despite low catabolism of plasma lipoproteins and low cholesterol synthesis. The same seems to apply to man, in whom thyroid activity is correlated negatively with the plasma cholesterol level and positively with cholesterol synthesis and cholesterol elimination as neutral sterols, the effect on bile acids being negligible. In hypothyroid patients the faecal bile acid excretion is slightly subnormal but only tends to be lower than in hyperthyroidism, the neutral sterol elimination and cholesterol synthesis being markedly reduced (MIETTINEN, 1968d, 1970c, 1973). In most of the hyperthyroid patients the bile acid excretion is within the normal limits, the production being clearly increased in those subjects in whom hyperthyroidism is associated with diarrhoea. Treatment of hypothyroid subjects with thyroid hormones increases the bile acid production inconsistently, while cholesterol elimination as neutral sterols and cholesterol synthesis are clearly increased. Furthermore, the increase of faecal bile acid excretion by cholestyramine appears to be of equal magnitude in hypo- and hyperthyroid subjects, no consistent change in this response being observed when the patients are treated to the euthyroid state (MIETTINEN, 1970c, 1972b).

The pool size of cholic acid is about the same in hypo- and hyperthyroid subjects though the half life is longer and the turnover slower in the former than the latter patients (HELLSTRÖM and LINDSTEDT, 1964). The treatment of hypothyroid patients increases the turnover of cholic acid and normalizes the increased glycine/taurine ratio of bile acid conjugates. In contrast to the rat, hyperthyroidism of man does not exhibit any striking increase of chenodeoxycholate at the expense of cholate (FAILEY et al., 1962; HELLSTRÖM and LINDSTEDT, 1964).

VII. Hyperlipidaemia

A. Chylomicronaemia (Type I)

The faecal bile acid excretion, determined in two children with type I hyperlipopro-teinaemia (GRUNDY et al., 1972b), is within the normal adult limits (2 to 4 mg/kg/day). No significant change is observed, in analogy to other hyperlipidaemic subjects, when switched from a fat-free (low-cholesterol) to fat-containing (219 to 307 mg/day of cholesterol) diet which provoked a marked hyperglyceridaemia. Thus the defective removal of chylomicrons may not alter bile acid production, though detailed studies are not available.

B. Hypercholesterolaemia (Type II)

This group is fairly heterogeneous and accordingly the cholesterol and bile acid metabolism may be variable, particularly because some of these patients, especially those with mixed type (type IIB), can be obese. The severe, usually xanthomatotic, clearly familial form can apparently be either 1) homozygous or 2) heterozygous; plasma triglycerides and pre-β-lipoprotein can be normal (type IIA) or sometimes slightly elevated (type IIB) and the abnormality manifests itself already in early childhood or even at birth; 3) in less severe (essential) pure hypercholesterolaemia (type IIA) the genetics may be unclear, xanthomata are infrequent and the preva-lence increases with age, while 4) in mixed hypercholesterolaemia (type IIB) the plasma triglycerides (and pre-β-lipoproteins) are also increased and the disorder is rarely seen below the age of 20 (MIETTINEN et al., 1972).

Homozygous subjects with familial hypercholesterolaemia, usually children, ap-pear to produce, according to the isotopic sterol balance, quite normal amounts of bile acids, and furthermore the increase of faecal bile acids in response to cholestyr-amine has been interpreted to indicate that the grossly elevated plasma cholesterol level is not due to inability to synthesize bile acids normally or to defective regula-tion of bile acid synthesis (MOUTAFIS and MYANT, 1971; MYANT, 1972). Relatively low faecal bile acid values were seen in the two homozygous children studied by GRUNDY et al. (1971). It is apparently owing to a markedly enhanced cholesterol synthesis that in the homozygous patients the interruption of the enterohepatic circulation of bile acids by cholestyramine or ileal by-pass has usually no effect on the plasma cholesterol level or the hypercholesterolaemia may even become worse (GRUNDY et al., 1971). Our chemical analysis of faecal bile acids in a homozygous and two heterozygous children revealed that the respective outputs were 2 mg/kg/day (low normal adult value) and 3 to 5 mg/kg/day under basal conditions, and 35 and 10 to 51 mg/kg/day during cholestyramine. A value of 49 mg/kg/day was found in the homozygous girl after an ileal by-pass operation, the procedure decreasing her serum cholesterol from 1200 to 928 mg%, yet cutaneous xanthomata continued to grow.

In heterozygous type II subjects the mean faecal bile acid excretion, measured from a fairly large number of subjects, has turned out to be subnormal and lower than in any other type of hyperlipidaemia, the relative catabolism of cholesterol by way of bile acids being also lower than normal (MIETTINEN, 1970b, 1973). The lack of correlation between faecal bile acids and serum triglycerides indicates that the bile acid production of type II B variants of the group was identical with that of type II A variants, and that the increased VLDL was not, in contrast to what was found in obese subjects (MIETTINEN, 1973b) associated with enhanced cholesterol catabolism as bile acids. The significant correlation between faecal bile acids and the plasma pool of cholesterol and triglycerides disappeared when the body weight was taken into account. Since, in addition, a more or less striking negative correlation is found between faecal bile acids and plasma cholesterol (MIETTINEN, 1973, 1973b; MIETTINEN et al., 1967) it has been suggested that in these subjects a defect in the catabolism of cholesterol as bile acids would contribute to the hypercholesterolaemia. The daily fractional removal of the plasma cholesterol pool as faecal bile acids (0.0139 ± 0.0008) is only about one third of that in normal subjects (0.0426 ± 0.0041).

The actual reason for the low bile acid synthesis by these patients is not apparent. The defect could be prehepatic associated with an abnormal catabolism of plasma LDL, though in hypothyroid patients the impaired removal of plasma lipoproteins has been suggested to reflect itself more as low neutral than acidic faecal steroid excretion (MIETTINEN, 1973a). The reason could be hepatic, i.e., the bile acid production itself could be defective or the availability of hepatic cholesterol for bile acid synthesis could be altered. As a matter of fact, analysis of bile acid kinetics by EINARSSON and HELLSTRÖM (1972) has revealed that in hypercholesterolaemic subjects the turnover and pool size of cholic acid are subnormal while those of chenodeoxycholic acid are normal. The small pool of deoxycholate and its occasional absence in hypercholesterolaemic subjects (BLOMSTRAND, 1961; HELLSTRÖM and LINDSTEDT, 1966; SJÖVALL, 1960) can be explained by the presence of a relatively small amount of cholic acid in the intestinal lumen when normal reabsorption allows only small quantities of cholate to escape into the colon for conversion to deoxycholate by colonic bacteria. KUDCHODKAR and SODHI (1972) discovered that lithocholic acid was the major faecal bile acid in type II A subjects and deoxycholic acid in type II B patients, indicating that chenodeoxycholic acid predominated in the bile acid synthesis of the former cases. These findings suggest that the low bile acid production in heterozygous type II subjects is due to an abnormally low synthesis of cholic acid. In connection with the action of thyroid hormones chenodeoxycholate was shown to predominate if side chain oxidation of cholesterol occurs before 12α-hydroxylation and/or if 12α-hydroxylation is inhibited. It remains to be shown whether these types of changes are detectable in the liver of hypercholesterolaemic subjects. Even a small defect, for instance in 12α-hydroxylation of cholic acid synthesis, could reduce the conversion of newly synthesized cholesterol or of cholesterol from catabolized lipoproteins to bile acids, allowing the release of more cholesterol into the plasma pool as lipoproteins. These phenomena may finally inhibit the total cholesterol synthesis by the negative feed-back mechanism. The overall cholesterol synthesis and the hepatic cholesterol synthesis tend actually to be low in these patients (MIETTINEN, 1970b, 1973b; SODHI and KUDCHODKAR, 1971). Under these conditions the inter-ruption of the enterohepatic circulation of bile acids, e.g. with cholestyramine, can be hypothesized to increase cholic acid production subnormally; the increase of cheno-deoxycholate synthesis, which in normal cholestyramine-treated subjects appears to be relatively less than that of cholate (GARBUTT and KENNEY, 1972), could be normal or perhaps compensatorily slightly greater than normal and that of overall choles-terol catabolism via bile acids subnormal. Thus, despite a markedly enhanced total bile acid production the basic defect would still allow an abnormal distribution between plasma lipoprotein and bile acids for increasingly synthesized cholesterol, the plasma cholesterol level being not completely normalized. As a matter of fact, an abnormally low increase of faecal bile acids has been found in hypercholesterolaemic subjects treated with cholestyramine (MIETTINEN, 1970d) even though, as compared to other hyperlipidaemic states, the difference appears to be small (Table 3). The contribution of cholic and chenodeoxycholic acids to this increase has not been studied.

Cholestyramine has been widely used in the treatment of hypercholesterolaemia, the decrease of plasma cholesterol ranging from zero to 70% (GRUNDY, 1972). The number of cholestyramine-treated patients studied for total bile acid elimination is quite limited. Therefore, factors influencing the magnitude of faecal bile acid increase and of serum cholesterol decrease have been incompletely explored. Our experience on the effects of cholestyramine in a fairly large number of patients with various hyperlipidaemias under comparable dietary and therapeutic conditions is presented in Table 2. These studies have shown that cholestyramine (32 g/day) reduces serum cholesterol and increases faecal bile acids in every heterozygous type II patient, the increment (range 302 to 2015 mg%) being correlated positively with body weight. Despite a negative correlation of initial faecal bile acids with serum cholesterol and a positive one with increase of faecal bile acids by cholestyramine, the latter showed a positive correlation with the absolute and relative decreases of serum cholesterol (Fig. 2). Since in addition the serum cholesterol concentration correlated negatively (MIETTINEN, 1971b) with the faecal bile acids in patients with ileal resection (appar-ently mostly normocholesterolaemic before manifestation of illnesses leading to ile-ectomy) it is reasonable to conclude that in general the greater the increase in bile acid elimination, the higher the reduction in the serum cholesterol level. Figure 2 shows that age correlated negatively with the cholestyramine-induced increase in faecal bile acids. This indicates that the older the subject is the lower is the increase in bile acid elimination and the smaller may also be the decrease in serum cholesterol. It is interesting to note that old rats appear to excrete cholesterol as bile acids and as cholesterol itself less effectively than the younger ones (HRUZA and ZBUZKOVÁ, 1973). It remains to be shown whether in man cholesterol elimination via bile acids and cholesterol itself is impaired with age in general and whether this impairment contributes to the well known increase of serum cholesterol with advancing age. Anyhow, the basal faecal bile acids of our adult heterozygous type II subjects ($n=81$) were not correlated significantly with age, while a slight negative correlation was found when all the adult type II patients and the control subjects were combined ($r = -0.189, n = 124$). Figure 2 also demonstrates that when age is taken into consideration the marked difference between the normocholesterolaemic control subjects and the hypercholesterolaemic patients is decreased, but even then the mean of the cholestyramine-induced increase in faecal bile acids is subnormal in heterozygous type II patients.

The increase of faecal bile acids appear to depend on the dose of cholestyramine. Thus, in our experiments 15 g/day enhanced bile acid output by a factor of four while the increase by 32 g/day was 7-fold (MIETTINEN, 1970 b). In the series of four patients by NAZIR et al. (1972) the increase of faecal bile acids by 12 g/day of cholestyramine ranges from 377 to 493 mg/day, a change for below that seen in Table 3 for the dose 32 g/day.

Earlier preliminary studies have indicated that cholestyramine, even in the large doses (32 g/day), may not elicit maximal bile acid excretion in hypercholesterolaemic patients because subsequent ileal by-pass further increased faecal bile acid output and further decreased serum cholesterol (MIETTINEN, 1969). Later on GRUNDY et al. (1971) were not able to detect any superior effect of the ileal by-pass as compared to cholestyramine on faecal bile acids and serum cholesterol. They proposed that the ileal exclusion may not offer any advantage over cholestyramine in the treatment of hypercholesterolaemia. Analysis of the data found in the literature by GRUNDY (1972) suggested that cholestyramine decreases serum cholesterol less effectively than ileal by-pass the measure which was mainly used by BUCHWALD and shown by MOORE et al. (1969) to markedly increase faecal bile acid elimination. Ten of our patients have been treated before the ileal by-pass operation with cholestyr-

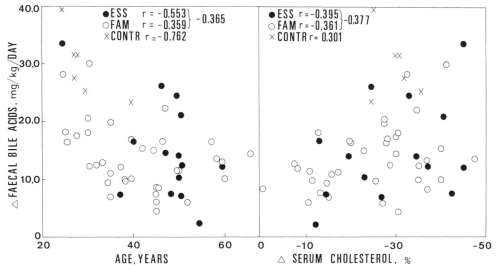

Fig. 2. Correlation of changes in faecal bile acids by cholestyramine with age (left panel) and changes in serum cholesterol (right panel) in normo- and hypercholesterolaemic patients. Cholestyramine (32 g/day) was given for 10 to 12 days. Low cholesterol (125 mg/2400 kcal) solid food diet. ● Ess = patients II Ess of Table 3 and ○ Fam = patients II Fam of Table 3; X controls; normocholesterolaemic subjects from MIETTINEN (1970d). Correlation coefficient for the whole material was $r = -0.515$ for the left panel and $r = -0.339$ for the right panel

Table 3. Serum lipids and faecal steroids prior to and during cholestyramine treatment in hyperlipidaemic subjects. Mean ± SE

Type of hyper-lipoproteinaemia	Treatment	Age	Weight kg	relative	Serum lipids, mmol/l Cholesterol	Triglyceride	Faecal steroids Bile acids mg/day	mg/kg/day	Neutral steroids mg/day	mg/kg/day	Total steroids mg/day	mg/kg/day
II Fam (36)	None	41	65	1.11	11.5 ± 0.35	1.57 ± 0.16	180 ± 12	2.8 ± 0.2	662 ± 35	10.3 ± 0.5	842 ± 39	13.1 ± 0.6
	Resin	± 2	± 2	± 0.001	8.6 ± 0.29[a]	1.58 ± 0.15	1070 ± 71[a]	16.6 ± 1.0[a]	652 ± 43	9.9 ± 0.5	1722 ± 94[a]	26.5 ± 1.2[a]
II Ess (14)	None	47[b]	69	1.13	7.6 ± 0.46[b]	1.13 ± 0.90	244 ± 20[b]	3.5 ± 0.2[b]	573 ± 66	8.0 ± 0.7[b]	817 ± 78	11.5 ± 0.8
	Resin	± 2	± 3	± 0.01	5.3 ± 0.31[a,b]	1.32 ± 0.12	1309 ± 194[a]	18.5 ± 2.4[a]	571 ± 37	8.2 ± 0.4[b]	1880 ± 209[a]	26.7 ± 2.5
MH (II B) (13)	None	49[b]	72	1.23	10.1 ± 1.63[a]	5.02 ± 1.86[b]	281 ± 41[b]	4.2 ± 0.6[b]	804 ± 83	11.4 ± 0.1	1085 ± 97[b]	15.6 ± 1.3
	Resin	± 3	± 7	± 0.11	8.5 ± 1.82	4.86 ± 1.74[b]	1031 ± 58[a]	15.8 ± 1.6[a]	772 ± 82	10.9 ± 0.7	1803 ± 74[a]	26.7 ± 1.9[a]
IV (7)	None	54[b]	72	1.21	7.0 ± 0.46[b]	4.90 ± 1.27[b]	337 ± 41[b]	4.7 ± 0.6[b]	997 ± 100[b]	14.0 ± 1.7	1334 ± 86[b]	18.7 ± 1.6[b]
	Resin	± 4	± 4	± 0.07	6.0 ± 0.68[b]	6.54 ± 1.67[b]	1537 ± 82[a,b]	21.6 ± 1.5[a,b]	842 ± 33[a]	11.7 ± 1.5[a]	2379 ± 116[a,b]	33.3 ± 2.0[a,b]

Number of patients in parenthesis; II FAM = familial type II hyper-β-lipoproteinaemia, II Ess = essential type II hyper-β-lipoproteinaemia and MH = mixed hyperlipoproteinaemia (see text); Resin = cholestyramine 32 g/day for 10–12 days; solid food diet (cholesterol content 125 mg/2400 kcal) was used in all experiments. [a] Statistically significant change ($P < 0.05$). [b] Statistically significant difference from II Fam.

amine (Miettinen, 1973c). The latter increased faecal bile acids by 1.2 g/day and subsequent ileal by-pass significantly more i.e. by 2.0 g/day. The serum cholesterol levels were reduced by 18% and 32%, respectively, indicating that ileal by-pass enhances cholesterol elimination as bile acids more effectively than cholestyramine and, in agreement what was presented above, this greater elimination is associated with a greater decrease in serum cholesterol. Furthermore, some experiments with cholestyramine in the patients with ileal by-pass indicated that bile acid excretion was further increased and serum cholesterol slightly decreased. However, even then the serum cholesterol level remained elevated in most of the cases, indicating that interruption of the enterohepatic circulation of bile acids rarely normalizes serum cholesterol in patients with familial hypercholesterolaemia, at least as far as adult subjects are concerned.

Bile acid production of patients with milder type II A abnormality appears to be less affected than in the severe familial form yet the response of bile acids to cholestyramine tends to be subnormal but slightly higher than in the familial form at the comparable age (Table 3, Fig. 2a negative correlation between however, found rather low faecal bile acid values and in agreement with Fig. 2a negative correlation between serum cholesterol and faecal bile acids. The figures reported by Ahrens' group (1972a) are apparently within the normal limits (Grundy et al., 1972b).

Patients with mixed hyperlipidaemia (type II B) have somewhat higher faecal bile acid production than the two type II A groups (Table 3). Similar results have been reported by Kudchodkar and Sodhi (1972) who showed, in contrast to Fig. 3, a positive correlation between faecal bile acids and serum cholesterol. Furthermore, they also found a positive correlation between serum triglycerides and faecal bile acids, suggesting that increased VLDL metabolism was associated with an enhanced bile acid synthesis. This type of correlation was not seen in the patients of Table 3 whose bile acid production was within the limits of the normoglyceridaemic controls (MIETTINEN, 1973). A negative correlation between faecal total steroids and serum cholesterol in hyperglyceridaemic patients have been interpreted to indicate that hypercholesterolaemia of these patients is due to defective cholesterol removal worsening of which leads finally to reduced cholesterol synthesis (MIETTINEN, 1971c). The negative correlation in Fig. 3 suggests that this worsening of removal defect is associated with worsening bile acid synthesis. Correction of the defect with cholestyramine caused a significant reduction of the serum cholesterol level which, as the increase in faecal bile acids, tended to be less than in the two other slightly younger hypercholesterolaemic groups of Table 3. Despite markedly increased cholesterol elimination by cholestyramine the majority of the patients still remained hypercholesterolaemic.

C. Familial Hyperlipoproteinaemia (Type III)

Bile acid production was measured by AHRENS' group (GRUNDY et al., 1972b) in three patients with the type III abnormality, the values ranging (2 to 5 mg/kg/day) within the normal limits. Furthermore, a marked reduction in the plasma values by clofibrate was not associated with any change in bile acid synthesis. In three of our type III patients normal or low normal faecal bile acid values have been recorded, a clearcut increase being seen during cholestyramine or after ileal by-pass. Though no detailed studies have been performed, the available data indicate that the suggested foulty conversion of VLDL to LDL (QUARFORDT et al., 1971) may not be associated in type III hyperlipoproteinaemia with any major abnormality in bile acid production.

D. Hypertriglyceridaemia (Type IV)

Faecal bile acid analysis have revealed that frequently but not constantly, patients with type IV hyperglyceridaemia exhibit increased faecal bile acid excretion (MIETTINEN, 1969, 1970b, 1971a, 1973). In terms of mg/kg/day the values are within the upper normal limits but even then higher than in hypercholesterolaemic patients (Table 3). It is interesting to note that in some lean hyperglyceridaemic patients faecal bile acid excretion may be high in some obese ones normal, resulting in lacking correlation between body weight and bile acids. This suggests that hyperglyceridaemia, i.e. increased VLDL concentration, can causally be related to enhanced catabolism of cholesterol by way of bile acids. The negative correlation of faecal bile acids with serum cholesterol (Fig. 3) in hyperglyceridaemic patients indicates that the more pure the type IV pattern is (clearly increased VLDL and low normal or even subnormal LDL) the higher is the bile acid production. That the latter is not associated in a simple way with the VLDL concentration is indicated by a lacking correlation of serum triglycerides with faecal bile acids in our patients with hyperglyceridaemia and is shown also in Table 2 which reveals that the carbohydrate-induced increase in serum triglycerides is not accompanied by any change in faecal bile acids.

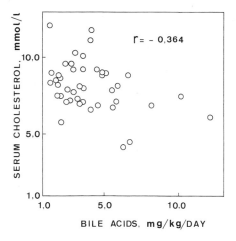

Fig. 3. Correlation of serum cholesterol with faecal bile acids in hyperglyceridaemic patients. Includes patients of Table 3 and earlier publications (MIETTINEN, 1971 a and c, 1973 a and b)

Faecal steroid analysis by AHRENS' group also indicate that the bile acid excretion is increased in hyperglyceridaemia. Thus, their normalized mean value for faecal bile acids of six normal control subjects (males and females) is 247 mg/day, of four hypertriglyceridaemic females 380 mg/day and of seven hyperglyceridaemic males 538 mg/day (cf. GRUNDY et al., 1972 a). Four type IV patients studied by HORLICCK et al. (1971) excreted quite normal amounts of bile acids into faeces (135 to 391 mg/day), clofibrate exhibiting no consistent effect despite decreased serum triglycerides. Occasionally, however, clofibrate inhibits bile acid elimination (GRUNDY et al., 1972 b).

Kinetic analysis of bile acid metabolism by KOTTKE (1969), WOLLENWEBER and STIEHL (1972), and EINARSSON and HELLSTRÖM (1972) have revealed markedly high production rates of bile acids in hyperglyceridaemic patients, the values in hypercholesterolaemic subjects being lower by a factor of four. The mean total bile acid production of those studies varied in type IV subjects from 1058 to 1336 mg/day the values markedly higher than those obtained by faecal analysis. The elevated formation of bile acids seemed mostly to be due to enhanced production of cholic acid while the increase in chenodeoxycholic acid is less marked or absent.

Cholestyramine usually has no marked effect on serum cholesterol in type IV hyperlipoproteinaemia yet a marked increase can be seen in faecal bile acids (Table 3). Under these conditions enhanced removal of cholesterol as bile acids may be solely balanced by increased synthesis because the unaltered serum cholesterol may not be associated with any enhanced mobilization of tissue cholesterol. The increased bile acid synthesis is partly balanced by decreased elimination as cholesterol itself, resulting in decreased faecal excretion of neutral sterols a phenomenon not seen in hypercholesterolaemic patients (Table 3). The high initial faecal bile acids in the type IV abnormality indicates as presented for hypercholesterolaemia, that the response of faecal bile acids to cholestyramine could also be high. Table III actually indicates that despite age difference the increase of faecal bile acids is greater in the type IV patients than in other groups and clearly greater than in the mixed hyperlipidaemia.

E. Hyperglyceridaemia (Type V)

Kinetic analysis have revealed that at the time of marked hyperglyceridaemia the turnover of bile acids is increased in patients with the type V abnormality (EINARSSON and HELLSTRÖM, 1972). The values (range of 3 subjects 655 to 1485 mg/day) are of the same magnitude as in type IV subjects, the turnover of cholic acid being predominantly increased. Faecal analysis by GRUNDY et al. (1972b) showed normal or slightly increased values (range of 5 subjects 249 to 421 mg/day). A decrease of plasma triglycerides by clofibrate was not associated with any consistent change in bile acid production.

Acknowledgements: Supported in part by grants from Sigrid Jusélius Foundation and Finnish State Council for Medical Research.

References

ABAURRE,R., GORDON,S.G., MANN,J.G., KERN,F.,JR.: Fasting bile salt pool size and composition after ileal resection. Gastroenterology **57**, 679—688 (1969).

ABELL,L.L., MOSBACH,E.H., KENDALL,F.E.: Cholesterol metabolism in the dog. J. biol. Chem. **220**, 527—536 (1956).

ADMIRAND,W.H., STIEHL,A., THALER,M.M.: Sulfation of bile salts: An important metabolic pathway in cholestasis. Gastroenterology **62**, 190 (1972).

ALSTRÖM,T., NORMAN,A.: Metabolism of cholic acid-24-^{14}C in patients with hepatobiliary diseases. Acta med. scand. **191**, 521—528 (1972).

ARIES,V.C., CROWTHER,J.S., DRASAR,B.S., HILL,M.J., ELLIS,F.R.: The effect of a strict vegetarian diet on the faecal flora and faecal steroid concentration. J. Path. **103**, 54—56 (1971).

AUSTAD,W.I., LACK,L., TYOR,M.P.: Importance of bile acids and of an intact distal small intestine for fat absorption. Gastroenterology **52**, 638—646 (1967).

AVERY,M.: In: These de Grade de Docteur es Sciences, Université Laval, Quebec 1970.

BACK,P.: Urinary profile of bile acids in liver disease. In: Bile acids in human diseases, pp. 53—55. Stuttgart—New York: F.K. Schattauer Verlag 1972.

BACK,P., HAMPRECHT,B., LYNEN,F.: Regulation of cholesterol biosynthesis in rat liver: Diurnal changes of activity and influence of bile acids. Arch. Biochem. Biophys. **133**, 11—21 (1969).

BADLEY,B.W.D., MURPHY,G.M., BOUCHIER,I.A.D.: Intraluminal bile-salt deficiency in the pathogenesis of steatorrhoea. Lancet **1969 II**, 400—402.

BADLEY,B.W.D., MURPHY,G.M., BOUCHIER,I.A.D., SCHERLOCK,S.: Diminished micellar phase lipid in patients with chronic nonalcoholic liver disease and steatorrhea. Gastroenterology **58**, 781—789 (1970).

BEHER,W.T., CASAZZA,K.K.: Effects of psyllium hydrocolloid on bile acid metabolism in normal and hypophysectomized rats. Proc. Soc. exp. Biol. (N.Y.) **136**, 253—256 (1971).

BEHER,W.T., BAKER,G.D., ANTHONY,W.L.: Effects of bile acids on fecal excretion of end products of cholesterol metabolism. Amer. J. Physiol. **199**, 736—740 (1960).

BEHER,W.T., BAKER,G.D., ANTHONY,W.L.: Feedback control of cholesterol biosynthesis in the mouse. Proc. Soc. exp. Biol. (N.Y.) **109**, 863—868 (1962).

BEHER,W.T., BEHER,M.E., SEMENUK,G.: The effect of pituitary and thyroid hormones on bile acid metabolism in the rat. Metabolism **15**, 181—188 (1966).

BEHER,W.T., CASAZZA,K.K., LIN,G.J.: Effects of age and sex on rat bile acid metabolism. Proc. Soc. exp. Biol. (N.Y.) **138**, 645—650 (1971).

BEHER,W.T., BAKER,G.D., ANTHONY,W.L., BEHER,M.E.: The feedback control of cholesterol biosynthesis. Henry Ford Hosp. Bull. **9**, 201—213 (1961).

BEHER,W.T., BAKER,G.D., BEHER,M.E., VULPETTI,A., SEMENUK,G.: Effects of hypophysectomy, thyroidectomy and thyroid hormones on steroid metabolism in the rat. Proc. Soc. exp. Biol. (N.Y.) **117**, 738—743 (1964).

BEHER,W.T., CASAZZA,K.K., FILUS,A.M., BEHER,M.E., BERTASIUS,J.: Effects of accumulated tissue cholesterol on bile acid metabolism in hypophysectomized rats and hamsters. Altherosclerosis **12**, 383—392 (1970).

BEHER, W. T., RAO, B., BEHER, M. E., SEMENUK, G., BERTASIUS, J., VULPETTI, N.: The accumulation of tissue cholesterol and its relationship to bile acid and sterol turnover. Henry Ford Hosp. med. J. **15**, 107—118 (1967).

BERGSTRÖM, S., DANIELSSON, H.: On the regulation of bile acid formation in rat liver. Acta physiol. scand. **43**, 1—7 (1958).

BERGSTRÖM, S., DANIELSSON, H., SAMUELSSON, B.: In: Lipid metabolism. New York: Wiley 1960.

BERSÉUS, O.: On the effect of thyroid hormones on the oxidation of these β-cholestane-3α, 7a, 12a-triol. Acta chem. scand. **19**, 2131—2135 (1965).

BILHEIMER, D. W., EISENBERG, S., LEVY, R. I.: The metabolism of very low density lipoprotein proteins. I. Preliminary *in vitro* and *in vivo* observations. Biochim. biophys. Acta (Amst.) **260**, 212—221 (1972).

BJÖRKHEM, I.: On the role of $\triangle^4$-3α-hydroxysterols in the biosynthesis of bile acids. Acta chem. scand. **21**, 2561—2564 (1967).

BLOMSTRAND, R.: Gas-liquid chromatography of human bile acids. Proc. Soc. exp. Biol. (N.Y.) **107**, 126—128 (1961).

BLUM, M., SPRITZ, N.: The metabolism of intravenously injected isotopic cholic acid in Laennec's cirrhosis. J. clin. Invest. **45**, 187—193 (1966).

BODE, CH., FRANZ, D.: Serum bile acid concentration in patients with chronic hepatitis and liver cirrhosis: Fasting values and effect of intraduodenal taurocholate administration. In: Bile acids in human diseases, pp. 57—60. Stuttgart-New York: F. K. Schattauer 1972.

BONGIOVANNI, A. M.: Bile acid content of gallbladder of infants, children and adults. J. clin. Endocr. **25**, 678—685 (1965).

BORGSTRÖM, B.: Studies on intestinal cholesterol absorption in the human. J. clin. Invest. **39**, 809—815 (1960).

BORGSTRÖM, B., LUNDH, G., HOFMANN, A.: The site of absorption of conjugated bile salts in man. Gastroenterology **45**, 229—238 (1963).

BOYD, G. S., PERCY-ROBB, I. W.: Enzymatic regulation of bile acid synthesis. Amer. J. Med. **51**, 580—587 (1971).

BOYD, G. S., EASTWOOD, M. A., MACLEAN, N.: Bile acids in the rat: Studies in experimental occlusion of the bile duct. J. Lipid Res. **7**, 83—94 (1966).

BRUNNER, H., HOFMANN, A. F., SUMMERSKILL, W. H. J.: Daily secretion of bile acids and cholesterol measured in health. Gastroenterology **62**, 188 (1972).

BRUUSGAARD, A., HESS THAYSEN, E.: Increased ratio of glycine/taurine conjugated bile acids in the early diagnosis of terminal ileopathy. Preliminary report. Acta med. scand. **188**, 547—548 (1970).

BURKE, C. W., LEWIS, B., PANVELIWALLA, D., TABAQCHALI, S.: The binding of cholic acid and its taurine conjugate to serum proteins. Clin. chim. Acta **32**, 207—214 (1971).

CAMPBELL, C. B., COWLEY, D. J., DOWLING, R. H.: Dietary factors affecting biliary lipid secretion in the rhesus monkey. A mechanism for the hypocholesterolaemic action of polyunsaturated fat? Europ. J. clin. Invest. **2**, 332—341 (1972).

CAREY, J. B., JR.: The serum trihydroxy-dihydroxy bile acid ratio in liver and biliary tract disease. J. clin. Invest. **37**, 1494—1503 (1958).

CAREY, J. B., JR.: Conversion of cholesterol to trihydroxycoprostanic acid and cholic acid in man. J. clin. Invest. **43**, 1443—1448 (1964).

CAREY, J. B., JR.: Bile salt metabolism in man. In: The bile acids, Vol. 2, pp. 55—82. New York-London: Plenum Press 1973.

CAREY, J. B., JR., HASLEWOOD, G. A. D.: Crystallization of trihydroxycoprostanic acid from human bile. J. biol. Chem. **238**, PC 855—856 (1963).

CAREY, J. B., JR., WILLIAMS, G.: Relief of the pruritus of jaundice with a bile-acid sequestering resin. J. Amer. med. Ass. **176**, 432—435 (1961).

CAREY, J. B., JR., WILLIAMS, G.: Lithocholic acid in human-blood serum. Science **150**, 620—622 (1965).

CAREY, J. B., JR., WILSON, I. D., ONSTAD, G., ZAKI, F. G.: Role of 12α hydroxylase deficiency in continuing liver injury. J. clin. Invest. **46**, 1042—1043 (1967).

CRONHOLM, T., SJÖVALL, J.: Bile acids in portal blood of rats fed different diets and cholestyramine. Bile acids and steroids 189. Europ. J. Biochem. **2**, 375—383 (1967).

CRONHOLM, T., NORMAN, A., SJÖVALL, J.: Bile acids and steroid sulphates in serum of patients with infectious hepatitis. Scand. J. Gastroenterol. **5**, 297—303 (1970).

DAM, H., PRANGE, I., JENSEN, M. K., KALLEHAUGE, H. E., FENGER, H. J.: Studies on human bile. IV. Influence of ingestion of cholesterol in the form of eggs on the composition of bile in healthy subjects. Z. Ernährungswiss. **10**, 178—187 (1971 a).

DAM, H., KRUSE, I., PRANGE, I., KALLEHAUGE, H. E., FENGER, H. J., KROGH JENSEN, M.: Studies on human bile. III. Composition of duodenal bile from healthy young volunteers compared with composition of bladder bile from surgical patients with and without uncomplicated gallstone disease. Z. Ernähungswiss. **10**, 160—177 (1971 b).

DANIELSSON, H.: Present status of research on catabolism and excretion of cholesterol. Advanc. Lipid Res. **1**, 335—385 (1963).

DANIELSSON, H.: Mechanisms of bile acid biosynthesis. In: The bile acids, Vol. 2, pp. 1—23. New York-London: Plenum Press 1973.

DANIELSSON, H., EINARSSON, K.: Formation and metabolism of bile acids. In: The biological basis of medicine, Vol. 5, pp. 279—315. London-New York: Academic Press Inc. 1969.

DANIELSSON, H., EINARSSON, K., JOHANSSON, G.: Effect of biliary drainage on individual reactions in the conversion of cholesterol to taurocholic acid. Europ. J. Biochem. **2**, 44—49 (1967).

DANIELSSON, H., ENEROTH, P., HELLSTRÖM, K., LINDSTEDT, S., SJÖVALL, J.: On the turnover and excretory products of cholic and chenodeoxycholic acid in man. J. biol. Chem. **238**, 2299—2304 (1963).

DANZINGER, R. G., HOFMANN, A. F., SCHOENFIELD, L. J., THISTLE, J. L.: Dissolution of cholesterol gallstones by chenodeoxycholic acid. New Engl. J. Med. **286**, 1—8 (1972).

DATTA, D. V., SHERLOCK, S.: Treatment of pruritus of obstructive jaundice with cholestyramine. Brit. med. J. **1963 I**, 216—219.

VAN DEEST, B. W., FORDTRAN, J. S., MORAWSKI, S. G., WILSON, J. D.: Bile salt and micellar fat. Concentration in proximal small bowel. Contents of ileectomy patients. J. clin. Invest. **47**, 1314—1324 (1968).

DIETSCHY, J. M.: Mechanism for the intestinal absorption of bile acids. J. Lipid Res. **9**, 297—309 (1968 a).

DIETSCHY, J. M.: The role of bile salts in controlling the rate of intestinal cholesterogenesis. J. clin. Invest. **47**, 286—300 (1968 b).

DIETSCHY, J. M.: The biology of bile acids. Arch. intern. Med. **130**, 473—474 (1972).

DIETSCHY, J. M., GAMEL, W. G.: Cholesterol synthesis in the intestine of man: Regional differences and control mechanisms. J. clin. Invest. **50**, 872—880 (1971).

DIETSCHY, J. M., WILSON, J. D.: Regulation of cholesterol metabolism. I, II, III New Engl. J. Med. **282**, 1128—1138, 1179—1183, 1241—1249 (1970).

DONALDSON, R. M., JR.: Studies on the pathogenesis of steatorrhea in the blind loop syndrome. J. clin. Invest. **44**, 1815—1825 (1965).

DOWLING, R. H.: The enterohepatic circulation. Gastroenterology **62**, 122—140 (1972).

EARNEST, D. L.: The effect of phenobarbital on pruritus and bile salt kinetics in patients with biliary cirrhosis and elevated serum bile salt concentrations. In: Bile acids in human diseases, pp. 145—151. Stuttgart-New York: F. K. Schattauer Verlag 1972.

EINARSSON, K., HELLSTRÖM, K.: The formation of bile acids in patients with three types of hyperlipoproteinaemia. Europ. J. clin. Invest. **2**, 225—230 (1972).

ELLIOTT, W. H., HYDE, P. M.: Metabolic pathways of bile acid synthesis. Amer. J. Med. **51**, 568—579 (1971).

ENCRANTZ, J.-C., SJÖVALL, J.: On the bile acids in duodenal contents of infants and children. Clin. chim. Acta **4**, 793—799 (1959).

ENEROTH, P., GORDON, B., SJÖVALL, J.: Characterization of trisubstituted cholanoic acids in human feces. J. Lipid Res. **7**, 524—530 (1966 a).

ENEROTH, P., GORDON, B., RYHAGE, R., SJÖVALL, J.: Identification of mono- and dihydroxy bile acids in human feces by gas-liquid chromatography and mass spectrometry. J. Lipid Res. **7**, 511—523 (1966 b).

ERIKSSON, S.: Influence of thyroid activity on excretion of bile acids and cholesterol in the rat. Proc. Soc. exp. Biol. (N.Y.) **94**, 582—584 (1957).

EYSSEN, H., PARMENTIER, G., COMPERNOLLE, F., BOON, J., EGGERMONT; E.: Trihydroxycoprostanic acid in the duodenal fluid of two children with intrahepatic bile duct anomalies. Biochim. biophys. Acta (Amst.) 273, 212—221 (1972).

FAILEY, R. B., JR., BROWN, E., HODES, M. E.: Bile acid excretion in man following administration of L 3:5:3′ triiodothyronine. Amer. J. clin. Nutr. 11, 4—11 (1962).

FORMAN, D. T., GARVIN, J. E., FORESTNER, J. E., TAYLOR, C. B.: Increased excretion of fecal bile acids by an oral hydrophilic colloid. Proc. Soc. exp. Biol. (N.Y.) 127, 1060—1063 (1968).

FRIEDMAN, M., ROSENMAN, R. H.: Type A behavior pattern: Its association with coronary heart disease. Ann. clin. Res. 3, 300—312 (1971).

FROMM, H., HOFMANN, A.: Breath test for altered bile-acid metabolism. Lancet II, 621—625 (1971).

FROSCH, B., WAGENER, H.: Konjugierte Serumgallensäuren bei akuter Hepatitis. Dtsch. med. Wschr. 93, 1754—1760 (1968 a).

FROSCH, B., WAGNER, H.: Methoden und Ergebnisse der quantitativen Bestimmung der konjungierten Serumgallensäuren bei Erkrankungen der Leber, Klin. Wschr. 46, 913—922 (1968 b).

GARBUTT, J. T., KENNEY, T. J.: Effect of cholestyramine on bile acid metabolism in normal man. J. clin. Invest. 51, 2781—2789 (1972).

GARBUTT, J. T., HEATON, K. W., LACK, L., TYOR, M. P.: Increased ratio of glycine- to taurine-conjugated bile salts in patients with ileal disorders. Gastroenterology 56, 711—720 (1969).

GARDINER, B. N., SMALL, D. M.: The effects of secretin (SEC) and cholycystokinin (CCK) on secretion of bile salts (BS) and biliary lipids. Clin. Res. 20, 454 (1972).

GIELEN, J., ROBAYE, B., VAN CANFORT, J., RENSON, J.: Facteurs endocriniens controlant le rhytme circadien de la biosynthése des acides biliaires. Arch. int. Pharmacodyn. 183, 403—405 (1970).

GINTER, E.: In: The role of ascorbic acid in cholesterol metabolism. Bratislava: Slovak Akad. Sci. 1970.

GINTER, E., NEMEC, R., BOBEK, P.: Stimulation of [26-^{14}C] cholesterol oxidation by ascorbic acid in scorbutic guinea-pigs. Brit. J. Nutr. a28, 205—211 (1972).

GINTER, E., CERVEN, J., NEMEC, R., MIKUS, L.: Lowered cholesterol catabolism in guinea pigs with chronic ascorbic acid deficiency. Amer. J. clin. Nutr. 24, 1238—1245 (1971).

GITLIN, D., CORNWELL, D. G., NAKASATO, D., ONCLEY, J. L., HUGHES, W. L., JR., JANEWAY, C. A.: Studies on the metabolism of plasma proteins in the nephrotic syndrome. II. The lipoproteins. J. clin. Invest. 37, 172—184 (1958).

GORBACH, S. L., NAHAS, L., WEISTEIN, L., LEVITAN, R., PATTERSON, J. F.: Studies of intestinal microflora. IV. The microflora of ileostomy effluent: a unique microbial ecology. Gastroenterology 53, 874—880 (1967).

GORDON, B. A., KUKSIS, A., BEVERIDGE, J. M. R.: Separation of bile acid conjugates by ion exchange chromatography. Canad. J. Biochem. 41, 77—89 (1963).

GREGG, J. A.: Urinary excretion of bile acids in patients with obstructive jaundice and hepatocellular disease. Amer. J. clin. Path. 49, 404—409 (1968).

GREIM, H., TRÜLZSCH, D., CZYGAN, P., RUDICK, J., HUTTERER, F., SCHAFFNER, F., POPPER, H.: Mechanism of cholestasis. 6. Bile acids in human livers with or without biliary obstruction. Gastroenterology 63, 846—850 (1972).

GRUNDY, S. M.: Treatment of hypercholesterolemia by interference with bile acid metabolism. Arch. intern. Med. 130, 638—648 (1972).

GRUNDY, S. M., AHRENS, E. H., JR.: An evaluation of the relative merits of two methods for measuring the balance of sterols in man: Isotopic balance versus chromatographic analysis. J. clin. Invest. 45, 1503—1515 (1966).

GRUNDY, S. M., METZGER, A. L.: A physiological method for estimation of hepatic secretion of biliary lipids in man. Gastroenterology 62, 1200—1217 (1972).

GRUNDY, S. M., AHRENS, E. H., JR., MIETTINEN, T. A.: Quantitative isolation and gas-liquid chromatographic analysis of total fecal bile acids. J. Lipid Res. 6, 397—410 (1965).

GRUNDY, S. M., AHRENS, E. H., JR., SALEN, G.: Dietary β-sitosterol as an internal standard to correct for cholesterol losses in sterol balance studies. J. Lipid Res. 9, 374—387 (1968).

GRUNDY, S. M., AHRENS, E. H., JR., SALEN, G.: Interruption of the enterohepatic circulation of bile acids in man: Comparative effects of cholestyramine and ileal exclusion on cholesterol metabolism. J. Lab. clin. Med. 78, 94—121 (1971).

GRUNDY, S. M., METZGER, A. L., ADLER, R. D.: Mechanisms of lithogenic bile formation in American Indian women with cholesterolgallstones. J. clin. Invest. **51**, 3026—3043 (1972a).

GRUNDY, S. M., HOFMANN, A. F., DAVIGNON, J., AHRENS, E. H., JR.: Human cholesterol synthesis is regulated by bile acids. J. clin. Invest. **45**, 1018—1019 (1966).

GRUNDY, S. M., AHRENS, E. H., JR., SALEN, G., SCHREIBMAN, P. H., NESTEL, P. J.: Mechanisms of action of clofibrate on cholesterol metabolism in patients with hyperlipidemia. J. Lipid Res. **13**, 531—551 (1972b).

GUCHAIT, R., GUHA, B. C., GANGULI, N. C.: Metabolic studies on scorbutic guinea pigs. 3. Catabolism of [4-^{14}C] cholesterol *in vivo* and *in vitro*. Biochem. J. **86**, 193—197 (1963).

GUSTAFSSON, B. E., NORMAN, A.: Physical state of bile acids in intestinal contents of germfree and conventional rats. Scand. J. Gastroenterol. **3**, 625—631 (1968).

HAMILTON, J. D., DYER, N. H., DAWSON, A. M., O'GRADY, F. W., VINCE, A., FENTON, J. C. B., MOLLIN, D. L.: Assessment and significance of bacterial overgrowth in the small bowel. Quart. J. Med. **39**, 265—285 (1970).

HAMPRECHT, B., NÜSSLER, C., LYNEN, F.: Rhytmic changes of hydroxymethylglutaryl coenzyme A reductase activity in livers of fed and fasted rats. FEBS Letters **4**, 117—121 (1969).

HAMPRECHT, B., NÜSSLER, C., WALTINGER, G., LYNEN, F.: Influence of bile acids on the activity of rat liver 3-hydroxy-3-methylglutaryl coenzyme A reductase. 1. Effect of bile acids *in vitro* and *in vivo*. Europ. J. Biochem. **18**, 10—14 (1971a).

HAMPRECHT, B., ROSCHER, R., WALTINGER, G., NÜSSLER, C.: Influence of bile acids on the activity of rat liver 3-hydroxy-3-methylglutaryl coenzyme A reductase. 2. Effect of cholic acid in lymph fistula rats. Europ. J. Biochem. **18**, 15—19 (1971b).

HASLEWOOD, G. A. D.: The biological significance of chemical differences in bile salts. Biol. Rev. **39**, 537—574 (1964).

HEATON, K. W., AUSTAD, W. I., LACK, L., TYOR, M. P.: Enterohepatic circulation of C^{14}-labeled bile salts in disorders of the distal small bowel. Gastroenterology **55**, 5—16 (1968).

HELLSTRÖM, K., LINDSTEDT, S.: Cholic-acid turnover and biliary bile-acid composition in humans with abnormal thyroid function. J. Lab. clin. Med. **63**, 666—679 (1964).

HELLSTRÖM, K., LINDSTEDT, S.: Studies on the formation of cholic acid in subjects given standardized diet with butter or corn oil as dietary fat. Amer. J. clin. Nutr. **18**, 46—59 (1966).

HEPNER, G. W., HOFMANN, A. F., THOMAS, P. J.: Metabolism of steroid and amino acid moieties of conjugated bile acids in man. I. Cholylglycine. J. clin. Invest. **51**, 1889—1897 (1972).

HILL, M. J., ARIES, V. C.: Faecal steroid composition and its relationship to cancer of the large bowel. J. Path. **104**, 129—139 (1971).

HISLOP, I. G., HOFMANN, A. F., SCHOENFIELD, L. J.: Determinants of the rate and site of bile acid absorption in man. J. clin. Invest. **46**, 1070—1071 (1967).

HOFMANN, A. F.: The function of bile salts in fat absorption. The solvent properties of dilute micellar solutions of conjugated bile salts. Biochem. J. **89**, 57—68 (1963).

HOFMANN, A. F.: A physicochemical approach to the intraluminal phase of fat absorption. Gastroenterology **50**, 56—64 (1966).

HOFMANN, A. F., BORGSTRÖM, B.: The intraluminal phase of fat digestion in man: The lipid content of the micellar and oil phases of intestinal content obtained during fat digestion and absorption. J. clin. Invest. **43**, 247—257 (1964).

HOFMANN, A. F., SCHOENFIELD, L. J., KOTTKE, B. A., POLEY, J. R.: Methods for the description of bile acid kinetics in man. In: Methods in medical research, Vol. 12, pp. 149—180. Chicago: Year Book Medical Publ. Inc. 1970.

HORLICK, L., KUDCHODKAR, B. J., SODHI, H. S.: Mode of action of chlorophenoxyisobutyric acid on cholesterol metabolism in man. Circulation **43**, 299—309 (1971).

HRUZA, Z., ZBUZKOVÁ, V.: Decrease of excretion of cholesterol during aging. Exp. Geront. **8**, 29—37 (1973).

VAN ITALLIE, T. B., HASHIM, S. A.: Clinical and experimental aspects of bile acid metabolism. Med. clin. N. Amer. **47**, 629—661 (1963).

JOHNSTON, J. M.: Mechanism of fat absorption. In: Handbook of physiology, Vol. III, sec. 6, pp. 1353—1375. Baltimore: Williams & Wilkins 1968.

KAPLOWITZ, N., KOK, E., JAVITT, N.: Postprandial serum bile acid: A sensitive test of liver function. Gastroenterology **62**, 768 (1972).

KEYS, A., GRANDE, F., ANDERSON, J. T.: Fiber and pectin in the diet and serum cholesterol concentration in man. Proc. Soc. exp. Biol. (N.Y.) **106**, 555—558 (1961).

KOTTKE, B. A.: Primary hypercholesteremia compared to combined hypercholesteremia and hypertriglyceridemia. Circulation **40**, 13—20 (1969).

KRITCHEVSKY, D.: In: Cholesterol. P. 203. New York: Wiley 1958.

KRITCHEVSKY, D., WHITEHOUSE, M. W., STAPLE, E.: Oxidation of cholesterol-26-C^{14} by rat liver mitochondria: effect of nicotinic acid. J. Lipid Res. **1**, 154—158 (1960).

KRITCHEVSKY, D., STAPLE, E., RABINOWITZ, J. L., WHITEHOUSE, M. W.: Differences in cholesterol oxidation and biosynthesis in liver of male and female rats. Amer. J. Physiol. **200**, 519—522 (1961).

KRITCHEVSKY, D., TEPPER, S. A., STAPLE, E., WHITEHOUSE, M. W.: Influence of sex and sex hormones on the oxidation of cholesterol-26-C^{14} by rat liver mitochondria. J. Lipid Res. a4, 188—192 (1963).

KUDCHODKAR, B. J., SODHI, H. S.: Enterohepatic metabolism of cholesterol in types II a and II b hyperlipoproteinemia. Circulation **46**, Suppl. II, II—267 (1972).

LEE, M. J., PARKE, D. V., WHITEHOUSE, M. V.: Regulation of cholesterol catabolism by bile salts and glycyrrhetic acid *in vivo*. Proc. Soc. exp. Biol. (N.Y.) **120**, 6—8 (1965).

LENGSFELD, H., GEY, K. F.: Mechanisms involved in the acute cholesterol-lowering effect of β-pyridylcarbinol in the starved rat. In: Metabolic effects of nicotinic acid and its derivatives, pp. 597—608. Bern-Stuttgart-Vienna: Hans Huber Publ. 1971.

LEWIS, B., PANVELIWALLA, D., TABAQCHALI, S., WOOTTON, I. D. P.: Serum-bile-acids in the stagnant-loop syndrome. Lancet **1969 I**, 219—224.

LIN, T. H., RUBINSTEIN, R., HOLMES, W. L.: A study of the effect of D- and L-triiodothyronine on bile acid excretion of rats. J. Lipid Res. **4**, 63—67 (1963).

LINDSTEDT, S.: The turnover of cholic acid in man. Acta physiol. scand. **40**, 1—9 (1957).

LINDSTEDT, S.: Catabolism of cholesterol by way of bile acids. In: Atherosclerosis, Proceedings of the Second International Symposium, pp. 262—271. Berlin-Heidelberg-New York: Springer 1970.

LINDSTEDT, S., NORMAN, A.: Turnover of bile acids in the rat. Acta physiol. scand. **38**, 121—128 (1956).

LOFLAND, H. B., JR., CLARKSON, T. B., ST. CLAIR, R. W., LEHNER, N. D. M.: Studies on the regulation of plasma cholesterol levels in squirrel monkeys of two genotypes. J. Lipid Res. **13**, 39—47 (1972).

LOTTSFELDT, F. I., KRIVIT, W., AUST, J. B., CAREY, J. B., JR.: Cholestyramine therapy in intrahepatic biliary atresia. Report of a case. New Engl. J. Med. **269**, 186—189 (1963).

LOW-BEER, T. S., POMARE, E. W., MORRIS, J. S.: Control of bile salt synthesis. Nature New Biol. **238**, 215—216 (1972).

LOW-BEER, T. S., POMARE, E. W., MORRIS, J. S.: Control of bile salt synthesis. Nature New Biol. terohepatic ciruculation of bile-salts in coeliac disease. Lancet **I**, 991—994 (1971).

MAKINO, I., NAKAGAWA, S., MASHIMO, K.: Conjugated and unconjugated serum bile acid levels in patients with hepatobiliary diseases. Gastroenterology **56**, 1033—1039 (1969).

MAKINO, I., SJÖVALL, J., NORMAN, A., STRANDVIK, B.: Excretion of 3β-hydroxy-5-cholenoic and 3α-hydroxy-5α-cholanoic acids in urine of infants with biliary atresia. FEBS Letters **15**, 161—164 (1971).

MAYER, D.: Some new aspects on the regulation of cholesterol-7α-hydroxylase activity. In: Bile acids in human diseases, pp. 103—109. Stuttgart-New York: F. K. Schattauer Verlag 1972.

MAYER, D., VOGES, A.: The role of the pituitary in control of cholesterol 7α-hydroxylase activity in the rat liver. Hoppe-Seyler's Zschr. Phys. Chem. **353**, 1187—1188 (1972).

McLEOD, G. M., WIGGINS, H. S.: Bile-salts in small intestinal contents after ileal resection and in other malabsorption syndromes. Lancet **1**, 873—876 (1968).

MEIHOFF, W. E., KERN, F., JR.: Bile salt malabsorption in regional ileitis, ileal resection, and mannitol-induced diarrhea. J. clin. Invest. **47**, 261—267 (1968).

MEKHJIAN, H. S., PHILLIPS, S. F., HOFMANN, A. F.: Conjugated bile salts block water and electrolyte transport by the human colon. Gastroenterology **54**, 1256 (1968).

MEKHJIAN, H. S., PHILLIPS, S. F., HOFMANN, A. F.: Determinants of the absorption of unconjugated bile acids (BA) in the human colon. Gastroenterology **62**, 783 (1972).

MERIMEE, T. J., HOLLANDER, W., FINEBERG, S. E.: Studies of hyperlipidemia in the HGH-deficient state. Metabolism **21**, 1053—1061 (1972).

MIDTVEDT, T., NORMAN, A.: Adsorption of bile acids to intestinal microorganisms. Acta path. microbiol. scand. **80 B**, 202—210 (1972).

MIDTVEDT, T., NORMAN, A., NYGAARD, K.: Metabolism of glycocholic acid in gastrectomized patients. Scand. J. Gastroenterol. **5**, 237—240 (1970).

MIETTINEN, T. A.: Effect of dietary cholesterol and cholic acid on cholesterol synthesis in rat and man. Progr. biochem. Pharmacol. **4**, 68—70 (1968a).

MIETTINEN, T. A.: Fecal steroid excretion during weight reduction in obese patients with hyperlipidemia. Clin. chim. Acta **19**, 341—344 (1968b).

MIETTINEN, T. A.: Fecal steroid excretion, liver lipids, and conversion of acetate and mevalonate to serum cholesterol during starvation and nicotinic acid treatment. Scand. J. clin. Lab. Invest. **21**, Suppl. 101, 20—21 (1968c).

MIETTINEN, T. A.: Mechanism of serum cholesterol reduction by thyroid hormones in hypothyroidism. J. Lab. clin. Med. **71**, 537—547 (1968d).

MIETTINEN, T. A.: Effect of nicotinic acid on catabolism and synthesis of cholesterol in man. Clin. chim. Acta **20**, 43—51 (1968e).

MIETTINEN, T. A.: Sterol balance in hypercholesterolemia. Scand. J. clin. Lab. Invest. **24**, Suppl. 110, 48—51 (1969).

MIETTINEN, T. A.: Enhanced cholesterol metabolism in obesity. Scand. J. clin. Lab. Invest. **25**, Suppl. 113, 28 (1970a).

MIETTINEN, T. A.: Detection of changes in human cholesterol metabolism. Ann. clin. Res. **2**, 300—320 (1970b).

MIETTINEN, T. A.: Drugs affecting bile acid and cholesterol excretion. In: Atherosclerosis, Proceedings of the Second International Symposium, pp. 508—515. Berlin-Heidelberg-New York: Springer-Verlag 1970c.

MIETTINEN, T. A.: Effect of cholestyramine on fecal steroid excretion and cholesterol synthesis in patients with hypercholesterolemia. In: Atherosclerosis, Proceedings of the Second International Symposium, pp. 558—562. Berlin-Heidelberg-New York: Springer-Verlag 1970d.

MIETTINEN, T. A.: Cholesterol production in obesity. Circulation **44**, 842—850 (1971a).

MIETTINEN, T. A.: Relationship between faecal bile acids, absorption of fat and vitamin B_{12}, and serum lipids in patients with ileal resections. Europ. J. clin. Invest. **1**, 452—460 (1971b).

MIETTINEN, T. A.: Cholesterol metabolism in patients with coronary heart disease. Ann. clin. Res. **3**, 313—322 (1971c).

MIETTINEN, T. A.: Effect of nicotinic acid on the fecal excretion of neutral sterols and bile acids. In: Metabolic effects of nicotinic acid and its derivatives, pp. 677—686. Bern-Stuttgart-Vienna: Hans Huber Publ. 1971d.

MIETTINEN, T. A.: Lipid absorption, bile acids, and cholesterol metabolism in patients with chronic liver disease. Gut **13**, 682—689 (1972a).

MIETTINEN, T. A.: Bile acid production in patients with thyroid dysfunction. In: Bile acids in human diseases, pp. 117—120. Stuttgart-New York: F. K. Schattauer 1972b.

MIETTINEN, T. A.: Removal of serum cholesterol in control and hyperlipidaemic subjects. Clin. chim. Acta **39**, 480—481 (1972c).

MIETTINEN, T. A.: Mode of action of a new hypocholesteraemic drug (DH-581) in familial hypercholesteraemia. Atherosclerosis **15**, 163—176 (1972d).

MIETTINEN, T. A.: Clinical implications of bile acid metabolism in man. In: The bile acids, pp. 191—247, Vol. 2. New York: Plenum Publ. Corp. 1973.

MIETTINEN, T. A.: Mechanisms of hyperlipidaemias in different clinical conditions. In: Early diagnosis of coronary heart disease. Adv. Cardiol., Vol. 8, pp. 85—99. Basel: Karger 1973a.

MIETTINEN, T. A.: Current views on cholesterol metabolism. In: Lipid metabolism, obesity and diabetes mellitus: Impact upon atherosclerosis, pp. 37—44, Stuttgart: Georg Thieme Publisher 1974.

MIETTINEN, T. A.: Effect of drugs on bile acid and cholesterol excretion. In: Lipid metabolism and atherosclerosis. International congress series n:o 283: pp. 77—89 Amsterdam; Excerpta Medica 1973.

MIETTINEN, T. A., ARO, A.: Faecal fat, bile acid excretion, and body height in familial hypercholesterolaemia and hyperglyceridaemia. Scand. J. clin. Lab. Invest. **30**, 85—88 (1972).

MIETTINEN, T. A., LESKINEN, E.: Glucuronic acid pathway. In: Metabolic conjugation and metabolic hydrolysis, pp. 157—237. New York: Academic Press Inc. 1970.

MIETTINEN, T. A., PELTOKALLIO, P.: Bile salt, fat, water, and vitamin B_{12} excretion after ileostomy. Scand. J. Gastroent. **6**, 543—552 (1971).

MIETTINEN, T. A., PERHEENTUPA, J.: Bile salt deficiency in fat malabsorption of hypoparathyroidism. Scand. J. clin. Lab. Invest. **27**, Suppl. **116**, 36 (1971).

MIETTINEN, T. A., SIURALA, M.: Distribution of lipids into micellar and oil phases during fat absorption under normal and pathological conditions. Scand. J. clin. Lab. Invest. **19**, Suppl. **95**, 69 (1967).

MIETTINEN, T. A., SIURALA, M.: Bile salts, sterols, sterol esters, glycerides and fatty acids in micellar and oil phases of intestinal contents during fat digestion in man. Z. klin. Chem. Biochem. **9**, 47—52 (1971a).

MIETTINEN, T. A., SIURALA, M.: Micellar solubilization of intestinal lipids and sterols in gluten enteropathy and liver cirrhosis. Scand. J. Gastroent. **6**, 527—535 (1971b).

MIETTINEN, T. A., PENTTILÄ, I. M., LAMPAINEN, E.: Familial occurrence of mild hyperlipoproteinaemias. Clin. Genet. **3**, 271—280 (1972).

MIETTINEN, T. A., PELKONEN, R., NIKKILÄ, E. A., HEINONEN, O.: Low excretion of fecal bile acids in a family with hypercholesterolemia. Acta med. scand. **182**, 645—650 (1967).

MITCHELL, W. D., MURCHISON, L. E.: The effect of clofibrate on serum and faecal lipids. Clin. chim. Acta **36**, 153—161 (1972).

MITROPOULOS, K. A., MYANT, N. B.: The formation of lithocholic acid, chenodeoxycholic acid and α- and β-muricholic acids from cholesterol incubated with rat-liver mitochondria. Biochem. J. **103**, 472—479 (1967).

MITROPOULOS, K. A., SUZUKI, M., MYANT, N. B., DANIELSSON, H.: Effects of thyroidectomy and thyroxine treatment on the activity of 12α-hydroxylase and of some components of microsomal electron transfer change in rat liver. FEBS Letters **1**, 13—15 (1968).

MIYAI, K., PRICE, V. M., FISHER, M. M.: Bile acid metabolism in mammals. Ultrastructural studies on the intrahepatic cholestasis induced by lithocholic and chenodeoxycholic acids in the rat. Lab. Invest. **24**, 292—302 (1971).

MODAI, M., THEODOR, E.: Intestinal contents in patients with viral hepatitis after a lipid meal. Gastroenterology **58**, 379—387 (1970).

MOORE, R. B., FRANTZ, I. D., JR., BUCHWALD, H.: Changes in cholesterol pool size, turnover rate, and fecal bile acid and sterol excretion after partial ileal bypass in hypercholesteremic patients. Surgery **65**, 98—108 (1969).

MOORE, R. B., ANDERSON, J. T., KEYS, A., FRANTZ, I. D., JR.: Effect of dietary fat on the fecal excretion of cholesterol and its degradation products in human subjects. J. Lab. clin. Med. **60**, 1000 (1962).

MOSBACH, E. H.: Regulation of bile acid synthesis. In: Bile acids in human diseases, pp. 89—96. Stuttgart-New York: F. K. Schattauer 1972.

MOSBACH, E. H., KENDALL, F. E.: Metabolism of bile acids in the dog. Circulation **16**, 490 (1957).

MOUTAFIS, C. D., MYANT, N. B.: Effects of nicotinic acid, alone or in combination with cholestyramine, on cholesterol metabolism in patients suffering from familial hyperbetalipoproteinaemia in the homozygous form. In: Metabolic effects of nicotinic acid and its derivatives, pp. 659—676. Bern-Stuttgart-Vienna: Hans Huber Publ. 1971.

MUKHERJEE, S., GUPTA, S.: Effects of gonadal hormones on cholesterol metabolism in the rat. J. Atheroscler. Res. **7**, 435—452 (1967).

MUPHY, G. M., BILLING, B. H.: The nature of monohydroxy bile acids in liver disease. In: Bile acids in human diseases, pp. 41—43. Stuttgart-New York: F. K. Schattauer Verlag 1972.

MURPHY, G. M., JANSEN, F. H., BILLING, B. H.: An abnormal bile salt in primary biliary cirrhosis. Gut **12**, 771 (1971).

MURPHY, G. M., JANSEN, F. H., BILLING, B. H.: Unsaturated monohydroxy bile acids in cholestatic liver disease. Biochem. J. **129**, 491—494 (1972a).

MURPHY, G. M., ROSS, A., BILLING, B. H.: Serum bile acids in primary biliary cirrhosis. Gut **13**, 201—206 (1972b).

MYANT, N. B.: Effects of drugs on the metabolism of bile acids. In: Pharmacological control of lipid metabolism, pp. 137—154. Adv. exp. Med. Biol., Vol. 26. New York-London: Plenum Press 1972.

MYANT, N. B., EDER, H. A.: The effect of biliary drainage upon the synthesis of cholesterol in the liver. J. Lipid Res. **2**, 363—368 (1961).

NAHRWOLD, D. L., GROSSMAN, M. I.: Effect of cholecystectomy on bile flow and composition in response to food. Amer. J. Surg. **119**, 30—34 (1970).

NAIR, P. P., GORDON, M., REBACK, J.: The enzymatic cleavage of the carbon-nitrogen bond in 3α, 7α, 12α-trihydroxy-5β-cholan-24-oylglycine. J. biol. Chem. **242**, 7—11 (1967).

NAZIR, D. J., HORLICK, L., KUDCHODKAR, B. J., SODHI, H. S.: Mechanisms of action of cholestyramine in the treatment of hypercholesterolemia. Circulation **46**, 95—102 (1972).

Neale, G., Lewis, B., Weaver, V., Panveliwalla, D.: Serum bile acids in liver disease. Gut **12**, 145—152 (1971).

Nikkilä, E. A., Kekki, M.: Polymorphism of plasma triglyceride kinetics in normal human adult subjects. Acta med. scand. **190**, 49—59 (1971).

Nikkilä, E. A., Kekki, M.: Plasma triglyceride metabolism in thyroid disease. J. clin. Invest. **51**, 2103—2114 (1972).

Nilsson, Å., Zilversmit, D. B.: Fate of intravenously administerd particulate and lipoprotein cholesterol in the rat. J. Lipid Res. **13**, 32—38 (1972).

Norman, A.: Metabolism of glycocholic acid in man. Scand. J. Gastroenterol. **5**, 231—236 (1970).

Norman, A., Strandvik, B., Zetterström, R.: Bile acid excretion and malabsorption in intrahepatic cholestasis of infancy ("Neonatal hepatitis"). Acta paediat. scand. **58**, 59—72 (1969).

Northfield, T. C., Condillac, E., McColl, I.: Bile salt metabolism in the normal human small intestine. Gut **11**, 1063 (1970).

Northfield, T. C., Drasar, B. S., Wrigth, J. T.: The value of small intestinal bile acid analysis in the diagnosis of the stagnant loop syndrome. Gastroenterology **62**, 790 (1972).

O'Maille, E. R. L., Richards, T. G.: The influence of conjugation of cholic acid on its uptake and secretion: Hepatic extraction of taurocholate and cholate in the dog. J. Physiol. **189**, 337—350 (1967).

Palmer, R. H.: The formation of bile acid sulfates: A new pathway of bile acid metabolism in humans. Proc. nat. Acad. Sci. (Wash.) **58**, 1047—1050 (1967).

Palmer, R. H.: Bile acids, liver injury, and liver disease. Arch. intern. Med. **130**, 606—617 (1972).

Palmer, R. H., Bolt, M. D.: Bile acid sulfates. I. Synthesis of lithocholic acid sulfates and their identification in human bile. J. Lipid Res. **12**, 671—679 (1971).

Peric-Golia, L., Socic, H.: Short communication. Free bile acids in sheep. Comp. Biochem. Physiol. **26**, 741—744 (1968).

Percy-Robb, I. W., Jalan, K. N., McManus, J. P. A., Sircus, W.: Bile-salt metabolism in patients with an ileostomy. Brit. J. Surg. **56**, 694—695 (1969 a).

Percy-Robb, I. W., Jalan, K. N., McManus, J. P. A., Sircus, W.: Effect of ileal resection on bile salt metabolism in patients with ileostomy following proctocolectomy. Clin. Sci. **41**, 371—382 (1971).

Percy-Robb, I. W., Telfer Brunton, W. A., Jalan, K. N., McManus, J. P. A., Sircus, W.: The relationship between the bacterial content of ileal effluent and the metabolism of bile salts in patients with ileostomies. Gut **10**, 1049 (1969 b).

Poley, J. R., Smith, J. D., Thompson, J. B.: Cholesterol-oversaturation of human gallbladder bile following treatment with human growth hormone. Gastroenterology **62**, 794 (1972 a).

Poley, J. R., Thompson, J. B., Smith, J. D.: Human growth hormone (HGH) and bile acid metabolism: Its influence upon the composition of the micellar phase during digestion. Biologie et Gastro-Enterologie **5**, 548 C (1972 b).

Poley, J. R., Dover, J. C., Owen, C. A., Jr., Stickler, G. B.: Bile acids in infants and children. J. Lab. clin. Med. **63**, 838—846 (1964).

Portman, O. W.: Nutritional influences on the metabolism of bile acids. Amer. J. clin. Nutr. **8**, 462—470 (1960).

Portman, O. W., Murphy, P.: Excretion of bile acids and β-hydroxysterols by rats. Arch. Biochem. Biophys. **76**, 367—376 (1958).

Quarfordt, S., Levy, R. I., Fredrickson, D. S.: On the lipoprotein abnormality in type III hyperlipoproteinemia. J. clin. Invest. **50**, 754—761 (1971).

Quintão, E., Grundy, S. M., Ahrens, E. H., Jr.: Effects of dietary cholesterol on the regulation of total body cholesterol in man. J. Lipid Res. **12**, 233—247 (1971).

Redgrave, T. G.: Formation of cholesteryl ester-rich particulate lipid during metabolism of chylomicrons. J. clin. Invest. **49**, 465—471 (1970).

Renson, J., van Canfort, J., Robaye, B., Gielen, J.: Mesures de la demi-vie de la cholesterol 7α-hydroxylase. Arch. int. Physiol. **77**, 972—973 (1969).

Roovers, J., Evrard, E., Vanderhaeghe, H.: An improved method for measuring human blood bile acids. Clin. chim. Acta **19**, 449—457 (1968).

Rosenberg, I. H., Hardison, W. G., Bull, D. M.: Abnormal bile-salt patterns and intestinal bacterial overgrowth associated with malabsorption. New Engl. J. Med. **276**, 1371—1397 (1967).

Rosenfeld, R. S., Hellman, L.: Excretion of steroid acids in man. Arch. Biochem. **97**, 406—410 (1962).

RUDMAN, D., KENDALL, F. E.: Bile acid content of human serum. I. Serum bile acids in patients with hepatic disease. J. clin. Invest. **36**, 530—537 (1957a).

RUDMAN, D., KENDALL, F. E.: Bile acid content of human serum. II. The binding of cholanic acids by human plasma proteins. J. clin. Invest. **36**, 538—542 (1957b).

SAMUEL, P., SAYPOL, G. M., MEILMAN, E., MOSBACH, E. H., CHAFIZADEH, M.: Absorption of bile acids from the large bowel in man. J. clin. Invest. **47**, 2070—2078 (1968).

SANDBERG, D. H., SJÖVALL, J., SJÖVALL, K., TURNER, D. A.: Measurement of human serum bile acids by gas-liquid chromatography. J. Lipid Res. **6**, 182—192 (1965).

SARLES, H., HAUTON, J., PLANCHE, N. E., LAFONT, H., GEROLAMI, A.: Diet, cholesterol gallstones, and composition of the bile. Amer. J. dig. Dis. **15**, 251—260 (1970).

SCHERSTÉN, T., NILSSON, S., CAHLIN, E., FILIPSON, M., BRODIN-PERSSON, G.: Relationship between the biliary excretion of bile acids and the excretion water, lecithin, and cholesterol in man. Europ. J. clin. Invest. **1**, 242—247 (1971).

SCHOENFIELD, L. J., SJÖVALL, J., PERMAN, E.: Bile acids on the skin of patients with pruritic hepatobiliary disease. Nature (Lond.) **213**, 93—94 (1967).

SHEFER, S., HAUSER, S., BEKERSKY, I., MOSBACH, E. H.: Feedback regulation of bile acid biosynthesis in the rat. J. Lipid Res. **10**, 646—655 (1969).

SHEFER, S., HAUSER, S., BEKERSKY, I., MOSBACH, E. H.: Biochemical site of regulation of bile acid biosynthesis in the rat. J. Lipid Res. **11**, 404—411 (1970).

SHEFER, S., HAUSER, S., LAPAR, V., MOSBACH, E. H.: HMG CoA reductase of intestinal mucosa and liver of the rat. J. Lipid Res. **13**, 402—412 (1972).

SHERR, H. P., SASAKI, Y., NEWMAN, A., BANWELL, J. G., WAGNER, H. N., JR., HENDRIX, T. R.: Detection of bacterial deconjugation of bile salts by a convenient breath-analysis technic. New Engl. J. Med. **285**, 656—661 (1971).

SHIMADA, K., BRICKNELL, K. S., FINEGOLD, S. M.: Deconjugation of bile acids by intestinal bacteria: Review of literature and additional studies. J. infect. Dis. **119**, 273—281 (1969).

SJÖVALL, J.: Dietary glycine and taurine on bile acid conjugation in man. Bile acids and steroids 75. Proc. Soc. exp. Biol. (N.Y.) **100**, 676—678 (1959).

SJÖVALL, J.: Bile acids in man under normal and pathological conditions. Clin. chim. Acta **5**, 33—41 (1960).

SJÖVALL, K., SJÖVALL, J.: Serum bile acid levels in pregnancy with pruritus. Clin. chim. Acta **13**, 207—211 (1966).

SMALL, D. M., DOWLING, R. H., REDINGER, R. N.: The enterohepatic circulation of bile salts. Arch. intern. Med. **130**, 552—573 (1972).

SODHI, H. S., KUDCHODKAR, B. J.: Relationship of hypertriglyceridemia and endogenous synthesis of cholesterol in man. Circulation **44**, Suppl. II, II—57 (1971).

SODHI, H. S., KUDCHODKAR, B. J.: Correlating metabolism of plasma and tissue cholesterol with that of plasma-lipoproteins. Lancet **1973** I, 513.

SOLOWAY, R. D., KELLY, K. A., SCHOENFIELD, L. J.: Meals and the enterohepatic circulation (EHC) of bile salts affect bile lithogenicity. Clin. Res. **19**, 403 (1971).

STANLEY, M. M.: Quantification of intestinal functions during fasting: Estimations of bile salt turnover, fecal calcium and nitrogen excretions. Metabolism **19**, 865—875 (1970).

STANLEY, M. M., NEMCHAUSKY, B.: Fecal C^{14}-bile acid excretion in normal subjects and patients with steroid-wasting syndromes secondary to ileal dysfunction. J. Lab. clin. Med. **70**, 627—639 (1967).

STANLEY, M., PAUL, D., GACKE, D., MURPHY, J.: Comparative effects of cholestyramine, metamucil and cellulose on bile salt excretion in man. Gastroenterology **62**, 816 (1972).

STAPLE, E., RABINOWITZ, J. L.: Formation of trihydroxycoprostanic acid from cholesterol in man. Biochim. biophys. Acta (Amst.) **59**, 735—736 (1962).

STIEHL, A.: Bile salt sulphates in intra- and extrahepatic cholestasis. In: Bile acids in human diseases, pp. 73—77. Stuttgart-New York: F. K. Schattauer 1972.

STIEHL, A., THALER, M. M., ADMIRAND, W. H.: The effects of phenobarbital on bile salts and bilirubin in patients with intrahepatic and extrahepatic cholestasis. New Engl. J. Med. **286**, 858—861 (1972).

STRAND, O.: Effects of D- and L-triiodothyronine and of propylthiouracil on the production of bile acids in the rat. J. Lipid Res. **4**, 305–311 (1963).

STRAND, O.: Influence of propylthiouracil and D- and L-triiodothyronine on excretion of bile acids in bile fistula rats. Proc. Soc. exp. Biol. (N.Y.) **109**, 668—672 (1962).

TABAQCHALI, S.: The pathophysiological role of small intestinal bacterial flora. Scand. J. Gastroenterol. **5**, Suppl. 6, 139—163 (1970).

TABAQCHALI, S., BOOTH, C. C.: Jejunal bacteriology and bile-salt metabolism in patients with intestinal malabsorption. Lancet **1966 II**, 12—15.

TABAQCHALI, S., HATZIOANNOU, J., BOOTH, C. C.: Bile-salt deconjugation and steatorrhoea in patients with the stagnant-loop syndrome. Lancet **1968 II**, 12—16.

THEODOR, E., SPRITZ, N., SLEISENGER, M. H.: Metabolism of intravenously injected isotopic cholic acid in viral hepatitis. Gastroenterology **55**, 183—190 (1968).

THISTLE, J. L., SCHOENFIELD, L. J.: Lithogenic bile among young Indian women. Lithogenic potential decreased with chenodeoxycholic acid. New Engl. J. Med. **284**, 177—181 (1971).

THUREBORN, E.: Human hepatic bile. Composition changes due to altered enterohepatic circulation. Acta chir. scand. Suppl. 303 (1962).

TREADWELL, C. R., VAHOUNY, G. V.: Cholesterol absorption. In: Handbook of physiology, Vol. III, sec. 6, pp. 1407—1438. Baltimore: Williams + Wilkins 1968.

TRÜLZSCH, D., GREIM, H., CZYGAN, P., ROBOZ, J., RUDICK, J., HUTTERER, F., SCHAFFNER, F., POPPER, H.: Hydroxylation of taurolithocholate by human liver microsomes. Gastroenterology **62**, 879 (1972).

TURNBERG, L. A., GRAHAME, G.: Bile salt secretion in cirrhosis of the liver. Gut **11**, 126—133 (1970).

VLAHCEVIC, Z. R., BELL, C. C., JR., SWELL, L.: Relationship of bile acid pool size and biliary lipid secretion in the formation of cholesterol gallstones in man. In: Bile acids in human diseases, pp. 161—165. Stuttgart-New York: F. K. Schattauer 1972 c.

VLAHCEVIC, Z. R., JUTTIJUDATA, P., BELL, C. C., SWELL, L.: Bile acid metabolism in patients with cirrhosis. II. Cholic and chenodeoxycholic acid metabolism. Gastroenterology **62**, 1174—1181 (1972 a).

VLAHCEVIC, Z. R., MILLER, J. R., FARRAR, J. T., SWELL, L.: Kinetics and pool size of primary bile acids in man. Gastroenterology **61**, 85—90 (1971 b).

VLAHCEVIC, Z. R., BELL, C. C., JR., BUHAC, I., FARRAR, J. T., SWELL, L.: Diminished bile acid pool size in patients with gallstones. Gastroenterology **59**, 165—173 (1970).

VLAHCEVIC, Z. R., BUHAC, I., FARRAR, J. T., BELL, C. C., SWELL, L.: Bile acid metabolism in patients with cirrhosis. I. Kinetic aspects of cholic acid metabolism. Gastroenterology **60**, 491—498 (1971 a).

VLAHCEVIC, Z. R., BELL, C. C., JR., GREGORY, D. H., BUKER, G., JUTTIJUDATA, P., SWELL, L.: Relationship of bile acid pool size to the formation of lithogenic bile in female Indians of the Southwest. Gastroenterology **62**, 73—83 (1972 b).

WALTON, K. W., SCOTT, P. J., DYKES, P. W., DAVIES, J. W. L.: The significance of alterations in serum lipids in thyroid dysfunction. II. Alterations of the metabolism and turnover of ^{131}I-low-density lipoproteins in hypothyroidism and thyrotoxicosis. Clin. Sci. **29**, 217—238 (1965).

WEINER, I. M., LACK, L.: Bile salt absorption; enterohepatic circulation. In: Handbook of physiology, Vol. III, sec. 6, pp. 1439—1455. Baltimore: Williams & Wilkins 1968.

WEIS, H. J., DIETSCHY, J. M.: Failure of bile acids to control hepatic cholesterogenesis: Evidence for endogenous cholesterol feedback. J. clin. Invest. **48**, 2398—2408 (1969).

WILSON, J. D.: The quantification of cholesterol excretion and degradation in the isotopic steady state in the rat: the influence of dietary cholesterol. J. Lipid Res. **5**, 409—417 (1964).

WILSON, J. D.: The relation between cholesterol absorption and cholesterol synthesis in the baboon. J. clin. Invest. **51**, 1450—1458 (1972).

WILSON, J. D., BENTLEY, W. H., CROWLEY, G. T.: Regulation of bile acid formation in intact animals. In: Bile salt metabolism, pp. 140—148. Springfield-Illinois: C. C. Thomas 1969.

WOLLENWEBER, J., STIEHL, A.: Größe des Pools und Turnover der primären Gallensäuren bei Hyperlipoproteinämien: Unterschiedliche Befunde bei Typ II und Typ IV Hyperlipoproteinämie. Klin. Wschr. **50**, 33—38 (1972).

WOLLENWEBER, J., KOTTKE, B. A., OWEN, C. A., JR.: Pool size and turnover of bile acids in six hypercholesteremic patients with and without administration of nicotinic acid. J. Lab. clin. Med. **69**, 584—593 (1967).

YOUSEF, I. M., FISHER, M. M.: Sex difference in bile acid composition of human bile. Gastroenterology **62**, 870 (1972).

YOUSEF, I. M., KAKIS, G., FISHER, M. M.: Bile acid metabolism in mammals. III. Sex difference in the bile acid composition of rat bile. Can. J. Biochem. **50**, 402—408 (1972).

Chapter 4

Mechanisms of Hyperlipidemia

J. M. FELTS and L. L. RUDEL

With 3 Figures

I. Introduction

Hyperlipidemia represents a spectrum of metabolic disorders, the manifestation of which includes an elevation of plasma cholesterol, triglyceride, or both above accepted normal limits. Primary lipid disorders are hereditary in nature, however, a number of plasma lipid disorders are secondary to an endocrine or nutritional imbalance or other disease processes. Although we allude to elevated cholesterol and/or triglycerides in plasma as criteria of defective lipid metabolism, a true understanding of the metabolic defects must reside in our understanding of the metabolism of the complex macromolecules which transport combinations of these lipids—i.e., the plasma lipoproteins. In the last decade we have learned a great deal about the synthesis, transport and catabolism of the various components of the lipoproteins. A completely integrated metabolic map is far from complete and in this review we will attempt to present a series of logical concepts which are supported by experimental data derived from experiments in man and other animals. At times we may indulge in speculation about possible mechanisms in areas where data are contradictory or missing. Unfortunately, few mechanisms seem fixed at the present time; instead they represent hypotheses based on limited data.

II. Normal Levels of Plasma Triglycerides and Cholesterol

To construct an accurate normal distribution curve for plasma lipid concentrations in a population, a set of standard conditions must be rigidly followed during plasma collection. These conditions are: (1) subjects should have no food or drink (except water) for a 12 to 16 hr period before the blood sample is drawn; (2) subjects should be on their normal diet for at least two weeks prior to sample collection, with no significant weight loss or gain; (3) subjects must have no family history of metabolic disease known to affect lipid levels; and (4) subjects must not be taking medications known to affect plasma lipid concentrations (FREDRICKSON and LEVY, 1972). Plasma (or serum) must be obtained promptly after blood collection and refrigerated. The lipid determinations must be done on fresh samples using methodology under good quality control, if comparisons between laboratories are to be meaningful. The usual manner of presentation is as the concentration (in mg/dl) of total triglycerides and total cholesterol in whole plasma. Lipoprotein concentrations are frequently expressed in terms of the cholesterol concentration, a practice which assumes that lipoprotein composition is comparable between individuals. Using these standard conditions, FREDRICKSON and LEVY (1972) published normal limits

Table 1. Plasma triglyceride and cholesterol concentrations in normal subjects

Age yr.	Triglycerides mg/dl	Total/Cholesterol mg/dl
0–19	65 (10–140)	175 (120–230)
20–29	70 (10–140)	180 (120–240)
30–39	75 (10–150)	205 (140–270)
40–49	85 (10–160)	225 (150–310)
50–59	95 (10–190)	245 (160–330)

Derived from Fredrickson and Levy (1972). Data from males and females were combined.

Table 2. Effect of selection on human serum lipid concentrations

Male subjects 41–73 years	Number studied	Cholesterol values		Triglyceride values	
		mean	+2 S.D.	mean	+2 S.D.
A. Random selection	151	260	358	124	283
B. After exclusion due to angina pectoris, hypertension etc.	121	256	340	119	233
C. After exclusion due to heredity	102	251	328	119	230
D. After exclusion due to abnormal EKG at rest and exercise	78	250	328	104	183

Modified from Carlson (1973)

for cholesterol and triglycerides obtained for a population of 279 males and 232 females grouped according to age. Table 1 shows their results. They have also reported an average distribution of cholesterol among lipoproteins (see Table 4) for all age groups of 9% in VLDL, 64% in LDL, and 27% in HDL. The age related trend was for LDL and VLDL cholesterol concentrations to increase, while HDL remained relatively constant.

The many difficulties in defining a "normal" plasma level has been discussed at length by Carlson (1973). Table 2 shows mean values and upper limits (95th percentile) in a small group of patients. It is clear that after exclusion of individuals on the basis of known risk factors for ischemic heart disease, the values for both cholesterol and triglycerides are lower and the reduced upper limit for triglyceride levels is most striking. It should be noted that these values are similar to the values reported by Fredrickson and Levy (1972) shown in Table 1.

III. The Plasma Lipoprotein Spectrum

The plasma lipoproteins are macromolecules composed of triglycerides, free cholesterol, cholesteryl esters, phospholipids and proteins, including some glycoproteins; relative proportions of these components are markedly different among lipoprotein classes. Description of the categories of lipoproteins is based on physicochemical techniques of isolation whereby lipoprotein species may be defined on the basis of particle density, particle charge, or particle size (Table 3).

Table 3. Lipoprotein species as established by several analytical techniques

Species	Synonyms	S_f value[a]	Flotation density[b]	Electrophoretic migration[c]	Agarose gel chromatography[d]	Particle size (Å)[e]
Chylomicrons	None	400–100000	$d < 1.006$	Remain at origin	Peak I, $K = 1.0$	800–5000
VLDL (Very low density lipoproteins)	Pre-β lipoproteins	20–400	$d < 1.006$	Pre-β or α_2 mobility	Peak I, $K = 0.94$[g]	250–800
ILDL[f] (Intermediate size low density lipoproteins)	Remnant?	? (12–20)	Not defined	? (pre-β and β)	Peak II, $K = 0.71$	?
LDL (Low density lipoproteins)	β-lipoproteins	0–12	$1.019 < d < 1.063$	β-mobility	Peak III, $K = 0.50$	215
HDL (High density lipoproteins)	α-lipoproteins	Not defined	$1.063 < d < 1.21$	α_1-mobility	Peak IV, $K = 0.30$	100
FFA (Free fatty acids)	Unesterified fatty acids	—	$d > 1.21$	albumin	—	—

[a] Svedberg flotation units (S_f) for NaCl solution of $d = 1.063$ at 26° C. HDL does not float at this density but may be isolated by flotation at $d = 1.21$ (for discussion see HATCH and LEES, 1968).

[b] Solvent density (g·ml^{-1}) at which species floats in a centrifugal field (HAVEL et al., 1955; HATCH and LEES, 1968) $d = 1.006$ is the solvent density of plasma.

[c] Migration on paper or agarose-gel electrophoresis.

[d] Agarose gel chromatography on Bio-Gel A–15 m (4%). Partition coefficients (K) calculated as follows: $K = \dfrac{V_e - V_T}{V_0 - V_T}$, where V_e = elution volume at center of peak, V_0 = void volume, and V_T = total column volume.

[e] Size as determined by electron microscopy (QUAN and JONES, personal communication).

[f] As detected using agarose gel chromatography on Bio-Gel A–15 m (4%).

[g] Chylomicrons and VLDL not resolved by chromatography

Table 4. Cholesterol distribution among serum lipoprotein of normal humans

Age	N	Serum lipoprotein cholesterol[a] distribution (mg/dl)		
		VLDL	LDL	HDL
0–19	143	12 ± 8	103 ± 27	52 ± 13
20–29	88	16 ± 10	112 ± 19	52 ± 12
30–39	67	17 ± 9	126 ± 33	51 ± 15
40–49	59	19 ± 11	134 ± 30	58 ± 16
50–59	24	25 ± 11	161 ± 30	45 ± 11

[a] Mean values $\pm$ standard deviation; nearly equal numbers of males and females are included at each age level. Derived from FREDERICKSON and LEVY (1972)

A. Techniques of Analysis

1. Separation on the Basis of Density

a) The Analytical Ultracentrifuge

The pioneering work of GOFMAN and colleagues laid the foundation for our understanding of plasma lipoproteins in normal and abnormal subjects. The relative flotation rates [expressed in SVEDBERG flotation units (S_f)] and density limits of individual lipoprotein classes were determined using analytical ultracentrifugation as the basic technique (DE LALLA and GOFMAN, 1954; DEL GATTO et al., 1959; EWING et al., 1965; and DE LALLA et al., 1967). This technique remains the standard for comparison, but it is expensive and is not available to many laboratories, thus other methods for lipoprotein characterization have been developed.

b) The Preparative Ultracentrifuge

Lipoprotein separations may be carried out in the preparative ultracentrifuge by selection of g forces and by sequentially increasing the solvent density of plasma. The original technique was described by DE LALLA and GOFMAN (1954). HAVEL et al. (1955) published a modified procedure which has been extensively used. With this technique, three species of lipoproteins are usually isolated: VLDL ($d < 1.006$), LDL ($1.006 < d < 1.063$) and HDL ($1.063 < d < 1.21$). Some laboratories isolate a subfraction of LDL ($1.006 < d < 1.019$). A small segment of the lipoprotein spectrum appears to have a density greater than $d = 1.21$ and may be recovered at a density of 1.250 (ALAUPOVIC et al., 1966). Chylomicrons are also $d < 1.006$ lipoproteins and can be separated from VLDL by an initial centrifugation at 1×10^6 g-min at $d < 1.006$ (DOLE and HAMLIN, 1962).

Almost all lipoprotein species isolated by ultracentrifugal techniques appear to be heterogenous, particularly VLDL and HDL (HATCH and LEES, 1968). Some of the apparent heterogeneity may be the result of the very high centrifugal forces involved in this technique (LEVY et al., 1965; ALAUPOVIC et al., 1966; SCANU and GRANDA, 1966; ALBERS and ALADJEM, 1971; HERBERT et al., 1973), but much of it is undoubtedly due to biological variation.

2. Separation on the Basis of Charge by Zonal Electrophoresis

Electrophoresis in a supporting medium has been often used for lipoprotein class separation. The movement of lipoproteins in an electric field is primarily due to the net charge although movement is modified if interaction with the support medium occurs. For instance, the migration of the larger lipoprotein molecules such as chylomicrons is prevented by many support media. In general, for most media, the other classes migrate and separate electrophoretically and their respective position of migration relative to plasma globulins is: VLDL, pre-β or α_2 mobility; LDL, β-mobility; HDL, α_1-mobility. Two of the most widely used and useful support media are filter paper and agarose gel. Electrophoresis using these systems is relatively inexpensive to carry out and has been used in screening large populations for abnormal lipoprotein patterns.

The use of filter paper (Table 3) as a support medium for lipoprotein electrophoresis was pioneered by FASOLI (1952) and DURRUM (1952). Subsequently, resolution of lipoprotein classes was greatly improved by addition of albumin to the buffer solution (SMITH, 1957). A standard paper electrophoresis system is described and discussed by HATCH and LEES (1968). More recently NOBLE (1968) described a system employing agarose gel as the support medium for lipoprotein electrophoresis. The separation of lipoprotein classes in this system is improved over paper since practically no charge interaction between lipoproteins and agarose occurs. In the authors' experience, agarose electrophoresis according to NOBLE (1968) is the most easily reproduced and interpreted of all forms of zonal electrophoresis of lipoproteins.

3. Gel Filtration Chromatography

The use of polymeric gels for the characterization of plasma lipoproteins was first reported by KILLANDER et al. (1964). Since then, several workers have found that individual lipoprotein species previously isolated by ultracentrifugation elute as discrete fractions from agarose gel columns (MARGOLIS, 1967; SATA et al., 1970; SATA et al., 1972; QUARFORDT et al., 1972). WERNER (1966) and MARGOLIS (1967) applied agarose gel chromatography to the estimation of the size of lipoproteins over a wide range of molecular weights. KALAB and MARTIN (1968) reported chromatographic separation of individual lipoprotein classes which had been simultaneously isolated from pig serum.

A detailed study of lipoproteins separated by agarose gel chromatography has been carried out by RUDEL et al. (1974). This technique has been extremely useful because of the time saved during lipoprotein purification. Another advantage is that the size distribution of plasma lipoprotein is recorded during separation. The spectrum of lipoproteins is quantitatively separated into three populations (peaks I, II, and III) using a 6% agarose column as shown in Fig. 1 (RUDEL et al., 1974). The column separated lipoprotein fractions were shown to be practically identical to VLDL, LDL, and HDL, respectively, which were separated from another aliquot of the same plasma samples by standard sequential ultracentrifugation procedures. Criteria used to establish identity included electrophoretic mobility in 0.5% agarose, immunoreactivity as determined by immunodiffusion and immunoelectrophoresis, size and homogeneity as seen by electron microscopy, apolipoprotein composition as seen after polyacrylamide disc gel electrophoresis and chemical composition

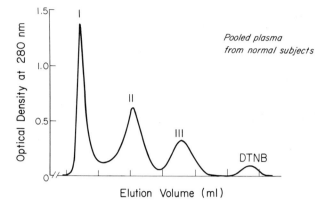

Fig. 1. Separation of plasma lipoprotein species by agarose column chromatography. Lipo-proteins from 10 ml of pooled plasma from two normal subjects were first isolated by ultracentri-fugation at $d = 1.225$, then applied to a Bio-Gel A −5 m agarose column (1.5 × 90 cm) and eluted with 0.15 M NaCl, 0.01% EDTA at 4° C. DTNB [5,5'-dithio (bis)-2-nitrobenzoic acid] was pre-sent in plasma as an inhibitor of the enzyme lecithin: cholesterol acyltransferase and serves as a marker for the total column volume (V_T). (Adapted from RUDEL et al., 1974)

(Table 5). The good agreement between the structure of column isolated and ultra-centrifugally isolated lipoprotein fractions is a significant finding since it probably represents the first such structural comparison with lipoprotein classes isolated by alternate techniques.

More recently we have used chromatography on 4% agarose columns to enhance the separation in the size range of the low density lipoproteins, i.e., those with density less than 1.063 g/ml. This procedure appears to give three subpopulations in this range. The largest are those particles which are nearly too large to enter the gel and elute near the void volume (Vo). They are the VLDL (partition coefficient, K, of 0.94). The smallest of the three is the LDL, $K = 0.50$. An unexpected finding for many plasma samples was the additional population of $d < 1.063$ lipoproteins which is intermediate in size between VLDL and LDL. It has been termed intermediate-size low density lipoprotein (ISL or ILDL), and has a partition coefficient of about 0.70. The ILDL appears to be present in many individuals with normal blood lipid values (Fig. 2a and 2b) and within the same individual relatively more material appears in the ILDL region in plasma collected shortly after a meal than in fasting plasma (RUDEL, unpublished data). In some patients with hyperlipidemia, ILDL may be the predominant lipoprotein (Fig. 2c). We know that at least two pathologic conditions, namely nephrosis and Type III hyperlipoproteinemia, can lead to elevated levels of ILDL. The chemical nature of ILDL has not yet been determined in a large number of individuals, but preliminary analyses have shown it is quite similar to LDL, except that it contains relatively more triglycerides and cholesteryl esters (RUDEL and FELTS, unpublished observations).

4. Precipitation with Polyanion-Metal Complexes

A technique useful when large numbers of samples are to be evaluated is the one in which classes of lipoproteins containing the apolipoprotein of LDL are precipitated using anionic polysaccharides (heparin or dextran sulfate) and divalent metal ions

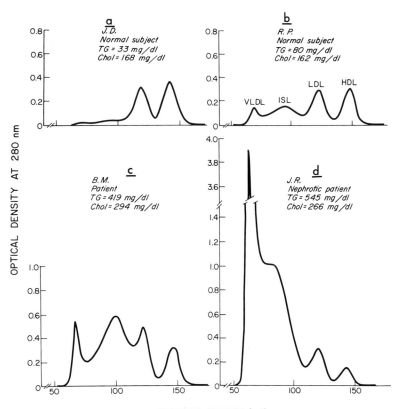

Fig. 2a—d. Chromatographic separation of plasma lipoprotein species on a Bio-Gel A-15 m (4%) agarose column. Lipoproteins from 30 ml of plasma were first isolated by ultracentrifugation at $d = 1.225$, then were applied to the agarose chromatography column (1.5 × 90 cm) and eluted with 0.15 M NaCl, 0.01% EDTA at 4° C (FELTS unpublished observations). (a) Male, normal subject, age 19. (b) Male, normal subject, age 21. (c) Male, hyperlipemic patient, age 53. (Variously classified by electrophoresis as Fredrickson Type II B, IV or V).(d) Male, nephrotic patient, age 32

(Ca^{++} or Mn^{++}) (BURSTEIN and SAMAILLE, 1960; CORNWELL and KRUGER, 1961; KRITCHEVSKY et al., 1963). The products of this type of separation are the HDL (α-lipoproteins), which remain in solution, and the VLDL + LDL (β + pre-β lipoproteins) which aggregate and precipitate as part of an ionic complex with the divalent metal and polyanionic polysaccharide. FREDRICKSON et al. (1967) have recommended a combination of ultracentrifugation at d 1.006 to isolate VLDL, combined with heparin-manganese precipitation to isolate HDL, as a means to determine the distribution of cholesterol among plasma VLDL, LDL, and HDL, The amount of cholesterol in LDL is determined by obtaining the difference between the VLDL + HDL cholesterol and whole plasma cholesterol. Mean values for lipoprotein cholesterol distribution obtained using this technique (FREDRICKSON and LEVY, 1972) are shown in Table 4.

Table 5. The chemical composition of human plasma lipoproteins isolated by agarose (6%) column chromatography (Col.) and by sequential ultracentrifugation (U.C.)

Lipo-protein fraction	Free choles-terol	% of total weight			Protein	Ratios	
		Choles-teryl ester	Phospho-lipid	Trigly-ceride		Total choles-terol/ phospho-lipid	Esterified/ total choles-terol
VLDL Col.	6.1 ±0.7	12.8 ± 3.3	19.6 ± 1.2	47.7 ± 6.2	13.5 ± 2.0	0.71	0.56
VLDL U.C.	5.4 ±0.7	12.6 ± 0.2	21.5 ± 1.8	48.1 ± 3.7	11.6 ± 0.7	0.62	0.58
LDL Col.	9.4 ±0.2	39.9 ± 1.2	22.6 ± 0.3	5.4 ± 0.3	21.6 ± 0.3	1.50	0.72
LDL U.C.	8.8 ±0.1	42.1 ± 1.4	23.7 ± 0.1	5.1 ± 1.7	19.9 ± 0.7	1.44	0.74
HDL Col.	3.2 ±0.2	20.8 ± 0.7	25.2 ± 0.6	7.7 ± 1.9	43.7 ± 1.5	0.64	0.79
HDL U.C.	3.0 ±0.4	21.4 ± 1.1	29.0 ± 0.9	2.1 ± 2.1	43.8 ± 3.9	0.55	0.81

Modified from Rudel et al. (1974).
Individual plasma samples were divided in half for lipoprotein isolation by both methods. Each value represents the mean ± SEM for determinations performed in duplicate on lipoprotein preparations from three individuals

B. Structure and Chemical Composition of Plasma Lipoproteins

Table 5 shows the chemical composition of the major classes of lipoproteins isolated by conventional ultracentrifugation methods and by the agarose column technique. Good agreement exists between the chemical composition of the lipoprotein species separated on the basis of density or particle size (Rudel et al., 1974). The density of the lipoprotein particles is inversely related to the total lipid content of the lipoprotein and is directly related to the protein content. The larger lipoproteins (VLDL and chylomicrons) are rich in triglyceride. Studies by Zilversmit (1965, 1968) suggest that chylomicrons probably consist of a core and a surface coat or shell. The core contains the most non-polar constituents—triglycerides and cholesteryl esters, while the coat consists of the more polar constituents—free cholesterol, phospholipids and the apolipoproteins. The same model probably applies to the VLDL. In this sense, these lipoproteins are similar to a triglyceride emulsion in an aqueous solution which is stabilized at the interface with molecules that possess both hydrophilic and hydrophobic groups.

The LDL are considerably smaller than the VLDL and are very rich in cholesteryl esters and poor in triglycerides. It has been suggested that LDL is a highly organized complex with sub-unit structure (Pollard et al., 1969). The HDL contains from 45 to 55% protein and significant amounts of cholesteryl ester and phospholipid. HDL may be a highly organized complex with sub-unit structure (Forte et al., 1968). By ultracentrifugal techniques, HDL is often divided into two sub-species, HDL_2 (95 Å) and HDL_3 (65 Å) (Forte et al., 1968).

In addition to the lipid constituents, plasma lipoproteins contain an array of different apolipoproteins which together constitute the protein component. Some apolipoproteins are glycoproteins and are distributed among several lipoprotein classes. Their movement from one lipoprotein to another during metabolism has been described (HAVEL et al., 1973; BILHEIMER et al., 1972; EISENBERG et al., 1972). The chemistry and distribution of the apolipoproteins has recently been reviewed (FREDRICKSON et al., 1972).

C. Free Fatty Acids (FFA)

The free fatty acids are long chain fatty acids which serve as an important source of calories for many tissues of the body during periods of fasting. They are transported between adipose tissue and other tissues as an ionic complex between serum albumin and the free (or unesterified) fatty acids. Albumin contains from 5 to 6 binding sites for fatty acids and is therefore a very efficient transport vehicle for free fatty acids (MASORO and FELTS, 1958). The concentration of FFA in plasma is relatively low compared to other plasma lipids; however, FFA turnover is much more rapid.

FFA concentrations in plasma are determined by the balance between adipose tissue esterification reactions which form triglycerides and lipolysis reactions which produce FFA. The mobilization of free fatty acids is dependent on the activation of hormone sensitive lipase contained in adipocytes. This lipase is under hormonal control and activation is carried out by a protein-kinase which is catalyzed by adenosine 3', 5'-monophosphate (Cyclic-AMP) (KHOO et al., 1973). The FFA liberated by hydrolysis of adipose tissue triglycerides are released by the adipocyte and become attached to plasma albumin for transport to sites of utilization. FFA are taken up by many tissues but a large fraction is removed by the liver. In the liver, the FFA may be oxidized or incorporated into triglycerides of VLDL (MAYES and FELTS, 1967). The fraction of FFA which gives rise to triglycerides in VLDL is under nutritional control.

IV. The Metabolism of Constituents of Plasma Lipoproteins

The concentration of each lipoprotein species in the circulation is the result of a balance between the rates of production and assimilation. Since each lipoprotein is a complex macromolecule consisting of several lipid classes and one or more apolipoproteins, the mechanisms involved in lipoprotein metabolism are necessarily complex and are incompletely understood. More of the details of synthesis and catabolism of VLDL are known than for LDL and HDL.

Two tissues appear to be responsible for the production of "nascent" VLDL which enter the circulation—the intestinal mucosa and the liver. The intestinal mucosa is responsible for the production of chylomicrons and VLDL (I-VLDL) primarily from exogenous or dietary lipids absorbed from the intestinal lumen. The liver produces VLDL (L-VLDL) primarily from endogenous sources of lipids. Once these "nascent" lipoproteins enter the circulation, assimilation begins immediately. What we observe in plasma is a spectrum of lipoprotein particles at all stages of degradation. The flux of plasma lipids through each of the lipoprotein pools at any point in time is related to the nutritional state of the subject, however, even under fasting conditions there is a continuing secretion of "nascent" VLDL from both the intestinal mucosa and from the liver.

The formation of LDL occurs as a part of the process of catabolism of VLDL (Eisenberg et al., 1973); that is to say LDL are apparently a product of intravascular VLDL catabolism. Some evidence suggests that LDL, *per se*, are also made in the liver (Marsh and Whereat, 1959) and intestine (Kessler et al., 1970). The site of LDL catabolism is presumed to be the liver. HDL appear to be synthesized and released, as such, by the intestine and the liver (Windmüller et al., 1973; Radding and Steinberg, 1960). At least some HDL catabolism appears to occur in the liver (Rachmilewitz et al., 1972).

A. Triglyceride Transport in Chylomicrons and VLDL

1. Intestinal Mucosal Cell

After breakdown in the intestinal lumen, dietary fat is absorbed primarily as monoglycerides and fatty acids whereupon it is resynthesized into triglyceride. It is then incorporated in combination with cholesteryl esters, free cholesterol, phospholipids, and apolipoproteins into chylomicrons and I-VLDL. These triglyceride-rich lipoproteins are then released into the intestinal lacteals for transport via the lymph system into the blood where metabolism of the triglyceride begins. The size of a fat meal appears to determine the amount of triglyceride absorbed and released by the cells in chylomicrons and I-VLDL; the more triglyceride absorbed, the higher the proportion of chylomicrons to VLDL (Windmüller et al., 1970). This arbitrary division of labor between chylomicrons and I-VLDL seems quite reasonable since these two lipoprotein classes appear to represent segments of a continuous spectrum of particles, the structure of which differs only on the basis of size (Rudel et al., 1973a). The intestinal mucosal cells continue to release I-VLDL long after the fat meal is absorbed and chylomicrons have disappeared (Ockner et al., 1969; Tytgat et al., 1971). In rats, the contribution of I-VLDL to the plasma pool of VLDL has been calculated to represent from 10% (Windmüller et al., 1970) to 40% (Ockner et al., 1969), and in rabbits, 20% (Rudel et al., 1973b).

2. Liver

In addition to the intestinal mucosa, the liver parenchymal cells synthesize and release triglyceride rich L-VLDL. Under normal conditions, the liver does not produce chylomicron-size particles. The driving force for L-VLDL production is analogous to that of the intestine, i.e., increased flux of fatty acids into the liver cells, or increased synthesis by the cells, which stimulates liver triglyceride formation and subsequent L-VLDL release. The origin of the fatty acids of L-VLDL triglyceride is not the same as for I-VLDL.

Some fatty acids of L-VLDL may arise from *de novo* fatty acid synthesis. During the post-prandial period, while dietary carbohydrate is being absorbed, lipogenesis in the liver is increased leading to *de novo* synthesis of fatty acids (Masoro et al., 1950) which could lead to an increased synthesis of triglycerides and of L-VLDL. However, dietary fat has an inhibitory effect on hepatic lipogenesis (Masoro, 1962) and the normal Western diet, which is a high fat diet, may have the effect of limiting *de novo* fatty acid synthesis in liver during the post-prandial period.

The most important source of fatty acids for L-VLDL triglyceride are the plasma free fatty acids (FFA). In fasting subjects, the plasma FFA are derived primarily from mobilization of adipose tissue fat stores. It has been estimated that in fasting man, FFA serve as virtually the sole precursors of L-VLDL triglycerides (HAVEL et al., 1970). However, during fat absorption after a meal, it has been shown in rabbits that at least a portion of plasma FFA are derived from the hydrolysis in plasma of chylomicron and I-VLDL triglycerides which is catalyzed by the enzyme lipoprotein lipase (HAVEL et al., 1962).

B. Cholesterol Transport in Chylomicrons and VLDL

1. Intestinal Mucosal Cell

Cholesterol absorption by the intestinal mucosa is the process by which cholesterol, solubilized by inclusion into mixed micelles in the intestinal lumen, is taken into the cell and incorporated into either chylomicrons or I-VLDL. These lipoproteins are subsequently released from the cell into the intestinal lacteals. It has been shown in the rat (TREADWELL et al., 1958) and in the rabbit (RUDEL et al., 1972) that 70 to 80% of the dietary (exogenous) cholesterol which appears in the lymph chylomicrons and I-VLDL is ester cholesterol, suggesting that the intestinal mucosal cell preferentially esterifies the exogenous cholesterol of chylomicrons and I-VLDL during absorption. Much less endogenous cholesterol than exogenous cholesterol was esterified in these two studies, a finding apparently in agreement with that of ZILVERSMIT (1965) for human chylomicrons.

The fact that dietary cholesterol may be preferentially esterified during absorption has often been overlooked but it may be an important aspect of the hypercholesterolemia which occurs in man and in many species of animals used in the study of experimental atherosclerosis. A characteristic of most of the animals which respond to dietary cholesterol with massive elevations of plasma cholesterol is the presence of cholesteryl ester-rich triglyceride-poor lipoproteins which span the size range from VLDL to LDL (CAMEJO et al., 1973; PAULA and RUDEL, 1974). These cholesteryl ester-rich lipoproteins may represent the "remnants" of chylomicron and I-VLDL metabolism by lipoprotein lipase.

In addition to the exogenous, or diet-derived cholesterol, much of that present in chylomicrons and I-VLDL is from endogenous sources, including bile, sloughed epithelial cells, and *de novo* synthesis by intestinal mucosal cells. RUDEL et al. (1972) have calculated that in rabbits fed meals containing 0.08% cholesterol, the percent of cholesterol appearing in lymph after a meal was about 60% from endogenous sources and 40% from exogenous sources. Further calculations showed that about 60% of the endogenous cholesterol of lymph chylomicrons and I-VLDL originated from the lumen and about 40% originated from the intestinal mucosal cell, probably via *de novo* synthesis.

The intestine has been shown to have a relatively high rate of cholesterol synthesis when compared to other tissues (DIETSCHY and WILSON, 1968). This synthesis is apparently not inhibited by cholesterol feeding, but is responsive to bile acids (DIETSCHY, 1968). It is not known if this represents synthesis of endogenous cholesterol of chylomicrons and I-VLDL *per se*, but this might be the case. In this circumstance, the endogeneous sources of chylomicrons and I-VLDL cholesterol might change, depending on the nutritional state of the animals.

2. Liver

The liver serves as the central clearing house for the cholesterol of the body (MORRIS and CHAIKOFF, 1959), i.e., the rate of synthesis in liver is higher than in other tissues; the liver is one of the few tissues which actively esterify cholesterol; and, the liver is the only tissue in which catabolism of significant amounts of cholesterol occurs. One of the means by which liver plays its central role is by synthesizing and releasing lipoproteins. Significant amounts of cholesterol are released as an integral part of L-VLDL and of HDL, although the absolute values for the amount released in each lipoprotein are open to debate. In addition, plasma VLDL are believed to give rise to plasma LDL. Thus, the liver seems directly responsible for the bulk of cholesterol which circulates in the plasma lipoproteins, the only other tissue of known significance being the intestine.

Factors that control the amount of cholesterol which is released into plasma include cholesterol synthesis and catabolism and protein synthesis and catabolism. The orchestration among all of these processes is not completely understood. We do know that chylomicrons and I-VLDL deliver cholesterol to the liver, probably in the form of cholesteryl ester-rich "remnant" lipoproteins (REDGRAVE, 1970), and in some way this signals the liver to decrease cholesterol synthesis (DIETSCHY and WILSON, 1970). Bile acids, which are the major products of cholesterol degradation in the liver, undergo enterohepatic circulation and apparently can exert a feedback effect on cholesterol synthesis (SHEFER et al., 1973). In these instances, presumably less cholesterol is available for release in the plasma lipoproteins. The exception is in animals fed cholesterol enriched diets when the amount of liver cholesterol may go up even while synthesis is depressed. In this case, more "remnant" lipoprotein cholesterol may be reaching the liver than is lost by cutbacks in synthesis. The liver may attempt to increase the mechanisms by which it can rid itself of excess cholesterol. In many species the rate of bile acid synthesis is turned up, and the rate of cholesterol excretion in bile is also increased. Increased amounts of cholesterol available for lipoprotein formation may also induce the formation of cholesteryl ester-rich very low density lipoproteins (SHORE et al., 1974). The extent to which cholesterol can direct the synthesis of L-VLDL is unknown but would seem limited since these lipoproteins are normally triglyceride rich and the primary stimulus for their formation is probably the FFA reaching the liver (see above).

C. Triglyceride Assimilation Mechanisms

1. Role of Liver

Until 1965 it was generally believed that the liver played a major role in the assimilation of triglycerides. Experiments carried out with a carefully designed liver perfusion technique demonstrated that the liver did not assimilate triglycerides in chylomicrons (FELTS and MAYES, 1965; FELTS, 1965) or in VLDL (MAYES and FELTS, 1967) at appreciable rates. These observations served to focus attention on peripheral mechanisms as primary in initiating the assimilation of triglycerides contained in circulating lipoproteins. Knowledge of peripheral mechanisms which could "clear" lipemic plasma had been developing over a period of years beginning with the observations of HAHN in 1943.

The assimilation of triglycerides contained in chylomicrons and VLDL is a complex interaction between these lipoprotein particles and the enzyme, lipoprotein lipase (LPL) which is located on capillary endothelial surfaces. Once chylomicrons, I-VLDL and L-VLDL enter the circulation, assimilation begins immediately, producing a diverse spectrum of particles at all stages of degradation. The role of the liver is in further metabolizing the triglyceride poor "remnant" lipoproteins resulting from the interaction with LPL. The reactants, products, and controlling factors for LPL are described below.

2. Role of Lipoprotein Lipase

In vivo and *in vitro* experiments carried out by HAHN (1943) and by ANDERSON and FAWCETT (1950) demonstrated that plasma from animals or human subjects previously injected with heparin (post-heparin plasma) had the property of clearing lipemic plasma when mixed with it *in vitro*. Heparin added directly to lipemic plasma *in vitro* had no clearing activity. These observations led to the concept that injected heparin releases a "clearing factor" from some tissue site in the body and that the "clearing factor" induced the degradation of chylomicrons in plasma. It is now recognized that the injection of heparin into the circulation releases lipolytic activity into the circulation, however, the lipolytic activity may be a mixture of lipases including at least one enzyme from the peripheral circulation and one enzyme from the liver. The lipase released from the peripheral circulation is LPL. This enzyme catalyzes the hydrolysis of triglycerides of chylomicrons and VLDL to FFA and free glycerol. An enzyme can be extracted from a number of tissues which has the characteristics of LPL and has been described by KORN (1955a) as a heparin-activated lipoprotein lipase. The localization of LPL activity released by heparin injection was investigated by ROBINSON and HARRIS (1959). They concluded that LPL was located on capillary endothelial surfaces and that heparin and other large negatively-charged polysaccharides are able to displace the enzyme from its binding sites (ROBINSON and HARRIS, 1959; KORN, 1959).

KORN (1955a) carried out studies of the lipase contained in acetone powder extracts of heart muscle and adipose tissue. In the presence of a fatty acid acceptor the enzyme in the tissue extracts actively hydrolyzed triglycerides contained in chylomicrons to free fatty acids and free glycerol. Little or no hydrolysis occurred when an artificial triglyceride emulsion was used as substrate, unless the artificial emulsion was preincubated with whole serum or serum lipoproteins. The reaction rate could be increased by the addition of small amounts of heparin to the assay system. On the basis of these and other observations, Korn postulated that the tissue enzyme was the same enzyme that was present in post-heparin serum. He described the tissue enzyme as a heparin-activated lipoprotein lipase, able to catalyze the clearing of lipemic plasma in identical fashion to plasma post-heparin lipoprotein lipase. The overall reaction may be represented as follows:

$$\text{Triglyceride-Lipoprotein Complex} + \text{Albumin} \xrightarrow{\text{LPL}} \text{Albumin-Fa} + \text{Free Glycerol} + \text{Lipoprotein Remnant}$$

LPL is characterized as follows: (1) it has lipolytic activity with "activated" trigly-ceride emulsions, chylomicrons and VLDL but is almost inactive with an artificial triglyceride emulsion; (2) it is stimulated by the addition of heparin to the assay system; (3) it is markedly inhibited by the addition of 0.5 to 1.0 M NaCl and by protamine.

In the plasma from normal fasting individuals, most investigators have found little or no LPL activity under the usual conditions of assay. However, after a fatty meal, LPL does appear in the plasma of rats (JEFFRIES, 1954; ROBINSON et al., 1954, 1955) and humans (ENGELBERG, 1957).

After the intravenous injection of heparin into normal fasting individuals, LPL rapidly appears in plasma. As the dose of heparin is increased more enzyme appears in the circulation until a maximum is reached. The activity is also related to the time lapse between the injection of heparin and collection of the blood sample (KORN, 1959). After injection, enzyme activity rapidly disappears from the circulation in an exponential manner (YOSHITOSHI et al., 1963) due to inactivation in the liver (NAITO and FELTS, 1970; WHAYNE et al., 1969). As stated above, the lipolytic activity appear-ing in plasma is in many cases a mixture of LPL from capillary surfaces and an enzyme from liver which is released by heparin (BOBERG et al., 1964; HAMILTON, 1965; KRAUSS et al., 1973). These latter studies have raised serious questions con-cerning the interpretation of post-heparin lipolytic activity. Recently KRAUSS et al. (1973) have described an approach to this problem which may be of benefit in differentiating the two types of activity in plasma. The magnitude of the contamina-tion of LPL with the liver enzyme may be related to the dose of heparin administered (FREDRICKSON et al., 1963). It should be noted that the liver enzyme does not have the same characteristics as LPL. It is relatively inactive against chylomicrons but will hydrolyze an artificial emulsion (HAMILTON, 1965); it is not inhibited by 1 M NaCl or protamine (MAYES and FELTS, 1968; KRAUSS et al., 1973).

LPL has been assayed in many tissues including heart muscle, skeletal muscle, adipose tissue, kidney, spleen, aorta and others (KORN, 1959). The enzyme is either absent in liver or is present in an inactive form (MAYES and FELTS, 1968). The enzyme is most active in heart muscle and adipose tissue where it appears to be under nutritional control (KORN, 1959; BEZMAN et al., 1962; GOUSIOS, 1963; BORENSTZ-TAJN and ROBINSON, 1970; ROBINSON, 1970). Robinson has postulated that LPL may be synthesized by tissue cells in a soluble form. It may then be translocated to binding sites on capillary endothelial surfaces. It is in this position that the solid state enzyme becomes effective in interacting with the large lipoprotein complexes to catalyze the hydrolysis of triglycerides (ROBINSON, 1970).

KORN was the first to recognize that the nature of the triglyceride substrate markedly influenced the rate of the LPL reaction (KORN, 1955b). He concluded that the "active" substrate must be a form of triglyceride-protein complex before an en-zyme-substrate interaction could be effected. Certain plasma lipoproteins were found to be effective activators, plasma HDL being most effective. More recent studies in the rat and human have shown that both VLDL and HDL are effective acti-vators while LDL and lipoprotein-free serum are ineffective (WHAYNE and FELTS, 1970b; BIER and HAVEL, 1970). Recent studies have been carried out in an attempt to define which of the numerous apolipoproteins shared by HDL and VLDL are most effective in the activation, in vitro, of lipoprotein lipase. The apolipo-

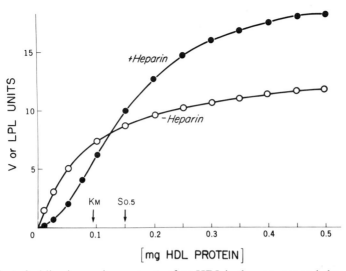

Fig. 3. The effect of adding increasing amounts of rat HDL in the presence and absence of heparin (1.0 U/ml) on the LPL activity in guinea pig postheparin serum. (Adapted from WHAYNE and FELTS, 1970)

protein referred to as apo-Lp-Glu (FREDRICKSON et al., 1972) or C–II (ALAUPOVIC, 1972), which contains C-terminal glutamic acid, has been shown in two laboratories to be the most effective activator (HAVEL et al., 1970; LA ROSA et al., 1970). It must be pointed out, however, that the *in vitro* system in which such studies are carried out is highly artificial, and it may not be that a single polypeptide is a simple activator, or cofactor, for the enzyme *in vivo*. Rather, it may be the combined effect of all of the apolipoproteins simultaneously present on a particular lipoprotein which determines the ability of lipoprotein lipase to catalyze hydrolysis. For example, LA ROSA et al. (1970) have found apo-Lp-ala to be an inhibitor of lipoprotein lipase, *in vitro*. Since this apolipoprotein appears to be present in high concentrations on all VLDL it probably does not completely inhibit LPL *in vivo*. It seems likely that the role of apolipoproteins is to confer structural specificity to triglyceride-rich lipoproteins which facilitates the action of lipoprotein lipase.

Heparin which was originally thought to be a cofactor for LPL, has a variable effect on the reaction rate in the assay system depending on the source of enzyme (WHAYNE and FELTS, 1970a). Recently, a kinetic study has been carried out on LPL in post-heparin serum from guinea pigs (WHAYNE and FELTS, 1970b). This animal has a very low level of circulating lipoproteins and its post-heparin serum contains a low concentration of apolipoproteins which activate triglyceride emulsions. The concentration of the "effective" substrate was increased stepwise by adding to the assay system rat HDL, which is rich in activator apolipoproteins. Thus, the velocity of the reaction could be plotted against increasing "effective" substrate concentrations. In the absence of heparin, a hyperbolic curve was found which conformed to Michaelis-Menten kinetics. In the presence of heparin an S-shaped curve was found with a marked increase in V_{max}. This curve conformed to the Hill equation which defines S-shaped kinetics (Fig. 3). These results strongly suggest that heparin acts as a specific ligand to produce a conformational change in LPL. This allosteric change in the enzyme may then allow cooperativity between "activated" areas of the substrate. At low "effective" substrate concentrations the reaction rate is decreased while at high "effective" substrate concentrations the reaction rate is accelerated. If the enzyme *in situ* were held in the heparin-configuration, it would serve a "lipostat" function to set the level of circulating triglycerides. In this connection, it is of interest that *in vivo* heparin is found in mast cells which are in close proximity to the capillaries where the active form of LPL is thought to reside. Experiments have shown that the affinity of LPL for heparin is very great, which supports the idea that it functions as a ligand for the enzyme (Olivecrona and Egelrud, 1971). Two forms of the enzyme have been demonstrated in adipose tissue (Garfinkel and Schotz, 1972). These may represent LPL in two different conformational states although their kinetic properties have not yet been investigated.

D. Cholesterol Assimilation Mechanisms

Chylomicrons, I-VLDL, and L-VLDL contain both free and esterified cholesterol. Cholesteryl esters have been shown to be present principally in the lipid core while much of the free cholesterol is found in association with the outer coat or "shell" (Zilversmit, 1965, 1968; Huang and Kuksis, 1967). Perhaps due in part to this configuration, cholesteryl ester does not readily exchange back and forth between chylomicrons, VLDL and other lipoproteins (Goodman, 1962; Minari and Zilversmit, 1963; Roheim et al., 1963). On the other hand, much of the free cholesterol is present near the surface and rapidly exchanges with free cholesterol of other lipoproteins and with that of cell membranes. (The use of the word "exchange" here implies a physical movement between sites, independent of energy-requiring metabolic processes.) These facts mean that biochemical study of the sequence of events in cholesteryl ester metabolism is quite feasible, whereas study of free cholesterol metabolism is more difficult.

Perhaps some of the most meaningful studies of lipoprotein cholesteryl ester metabolism are derived from reinjection studies of labeled chylomicrons. Biggs (1957) was first to show that the ^{3}H-cholesterol of labeled chylomicrons is selectively taken up by the liver. The uptake by liver has been further investigated in a number of laboratories. Goodman (1962) carried out a study of chylomicron ^{14}C-cholesteryl esters after injection into rats. The chylomicrons were pre-incubated with red blood cells before injection to reduce the amount of radioactivity in the free cholesterol moiety. After injection, tissue distribution was determined over intervals ranging from 5 min to 24 hrs. After 20 min, 85% of the ^{14}C-cholesterol had disappeared from blood. Most of the labeled cholesteryl ester was recovered in the liver and was apparently taken up or sequestered in the liver without prior hydrolysis of the ester. In the liver, a slow net hydrolysis of cholesteryl ester took place over a period of hours. By 3.5 hrs 80% of the cholesteryl ester had been hydrolyzed. Concomitant with hydrolysis, there was a progressive slow loss of ^{14}C-cholesterol from the liver as the released free cholesterol equilibrated between the cholesterol pools of liver, blood, and peripheral tissues. The central role of the liver in removal of chylomicron cholesterol was further emphasized by the studies of Nestel et al. (1963). In intact dogs, the $T_{\frac{1}{2}}$ for removal of labeled cholesteryl ester contained in injected chylomicrons averaged approximately 19 min. Total exclusion of the liver from the circulation in one dog increased the $T_{\frac{1}{2}}$ to 140 min. The effect of hepatectomy on triglyceride and phospholipid removal was much less marked.

In contrast to the rapid uptake of chylomicron cholesteryl ester seen *in vivo*, limited uptake occurs in perfused livers. HILLYARD et al. (1959) perfused livers with nonheparinized blood containing ^{14}C-cholesterol labeled chylomicrons. Only about 10% of the radioactivity was removed by the liver in 60 min. An increase to 30% removed in 60 min was observed when livers were perfused with blood from heparin-ized rats. QUARFORDT and GOODMAN (1969) studied uptake by liver of doubly-labeled cholesteryl esters of chylomicrons. These authors compared liver cholesteryl ester uptake when chylomicrons were injected into intact rats (after which the livers were removed for perfusion) to that observed when chylomicrons were administered directly to isolated perfused livers. The uptake of labeled cholesteryl ester by liver was increased several fold when the chylomicrons were administered to the intact animal before perfusion. In reinjection studies, LOSSOW et al. (1963) found that the rate of removal from plasma of ^{14}C-cholesterol of chyle injected into rats was in-creased significantly after the injection of heparin.

The discrepancies in the affinity by the liver for chylomicron cholesteryl ester as seen by comparing these results seem to have a common origin. Chylomicrons apparently need first to be acted upon by lipoprotein lipase before uptake of choles-teryl ester by the liver can occur. In this way mechanisms for the assimilation of triglycerides and cholesteryl esters are interrelated, although the events which occur are not yet understood at the molecular level. Hepatic uptake of cholesteryl esters could be dependent on the physicochemical composition of the particle. When the chylomicron or I-VLDL particles first enter the circulation, triglyceride removal may be initiated by peripheral LPL which leads to a smaller particle enriched with cholesteryl ester, which in turn may reduce the affinity of the particle for LPL. The particle may then recirculate to the liver where it discharges a fraction of its choles-teryl ester at specific loci on the hepatocyte. The particle with a lowered cholesteryl ester content may then recirculate and further interact with LPL in peripheral capil-lary beds. This process may continue until a much smaller "remnant" particle has been produced (REDGRAVE, 1970) which in the final stages of its degradation may give rise to LDL and HDL.

The transport of lipoprotein cholesteryl esters has also been studied in rabbit plasma after feeding a single meal containing ^{3}H-cholesterol (RUDEL et al., 1973b). Earlier studies of lymph lipoproteins by these authors (RUDEL et al., 1972) showed that the I-VLDL were the major transport form for exogenous ^{3}H-cholesterol, 80% of which was esterified, while chylomicrons transported the remainder. In plasma, the specific activity of the cholesteryl ester of chylomicrons and VLDL peaked at approximately 7 and 10 hrs, respectively. The HDL and LDL cholesteryl ester spe-cific activity increased more gradually, but the rate of increase for these two lipopro-teins was exactly the same. Since cholesteryl ester has been shown not to exchange between lipoprotein classes, this observation is strong evidence for a common origin of at least the core constituents of LDL and HDL and lends credance to the model proposed above. In all four major lipoprotein classes, the cholesteryl ester specific activity exceeded the free cholesterol specific activity at all times studied during the first 24 hrs after the meal. These results suggest that at least some of the cholesteryl esters of LDL and HDL arise from intravascular metabolism and do not transverse the liver free cholesterol pool in the process of their formation. The fact that the specific activity of the cholesteryl esters of all lipoproteins significantly exceeded the free cholesterol specific activity makes it highly unlikely that the labeled cholesteryl esters of LDL and HDL were derived from the lecithin: cholesterol acyl transferase (LCAT) reaction. However, the proposed central role of LCAT in the metabolism of lipoprotein surfaces, which was first suggested by SCHUMAKER and ADAMS (1969) and which has been recently reviewed by GLOMSET and NORUM (1973), seems consistent with the present hypothesis.

The evidence presently available, therefore, suggests that assimilation of cholesteryl ester of chylomicrons and VLDL may be a complex sequential interaction of the primary chylomicron (or VLDL) with lipoprotein lipase to initiate metabolism by triglyceride removal. Subsequently, the particle may interact with the hepatocyte where cholesteryl esters are taken into the liver. In addition, the particle may interact with the enzyme LCAT which may then modify the surface of the particle by removing some free cholesterol and lecithin. Any one particle may undergo one or several of each of these interactions before metabolism of the particle is complete. The apolipoproteins may serve as activators for any or all of these interactions by providing the correct conformation on the surface of the particle. Present evidence suggests that initial uptake by the liver of labeled cholesteryl esters which have entered the circulation in chylomicrons or VLDL is a relatively rapid process. After initial uptake, however, cholesteryl esters appear to be slowly hydrolyzed and further metabolized. The released free cholesterol apparently has several fates, but ultimately it equilibrates with free cholesterol pools throughout the body. The elimination of label from the whole body compartment is a gradual process, the time frame of which is several orders of magnitude slower than the biochemical processes discussed above. The liver is the primary site in the body for cholesterol catabolism but the means by which the liver balances uptake, synthesis, and catabolism remains unclear. Evidence cited above implies that cholesteryl esters of the partially metabolized "remnant" lipoproteins are in the form in which cholesterol is most effectively removed from plasma by the liver. In this sense, our attention is again focused on the interactions which occur between the intestine and the liver in controlling plasma cholesterol concentrations.

V. Classification of Hyperlipidemias

The search for systems with which to classify hyperlipidemias has been long and difficult. It is hampered by the fact that many of the individual steps of lipid metabolism and their controlling factors are incompletely understood. A large step forward was taken when it was recognized that all lipids are present in plasma in the form of lipid-protein complexes, or lipoproteins, and that any one plasma lipid is present in several types of lipoproteins. Thus, it is important to consider hyperlipidemia as hyperlipoproteinemia. Most of the recent attempts at classification have been directed at the lipoprotein level of plasma lipid organization.

Primary forms of hyperlipoproteinemia are generally defined as those which result from a genetic defect and are not a result of a separate endocrine or metabolic

Table 6. Classification of hyperlipoproteinemias[a]

Type	Synonym	Lipoprotein Abnormality[b]				Plasma lipid changes	
		Chylo	VLDL	LDL	HDL	Cholesterol	Triglyceride
I	Familial hyperchylo-micronemia	↑	↔	↓	↓	↑	↑
IIa	Familial hypercholes-terolemia	—	↔	↑	↓	↑	↔
IIb	Combined hyperlipo-proteinemia	—	↑	↑	↔	↑	↑
III	Broad-beta disease	—	↑[c]	↑	↔	↑	↑
IV	Familial hypertrigly-ceridemia	—	↑	↔	↕	↔	↑
V	Familial mixed hyperlipemia	↑	↑	↔	↕	↑	↑

[a] Based on work of FREDRICKSON and LEVY (1972).
[b] ↑ = increased concentration, ↓ = decreased concentration, ↔ = no change, — = absent.
[c] Abnormal composition and electrophoretic migration.

disorder. Those hyperlipoproteinemias which result from other disorders are termed *secondary*. For example, marked hyperlipoproteinemia exists in uncontrolled diabetes, in patients with the nephrotic syndrome, and in hypothyroid patients.

Since many types of hyperlipoproteinemia exist, a classification system is needed to help distinguish between types. The ultimate goal is to identify particular abnormalities, define the distinguishing characteristics (the phenotype), then to establish the trait as heritable and indicative of genotype. The most widely accepted classification system of the hyperlipoproteinemias was originally proposed by FREDRICKSON and LEES (1965) and is based on an electrophoretic separation of plasma lipoproteins by the paper electrophoretic method of LEES and HATCH (1963). The four major classes of plasma lipoproteins, chylomicrons (which remain on origin), VLDL (pre-β), LDL (β), and HDL (α) are separated by this procedure. Using this procedure with a large number of selected hyperlipoproteinemic patients, FREDRICKSON et al. (1967) described five different phenotypes to classify the hyperlipoproteinemias which they designated as types I, II, III, IV, and V. The basis of their classification is presented in Table 6. This system has been very useful in organizing the various hyperlipoproteinemias into meaningful categories for treatment and for further study. In many cases, the phenotype has been shown to be a familial trait (FREDRICKSON and LEVY, 1972). With time, it has become apparent that all of these proposed phenotypes do not sort out into distinct genotypes (GOLDSTEIN et al., 1973; HAZZARD et al., 1973; ROSE et al., 1973, 1974; BROWN, LEWIS, and PAGE, 1974). Unfortunately, it seems to have been a natural tendency of many people to oversimplify and presume phenotype would specify genotype. What appears consistent from viewing the many kindreds (pedigrees) which have appeared in the literature on the subject, is that the genotype of various individuals can be expressed as one of several phenotypes of the Fredrickson classification. This implies that a refinement of the classification system will be needed as additional new information is obtained, a fact acknowledged by Fredrickson and Levy (1972). The most comprehensive classification system presently available is the one presented in Table 6.

A. Primary Hyperlipoproteinemias

Increased concentrations of lipoproteins in plasma are a result of altered rates of metabolism, be it synthesis, release from cells into the blood stream, or catabolism. Translating an alteration in kinetics into a defect at the molecular level requires a more detailed knowledge of lipoprotein metabolism than is presently available for most of the hyperlipoproteinemias. Brown and Goldstein (1974) have provided information at this level for Type II hyperlipoproteinemia. Havel (1956) and Havel and Gordon (1960) have provided evidence that the defect in Type I hyperlipoproteinemia is a deficiency in lipoprotein lipase. Less information is available for the other types. A breakthrough awaits more detailed studies of lipid and lipoprotein metabolism.

1. Familial Type I Hyperlipoproteinemia (Familial Hyperchylomicronemia, Fat Induced Hyperlipidemia, Idiopathic Hyperlipemia)

This disease is characterized by a marked elevation of triglyceride-rich chylomicrons even in fasting plasma. While the patient is on a normal diet the plasma triglyceride/cholesterol ratio may exceed 10. When these patients are placed on a fat-free diet the chylomicrons disappear within a few days. Clinical findings commonly associated with this disease include episodic abdominal pain, hepatosplenomegaly, eruptive xanthomas, and pancreatitis apparently caused by the lipemia (Klatskin and Gordon, 1952).

   Havel and Gordon (1960) found that chylomicron clearance as measured after heparin injection was 20 to 25% of normal in this disease. The decrease in post-heparin lipolytic activity was not due to an inhibitor present in the patient's plasma. Normally post-heparin lipolytic activity is primarily a measure of lipoprotein lipase, but a liver lipase is also released into plasma by heparin (see above). In Type I patients, the post-heparin lipolytic activity is probably principally from the liver lipase (Schreibman et al., 1973; Steiner, 1968), and an active lipoprotein lipase may not be present to a significant extent in post-heparin plasma of Type I patients, nor does there appear to be lipoprotein lipase activity in adipose tissue of affected individuals (Harlan, 1967). The evidence is good, therefore, that the molecular defect in Type I hyperlipoproteinemia is in the enzyme lipoprotein lipase, *per se* or in one of the steps leading to its synthesis. This being the case, it is likely that the rate of removal of VLDL may also be decreased in this disorder, which may explain the occasional elevation of VLDL (Fredrickson and Levy, 1972) although it is somewhat puzzling that VLDL levels do not rise more significantly. In line with the proposed role of lipoprotein lipase in the assimilation of chylomicrons and VLDL (see above), the decreased rate of metabolism of these lipoproteins could in part explain the decreased concentrations of LDL and HDL in the plasma of these patients. Further studies on this point would be instructive, however, since HDL and LDL concentrations do not normalize in patients on fat-free diets in which chylomicrons have disappeared from plasma.

The cause of the most serious clinical complications, namely abdominal pain and pancreatitis, are unknown. The prognosis in familial Type I is not normal because of recurrent pancreatitis. The enlargement of the liver and spleen is apparently due to the fact that the reticuloendothelial cells take up lipid and become foam cells, but liver function appears to remain normal and hypersplenism has not been reported. The available genetic data, compiled by FREDRICKSON and LEVY (1972) suggests that the Type I disorder results from inheritance of a pair of autosomal alleles. The possibility can not be excluded that there exists more than one mutation leading to the Type I phenotype. Presumed heterozygous individuals may have reduced lipoprotein lipase activity, but this is not yet firmly established.

A pseudo Type I disorder has been reported in two patients with systemic lupus erythematosis and in one with lymphoma by GLUECK et al. (1969a). The lipolytic response after heparin injection in these individuals is low when the standard dose of heparin is given, but larger doses of heparin normalized the response. Immunoglobulins isolated from the plasma of the patients were shown to preferentially bind heparin. These findings illustrate the physiological importance of heparin as a cofactor for lipoprotein lipase, since in their "heparin-deficient" state, these patients exhibited a hyperchylomicronemia.

2. Familial Type II Hyperlipoproteinemia (Familial Hypercholesterolemia; Familial Hypercholesterolemic Xanthomatosis)

Familial Type II hyperlipoproteinemia is characterized by an increased concentration of LDL. Since LDL are cholesterol-rich lipoproteins it follows that plasma cholesterol levels are also elevated. The degree of elevation depends on whether the patient is homozygous or heterozygous, the absolute LDL (and cholesterol) concentration being almost twice as high in homozygotes as in heterozygotes. In homozygotes, the plasma VLDL and triglyceride values are usually normal, whereas in some heterozygotes VLDL and triglycerides are moderately elevated. FREDRICKSON and LEVY (1972) reported that by March 1971, they had examined 620 Type II patients in 225 kindreds. In 79 of the kindreds, there were both patients with normal and with abnormal VLDL concentrations. The designations Type IIa and Type IIb have been used to distinguish between those individuals with elevated LDL in the absence or presence, respectively, of elevated VLDL.

FREDRICKSON and LEVY (1972) state that Type II is the most common hyperlipoproteinemia based on their extensive experience (966 hyperlipoproteinemic patients in 421 kindreds in 1971). GLUECK et al. (1971) have estimated the frequency of Type II in a population derived from observing cord blood samples of 1800 children. The estimated frequency of Type II among the population was between 1:100 and 1:200. BROWN and DAUDISS (1973) studied the prevalence of the lipoprotein phenotypes in a free-living population in Albany, New York. They found the frequency of Type II was similar for males and females. In their study, they observed Type IV in females as often as Type II but Type IV hyperlipoproteinemia was more than twice as frequent in males as Type II.

Increased concentrations of LDL are present throughout the life of a Type II individual. The disorder is detectable at birth by analysis of cord blood cholesterol (KWITTEROVICH et al., 1970; GLUECK et al., 1971; and LEE et al., 1969), but analysis of cord blood LDL proves to be a better discriminant at this age (KWITTEROVICH et al., 1970), just as it is in older individuals. The progressive increase in LDL concentrations with age in Type II individuals parallels that of normals. There is a sharp rise after birth and another marked rise at maturity (FREDRICKSON and LEVY, 1972). Type II individuals respond to dietary treatment with a decrease in plasma cholesterol. GLUECK and TSANG (1972) report that plasma cholesterol levels can be normalized in the first year of life by diets poor in cholesterol and relatively rich in polyunsaturates. In Type II adults, the cholesterol and LDL levels are not normalized by dietary treatment, but significant decreases do occur (BROWN et al., 1974; FREDERICKSON and LEVY, 1972). Further lowering of plasma LDL in Type II heterozygotes can be effected by treatment with cholestyramine, although in some patients the LDL levels may still not reach normal levels (LEVY and FREDRICKSON, 1970). Clofibrate has not been found effective in treating patients with Type II hyperlipoproteinemia (LEVY et al., 1969).

Clinical findings associated with Type II hyperlipoproteinemia include frequent tendonous xanthomas, arcus cornea in as many as 50% of the patients over age 30, and most importantly, premature coronary artery atherosclerosis. In Type II homozygotes, death by myocardial infarction may often occur in the first decade of life (LEES et al., 1973), and most of these patients fail to survive into the fourth decade. SLACK and NEVIN (1968) found that in Type II heterozygotes, the mean age of onset of symptomatic ischemic heart disease was 43 and 53 years in men and women, respectively. STONE et al. (1973) have reported a study of 116 kindreds in which coronary artery disease was diagnosed in 30% of the relatives with Type II disease and 10% in relatives without disease. Death due to coronary artery disease was 10% in Type II relatives, compared to 2% in normal relatives.

The molecular defect responsible for Type II hyperlipoproteinemia has been suggested by the studies of BROWN and co-workers. These authors have worked on the *in vitro* binding of LDL (and VLDL) to cultured skin fibroblasts, and the subsequent effect on the activity of the enzyme 3-hydroxy-3-methylglutaryl-coenzyme A reductase (HMG-CoA reductase) which is the rate limiting enzyme in cholesterol synthesis. Of the plasma lipoprotein classes, LDL and VLDL inhibit HMG-CoA reductase activity in normal cells, whereas HDL are 40-fold less effective (BROWN et al., 1973). In cells from homozygous Type II patients (familial hypercholesterolemia in the author's terminology) there was a 40- to 60-fold higher activity of HMG-CoA reductase, and an absence of regulation of this enzyme by LDL added *in vitro* (GOLDSTEIN and BROWN, 1973). Over-production of the enzyme occurred and led to over-production of cholesterol. When ^{125}I-LDL were incubated with fibroblasts, the amount of labeled LDL bound to the cultured fibroblasts was proportional to the decrease of HMG-CoA reductase activity, indicating that the fibroblasts from homozygous Type II patients had an altered receptor on the cell surface with decreased affinity for LDL binding (BROWN and GOLDSTEIN, 1974). In addition, LDL was degraded in proportion to the amount of binding. Cultured fibroblasts from heterozygous patients responded with a 60% reduction from normal in binding and degradation, compared to 97% in homozygotes, and the genetic defect was identified as autosomal dominant. Further studies demonstrated that the relationship between LDL binding and the decrease in HMG-CoA reductase activity was in the transfer of LDL cholesterol from the bound apolipoprotein-B to its presumed site of action within the cell (BROWN et al., 1974).

One can only speculate about how the identified receptor defect could translate into the increased plasma LDL concentrations in Type II hyperlipoproteinemic patients, but it seems likely it could be a result of a defect in the liver analogous to that in fibroblasts, resulting in both overproduction of endogenous cholesterol and decreased rates of binding and subsequent catabolism of LDL. Presumably the liver is the tissue responsible for LDL catabolism since it is the only tissue in the body that can catabolize significant amounts of cholesterol. The liver is also the tissue believed to be responsible for much of the plasma LDL synthesis, albeit in the form of VLDL, and could synthesize more LDL due to an increased endogenous synthesis of cholesterol. The possibility that both increased synthesis and decreased catabolism of LDL could result from the receptor defect may, in part, help explain findings in the literature seemingly at opposition. Based on the die-away of radio-iodinated LDL in normal and Type II patients, LANGER et al. (1972) concluded that catabolism of LDL was defective in Type II patients while SCOTT and HURLEY (1969) concluded that the defect was in synthesis.

The weight of the evidence currently available suggests that LDL of Type II hyperlipoproteinemic patients is structurally identical to normal LDL (FREDRICKSON and LEVY, 1972; FISHER et al., 1972), and that metabolism of LDL isolated from normal and Type II individuals is the same *in vivo* (LANGER et al., 1972) and *in vitro* (GOLDSTEIN and BROWN, 1973). However, several reports have suggested that the chemical composition of LDL from Type II individuals is not identical with that of LDL from normal individuals (SLACK and MILLS, 1970; BROWN, LEWIS, and PAGE, 1974; BAGNALL, 1972). This is an important consideration relative to the atherosclerotic complications resulting from Type II hyperlipoproteinemia. It is possible that slightly modified LDL may be more (or less) atherogenic than normal LDL. Such modifications might help explain unusual findings, such as those of HARLAN et al. (1966) in which a large kindred of 659 members was studied, 79 of whom had heterozygous Type II hypolipoproteinemia and in which no decrease in longevity and no increased incidence of coronary artery disease was apparent. The possibility of a relationship between modified LDL structure and increased atherosclerosis has been suggested by analysis of LDL isolated from nonhuman primates in which experimental atherosclerosis was induced by feeding cholesterol (RUDEL and LOFLAND, 1974).

The observed variation among patients studied in different laboratories creates the impression that more than one genotype may result in the expression of the Type II phenotype. However, this may simply be due to the lack of information presently available concerning the molecular defect in Type II hyperlipoproteinemia and the influence of environment on the expression of the phenotype. Several modifications in the classification of Type II hyperlipoproteinemia have been suggested. ROSE et al. (1973) have identified individuals with elevations of both VLDL and LDL which they have termed Combined Hyperlipoproteinemia as a separate phenotype from Type II. They have reported three kindreds to show that this pattern is heritable. Features which distinguish this phenotype from Type II were the occurrence of a low frequency of LDL elevation in the absence of VLDL elevation among the kindreds, the absence of the abnormality in childhood members at risk, and an absence of xanthomas. Characteristics such as impaired glucose tolerance, obesity, and hyperuricemia were prevalent in the Combined Hyperlipoproteinemic individuals, findings not uncommon in Type IV patients as well. However, Rose et al. (1974) have shown that a clean discrimination between individuals with Type IV and Combined Hyperlipoproteinemia can be made on the basis of LDL cholesterol concentrations. Brown, Lewis, and Page (1974) also feel that the phenotype for some individuals with Combined Hyperlipoproteinemia should be distinguished from Type II, and they have suggested it be called Type VI. They have made the important observation that plasma LDL and VLDL concentrations of individuals with Combined Hyperlipoproteinemia can be normalized by proper dietary therapy, namely, by placing them on a diet containing 38% of the calories from fat, with 17% of total calories from polyunsaturated fatty acids, no more than 11% from saturated fatty acids, and less than 300 mg of cholesterol per day. They agree with Fredrickson and Levy (1972) that Type II patients cannot normalize their LDL concentrations by diet therapy alone.

Hazzard et al. (1973) have stated that the phenotypes described by Fredrickson et al. (1967) do not describe the genetic disorders they have identified among the pedigrees of several survivors of myocardial infarction (Goldstein et al., 1973). However, there seems to be good correlation between the Type II phenotype and the monogenic disorder of familial hypercholesterolemia which they describe (Hazzard et al., 1973). The discrepancy appears to be highest in the group with combined hyperlipidemia in that some kindred members can have phenotypes for Type IIa, IIb, and IV hyperlipoproteinemia. This appears to be a similar finding to that of Rose et al. (1973) and Brown et al. (1974) and appears to support the viewpoint that more than one genetic defect can be expressed as the Type II phenotype, and that an alternate phenotype (IIb) should be considered separately from IIa. This and other problems in phenotyping hyperlipoproteinemias do not seem unreasonable based on the original intent of categorizing hyperlipidemia as hyperlipoproteinemia, i.e., that of clarifying differences among types of hyperlipidemia. Nor does it seem to be sufficient justification to disregard the classification of hyperlipidemia as hyperlipoproteinemia. As pointed out in the work of Brown et al. (1973) it was not the plasma cholesterol, *per se*, that interacted *in vitro* with the fibroblasts, rather it was only the cholesterol of plasma associated with LDL and VLDL. This type of finding seems to further emphasize the importance of approaching the understanding of primary hyperlipidemia by thinking of it as hyperlipoproteinemia and by considering the possible defects in the synthesis or catabolism of lipoproteins that could lead to the disease.

3. Familial Type III Hyperlipoproteinemia (Broad-Beta Disease, Remnant Disease)

This lipoprotein disorder is characterized by the presence of an unusual class of lipoproteins, the properties of which include a density less than 1.006 g/ml, β-mobility on agarose and paper electrophoresis, a relatively high concentration of cholesteryl esters and low concentration of triglycerides (FREDRICKSON and LEVY, 1972) and a relatively high proportion of an arginine-rich apolipoprotein (HAVEL and KANE, 1973). This lipoprotein is often called an "abnormal" VLDL, but in other ways it is like an "abnormal" triglyceride-rich LDL. The most certain diagnosis of Type III hyperlipoproteinemia can be made by finding a β-migrating lipoprotein which floats during ultracentrifugation at d 1.006. Electrophoresis of whole plasma usually shows a single broad band which extends from the β into the pre-β region. Chylomicrons are sometimes visible in these patients (HAZZARD et al., 1970b).

As a result of the elevated concentration of the "abnormal" lipoprotein, the plasma triglycerides and cholesterol are both elevated often into the 300 to 600 mg/dl range although in any one patient the variation from time to time is pronounced (LEES et al., 1973). Part of the variation is apparently diet-induced. As a group, the patients with Type III hyperlipoproteinemia respond to diet manipulation better than those with any other type of primary hyperlipoproteinemia. Cutaneous and subcutaneous xanthomas often accompany the Type III disorder, most typically on the palms of the hands. About half of the patients seen have shown xanthomas (FREDRICKSON and LEVY, 1972; LEES et al., 1973) but when the plasma lipids are controlled with diet these lesions disappear. Some 40% of the patients seen by FREDRICKSON and LEVY (1972) have had diabetic responses to glucose tolerance tests. GLUECK et al. (1969b) found immunoreactive insulin responses to be abnormal in 45% of the patients, about half with high and half with low responses, but frank diabetes was not seen.

The incidence of premature vascular disease in Type III hyperlipoproteinemia is high. FREDRICKSON and LEVY (1972) found that over 80% of the males and in 25% of the females in a population of 51 patients had signs of arterial degeneration by age 50, even though the mean age for appearance of the phenotype is over 20. BORRIE (1969) found that the prevalence of coronary disease was not as high as that of peripheral vascular disease in 18 Type III patients. ZELIS et al. (1970) have suggested that the peripheral atherosclerosis may regress in Type III patients which successfully respond to diet and drug therapy.

Because of the metabolic relationships of the VLDL as a precursor to LDL, and the chemical and physical properties of the "abnormal" lipoprotein of Type III, the observation has been made that this lipoprotein may be a "remnant" of VLDL catabolism for which triglyceride removal is incomplete. It is uncertain whether it is an abnormal lipoprotein or an abnormal accumulation of an intermediate of lipoprotein metabolism. Normal chylomicrons (HAZZARD et al., 1970a) and normal VLDL (QUARFORDT et al., 1971) are present in Type III patients, and the unusual lipoproteins of Type III appear to have the core and coat structure typical of normal very low density lipoproteins (SATA et al., 1972). HAVEL and KANE (1973) have studied the apolipoproteins of the chylomicrons of a Type III patient, and have found a normal distribution. In contrast, the VLDL contained a disproportionately high amount of an arginine-rich apolipoprotein, which other workers have shown also to be true for other very low density lipoproteins relatively rich in cholesteryl esters (SHORE and SHORE, 1973; SHORE et al., 1974). These findings suggest that the degradation of VLDL is stopped at a point after triglyceride assimilation before cholesteryl ester assimilation (see above). In Type III hyperlipoproteinemia, cholesteryl ester uptake by the liver is apparently abnormal either due to structural mutations in the lipoproteins, *per se*, or to a defect in one or several of the individual steps of cholesteryl ester uptake by the liver. Our incomplete understanding of these complex metabolic processes does not permit further definition of the molecular defect at this time.

The mode of genetic inheritance in Type III hyperlipoproteinemia has been reviewed by Fredrickson and Levy (1972). Both Type III and Type IV phenotypes appear frequently in the kindreds of Type III individuals, whereas Type II appears infrequently. It seems possible that the Type IV phenotype in these kindreds may result from a gene defect separate from that for the Type IV individuals in kindreds with no Type III relatives. Verticle transmission of the Type III phenotype has been observed in 5 of 36 kindreds and in most kindreds large enough, more than one affected sibling was identified. Although the familial nature of Type III seems firmly established, the mode of inheritance is presently unexplained.

4. Familial Type IV Hyperlipoproteinemia (Hyperprebetalipoproteinemia, Familial Hyperlipemia, Carbohydrate-Induced Hyperlipemia, Endogenous Hyperglyceridemia)

Type IV hyperlipoproteinemia is characterized by an elevation in concentration during fasting of plasma VLDL or pre-beta lipoproteins. Since these lipoproteins are triglyceride-rich, plasma triglycerides are elevated. Some elevation in plasma cholesterol concentration is usually seen due to the increased amount of VLDL cholesterol in plasma, however, LDL concentrations are normal or slightly decreased in Type IV hyperlipoproteinemia which distinguishes the Type IV phenotype from Type II b. The Type IV phenotype frequently appears to be present in the kindreds for Type II b, III, and V, however, the pattern of association of the Type IV phenotype with these other phenotypes suggests that in each of these cases, different genetic defects are present. In primary familial Type IV hyperlipoproteinemia, a prerequisite to this classification is that no relative with another type of hyperlipoproteinemia is found (Fredrickson and Levy, 1972). These authors report 189 individuals in which primary Type IV has been found; the mean ($\pm$ standard deviation) plasma cholesterol and triglyceride concentrations were 257 ± 36 mg/dl and 445 ± 37 mg/dl, respectively. In the kindreds of 53 propositi, 85 parents and adult siblings had Type IV hyperlipoproteinemia, 90 were normal and no other form of hyperlipoproteinemia was present.

The prevalence of Type IV phenocopies among the other types of hyperlipoproteinemia makes difficult the assessment of frequency of the primary Type IV disorder among the population in general. The phenotype of elevated VLDL with normal LDL, is one of the most prevalent patterns encountered (Brown and Daudiss, 1973). However, the need to rule out other hyperlipoproteinemias in the family and the need for repeated sampling of suspected individuals make population frequency studies for primary Type IV very difficult. Primary Type IV is infrequently identified in patients below 21 years of age. Children which have been identified are obese and both parents have hyperglyceridemia (Fredrickson and Levy, 1972), but obesity is not highly correlated with Type IV hyperlipoproteinemia in adults. Abnormal glucose tolerance and abnormal insulin levels are seen frequently in Type IV individuals (Glueck et al., 1969 b). Xanthomas only appear to occur in Type IV individuals with severe hyperglyceridemia. Hyperuricemia has appeared in 9 of 22 Type IV individuals studied by FREDRICKSON and LEVY (1972). Premature coronary artery disease has been described in 38% of the 78 Type IV patients studied by FREDRICKSON and LEVY (1972). The risk seems high, but accurate estimation awaits further study. Carbohydrate-induced hypertriglyceridemia is often exaggerated in Type IV individuals when the patient's diet is changed from normal to one of high carbohydrate composition (LEES et al., 1973).

The metabolic defect in Type IV hyperlipoproteinemia is still unknown. The possible areas in which the defect may lie are: 1) in VLDL structure, 2) in the synthetic pathway for VLDL, and 3) in the catabolic pathway for VLDL. No abnormalities in the structure of VLDL of Type IV individuals have become apparent. The chemical composition of VLDL were comparable to those of normals, and to those of patients with other types of hyperlipoproteinemia (FREDRICKSON and LEVY, 1972), however, complete chemical comparisons do not appear in the literature. The apolipoproteins of normal VLDL have not been as well studied as those of Type IV patients, thus differences could occur here which are unknown.

Increased VLDL synthesis could result from increased FFA flux to the liver or to step-up in the rate of lipogenesis in the liver. Decreased rates of catabolism of VLDL could be a result of alterations in apolopoprotein structure of VLDL. Equally likely is that this decrease results from abnormalities in the synthesis of lipoprotein lipase, in the activation of the enzyme by cofactors and by various physiological stimuli, or in the structure of the enzyme *per se* (see Triglyceride Assimilation section). Evidence in the literature concerning which of these mechanisms are operable in primary Type IV is not available. One difficulty in this area is the lack of suitable animal models in which this phenomenon can be studied. Primary hypertriglyceridemia, i.e. not associated with diabetes or other diseases, is very rare in experimental animals.

5. Familial Type V Hyperlipoproteinemia [Familial Mixed (Endogenous and Exogenous) Hyperlipemia, Familial Hyperprebetalipoproteinemia with Hyperchylomicronemia]

The characteristics of this disorder include the presence of elevated levels of VLDL and chylomicrons in fasting plasma. The LDL and HDL concentrations are normal or slightly decreased. The plasma cholesterol and triglycerides levels in Type V individuals are markedly elevated. The mean values ($\pm$ standard deviation) for 36 primary Type V patients reported by FREDRICKSON and LEVY (1972) was cholesterol, 452 ± 47 mg/dl, and triglyceride, 2425 ± 319 mg/dl. These levels establish the Type V patients as the most lipemic of all the types of hyperlipoproteinemia.

The clinical signs and symptoms of Type V patients are similar but often more pronounced than those with Type IV. For example, 82% of the 22 Type V probands of FREDRICKSON and LEVY (1972) had abnormal glucose tolerance tests, and 73% complained of abdominal pain. Hyperinsulinemia was present in a majority of the Type V patients studied by GLUECK et al. (1969) whereas they found only 22% of Type IV patients with a high insulin level. In neither of these two diseases was obesity especially prevalent although when it was present it seemed to accentuate the hyperlipoproteinemia. As in Type I hyperlipoproteinemic patients, abdominal pain is frequently encountered in Type V individuals although here the general age of onset of this complaint is in the third decade of life. Pancreatitis is also often present and in some individuals severe attacks can occur. In contrast to the high frequency of ischemic heart disease prevalent among Type II, III, and IV patients, a relatively low frequency was shown in Type V patients by Fredrickson and Levy (1972). Their experience with Type I and V hyperlipoproteinemia led them to wonder if an excess of circulating chylomicrons might in some way retard the rate of development of atherosclerosis (Fredrickson and Levy, 1972).

The biochemical defect in Type V hyperlipoproteinemia is not understood. Clearance of dietary fat is impaired, and post-heparin lipolytic activity may be low in some individuals, although this is not necessarily a measure of lipoprotein lipase as previously pointed out. Many of the possible malfunctions in triglyceride metabolism mentioned earlier could occur in Type V, and it is possible that perhaps more than one occurs in Type V since both endogenous and exogenous triglycerides are elevated. No conclusions about the mode of transmission of the genetic defect have been reached (Fredrickson and Levy, 1972). The most that can be said presently is that familial Type V hyperlipoproteinemia appears to be genotypically separate from familial Type IV hyperlipoproteinemia based on analysis of 22 Type V kindreds.

B. Secondary Hyperlipoproteinemias

In a number of diseases, an associated finding is secondary hyperlipoproteinemia. Frequently, a characteristic pattern of hyperlipoproteinemia is found for a particular disease. By studying the reasons for this association we may learn more about the mechanisms of hyperlipoproteinemia, in addition to more completely understanding the primary disease. In this context, we present a brief review of some secondary hyperlipoproteinemias.

1. Alcoholic Hyperlipoproteinemia

This abnormality is among the most prevalent of the secondary hyperlipoproteinemias (Lees et al., 1973) and is one in which triglycerides are the lipid class most often elevated, with the triglyceride to cholesterol ratio often reaching as high as four to one (Skipski, 1972). The pattern of hyperlipoproteinemia is similar to Type IV or Type V although some alcoholics are seen which are not markedly hyperlipoproteinemic (Lewis et al., 1973). The extent of the response is related to the nutritional state of the individual and to the amount of ethanol consumed.

Studies in both experimental animals and man suggest that over-production of VLDL by the liver is the major defect in the hyperlipoproteinemia induced by alcohol, apparently due to an alteration in liver metabolism. Post-heparin lipoprotein lipase appears to be normal (Lewis et al., 1973). When the liver oxidizes ethanol to acetaldehyde and acetate, the oxidation of FFA is decreased in proportion to plasma ethanol levels (Havel, 1972), and more of the influx of FFA are converted by esterification into triglycerides and secreted as part of L-VLDL. Experiments have shown that livers of rabbits given ethanol incorporate an average of two to three times more labeled FFA into triglycerides of VLDL than do control animals (Bez-man-Tarcher et al., 1966). This effect is modified by the effect of acetate which inhibits the mobilization of FFA from adipose tissue (Crouse et al., 1968; Abram-

SON and ARKY, 1968), but the overall effect is increased production of VLDL, particularly in fasting. Further evidence that alcohol induces overproduction of VLDL
was presented by LEWIS et al. (1973) who studied a series of alcoholic patients using
an intravenous fat tolerance test. Before alcohol withdrawal, the mean triglyceride
levels were 746 mg/dl and the fractional removal rate was 0.027 per minute. After
alcohol withdrawal for 7 to 12 days, mean triglyceride levels were reduced to 184 mg/
dl but the fractional removal rate was unchanged at 0.028 per minute. Although the
fractional removal rates were below normal for the patients, alcohol withdrawal did
not increase this value, and triglyceride removal mechanisms appeared not to be
influenced by alcohol.

2. Diabetic Hyperlipoproteinemia

The severity of hyperlipoproteinemia associated with diabetes mellitus is dependent
on the severity of the disturbance in carbohydrate metabolism and the degree to
which the disease is controlled in the patient in question. LINDGREN and NICHOLS
(1960) reported that a severely diabetic patient in ketoacidosis had grossly elevated
S_f 100 to 400 and 20 to 100 lipoproteins (VLDL) with low levels of LDL and normal
HDL concentrations. Normal electrophoretic patterns have been observed in juvenile diabetic patients that were under good control with insulin (BACON and SANBAR,
1968). It is well known that in uncontrolled diabetes there is an increased mobilization of FFA from adipose tissue which is reflected in an increased plasma FFA level.
The increased mobilization is due to an absolute or relative deficiency of insulin
which activates hormone sensitive lipase in adipose tissue through cyclic AMP
(STEINBERG, 1972). In addition, LPL and hormone-sensitive lipase activities in adipose tissue are reciprocally related (ROBINSON, 1970). A combination of overproduction of triglyceride in VLDL by the liver and a defect in removal mechanisms due to
lower levels of available LPL in extrahepatic tissues may potentiate the hypertriglyceridemia.

In a study of vascular disease and serum lipids in diabetes ALBRINK et al. (1963)
compiled data on patients seen in clinic at New Haven, Connecticut from 1931 to
1961. When patients were instructed to eat a high fat diet in the 1930's, mean
triglyceride levels were approximately 160 mg/dl. In the 1940's and 50's carbohydrate
intake was increased and the triglyceride levels increased to a mean of 231 mg/dl.
The mechanism for this effect of diet is not established but may be similar to the one
suggested by HARRIS and FELTS (1973) who observed that triglyceride clearance is
inhibited, probably by a decrease in available LPL activity, when rats are maintained
on high carbohydrate diets. The effect of carbohydrate intake may apply to normal
subjects and diabetic patients alike.

BIERMAN et al. (1966) carried out a careful study of four diabetic patients with
severe lipidemia. These patients had several features in common. They were younger
patients and had experienced uncontrolled diabetes for weeks or months. Ketoacidosis, if present was mild. The patients had massive hypertriglyceridemia on a 40% fat
diet with plasma triglycerides as high as 7,500 mg-%, but on a 0% fat diet triglyceride levels returned to normal values within a few days. Post-heparin lipolytic activity
was subnormal. These investigators have classified this type of diabetic as a form of
fat-induced lipemia secondary to chronic insulin deficiency as seen in some forms of

juvenile diabetes. Not only diet control but appropriate insulin therapy was effective in clearing the hyperlipoproteinemia. Three patients of this type were also studied by SHIPP et al. (1964). Hypertriglyceridemia appears to result from decreased rates of triglyceride clearance by lipoprotein lipase, the decreased activity of which apparently is caused by insulin deficiency.

In another study by BAGDADE et al. (1968a) insulin was acutely withdrawn in seven insulin dependent diabetic subjects. After 48 hrs plasma triglyceride levels were increased and post-heparin lipolytic activity was diminished. It was concluded that insulin is required for maintaining normal LPL activity and adequate triglyceride removal. Direct measurement of the $T_{\frac{1}{2}}$ of removal of labeled $S_f > 400$ lipoproteins from the circulation fully supported these conclusions.

These explanations of potential mechanisms to explain the hyperlipoproteinemia associated with the insulin deficiency of juvenile onset diabetes do not apply to maturity onset diabetes in which insulin levels are often elevated. No satisfactory explanations are presently available in the latter case.

3. Hyperlipoproteinemia of the Nephrotic Syndrome

In 1953, LEWIS and PAGE stated: "The nephrotic syndrome has been associated in the minds of most clinicians with severe lipemia, indeed it has been called on occasion a lipid diabetes. Vascular disease of the atherosclerotic type is hastened by appearance of the syndrome." In a group of 16 nephrotic patients, these investigators noted an elevation of the lighter, larger molecular weight lipoproteins. GOFMAN et al. (1954) stated that "The diagnosis of nephrotic syndrome can almost always be made by the serum lipoprotein spectrum alone." They reported an elevation in the S_f 20 to 100 and the S_f 100 to 400 range. BAXTER et al. (1960) examined a series of 44 patients with symptoms of nephrosis from mild to severe. They found a nonlinear inverse correlation between plasma albumin levels and plasma lipid levels. In this and other studies (GITLIN et al., 1958) it was also observed that there was a reduced concentration of plasma high density lipoproteins (HDL) in those patients with the greatest lipid elevations, however, little note was taken of this fact. LEWIS et al. (1966) suggested that alpha-lipoproteins (HDL) were regulated by the kidney by some unknown mechanism, but the relationship of these observations to the hyperlipidemia was not elucidated.

The mechanism of the hyperlipoproteinemia in both nephritis and nephrosis is not established, although several hypotheses have been presented. BRAUN et al. (1962) postulated that due to the lowered plasma albumin, all protein synthesis may be stimulated including the synthesis of VLDL by the liver. This may be related to an increased level of circulating insulin in these patients (BAGDADE et al., 1968b). However, there is evidence that a lowered post-heparin lipolytic activity could also contribute to a defect in the removal of very low density lipoproteins (VLDL) from the circulation (BAGDADE et al., 1968b).

Our recent observations on two patients have led us to the hypothesis that there may be an important connection between the lowered plasma level of HDL and the elevated level of circulating plasma VLDL (FELTS, unpublished observations). Previous work has established that VLDL and HDL contain activators which convert artificial triglyceride emulsions into active substrates for LPL

(WHAYNE and FELTS, 1970b; HAVEL et al., 1970). Apparently, the activators are apolipoproteins common to HDL and VLDL which exchange onto the surface of the triglyceride emulsion (HAVEL et al., 1970; HAVEL et al., 1973). These findings have led to the postulate that the HDL is the reservoir in plasma of activator apolipoproteins which must transfer onto newly formed chylomicrons and VLDL so that lipoprotein lipase can begin triglyceride clearance. With this in mind, we studied the lipoprotein spectrum of two nephrotic patients using agarose gel chromatography (FELTS, unpublished observations). Both patients had markedly reduced levels of plasma HDL and markedly elevated VLDL. Although it is not generally recognized, the molecular dimensions of albumin (37×150 Å) and HDL (100 Å) are quite similar, and both molecules elute almost simultaneously during gel filtration. In patients with severely damaged glomerular capillary basement membranes, it is reasonable to postulate that not only albumin but also HDL could be filtered and lost in the urine. We have concentrated a 24-hour urine sample from one patient and examined it for HDL. HDL was positively identified by flotation in the ultracentrifuge and by gel filtration. It is possible that urinary loss of HDL may lead to a lowered level of plasma HDL, which may then result in a deficiency of activator apolipoproteins needed for the metabolism of VLDL by lipoprotein lipase.

4. Hyperlipoproteinemia Associated with Myxedema

One of the cardinal signs of hypothyroidism is hypercholesterolemia. The cholesterol elevation is usually in the LDL, and a Type IIa phenotype results although in many patients VLDL elevations also occur and the Type IIb phenotype is present (KOPPERS and PALUMBO, 1972). Some patients appear to have a Type III electrophoretic pattern, although this appears infrequently. The hyperlipoproteinemia in hypothyroid patients can be treated with dextrothyroxine and lipoprotein levels are normalized.

The mechanism of this hyperlipoproteinemia is likely to be related to the metabolic effects of thyroxine on lipid metabolism. Thyroxine stimulates cholesterol synthesis and degradation, so that in its absence as in hypothyroid patients, a decrease in catabolism may give rise to an elevation in plasma cholesterol (LDL) concentration. PORTE et al. (1966) showed that post-heparin lipolytic activity is low in hypothyroid patients, which probably helps explain the elevated level of plasma triglycerides which occurs in the face of the decreased rate of FFA mobilization (CREPALDI et al., 1973). NIKKILA (1972) has reported findings consistent with this conclusion, since he was able to demonstrate reduced rates of triglyceride removal in the presence of normal rates of production in hypothyroid patients. The conclusion to be drawn from these studies is that in the absence of adequate amounts of thyroxine, decreased rates of cholesterol and triglyceride catabolism occur, which in turn leads to the hyperlipoproteinemia of myxedema.

5. Hyperlipoproteinemia Associated with Obesity and Excess Caloric Intake

Obesity is frequently accompanied by hyperlipoproteinemia which is reflected in an increase in VLDL triglycerides (BARTER and NESTEL, 1973). In some individuals only moderate increases or decreases in body weight may have dramatic effects on the levels of circulating lipoproteins. Obesity is sometimes seen in familial Types III, IV, and V and reduction to ideal body weight has the beneficial effect of lowering plasma lipoprotein levels (Fredrickson and Levy, 1972).

A direct relationship between body weight and plasma FFA levels was first shown by Dole (1956). Nestel and Whyte (1968) have shown that obese subjects have an increase in plasma FFA turnover which correlates well with the degree of adiposity. They also observed that plasma FFA turnover rate was significantly related to plasma FFA concentration. These studies also showed a significant correlation between triglyceride concentrations in VLDL and triglyceride turnover. Barter and Nestel (1973) have attempted to establish the origin of the precursor fatty acids of plasma triglycerides in lean and obese subjects by using a constant infusion of labeled FFA. In the lean individuals 80 to 90% of the triglyceride fatty acids were derived from plasma FFA. In the obese subjects only 22 to 64% of the triglyceride fatty acids in VLDL were derived from plasma FFA. The remainder of the triglyceride fatty acids apparently were not derived from blood glucose. These workers postulate that, in the postprandial state, the extra triglyceride fatty acids are not derived from hepatic lipogenesis but probably from stored hepatic triglycerides. However, studies of this type are difficult to interpret unless the triglyceride pools in liver have come into isotopic equilibrium. In obese subjects the liver pools are likely to be increased and require much longer periods to reach isotopic equilibrium.

Obesity is also known to be accompanied by a decreased sensitivity of adipose tissue cells to insulin (Salans et al., 1968). This could lead to an increase in the activity of hormone sensitive lipase in adipose tissue which would contribute increased levels of plasma FFA. As noted above hormone sensitive lipase and LPL are reciprocally related, therefore, it is likely that clearance mechanisms are reduced in obese subjects. These mechanisms may operate in concert to delimit the increased VLDL levels in obese subjects. The insulin resistence of adipose tissue may lead to an increased mobilization of FFA which stimulates increased production of VLDL by the liver. During periods of active absorption of a meal, especially if it is high in carbohydrate, hepatic lipogenesis may also contribute to a greater output of VLDL by the liver (Barter et al., 1972; Mayer, 1964). At the same time, LPL clearance mechanisms may be reduced when the diet is high in carbohydrate (Harris and Felts, 1973).

References

Abramson, E. A., Arky, R. A.: Acute antilipolytic effects of ethyl alcohol and acetate in man. J. Lab. clin. Med. **72**, 105—117 (1968).

Alaupovic, P., Sanbar, S. S., Furman, R. H., Sullivan, M. L., Walraven, S. L.: Studies of the composition and structure of serum lipoproteins. Isolation and characterization of very high density lipoproteins of human serum. Biochemistry **5**, 4044—4053 (1966).

Alaupovic, P.: Conceptual development of the classification systems of plasma lipoproteins. In: Peeters, H. (Ed.) Proceedings of the XIX Annual Colloquium of the Protides of Biological Fluids. New York: Pergamon Press 1972.

Albers, J. J., Aladjem, F.: Precipitation of ^{125}I-labeled lipoproteins with specific polypeptide antisera. Evidence for two populations with differing polypeptide compositions in human high density lipoproteins. Biochemistry **10**, 3436—3442 (1971).

Albrink, M. J., Lavietes, P. H., Mann, E. B.: Vascular disease and serum lipids in diabetes mellitus. Ann. intern. Med. **58**, 305—323 (1963).

Anderson, N. G., Fawcett, B.: An antichylomicronemic substance produced by heparin injection. Proc. Soc. exp. Biol. (N.Y.) **74**, 768—771 (1950).

BACON, G. E., SANBAR, S. S.: Serum lipids and lipoproteins in diabetic children. Univ. Mich. Med. Centr. J. **34**, 84—87 (1968).

BAGDADE, J. D., PORTE, D., JR., BIERMAN, E. L.: Acute insulin withdrawal and the regulation of plasma triglyceride removal in diabetic subjects. Diabetes **17**, 127—132 (1968a).

BAGDADE, J. D., PORTE, D., JR., BIERMAN, E. L.: Hypertriglyceridemia. A metabolic consequence of chronic renal failure. New Engl. J. Med. **279**, 181—185 (1968b).

BAGNALL, T. F.: Composition of low density lipoprotein in children with familial hyperbetalipoproteinemia and the effect of treatment. Clin. chim. Acta **42**, 229—233 (1972).

BARTER, P. J., NESTEL, P. J., CARROLL, K. F.: Precursors of plasma triglyceride fatty acid in humans. Effects of glucose consumption, clofibrate administration, and alcoholic fatty liver. Metabolism **21**, 117—124 (1972).

BARTER, P. J., NESTEL, P. J.: Precursors of plasma triglyceride fatty acids in obesity. Metabolism **22**, 779—785 (1973).

BAXTER, J. H., GOODMAN, H. C., HAVEL, R. J.: Serum lipid and lipoprotein alterations in nephrosis. J. clin. Invest. **39**, 455—465 (1960).

BEZMAN, A., FELTS, J. M., HAVEL, R. J.: Relation between incorporation of triglyceride fatty acids and heparin-released lipoprotein lipase from adipose tissue slices. J. Lipid Res. **3**, 427—431 (1962).

BEZMAN-TARCHER, A., NESTEL, P. J., FELTS, J. M., HAVEL, R. J.: Metabolism of hepatic and plasma triglycerides in rabbits given ethanol or ethionine. J. Lipid Res. **7**, 248—257 (1966).

BIER, D. M., HAVEL, R. J.: Activation of lipoprotein lipase by lipoprotein fractions of human serum. J. Lipid Res. **11**, 565—570 (1970).

BIERMAN, E. L., BAGDADE, J. D., PORTE, D., JR.: A concept of the pathogenesis of diabetic lipemia. Trans. Ass. Amer. Physicns **79**, 348—360 (1966).

BIGGS, M. W.: Studies on exogenous cholesterol metabolism in human atherosclerosis with the aid of isotopes. Advanc. Biol. med. Physics **5**, 357—384 (1957).

BILHEIMER, D. W., EISENBERG, S., LEVY, R. I.: The metabolism of very low density lipoprotein proteins. I. Preliminary *in vitro* and *in vivo* observations. Biochim. biophys. Acta (Amst.) **260**, 212—221 (1972).

BOBERG, J., CARLSON, L. A., NORMELL, L.: Production of lipolytic activity by the isolated, perfused dog liver in response to heparin. Life Sci. **3**, 1011—1019 (1964).

BORENSZTAJN, J., ROBINSON, D. S.: The effect of fasting on the utilization of chylomicron triglyceride fatty acids in relation to clearing factor lipase (lipoprotein lipase) releasable by heparin in the perfused rat heart. J. Lipid Res. **11**, 111—117 (1970).

BORRIE, P.: Type III hyperlipoproteinemia. Brit. med. J. **1969 II**, 665—667.

BRAUN, G. A., MARSH, J. B., DRABKIN, D. L.: Stimulation of protein and plasma albumin synthesis in a cellfree system from livers of nephrotic rats. Biochem. Res. Commun. **8**, 28—32 (1962).

BROWN, D. F., DAUDISS, K.: Hyperlipoproteinemia prevalence in a free living population in Albany, New York. Circulation **47**, 558—566 (1973).

BROWN, M. S., DANA, S. E., GOLDSTEIN, J. L.: Regulation of 3-hydroxy-3-methylglutaryl coenzyme A reductase activity in human fibroblasts by lipoproteins. Proc. nat. Acad. Sci. (Wash.) **70**, 2162—2166 (1973).

BROWN, M. S., DANA, S. E., GOLDSTEIN, J. L.: Regulation of 3-hydroxy-3-methylglutaryl coenzmye A reductase activity in cultured human fibroblasts comparison of cells from a normal subject and from a patient with homozygous familial hypercholesterolemia. J. biol. Chem. **249**, 789—796 (1974).

BROWN, M. S., GOLDSTEIN, J. L.: Expression of the familial hypercholesterolemia gene in heterozygotes: mechanism for a dominant disorder in man. Science **185**, 61—63 (1974).

BROWN, H. B., LEWIS, L. A., PAGE, I. H.: Mixed hyperlipemia, a sixth type of hyperlipoproteinemia. Atherosclerosis **17**, 181—196 (1974).

BURSTEIN, M., SAMAILLE, J.: Sur un dosage rapide du cholesterol lie aux α- et aux β-lipoproteines du serum. Clin. chim. Acta **5**, 609 (1960).

CAMEJO, G., BOSCH, V., ARREAZA, C., MENDEZ, H. C.: Early changes in plasma lipoprotein structure and biosynthesis in cholesterol-fed rabbits. J. Lipid Res. **14**, 61—68 (1973).

CARLSON, L. A.: Clinical aspects of classification of primary hyperlipoproteinemias. In: Human Hyperlipoproteinemias Principles and Methods. FUMAGALLI, R., RICCI, G., GORINI, S. (Eds.) Advanc. exp. Med. Biol. **38**, 89—104 (1973).

CORNWELL,D.G., KRUGER,F.A.: Molecular complexes in isolation and characterization of plasma lipoproteins. J. Lipid Res. **2**, 110—134 (1961).

CREPALDI,G., FELLIN,R., TIENGO,A.: Hyperlipoproteinemias and endocrine diseases. In: FUMA-GALLI,R., RICCI,G., GORINI,S. (Eds.): Human Hyperlipoproteinemias Principles and Methods. Advanc. Exp. Med. Biol. **38**, 113—132 (1973).

CROUSE,J.R., GERSON,C.D., DE CARLI,L.M., LIEBER,C.S.: Role of acetate in the reduction of plasma free fatty acids produced by ethanol in man. J. Lipid Res. **9**, 509—512 (1968).

DEL GATTO,L., LINDGREN,E.T., NICHOLS,A.V.: Ultracentrifugal methods for the determination of serum lipoproteins. Anal. Chem. **31**, 1397—1399 (1959).

DE LALLA,O., GOFMAN,J.: Ultracentrifugal analysis of serum lipoproteins. Methods Biochem. Anal. **1**, 459—478 (1954).

DE LALLA,O.F., TANDY,R.K., LOEB,H.G.: A simplified method for the analysis of ultracentrifuge film records of low density lipoproteins of human serum. Clin. Chem. **13**, 85—100 (1967).

DIETSCHY,J.M.: The role of bile salts in controlling the rate of intestinal cholesterogenesis. J. clin. Invest. **47**, 286—300 (1968).

DIETSCHY,J.M., WILSON,J.D.: Cholesterol synthesis in the squirrel monkey: relative rates of synthesis in various tissues and mechanisms of control. J. clin. Invest. **47**, 166—174 (1968).

DIETSCHY,J.M., WILSON,J.M.: Regulation of cholesterol metabolism. New Engl. J. Med. **282**, 1179—1183 (1970).

DOLE,V.P.: A relation between non-esterified fatty acids in plasma and the metabolism of glucose. J. clin. Invest. **35**, 150—154 (1956).

DOLE,V.P., HAMLIN,J.T.III: Particulate fat in lymph and blood. Physiol. Rev. **42**, 674—701 (1962).

DURRUM,E.L., PAUL,M.H., SMITH,E.R.B.: Lipid detection in paper electrophoresis. Science **116**, 428—430 (1952).

EISENBERG,S., BILHEIMER,D.W., LEVY,R.I.: The metabolism of very low density lipoprotein proteins. II. Studies on the transfer of apoproteins between plasma lipoproteins. Biochim. biophys. Acta (Amst.) **280**, 94—104 (1972).

EISENBERG,S., BILHEIMER,D.W., LEVY,R.I., LINDGREN,F.T.: On the metabolic conversion of human plasma very low density lipoprotein to low density lipoprotein. Biochim. biophys. Acta (Amst.) **326**, 361—377 (1973).

ENGELBERG,H.: *In vitro* studies of human plasma lipolytic activity before and after oral fat intake. J. appl. Physiol. **11**, 155—160 (1957).

EWING,A.M., FREEMAN,N.K., LINDGREN,F.T.: The analysis of human serum lipoprotein distributions. Advanc. Lipid Res. **3**, 25—61 (1965).

FASOLI,A.: Electrophoresis of serum lipoproteins of filter paper. Lancet **1952 I**, 106.

FELTS,J.M.: The metabolism of chylomicron triglyceride fatty acids by perfused rat livers and by intact rats. Ann. N.Y. Acad. Sci. **131**, 24—33 (1965).

FELTS,J.M., MAYES,P.A.: Lack of uptake and oxidation of chylomicron triglyceride to carbon dioxide and ketone bodies by the perfused rat liver. Nature (Lond.) **206**, 195—196 (1965).

FISHER,W.R., HAMMOND,M.G., WARMKE,G.L.: Measurements of the molecular weight variability of plasma low density lipoproteins among normals and subjects with hyper-β-lipoproteinemia. Demonstration of macromolecular heterogeneity. Biochemistry **11**, 519—525 (1972).

FORTE,G.M., NICHOLS,A.V., GLAESER,R.M.: Electron microscopy of human serum lipoproteins using negative staining. Chem. Phys. Lipids **2**, 396—408 (1968).

FREDRICKSON,D.S., ONO,K., DAVIS,L.L.: Lipolytic activity of postheparin plasma in hyperglyceridemia. J. Lipid Res. **4**, 24—33 (1963).

FREDRICKSON,D.S., LEES,R.S.: System for phenotyping hyperlipoproteinemia. Circulation **31**, 321—327 (1965).

FREDRICKSON,D.S., LEVY,R.I., LEES,R.S.: Fat transport in lipoproteins—an integrated approach to mechanisms and disorders. New Engl. J. Med. **276**, 32—44; 94—103; 148—156; 215—226; 273—281 (1967).

FREDRICKSON,D.S., LEVY,R.I.: Familial hyperlipoproteinemia. In: STANBURY,J.B., WYNGAARDEN,J.B., FREDRICKSON,D.B. (Eds.): The Metabolic Basis of Inherited Disease. New York: McGraw-Hill 1972.

FREDRICKSON,D.S., LUX,S.E., HERBERT,P.N.: The apolipoproteins. Advanc. exp. Med. Biol. **26**, 25—56 (1972).

GARFINKEL, A. S., SCHOTZ, M. C.: Separation of molecular species of lipoprotein lipase from adipose tissue. J. Lipid Res. **13**, 63—68 (1972).

GILTIN, D., CORNWELL, D. G., NAKASATO, D., ONCLEY, J. L., HUGHES, W. L., JR., JANEWAY, C. A.: Studies on the metabolism of plasma proteins in the nephrotic syndrome. II. The lipoproteins. J. clin. Invest. **37**, 172—184 (1958).

GLOMSET, J. A., NORUM, K. R.: The metabolic role of lecithin: cholesterol acyltransferase: perspectives from pathology. Advanc. Lipid. Res. **11**, 1—65 (1973).

GLUECK, C. J., LEVY, R. I., GLUECK, H. I., GRALNICK, H. R., GRETEN, H., FREDRICKSON, D. S.: Acquired Type I hyperlipoproteinemia with systemic lupus erythematosus, dysglobulinemia, and heparin resistance. Amer. J. Med. **47**, 318—324 (1969 a).

GLUECK, C. J., LEVY, R. I., FREDRICKSON, D. S.: Immunoreactive insulin, glucose tolerance, and carbohydrate inducibility in Types II, III, IV, and V hyperlipoproteinemia. Diabetes **18**, 739—747 (1969 b).

GLUECK, C. J., HECKMAN, F., SCHOENFELD, M., STEINER, P., PEARCE, W.: Neonatal familial Tape II hyperlipoproteinemia; cord blood cholesterol in 1800 live births. Metabolism **20**, 597—608 (1971).

GLUECK, C. J., TSANG, R. C.: Neonatal familial Type II hyperlipoproteinemia: Effects of diet on plasma cholesterol in the first year of life. Amer. J. clin. Nutr. **25**, 224—230 (1972).

GOFMAN, J. W., RUBIN, L., McGINLEY, J. P., JONES, H. B.: Hyperlipoproteinemia. Amer. J. Med. **17**, 514—520 (1954).

GOLDSTEIN, J. L., BROWN, M. S.: Familial hypercholesterolemia identification of a defect in the regulation of 3-hydroxy-3-methyl glutaryl coenzyme. A reductase activity associated with over production of cholesterol. Proc. nat. Acad. Sci. (Wash.) **70**, 2804—2808 (1973).

GOLDSTEIN, J. L., SCHROTT, H. G., HAZZARD, W. R., BIERMAN, E. L., MOTULSKY, A. G.: Hyperlipidemia in coronary heart disease. II. Genetic analysis of lipid levels in 176 families and delineation of a new inherited disorder, combined hyperlipidemia. J. clin. Invest. **52**, 1544—1568 (1973).

GOODMAN, D. S.: The metabolism of chylomicron cholesterol ester in the rat. J. clin. Invest. **41**, 1886—1896 (1962).

GOUSIOS, A., FELTS, J. M., HAVEL, R. J.: The metabolism of serum triglycerides and free fatty acids by the myocardium. Metabolism **12**, 75—80 (1963).

HAHN, P. F.: Abolishment of alimentary lipemia following injection of heparin. Science **98**, 19—20 (1943).

HAMILTON, R. L.: Postheparin plasma lipase from the hepatic circulation. Dissertation Abs. **26**, 24 (1965).

HARLAN, W. R., JR., GRAHAM, J. B., ESTES, E. H.: Familial hypercholesterolemia: a genetic and metabolic study. Medicine **45**, 77—110 (1966).

HARLAN, W. R., WINESETT, P. S., WASSERMAN, A. J.: Tissue lipoprotein lipase in normal individuals and in individuals with exogenous hypertriglyceridemia and the relationship of this enzyme to assimilation of fat. J. clin. Invest. **46**, 239—247 (1967).

HARRIS, K., FELTS, J. M.: Kinetics of chylomicron triglyceride removal from plasma in rats: the effect of diet. Biochim. biophys. Acta (Amst.) **316**, 288—295 (1973).

HATCH, F. T., LEES, R. S.: Practical methods for plasma lipoprotein analysis. Advanc. Lipid Res. **6**, 1—68 (1968).

HAVEL, R. J., EDER, H. A., BRAGDON, J. H.: The distribution and chemical composition of ultra-centrifugally separated lipoproteins in human serum. J. clin. Invest. **34**, 1345—1353 (1955).

HAVEL, R. J.: Evidence for the participation of lipoprotein lipase in the transport of chylomicrons. In: Blood Lipids and the Clearing Factor. Third International Conference on Biochemical Problems of Lipids. Brussels: K. Vlaamse Acad. 1956.

HAVEL, R. J., GORDON, R. S., JR.: Idiopathic hyperlipemia: metabolic studies in an affected family. J. clin. Invest. **39**, 1777—1790 (1960).

HAVEL, R. J., FELTS, J. M., VAN DUYNE, C. M.: Formation and fate of endogenous triglycerides in blood plasma of rabbits. Lipid Res. **3**, 297—308 (1962).

HAVEL, R. J., SHORE, V. G., SHORE, B., BIER, D. M.: Role of specific glycopeptides of human serum lipoproteins in the activation of lipoprotein lipase. Circulation Res. **27**, 595—600 (1970).

HAVEL, R. J.: Mechanisms of hyperlipoproteinemia. Advanc. exp. Biol. **26**, 57—70 (1972).

Havel,R.J., Kane,J.P.: Primary dysbetalipoproteinemia: a predominance of a specific apoprotein species in triglyceride-rich lipoproteins. Proc. nat. Acad. Sci. (Wash.) **70**, 2015—2019 (1973).

Havel,R.J., Kane,J.P., Kashyap,M.L.: Interchange of apolipoproteins between chylomicrons and high density lipoproteins during alimentary lipemia in man. J. clin. Invest. **52**, 32—38 (1973).

Hazzard,W.R., Lindgren,F.T., Bierman,E.L.: Very low density lipoprotein subfractions in a subject with broad-β disease (Type III hyperlipoproteinemia) and a subject with endogenous lipemia (Type IV). Chemical composition and electrophoretic mobility. Biochim. biophys. Acta (Amst.) **202**, 517—525 (1970a).

Hazzard,W.R., Porte,D.,Jr., Bierman,E.L.: Abnormal lipid composition of chylomicrons in broad-β disease (Type III hyperlipoproteinemia). J. clin. Invest. **49**, 1853—1858 (1970b).

Hazzard,W.R., Goldstein,J.L., Schrott,H.G., Motulsky,A.G., Bierman,E.L.: Hyperlipidemia in coronary heart disease. III. Evaluation of lipoprotein phenotypes of 156 genetically defined survivors of myocardial infarction. J. clin. Invest. **52**, 1569—1577 (1973).

Herbert,P.N., Forte,T.M., Schulman,R.S., Gong,E.L., Lapiana,M.J., Nichols,A.V., Levy,R.I., Fredrickson,D.S.: Selective loss of apolipoproteins upon ultracentrifugation of very low density lipoproteins (VLDL). Federation Proc. **32**, 548a (1973).

Hillyard,L.A., Cornelius,C.E., Chaikoff,I.L.: Removal by the isolated rat liver of palmitate-1-C^{14} bound to albumin and of palmitate-1-C^{14} and cholesterol-4-C^{14} in chylomicrons from perfusion fluid. J. biol. Chem. **234**, 2240—2245 (1959).

Huang,T.C., Kuksis,A.: A comparative study of the lipids of chylomicron membrane and fat core and of the lymph serum of dogs. Lipids **2**, 443—452 (1967).

Jeffries,G.H.: The effect of fat absorption on the interaction of chyle and plasma in the rat. Quart. J. exp. Physiol. **39**, 77—81 (1954).

Kalab,M., Martin,W.G.: Gel filtration of native and modified pig serum lipoproteins. J. Chromatogr. **35**, 230—233 (1968).

Kessler,J.I., Stein,J., Dannacker,D., Narcessian,P.: Biosynthesis of low density lipoprotein by cell-free preparations of rat intestinal mucosa. J. biol. Chem. **245**, 5281—5288 (1970).

Khoo,J.C., Steinberg,D., Thompson,B., Mayer,S.E.: Hormone regulation of adipocyte enzymes. J. biol. Chem. **248**, 3823—3830 (1973).

Killander,J., Bengtsson,S., Philipson,L.: Fractionation of human plasma macroglobulins by gel filtration on pearl-condensed agar. Proc. Soc. exp. Biol. (N.Y.) **115**, 861—865 (1964).

Klatskin,G., Gordon,M.: Relationship between relapsing pancreatitis and essential hyperlipemia. Am. J. Med. **12**, 3—23 (1952).

Koppers,L.E., Palumbo,P.J.: Lipid disturbances in endocrine disorders. Med. Clin. N. Am. **56**, 1013—1020 (1972).

Korn,E.D.: Clearing factor, a heparin-activated lipoprotein lipase. I. Isolation and characterization of the enzyme from normal rat heart. J. biol. Chem. **215**, 1—14 (1955a).

Korn,E.D.: Clearing factor, a heparin-activated lipoprotein lipase. II. Substrate specificity and activation of coconut oil. J. biol. Chem. **215**, 15—26 (1955b).

Korn,E.D.: The assay of lipoprotein lipase *in vivo* and *in vitro*. Methods Biochem. Anal. **7**, 145—192 (1959).

Krauss,R.M., Windmueller,H.G., Levy,R.I., Fredrickson,D.S.: Selective measurement of two different triglyceride lipase activities in rat postheparin plasma. J. Lipid Res. **14**, 286—295 (1973).

Kritchevsky,D., Tepper,S.A., Alaupovic,P., Furman,R.H.: Cholesterol content of human serum lipoproteins obtained by dextran sulfate precipitation and by preparative ultracentrifugation. Proc. Soc. exp. Biol. (N.Y.) **112**, 259—262 (1963).

Kwiterovich,P.O., Levy,R.I., Fredrickson,D.S.: Early detection and treatment of familial Type II hyperlipoproteinemia. Circulation **42**, III—11 (1970).

Langer,T., Strober,W., Levy,R.I.: The metabolism of low density lipoprotein in familial Type II hyperlipoproteinemia. J. clin. Invest. **51**, 1528—1536 (1972).

Larosa,J.C., Levy,R.I., Herbert,P., Lux,S.E., Fredrickson,D.S.: A specific apoprotein activator for lipoprotein lipase. Biochem. Biophys. Res. Commun. **41**, 57—62 (1970).

Lee,G.B., Culley,G.A., Lawson,M.J., Adcock,L.L., Krivit,W.: Type II hyperlipoproteinemia in mother and twins. Circulation **39**, 183—188 (1969).

LEES,R.S., HATCH,F.T.: Sharper separation of lipoprotein species by paper electrophoresis in albumin-containing buffer. J. Lab. clin. Med. **61**, 518—528 (1963).

LEES,R.S., WILSON,D.E., SCHONFELD,G., FLEET,S.: The familial dyslipoproteinemias. Prog. Med. Genet. **9**, 237—290 (1973).

LEVY,R.I., QUARFORDT,S.H., BROWN,W.V.., SLOAN,H.R., FREDRICKSON,D.S.: The efficacy of clofibrate (CPlB) in familial hyperlipoproteinemias. In: HOLMES,W.L., CARLSON,L.A., PAOLETTI,R. (Eds.): Drugs Affecting Lipid Metabolism. New York: Plenum 1969.

LEVY,R.I., LEES,R.S., FREDRICKSON,D.S.: The nature of pre-beta (very low density) lipoproteins. J. clin. Invest. **45**, 63—77 (1965).

LEVY,R.I., FREDRICKSON,D.S.: The current status of hypolipidemic drugs. Postgrad. Med. **47**, 130—136 (1970).

LEWIS,L.A., PAGE,I.H.: Electrophoretic and ultracentrifugal analysis of serum lipoproteins of normal, nephrotic, and hypertensive persons. Circulation **7**, 707—717 (1953).

LEWIS,L.A., ZUEHLKE,V., NAKAMOTO,S., KOLFF,W.J., PAGE,I.H.: Renal regulations of serum α-lipoproteins. Decrease of α-lipoproteins in the absence of renal function. New Engl. J. Med. **275**, 1097—1105 (1966).

LEWIS,B., CHAIT,A., SISSONS,P.: Lipid abnormalities in alcoholism and chronic renal failure. Advanc. exp. Med. Biol. **38**, 155—159 (1973).

LINDGREN,F.T., NICHOLS,A.V.: Structure and function of human serum lipoproteins. In: PUTMAN,F.W. (Ed.): Plasma Proteins. New York: Academic Press 1960.

LOSSOW,W.J., NAIDOO,S.S., CHAIKOFF,I.L.: Effect of heparin on disappearance of the cholesterol moiety of an injected cholesterol-C^{14}-labeled, very low density chyle lipoprotein fraction from the circulation of the rat. J. Lipid Res. **4**, 419—423 (1963).

MARGOLIS,S.: Separation and size determination of human serum lipoproteins by agarose gel filtration. J. Lipid Res. **8**, 501—507 (1967).

MARSH,J.B., WHEREAT,A.F.: The synthesis of plasma lipoprotein by rat liver. J. biol. Chem. **234**, 3196—3200 (1959).

MASORO,E.J., CHAIKOFF,I.L., CHERNICK,S.S., FELTS,J.M.: Previous nutritional state and glucose conversion to fatty acids in liver slices. J. biol. Chem. **185**, 845—856 (1950).

MASORO,E.J., FELTS,J.M.: Role of carbohydrate metabolism in promoting fatty acid oxidation. J. biol. Chem. **231**, 347—356 (1958).

MASORO,E.J.: Biochemical mechanisms related to the homeostatic regulation of lipogenesis in animals. J. Lipid Res. **3**, 149—164 (1962).

MAYER,J.: Metabolism of the adipose tissue in the hereditary obese-hyperglycemic syndrome. In: RODAHL,K., ISSEKUTZ,B. (Eds.): Fat as a Tissue. New York: McGraw-Hill 1964.

MAYES,P.A., FELTS,J.M.: Lack of uptake and metabolism of the triglyceride of serum lipoproteins of density less than 1.006 by the perfused rat liver. Biochem. J. **105**, 18c—20c (1967).

MAYES,P.A., FELTS,J.M.: The functional status of lipoprotein lipase in rat liver. Biochem. J. **108**, 483—487 (1968).

MINARI,O., ZILVERSMIT,D.B.: Behavior of dog lymph chylomicron lipid constituents during incubation with serum. J. Lipid Res. **4**, 424—436 (1963).

MORRIS,M.D., CHAIKOFF,I.L.: The origin of cholesterol in liver, small intestine, adrenal gland, and testis of the rat: dietary versus endogenous contributions. J. biol. Chem. **234**, 1095—1097 (1959).

NAITO,C., FELTS,J.M.: Influence of heparin on the removal of serum lipoprotein lipase by the perfused liver of the rat. J. Lipid Res. **11**, 48—53 (1970).

NESTEL,P.J., HAVEL,R.J., BEZMAN,A.: Metabolism of constituent lipids of dog chylomicrons. J. clin. Invest. **42**, 1313—1321 (1963).

NESTEL,P.J., WHYTE,H.M.: Plasma free fatty acid and triglyceride turnover in obesity. Metabolism **17**, 112—118 (1968).

NIKKILA,N.A.: Metabolic typing of hypertriglyceridemia. Scand. J. clin. Lab. Invest. **29**, 126—3.3a (1972).

NOBLE,R.P.: Electrophoretic separation of plasma lipoproteins in agarose gel. J. Lipid Res. **9**, 693—700 (1968).

OCKNER,R.K., HUGHES,F.B., ISSELBACHER,K.J.: Very low density lipoproteins in intestinal lymph: role in triglyceride and cholesterol transport during fat absorption. J. clin. Invest. **48**, 2367—2373 (1969).

Olivecrona, T., Egelrud, T.: Evidence for an ionic binding of lipoprotein lipase to heparin. Biochem. Biophys. Res. Commun. **43**, 524—529 (1971).

Paula, R. K., Rudel, L. L.: Influence of dietary cholesterol on plasma lipoprotein structure and distribution in *Macaca nemestrina*. Circulation **49, 50**, III—269 (1974).

Pollard, H., Scanu, A. M., Taylor, E. W.: On the geometrical arrangement of the protein subunits of human serum low density lipoprotein: evidence for a dodecahedral model. Proc. nat. Acad. Sci. (Wash.) **64**, 304—310 (1969).

Porte, D., O'Hara, D. D., Williams, R. H.: The relationship between postheparin lipolytic activity and plasma triglyceride in myxedema. Metabolism **15**, 107—113 (1966).

Quarfordt, S. H., Goodman, D. S.: Chylomicron cholesteryl ester metabolism in the perfused rat liver. Biochim. Biophys. Acta (Amst.) **176**, 863—872 (1969).

Quarfordt, S., Levy, R. I., Fredrickson, D. S.: On the lipoprotein abnormality in Type III hyperlipoproteinemia. J. clin. Invest. **50**, 754—761 (1971).

Quarfordt, S., Nathans, A., Dowdee, M., Hilderman, H. L.: Heterogeneity of human very low density lipoproteins by gel filtration chromatography. J. Lipid Res. **13**, 435—444 (1972).

Rachmilewitz, D., Stein, O., Roheim, P. S., Stein, Y.: Metabolism of iodinated high density lipoproteins in the rat. II. Autoradiographic localization in the liver. Biochim. biophys. Acta (Amst.) **270**, 414—425 (1972).

Radding, C. M., Steinberg, D.: Studies on the synthesis and secretion on serum lipoproteins by rat liver slices. J. clin. Invest. **39**, 1560—1569 (1960).

Redgrave, T. B.: Formation of cholesteryl ester-rich particulate lipid during metabolism of chylomicrons. J. clin. Invest. **49**, 465—471 (1970).

Robinson, D. S., Jeffries, G. H., French, J. E.: Studies on the interaction of chyle and plasma in the rat. Quart. J. exp. Physiol. **39**, 165—176 (1954).

Robinson, D. S., Jeffries, G. H., Poole, J. C. F.: Further studies on the interaction of chyle and plasma in the rat. Quart. J. exp. Physiol. **40**, 297—308 (1955).

Robinson, D. S., Harris, P. M.: The production of lipolytic activity in the circulation of the hind limb in response to heparin. Quart. J. exp. Physiol. **44**, 80—90 (1959).

Robinson, D. S.: The function of the plasma triglycerides in fatty acid transport. In: Florkin, M., Stotz, E. H. (Eds.): Comprehensive Biochemistry. New York: Elsevier Publishing Company 1970.

Roheim, P. S., Haft, D. E., Gidez, L. I., White, A., Eder, H. A.: Plasma lipoprotein metabolism in perfused rat livers. II. Transfer of free and esterified cholesterol into the plasma. J. clin. Invest. **42**, 1277—1285 (1963).

Rose, H. G., Kranz, P., Weinstock, M., Juliano, J., Haft, J. I.: Inheritance of combined hyperlipoproteinemia: Evidence for a new lipoprotein phenotype. Amer. J. Med. **54**, 148—159 (1973).

Rose, H. G., Kranz, P., Weinstock, M., Juliano, J., Haft, J. I.: Combined hyperlipoproteinemia—evidence for a new lipoprotein phenotype. Atherosclerosis **20**, 51—64 (1974).

Rudel, L. L., Morris, M. D., Felts, J. M.: The transport of exogenous cholesterol in the rabbit. I. Role of cholesterol ester of lymph chylomicra and lymph very low density lipoproteins in absorption. J. clin. Invest. **51**, 2686—2692 (1972).

Rudel, L. L., Mitamura, T., Felts, J. M.: Characterization of rabbit lymph chylomicra and very low density lipoproteins. Circulation **47, 48**, IV-252 (1973a).

Rudel, L. L., Felts, J. M., Morris, M. D.: Exogenous cholesterol transport in rabbit plasma lipoproteins. Biochem. J. **134**, 531—537 (1973b).

Rudel, L. L., Lee, J. A., Morris, M. D., Felts, J. M.: Characterization of plasma lipoproteins separated and purified by agarose-column chromatography. Biochem. J. **139**, 89—95 (1974).

Rudel, L. L., Lofland, H. B., Jr.: Circulating lipoproteins in nonhuman primates. In: Strong, J. P. (Ed.): Atherosclerosis in Primates. New York: Karger. In Press.

Salans, L. B., Knittle, J. L., Hirsch, J.: The role of adipose cell size and adipose tissue insulin sensitivity in carbohydrate intolerance of human obesity. J. clin. Invest. **47**, 153—165 (1968).

Sata, T., Estrich, D. L., Wood, P. D. S., Kinsell, L. W.: Evaluation of gel chromatography for plasma lipoprotein fractionation. J. Lipid Res. **11**, 331—340 (1970).

Sata, T., Havel, R. J., Jones, A. L.: Characterization of subfractions of triglyceride-rich lipoproteins separated by gel chromatography from blood plasma of normolipemic and hyperlipemic humans. J. Lipid Res. **13**, 757—768 (1972).

SCANU, A. M., GRANDA, J. L.: Effects of ultracentrifugation of the human serum high density (1.063 < d < 1.21 g/ml) lipoprotein. Biochemistry 5, 446—454 (1966).

SCHREIBMAN, P. H., ARONS, D. L., SAUDEK, C. D., ARKY, R. A.: Abnormal lipoprotein lipase in familial exogenous hypertriglyceridemia. J. clin. Invest. 52, 2075—2082 (1973).

SCHUMAKER, V. N., ADAMS, G. H.: Circulating lipoproteins. Ann. Rev. Biochem. 38, 113—136 (1969).

SCOTT, P. J., HURLEY, P. J.: Effect of clofibrate on low density lipoprotein turnover in essential hypercholesterolaemia. J. Atheroscler. Res. 9, 25—34 (1969).

SHEFER, S., HAUSER, S., LAPAR, V., MOSBACH, E. H.: Regulatory effects of sterols and bile acids on hypercholesterolemia. J. Atheroscler. Res. 9, 25—34 (1969). J. Lipid Res. 14, 573—580 (1973).

SHIPP, J. C., WOOD, F. C., JR., MARBLE, A.: Hyperlipemia following sulfonylurea therapy in young diabetics. J. Amer. med. Ass. 188, 468—471 (1964).

SHORE, V. G., SHORE, B.: Heterogeneity of human plasma very low density lipoproteins. Separation of species differing in protein components. Biochemistry 12, 502—507 (1973).

SHORE, V. G., SHORE, B., HART, R. G.: Changes in apolipoproteins and properties of rabbit very low density lipoproteins on induction of cholesteremia. Biochemistry 13, 1579—1584 (1974).

SKIPSKI, V. P.: Lipid composition of lipoproteins in normal and diseased states. In: NELSON, G. J., (Ed.): Blood Lipids and Lipoproteins: Quantitation, Composition, and Metabolism. New York: Wiley-Interscience 1972.

SLACK, J., NEVIN, N. C.: Hyperlipidaemic xanthomatosis. I. Increased risk of death from ischaemic heart disease in first degree relatives of 53 patients with essential hyperlipidaemia and xanthomatosis. J. med. Genet. 5, 4—28 (1968).

SLACK, J., MILLS, G. L.: Anomalous low density lipoproteins in familial hyperbetalipoproteinemia. Clin. chim. Acta 29, 15—25 (1970).

SMITH, E. B.: Lipoprotein patterns in myocardial infarction. Lancet 1957 II, 910—914.

STEINBERG, D.: Hormonal control of lipolysis in adipose tissue. Advanc. Exp. med. Biol. 26, 77—88 (1972).

STEINER, G.: Lipoprotein lipase in fat induced hyperlipidemia. New Engl. J. Med. 279, 70—74 (1968).

STONE, N., LEVY, R., FREDRICKSON, D., VERTER, J.: Coronary artery disease in familial Type II hyperlipoproteinemia: Study of 116 kindreds. Third International Symposium on Atherosclerosis, Berlin 1973. SCHETTLER, G., SCHLIERF, G. (Eds.). Berlin: Karger, In Press.

TREADWELL, C. R., SWELL, L., VAHOUNY, G. V., FIELD, H., JR.: Observations on the mechanism of cholesterol absorption. J. Amer. Oil chem. Soc. 36, 107—111 (1958).

TYTGAT, G. N., RUBIN, C. E., SAUNDERS, D. R.: Synthesis and transport of lipoprotein particles by intestinal absorptive cells in man. J. clin. Invest. 50, 2065—2078 (1971).

WERNER, M.: Fractionation of lipoproteins from blood by gel filtration. J. Chromatogr. 25, 63—70 (1966).

WHAYNE, T. F., JR., FELTS, J. M., HARRIS, P. A.: Effect of heparin on the inactivation of serum lipoprotein lipase by the liver in unanesthetized dogs. J. clin. Invest. 48, 1246—1251 (1969).

WHAYNE, T. F., JR., FELTS, J. M.: Activation of lipoprotein lipase. Comparative study of man and other mammals. Circulation Res. 26, 545—551 (1970a).

WHAYNE, T. F., JR., FELTS, J. M.: Activation of lipoprotein lipase. Effects of rat serum lipoprotein fractions and heparin. Circulation Res. 27, 941—951 (1970b).

WINDMUELLER, H. G., LINDGREN, F. T., LOSSOW, W. J., LEVY, R. I.: On the nature of circulating lipoproteins of intestinal origin in the rat. Biochim. biophys. Acta (Amst.) 202, 507—516 (1970).

WINDMUELLER, H. G., HERBERT, P. N., LEVY, R. I.: Biosynthesis of lymph and plasma lipoprotein apoproteins by isolated perfused rat liver and intestine. J. Lipid Res. 14, 215—223 (1973).

YOSHITOSHI, Y., NAITO, C., OKANIWA, H., USUI, M., MOGAMI, T., TOMONO, T.: Kinetic Studies on metabolism of lipoprotein lipase. J. clin. Invest. 42, 707—713 (1963).

ZELIS, R., MASON, D. T., BRAUNWALD, E., LEVY, R. I.: Effects of hyperlipoproteinemias and their treatment on the peripheral circulation. J. clin. Invest. 49, 1007—1015 (1970).

ZILVERSMIT, D. B.: The composition and structure of lymph chylomicrons in dog, rat, and man. J. clin. Invest. 44, 1610—1622 (1965).

ZILVERSMIT, D. B.: The surface coat of chylomicrons: lipid chemistry. J. Lipid Res. 9, 180—186 (1968).

CHAPTER 5

Lipoproteins and Lipoprotein Metabolism

S. Eisenberg and R. I. Levy

With 6 Figures

The plasma lipoproteins provide the body with a transport system for the otherwise insoluble lipids. All lipids except for free fatty acids and lysolecithin, circulate in plasma from their site of origin to their site of utilization in association with these lipid-protein complexes, the lipoproteins. In healthy humans, more than 100 g of triglycerides, phospholipids and cholesterol are transported each day in lipoproteins; under certain pathological conditions, the human plasma lipoprotein system may contain more than 500 g of lipids. The aim of the present review is to define the various lipoproteins, describe their routes of metabolism and identify the possible mechanisms by which drugs may affect lipoprotein metabolism.

I. Structure and Functions of Lipoproteins

A. Physical Properties

Lipoproteins, first described in 1929 by Macheboeuf, represent a wide spectrum of particles, varying in weight from many billions to about one hundred thousand daltons, and varying in diameter from 10000 to 50 Å. They are customarily divided into four major families on the basis of their physical characteristics and chemical composition: chylomicrons; very low density lipoprotein (VLDL), low density lipoprotein (LDL) and high density lipoprotein (HDL). Two procedures are commonly used to separate lipoproteins: analytical ultracentrifugation and electrophoresis. Lipoproteins are separated in the analytical ultracentrifuge according to their density (Fig. 1) and are defined in this system following either density units (g/ml) or flotation units—S_f (10^3 cm/sec/dyne/g in a sodium chloride solution of density 1.063 g/ml at 26° C) (Delalla and Gofmann, 1954; Ewing et al., 1965; Nichols, 1967; Lindgren et al., 1972). The electrophoretic migrations of lipoproteins on different media (Fig. 1) is carried out usually at a basic pH (8.6) and is dependent primarily on their charge (Hatch and Lees, 1968). With both methods, however, lipoproteins size and shape may influence some of the resulting pattern of separation. Both of these systems are clearly operational rather than fuctional. A functional approach towards lipoprotein separation is obviously needed. Unfortunately, such an approach is still not available.

1. Chylomicrons

Defined originally as fat particles of intestinal origin (Gage, 1920; Gage and Fish, 1924), chylomicrons are lipoproteins of density less than 0.95 g/ml (S_f greater than 400) synthesized in the intestine during active fat absorption and carrying triglycer-

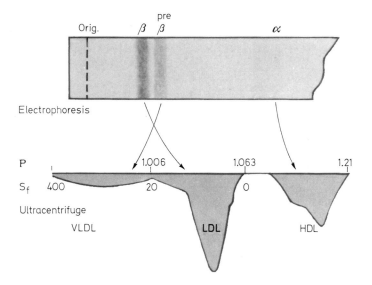

The normal lipoprotein spectrum

Fig. 1. Schematic presentation of the ultracentrifugal and electrophoretic distribution of the human plasma lipoproteins

Table 1. Human plasma lipoproteins: physical characteristics

Lipoprotein	S_f[a]	Density g/ml	Molecular weight daltons	Size Å	Electrophoretic mobility (paper, agarose gel)
Chylomicrons	>400	<0.95	$10^3-10^4 \times 10^6$	$750-10^4$	Origin
VLDL	20–400	0.95–1.006	$5-100 \times 10^6$	300–800	pre-β
LDL	0–12	1.019–1.063	$2-4 \times 10^6$	200–250	β
HDL	—	1.063–1.210	$2-4 \times 10^5$	75–100	α

[a] Lipoprotein flotation rate in Svedberg units (10^{-13} cm/sec/dyne/gm) in a sodium chloride solution of density 1.063 gm/ml (26° C).

ides of exogenous origin (Zilversmit, 1969). They represent a spectrum of particles varying in diameter between 0.1 to 1 micron and of molecular weight 100 to 1000 million (Table 1). Their light scattering properties cause the blood and plasma to appear "cloudy" or "milky" and they float to the top of a test-tube within 12 to 24 hrs to form a "creamy" layer. Chylomicrons do not migrate on paper or agarose gel electrophoresis and are found at the line of sample application ("origin"); they exhibit α_2-mobility in free electrophoresis on starch and cellulose acetate systems (Fredrickson and Levy, 1972b). The presence of chylomicrons in plasma after an overnight fast (12 to 16 hrs) is pathological.

2. Very Low Density Lipoprotein

Very low density lipoproteins (VLDL) occupy a density range of 0.95 to 1.006 g/ml or S_f interval of 20 to 400. Their diameter varies between 300 and 800 Å and molecular weight from 5 to 130 million daltons (LINDGREN et al., 1972). As observed through the electron microscope, they are surrounded by a "hallow", which may represent a surface coat (HAMILTON, 1968). They do not float to the top of a test-tube on standing, but when present in plasma in excessive amounts, will cause the plasma to appear "cloudy" or even "milky". VLDL migrate in most electrophoretic media towards the anode with a prebeta (α_2) mobility, and are frequently referred to as "prebeta lipoproteins". VLDL is present normally in fasting plasma where it carries triglycerides of endogenous origin.

3. Low Density Lipoprotein

Low density lipoproteins (LDL) are defined as lipoproteins of density 1.006 to 1.063 g/ml, or S_f 0 to 20. This density range is often subdivided into lipoproteins of density 1.006 to 1.019 g/ml (S_f 12 to 20) and 1.019 to 1.063 g/ml (S_f 0 to 12). The bulk of LDL is present in the fraction of density 1.019 to 1.063 g/ml. This fraction is of an average S_f rate of 6.2 to 7.1, hydrated density of 1.028 to 1.030 and molecular weight of 2.12 to 2.36×10^6 daltons (LINDGREN et al., 1972). The diameter of the lipoproteins varies between 200 to 250 Å and they do not cause turbidity of plasma even when present in grossly excessive amounts. LDL migrates in electrophoretic media with the β-globulins, and is therefore also referred to as "beta lipoprotein".

4. High Density Lipoprotein

High density lipoproteins (HDL) occupy a density interval of 1.063 to 1.21 g/ml, and are frequently subdivided into HDL_2 ($d = 1.063$ to 1.125 g/ml) and HDL_3 ($d = 1.125$ to 1.210 g/ml). The physiological significance of the HDL subfraction is yet unclear. HDL represents the smallest lipoprotein particle, of diameter 50 to 100 Å and molecular weight range of 150000 to 400000 (FORTE et al., 1968). HDL migrates in electrophoretic systems with α_1 mobility and is also referred to as "alpha lipoproteins".

Several other lipoproteins have been described in normal plasma or in plasma obtained from patients with different diseases. Of the former are a group of lipoproteins—the Lp(a), or "sinking prebeta" lipoproteins which have a mean density of between 1.055 to 1.075 g/ml, do not produce turbidity and have an α_2 or prebeta mobility (SIMONS et al., 1970; LEVY et al., 1972b). Of the latter, perhaps the most interesting is the lipoprotein complex of biliary obstruction—"LpX". This lipoprotein with a mean density of 1.019 to 1.040 g/ml has a slow β mobility by electrophoresis, and is composed primarily of free cholesterol and lecithin (SEIDEL et al., 1969).

B. Lipid Composition

The major function of lipoproteins is to transport triglycerides from their site of synthesis—liver and intestine—to their site of utilization, primarily in the muscle and adipose tissue. The role of lipoproteins in cholesterol transport, possibly from extra-hepatic tissues to the liver, is yet to be established.

Table 2. Human plasma lipoproteins: chemical composition

Lipoprotein	Protein	TG	CE	FC	PL
	mg/100 mg lipoprotein				
Chylomicrons	1– 2	85–90	2– 5	1– 3	4– 8
VLDL	10	55–65	10–15	5–10	15–20
LDL	25	5–10	35–45	5–10	20–25
HDL	45–55	3– 5	15–25	5–10	25–30

TG = Triglyceride, CE = Cholesteryl esters, FC = Free cholesterol, PL = Phospholipid.

Chylomicrons and VLDL are the two major triglyceride transport lipoproteins carrying respectively glycerides of either exogenous (dietary) or endogenous origin. Triglycerides constitute more than 90% of chylomicron lipids and more than 70% of VLDL lipids (Table 2). Cholesterol, esterified and unesterified, and phospholipids constitute the remainder of the lipids (Levy et al., 1966, 1971; Skipski, 1972). Both free cholesterol and phospholipid may be present primarily in the surface coat of the two lipoproteins (Yokoyama and Zilversmit, 1965; Zilversmit, 1968). Recently, using salt density gradients and swinging bucket rotors, chylomicrons and VLDL have been separated into subfractions of different densities, S_f rates, size, and molecular weight (Lossow et al., 1969; Lindgren et al., 1972). With decreasing density, the lipoprotein subfractions contained less triglycerides but were relatively enriched with protein, cholesterol and phospholipids.

LDL is the major cholesterol carrying lipoprotein of human plasma, and cholesteryl esters constitute about one-half of its total mass. As much as 70 to 80% of total plasma cholesterol is associated with LDL. LDL cholesteryl esters contain predominantly unsaturated fatty acids, the more prevalent one being linoleic acid (18:2), about 40% of total fatty acids. The content of unesterified cholesterol and triglyceride in LDL is less than 10% of its total lipids, whereas phospholipids comprise about one-fourth of LDL mass. When the phospholipid composition of LDL was determined, it was found to be relatively enriched with sphingomyelin as compared to other plasma lipoproteins with a lecithin to sphingomyelin ratio of two to three (Skipski, 1972; Eisenberg et al., 1973a). The significance of this observation is yet unknown.

About one-half of the HDL mass is protein; phospholipids and cholesterol (mainly in esterified form) constitute 30% and 20% of the HDL respectively (Table 2). As discussed below, HDL may play an important role in the generation of cholesteryl esters in plasma, being a preferable substrate for the enzyme system lecithin:cholesterol acyltransferase (LCAT).

C. The Apoprotein Moiety of Lipoproteins

Proteins are an integral part of the lipoproteins, and though they may constitute less than 1% of the total lipoprotein mass (as in chylomicrons), they are essential for the assembly and secretion of lipoproteins (see II C).

Several methods have been developed in the last decade for the preparation, isolation and characterization of apolipoproteins. These were recently reviewed (Fredrickson et al., 1972c; Shore and Shore, 1972). The pattern of apoproteins

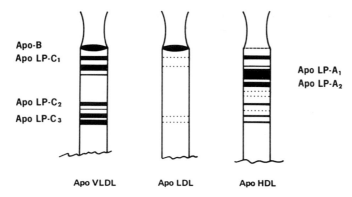

Apo-B
Apo LP-C₁

Apo LP-C₂
Apo LP-C₃

Apo LP-A₁
Apo LP-A₂

Apo VLDL   Apo LDL   Apo HDL

Fig. 2. Schematic view of polyacrylamide gel patterns of the apolipoproteins from VLDL, LDL, and HDL

Table 3. Human plasma Apolipoproteins: Characteristics

Apo-protein	Synonym	Characteristics of Human Apolipoproteins				
		C-terminal	N-terminal	Missing AA	Molecular weight	Carbo-hydrates
A_1	R-"thr", apoLP-glnI, fraction III	Glutamine	Aspartic acid	Isoleucine	27000	+
A_2	R-gln, apoLP-glnII, fraction IV	Glutamine	Pyrrolidone carboxylic acid	Histidine, arginine, tryptophane	8600	±
B	R-ser, apoLDL,	—	Glutamic acid	—	—	5%
C_1	R-val, apoLP-ser, D_1, fraction V	Serine	Threonine	Histidine, tyrosine, cysteine	7000	0
C_2	R-glu, apoLP-glu, D_2, fraction V	Glutamic acid	Threonine	Histidine, cysteine	10000	0
C_3	R-ala, apoLP-ala, $D_{3,4}$, fraction V	Alanine	Serine	Cysteine, isoleucine	8764	+

obtained from human lipoproteins and separated on polyacrylamide gels in shown in Fig. 2. A proposed nomenclature for these proteins, their more important properties and their average content in lipoproteins is presented in Tables 3 and 4. As is evident from the figure and tables, each lipoprotein contains a specific pattern of apoproteins. However, many of these proteins are present in more than one lipoprotein family.

The A proteins (A_1 and A_2) are the major apoproteins of human plasma HDL (SHORE and SHORE, 1968; KOSTNER and ALAUPOVIC, 1971). They may be present in small amounts in chylomicrons (KOSTNER and HOLASEK, 1972) and in trace amounts in VLDL (PEARLSTEIN et al., 1971). Both were isolated from human HDL, and their

Table 4. Human plasma apolipoproteins: distribution

Lipoprotein	A_1	A_2	B	C_1	C_2	C_3
	Percent of total lipoprotein protein					
Chylomicrons	?	?	5–20	15+	15+	40+
VLDL	Trace	?	40^a	10^a	10^a	30^a
LDL	—	—	>95	Trace	Trace	Trace
HDL	65–70	20–25	Trace	1–3	1–3	5–10

[a] See text for detailed description of the changing pattern of VLDL apoproteins.

structure has been studied in detail. They are soluble in water and urea solutions; contain glutamine at their carboxyterminal end but differ in amino acid composition, N-terminal amino acid, secondary structure, immunological properties, etc. (Fredrickson et al., 1972c). The A_2 protein can be cleaved by reduction of its single –S–S– bridge into two identical polypeptides, of about 8500 molecular weight. The primary sequence of this polypeptide has been recently reported (Brewer et al., 1972b). Immunological studies employing specific antisera have indicated that most HDL particles contain both the A_1 and A_2 proteins; a fraction of HDL, however, may contain only the A_1 proteins (Albers and Aladjem, 1971).

The B protein is the major human plasma LDL apoprotein, accounting for about 25% of total LDL mass. It constitutes more than 95% of the LDL apoproteins, and is present in constant amounts in LDL particles of different molecular weights (Hammond and Fisher, 1971). The B protein is also a major apoprotein constituent of chylomicrons and VLDL. In average, about 40% of VLDL (Shore and Shore, 1969; Gotto et al., 1972) and 20% of chylomicron (Kostner and Holasek, 1972) apoproteins are the B protein. After removal of lipids from lipoproteins, the B protein is obtained in a water insoluble form. The number and nature of protein subunits present in B protein are unknown.

A group of small molecular weight proteins (M.W. 10000 or less) were originally described in VLDL by Gustafson et al. (1966) and collectively designated apoC. Apoprotein C has subsequently been shown to consist of at least three different proteins, C_1, C_2, and C_3 (see Table 3), the latter appearing in two forms containing 1 and 2 moles of sialic acid per mole of protein respectively (Brown et al., 1969, 1970a, 1970b; Herbert et al., 1971). They constitute 40 to 80% of the VLDL apoproteins and 70 to 90% of the apoprotein moiety of chylomicrons. The relative content of B and C proteins in subfractions of VLDL was shown recently to be dependent on their density. VLDL subfractions of higher S_f rates contain relatively more C protein than subfractions of lower density (Eisenberg et al., 1972b). C proteins are also present in small amounts in HDL (5 to 10% of total HDL proteins), and in trace amounts in LDL. In normal fasting human plasma the absolute content of apoHDL is about 10 times that of apoVLDL, and therefore the absolute amount of C protein in HDL is comparable to that in VLDL. The three C proteins each have different physical, chemical and immunological properties, and each represent a discernible protein moiety. The primary sequence of C_1 and C_3 has been recently reported (Brewer et al., 1972a; Shulman et al., 1972).

The C proteins play an important physiological role in the transport of fat, acting as cofactors for the enzyme system lipoprotein lipase. C_2, together with phospholipids, is a specific and obligatory activator of the enzyme from post-heparin plasma, milk and adipose tissue (LAROSA et al., 1970; FREDRICKSON et al., 1972c). C_1 has also been reported to be an activator for the enzyme in post-heparin plasma but this observation remains to be confirmed (GANESEN et al., 1971).

Several other apoprotein fractions are encountered in either VLDL or HDL (FREDRICKSON et al., 1972c). These fractions are present in lipoproteins in relatively small amounts (less than 5% of total protein), have not been isolated free of other proteins and are poorly characterized. Several of them now appear to be artifacts of the isolation procedure. Nevertheless, one or more additional apoproteins may prove to be of importance in the physiology of fat transport, and further studies concerned with their isolation and characterization are needed.

D. Conclusion

From the foregoing discussion, it is apparent that lipoproteins, the vehicles for fat transport, exist in plasma as discrete entities. They may be grouped into families following their physical properties and lipid and protein composition. Yet, they share many lipid and protein constituents and thus appear to be metabolically related.

II. Synthesis of Lipoproteins

A. Assembly, Intracellular Transport, and Release

Lipoproteins are synthesized and secreted into the blood stream by the liver and the small intestine. Chylomicrons (by definition) are produced in the intestine; VLDL and HDL are synthesized in both liver and intestine. Most of the available information on lipoprotein synthesis and secretion has been obtained using the intact rat or isolated, perfused organs of the rat (MARSH, 1971; HAMILTON, 1972). There is some doubt as to the relevance of these data to the human.

The protein moiety of lipoproteins is formed most probably in ribosomes of the rough endoplasmic reticulum (BUNGENBERG/DEJONG and MARSH, 1968; LO and MARSH, 1970), and the lipids are synthesized in both the rough and smooth endoplasmic reticulum (STEIN and STEIN, 1967). Lipoprotein particles of size and shape similar to VLDL (liver and intestine) or chylomicrons (intestine) are identified first in the smooth endoplasmic reticulum. The exact site and mechanism of assembly of lipoproteins is not known. Detailed morphological studies of intracellular transport and secretion of lipoproteins by human intestinal absorptive cells (TYTGAT et al., 1971) has indicated the following sequence: lipoproteins are first observed in smooth vesicles of the endoplasmic reticulum, are transferred to golgi cisternae, and probably accumulate there. They can be identified in the golgi area even when they are not found in any other cell organelle. Lipoproteins then are found within smooth vesicles, extending towards the lateral and basal portion of the intestinal cell membrane. They then may leave the cell by reverse pinocytosis, and are found in the intercellular space. A similar sequence of events takes place in the rat liver (STEIN and STEIN, 1967; HAMILTON, 1968, 1972). The presence of secretory vesicles, of golgi origin, in the liver has been postulated in both studies. As all of the above mentioned cell organelles are probably interconnected, this system of intracellular transport may direct lipoproteins from the site of synthesis of their individual lipid and protein constituents to their ultimate site of release to extracellular spaces. The assembly of lipids and proteins probably occurs in the region of the endoplasmic reticulum; the attachment of carbohydrates to proteins may begin in smooth endoplasmic reticulum (Molnar, 1967), but takes place mainly in the golgi area (Wagner and Cynkin, 1971). A group of enzymes, the nucleotide glycoprotein glycosyltransferases, present in the golgi, were recently shown to use lipoproteins as one of their hexoseamine acceptors (Lo and Marsh, 1970). In analogy to other plasma glycoproteins, the addition of carbohydrates to lipoproteins may play an important role in the mechanism of their release from the cell.

Organ perfusion studies have demonstrated that VLDL and HDL are secreted into the perfusate by either liver or intestine. No release of LDL from either organ has been found (Hamilton, 1972), and it is therefore not clear that apo-B is ever produced in rats independent of chylomicrons and VLDL synthesis. Of interest is the fact that particles the size of LDL or HDL have not been found in any of the morphological studies concerned with lipoprotein synthesis by liver and intestine. Nevertheless, HDL is consistently found in perfusate, and its production is independent, at least in part, of that of other lipoproteins.

Lipoproteins isolated from golgi cisternae, or liver perfusate, are generally similar to circulating lipoproteins (Mahley et al., 1970). However, several differences have been recently described (Hamilton, 1972). Both nascent VLDL and chylomicrons contain more phospholipids and less proteins as compared to plasma lipoproteins and they have slower electrophoretic mobility. Some of these differences disappear following incubation with HDL. Nascent HDL also is different from plasma HDL, and has been reported to resemble the "abnormal HDL" of LCAT deficient patients or the "lipoprotein of obstructive jaundice". The difference between perfusate and plasma HDL is probably due to the esterification of free cholesterol in plasma by the LCAT system (See III D).

B. Synthesis of Apoproteins

Several studies during the last 15 years have demonstrated that radioactive amino acids are incorporated into the protein moiety of newly synthesized lipoproteins of liver (Radding et al., 1958; Haft et al., 1962; Windmueller et al., 1973) or intestinal (Roheim et al., 1966; Windmueller and Spaeth, 1972; Windmueller et al., 1973) origin. However, only very recently was the synthesis of individual apoproteins studied. Windmueller et al. (1973) have studied the incorporation of amino acids into lipoprotein apoproteins isolated following liver or intestinal perfusion. With either organ, significant amounts of radioactivity were associated with VLDL and HDL, and neither tissue produced any detectable amount of labeled LDL. VLDL and HDL of liver origin contained radioactivity in three protein groups. However, the amount of radioactivity associated with VLDL proteins analogous to the human B-protein were considered to be disproportionately high, and that associated with proteins analogous to the human C proteins disproportionately low. Intestinal lymph VLDL and HDL did not contain any appreciable amount of radioactivity associated with their C proteins. The results, therefore, suggest that the C proteins were not synthesized in the intestinal cells, and that their presence in the lymph is due to a transfer of C protein from HDL. These conclusions are corroborated by the qualitative data obtained from lipoproteins isolated from golgi cisternae of rat liver (MAHLEY et al., 1970) and intestine (MAHLEY et al., 1971), and by the experiments cited by HAMILTON (1972) on the lipoprotein lipase activation properties of VLDL isolated from rat golgi apparatus.

C. Regulation of Lipoprotein Synthesis

Availability and flux of fatty acids (or partial glycerides), has been documented to affect VLDL and chylomicron formation in liver and intestine (MARSH, 1971). Chylomicrons are formed and released only during active absorption of lipids from the intestinal lumen. The amount of VLDL in the intestinal absorptive cells is decreased considerably following bile diversion or cholestyramine administration, bile lecithin being an important source of intestinal fatty acids during fasting periods (PORTER et al., 1971). The release of VLDL by liver increases when the amount of fatty acids in the perfusate increases (RUDERMAN et al., 1968). This same mechanism may explain the increase in VLDL production seen in diabetics (BIERMAN, 1972). Carbohydrate feeding and insulin may stimulate liver VLDL synthesis by affecting fatty acid synthesis by this organ (NIKKILA, 1969; FREDRICKSON and LEVY, 1972b). The decrease of plasma VLDL levels seen following nicotinic acid administration may be due to decreased flux of free fatty acids from adipose tissue to the liver. Though many of these cited examples may have other effects on lipoprotein metabolism, all are compatible with the assumption that the flux and availability of fatty acids to liver and intestine affects lipoproteins synthesis. The possible role of lipids other than triglycerides and triglyceride precursors in regulating lipoprotein synthesis is uncertain, at least under normal conditions. Lipoproteins of abnormal composition are seen in animals fed high cholesterol diets (SARDET et al., 1972) but similar lipoproteins have not as yet been described in humans.

The possible role of apoprotein synthetic rates on the formation of lipoproteins is also uncertain. Increased apoprotein synthesis has been postulated to cause increased lipoprotein synthesis in the nephrotic syndrome, after partial hepatectomy, and in alcohol-induced hyperlipemia (MARSH, 1971). Apoprotein synthesis may play a role in the difference observed in the lipoprotein levels of males and females. Normal synthesis of apoproteins is obligatory for the formation of lipoproteins, and the administration of protein-synthesis inhibitors to rats results in complete inhibition of lipoprotein formation in liver (JONES et al., 1967) or intestine (SABESIN and ISSELBACHER, 1969). The essentiality of the apoproteins for plasma lipoprotein formation is most dramatically illustrated in the two rare congenital diseases: abetalipoproteinemia and Tangier disease (FREDRICKSON et al., 1972a).

In abetalipoproteinemia the B protein is completely absent from the plasma. Both A proteins and the C proteins are present (GOTTO et al., 1971). Apparently secondary to this inability to synthesize or release B protein, glycerides accumulate in vesicles in the liver and intestine but do not enter into the plasma. Neither chylomicrons, VLDL or LDL are released. Patients with abetalipoproteinemia have extremely low levels of plasma lipids, all bound to HDL, and exhibit malabsorption of fat and fat soluble vitamins essentially from birth (FREDRICKSON et al., 1972a).

This experiment of nature clearly suggests the importance of the B protein in lipoprotein formation. In contrast in another inheritable disorder, Tangier disease, (Familial HDL Deficiency) where the A_1 protein is markedly deficient and possibly abnormal (Lux et al., 1972), and the concentration of A_2, B and C seem somewhat reduced, there is no evidence of any defect in the formation of glyceride rich particles. In Tangier disease, in fact, chylomicrons and VLDL tend to accumulate in the plasma and this disorder is usually characterized by a very low cholesterol concentration (less than 90 mg-%) in the face of elevated plasma triglycerides (Fredrickson et al., 1972a). These observations suggest that the A_1 protein may be involved in lipoprotein clearence, for not only does the concentration of VLDL and chylomicrons tend to be high, but in Tangier disease cholesteryl esters tend to accumulate in all the reticuloendothelial system (liver, spleen, tonsils, and lymph nodes).

III. Lipoprotein Metabolism

The fate of lipoprotein lipids has been studied extensively in humans and experimental animals. The results of most studies, however, do not reflect the fate of the lipoprotein particle because of the rapid exchange of lipid between the lipoproteins themselves, between lipoproteins and cells, and the reutilization of the labeled lipids for synthesis of new lipoproteins.

A. Chylomicrons

The disappearance rate of chylomicron-triglycerides from the circulation is extremely rapid. Chylomicrons labeled in their triglycerides disappear from plasma with a half-life time of less than an hour (human) (Nestel, 1966), and as short as a few minutes (rat) (Olivecrona and Belfrage, 1965). Studies in rats have demonstrated that the fate of chylomicron lipids is heterogeneous, and involves two separate steps. About 80% of chylomicron triglyceride fatty acids are taken up by muscle and adipose tissues, and only a small fraction is recovered in other tissues (Fredrickson et al., 1958; Olivecrona, 1962; Olivecrona and Belfrage, 1965). Most of the chylomicron cholesteryl esters and phospholipids, in contrast, are catabolized in the liver (Quarfordt and Goodman, 1967), where they are found within the parenchymal liver cells (Stein et al., 1969). These two steps can be dissociated by using hepatectomized rats (Redgrave, 1970). Injection of labeled chylomicrons in such animals results in a particle relatively rich in cholesteryl esters and phospholipids. This particle, designated "remnant" by Redgrave (1970), then persists in the plasma in the absence of the liver (Fig. 3). The fate of chylomicron proteins is unknown. In a single study published in 1960, Hoffman described transfer of chylomicron proteins to other lipoproteins in vitro, a phenomenon which may be analogous to that occurring with VLDL proteins (see below).

The hydrolysis of chylomicron-triglycerides is mediated through the activity of the enzyme called lipoprotein lipase. The enzyme present on the surface of endothelial cells, especially in adipose tissue, skeletal muscle and heart, hydrolizes triglycerides to free fatty acid, partial glycerides and glycerol which are then recovered in lipids of the tissue cells (Robinson, 1970; Scow, 1970). In the absence of this enzyme,

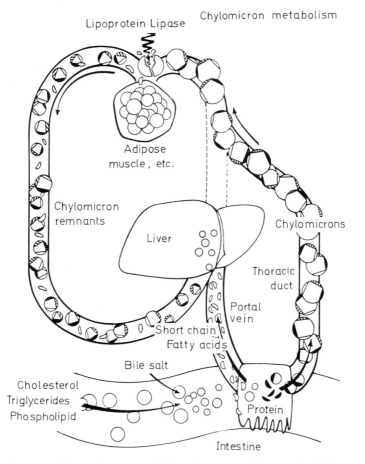

Fig. 3. Schematic view of chylomicron metabolism. (Courtesy of LEVY et al., 1971)

the clearance of chylomicrons from circulation is delayed, they accumulate in plasma and are removed by reticuloendothelial cells. This situation is dramatically illustrated in humans with the rare congenital disease, familial Type I hyperlipoproteinemia (see Section IV). Recent studies have demonstrated that lipoprotein lipase may include at least two species of enzymes, one of adipose tissue and the other of hepatic origin (LA ROSA et al., 1972). The adipose tissue enzyme may also contain several species of enzymes with preferential activities against triglycerides, diglycerides and monoglycerides (GRETEN et al., 1969). All these enzymes are released into the circulation following intravenous injection of heparin and result in a rapid hydrolysis of chylomicron and VLDL triglycerides. Of particular interest is the obligatory role of phospholipids and an apolipoprotein cofactor for non-lipoprotein triglyceride hydrolysis by adipose tissue lipoprotein lipase (LA ROSA et al., 1970). Since this protein cofactor, identified recently as apolipoprotein glutamic acid (C_2), is abundant in chylomicrons and VLDL, these two lipoproteins provide the enzyme with both the substrate and the cofactors necessary for its activity.

B. Very Low Density Lipoproteins

The fate of VLDL triglycerides in circulation has been the subject of numerous investigations during the last decade. The interpretation of these studies, however, necessitates the use of complex mathematical models, none of which is as yet satisfactory (see for discussion Quarfordt et al., 1970). Thus, the information gathered from these studies is still of limited value. The estimated half life time of VLDL triglycerides in circulation in normal humans ranges between two to four hours. VLDL triglyceride clearance is greatly accelerated following injection of heparin, as much as 80% of VLDL triglyceride may be hydrolized within 10 to 30 min of the injection. Similar to chylomicrons, the larger VLDL particles are more susceptible to lipoprotein lipase enzyme and give rise to smaller VLDL particles (Barter and Nestel, 1972). VLDL triglycerides are precursors of the small amount of plasma LDL triglycerides (Havel et al., 1962; Quarfordt et al., 1970).

A different approach to the study of VLDL metabolism, that of following the fate of its apoproteins, was originally suggested in 1957 to 1958 (Gitlin et al., 1958), and used recently by us (Bilheimer et al., 1972; Eisenberg et al., 1972a, 1972b, 1973a). VLDL labeled with ^{125}I in its protein moiety was prepared, and the fate of individual apoproteins was studied. About 50% of the radioactivity was associated with the B protein and about 40% with two of the C proteins (C_2 and C_3). When ^{125}I-labeled VLDL was incubated *in vitro* with plasma or isolated lipoproteins, the labeled C proteins of VLDL were found to equilibrate with the unlabeled C proteins of HDL. Since the C proteins are also readily transferrable back to VLDL from HDL, it was suggested that this bidirectional transfer represents free exchange of C proteins between VLDL and HDL (Eisenberg et al., 1972a). Similar transfer of C proteins between VLDL and HDL was also described recently in rats (Eisenberg et al., 1973a). In these latter studies it was also shown that following injection of either ^{125}I-VLDL or ^{125}I-HDL, the decay of C protein from VLDL and HDL was parallel, and similar to that found following injection of isolated labeled C proteins (Eisenberg and Rachmilewitz, 1973b). These observations suggest that the C proteins of different lipoproteins represent one single pool which is distributed among chylomicrons, VLDL and HDL in proportion to their relative concentration in plasma.

The metabolic fate of the B protein of VLDL was found to be different from that of the C protein (Fig. 4). The B protein was always recovered with VLDL following *in vitro* incubations or immediately after injection of ^{125}I-VLDL to humans. However, 6 to 12 hrs after the injection of ^{125}I-VLDL to humans, the B protein disappeared from the VLDL density range and was found in association with lipoproteins of intermediate density ($d = 1.006$ to 1.019 g/ml). During the next 12 hrs, radioactivity associated with the intermediate density lipoproteins declined rapidly and the B protein transferred to LDL. The study indicated that the B protein moiety of VLDL is a precursor of the B protein of LDL, and that plasma LDL is therefore a "remnant" of VLDL metabolism (Fig. 5). Studies on the effect of heparin on ^{125}I-VLDL metabolism demonstrated that the formation of intermediate lipoproteins from VLDL is dependent on lipoprotein lipase activity and involves triglyceride hydrolysis as well as removal of C proteins and some cholesterol and phospholipids from VLDL. These proteins, and the cholesterol and phospholipids are recovered, at least in part, in HDL (La Rosa et al., 1971; Eisenberg et al., 1973a). The formation of LDL from

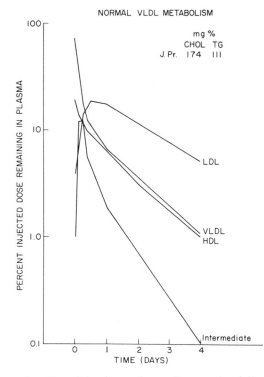

Fig. 4. Disappearance of radioactivity from plasma lipoproteins following injection of ^{125}I-VLDL into a normal human. ^{125}I-apoB comprised more than 80% of the radioactivity of intermediate and low density (LDL) lipoproteins and ^{125}I-apoC was the predominant labeled apoprotein of HDL at all time intevals. The contribution of ^{125}I-apoB to labeled proteins in VLDL decreased during the first 24 hours after the injection from 50—60% to less than 10% of protein bound radioactivity and that of ^{125}I-apoC increased from 20—30% to more than 80%. ^{125}I-apoC comprised more than 80% of labeled apoproteins in VLDL after the first day

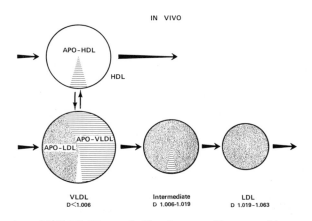

Fig. 5. Schematic view of ^{125}I-VLOL metabolism in normal human subjects

intermediate lipoproteins occurred later and was independent of lipoprotein lipase activity (Eisenberg et al., 1973a). Moreover, when the quantities of the various VLDL protein and lipid constituents which form an LDL particle were calculated, it was found that each VLDL particle contained all the B protein moiety of the original VLDL particle, only traces of its C protein, and 15 to 25% of the original VLDL cholesterol and phospholipids.

These studies have thus established a relationship between all major plasma lipoproteins, and indicate that at least one lipoprotein, LDL, is formed in plasma.

C. Low Density Lipoprotein

Studies on the metabolism of LDL lipids were concerned mainly with the fate of LDL cholesterol. However, since free cholesterol is readily exchangeable and since the bulk of plasma esterified cholesterol is formed in plasma (see III D), these studies measure total body cholesterol turnover rather than lipoprotein turnover.

Relative to other lipoproteins, the fate of LDL protein has been studied in detail. Most studies have utilized LDL labeled with radioactive iodine in its B protein moiety. The decay of LDL protein from plasma is biexponential, and its distribution between intravascular and extravascular compartments, half-life time in circulation, fractional catabolic rate and synthetic rate can be calculated by using simple mathematical equations commonly applied to turnover studies of other plasma proteins (Waldman and Strober, 1969). Such measurements were carried out by Langer et al. (1972) in a group of normal humans and patients with Type II hyperlipoproteinemia. These authors also studied the effects of diet and drugs on LDL metabolism in humans (Levy et al., 1972a). In normal humans the biological half-life of LDL protein varied between 2.25 to 3.58 days, the fractional catabolic rate (fraction of intravascular pool cleared/day) varied between 0.385 and 0.633 and the synthetic rate (mg LDL protein/kg/day) between 12.0 and 18.2. Sixty-two to seventy-five percent of the LDL protein was found in the intravascular compartment. A linear correlation was found between the fractional catabolic rates and plasma LDL concentrations of individual subjects suggesting that the physiologic control of plasma LDL concentration may be mediated by its rate of catabolism. In patients with Type II hyperlipoproteinemia, the only defect discovered was a greatly reduced fractional catabolic rate, indicating that this disorder is most probably due to defective removal of LDL from circulation. Diet, low in cholesterol and enriched with polyunsaturated fatty acids decreased the LDL pool size and increased LDL catabolic rates, as did the administration of cholestyramine. Administration of nicotinic acid, in contrast, did not affect the fractional catabolic rate of LDL but did decrease its synthetic rate and concentration in plasma (Langer et al., 1969; Levy et al., 1972a).

These results are consonant with the hypothesis that LDL catabolism is determined mainly by the utilization of LDL in tissues. Since several recent studies in rats have indicated that the liver may play a predominant role in lipoprotein catabolism (Hay et al., 1971; Roheim et al., 1971; Rachmilewitz et al., 1972; Eisenberg et al., 1973b; Eisenberg and Rachmilewitz, 1973d), the rate of disappearance of LDL from circulation may depend upon its removal by the liver. This, in turn, may be dependent upon the need for LDL cholesterol in the liver. The exact mechanisms governing LDL removal from the plasma and their uptake by the liver cells remains to be clarified.

D. High Density Lipoprotein

Virtually nothing is known about the fate of human HDL in circulation. One study, published in 1964, demonstrated that the half-life time of total HDL proteins in circulation was about five days, and that more than 90% of the injected labeled proteins were recovered within the HDL density range (FURMAN et al., 1964). Several studies, carried out in dogs, rats and mice, have measured the rate of disappearance of HDL protein from the plasma space and showed that in these species also most of the injected radioactive proteins were associated with HDL (SCANU and HUGHES, 1962; ROHEIM et al., 1971). Studies on the fate of individual apoproteins have been carried out only in rats. Two such studies, published recently have shown that the fate of the C proteins of HDL is different from that of the A proteins, and that they equilibrate with the C proteins in VLDL (ROHEIM et al., 1972; EISENBERG et al., 1973b). The fate of several other rat HDL proteins may also be heterogenous. The role of the liver in the catabolism of rat HDL was emphasized in the two studies. EISENBERG et al. (1973b) have recently determined the fate of the two human A proteins in rats. The study demonstrated a striking difference in the half-life time of the two; the rate of disappearance of the A_2 protein exceeding that of A_1 protein by about 50%. It is yet unknown whether these two proteins are metabolized in the human as a unit or as two different and distinct entities.

The fate of HDL lipids is even less certain. Both phospholipids and free cholesterol are rapidly exchangeable between HDL and other plasma lipoproteins and between HDL and tissue cells. In addition, there is a constant change in HDL lipid composition due to generation of cholesteryl esters from free cholesterol and lecithin within the HDL molecule. This reaction is performed by a transfer of the fatty acid of the two position of lecithin to free cholesterol, and is activated by the enzyme lecithin: cholesterol acyl transfer (GLOMSET, 1968). The enzyme, synthesized in the liver, circulates in plasma in association with HDL, and may specifically be activated by the A_1 protein of HDL (FIELDING et al., 1972). Early studies have shown that of the various plasma lipoproteins, HDL is the preferable substrate for the enzyme, and that HDL cholesteryl esters may be transferred to other lipoproteins, though at a relatively slow rate (NICHOLS and SMITH, 1965). A human disease, due to absence of the enzyme, has been described in three families in Scandinavia (NORUM and GJONE, 1967; NORUM et al., 1972). More than 80 to 90% of plasma lipoprotein cholesterol in these patients was found to be in the unesterified cholesterol fraction. In addition to a pleomorphic clinical picture, the structure, shape, composition and distribution of plasma lipoproteins was abnormal (NORUM et al., 1971; FORTE et al., 1971). These observations suggest that generation of cholesteryl esters is of importance for lipoprotein integrity and metabolism.

E. Conclusions

The studies described above, especially those using radioactive apoproteins, have demonstrated that all plasma lipoproteins are interrelated (Fig.6). The plasma lipoproteins represent a system of "units" in a dynamic equilibrium, with transfer, trans-

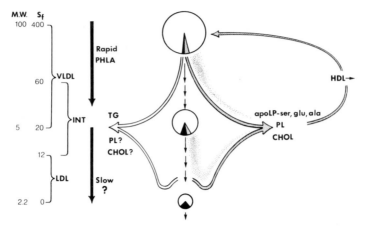

METABOLIC RELATIONSHIPS OF HUMAN PLASMA LIPOPROTEINS

Fig. 6. Schematic view of *in vivo* lipoprotein metabolism demonstrating the interrelationship of the different lipoprotein families

port, and exchange of subunits among lipoproteins. Many of these processes are mediated through the activity of enzymes and they may play an important role in the regulation of plasma lipoprotein levels. Moreover, since these phenomena occur while lipoproteins are in the circulation, the plasma compartment has to be regarded as an important site of lipoprotein metabolism and not merely as a passive transport system for fats.

IV. The Hyperlipoproteinemias (Fredrickson and Levy, 1972; Levy et al., 1972b)

Insight into the mechanisms governing normal lipoprotein metabolism now makes it easier to understand the pathophysiology behind the hyperlipoproteinemias.

Type I. Type I hyperlipoproteinemia is characterized by massive fasting chylomicronemia. When primary and genetic, this rare recessively transmitted disorder has been shown to result from the near absence of releasable extra-hepatic lipoprotein lipase. Without intravascular lipolysis, chylomicrons persist in the plasma and are removed only by the reticuloendothelial system. In the secondary forms of type I both a deficiency of enzyme (insulinopenic diabetes mellitus) and its heparin-like plasma releaser (lymphoma, lupus erythematosis) have been reported. With an inability to clear chylomicrons, patients with type I are markedly intolerant to dietary fat and develop massive hypertriglyceridemia often associated with eruptive xanthomas, abdominal pains and pancreatitis on fat feeding.

Type IV. Type IV hyperlipoproteinemia is characterized by increased concentrations of VLDL. The mechanism behind the primary inheritable form of type IV is unclear; both overproduction and decreased clearance of VLDL have been proposed (Quarfordt et al., 1970). In the secondary forms of type IV (nephrosis, glycogen storage disease, diabetes mellitus, alcoholism, stress) both increased production and decreased clearance have also been reported. Lipoprotein lipase is usually normal in type IV. Subjects with type IV often exhibit evidence of glucose intolerance and hyperuricemia. Increased flux of glyceride precursors in the liver secondary to stress, hyperinsulinemia, carbohydrate and alcohol ingestion will increase VLDL concentrations in normals and usually significantly increase triglyceride levels in type IV subjects.

Type V. Type V hyperlipoproteinemia is associated with a mixed hypertriglyceridemia, both exogenous triglyceride (chylomicrons) and endogenous triglyceride (VLDL) accumulate. The mechanism behind the relatively uncommon familial form of type V is unclear. It appears to involve an inability of the periphery to assimilate or clear glyceride rich particles. In secondary type V (alcoholism, nephrosis, diabetic acidosis) similar problems in glyceride-rich particle clearance occurs. The nature of the clearance defect or defects that results in the type V pattern is unclear. Both extra-hepatic and hepatic lipase activity appear normal and defects in the adipose cell itself have been proposed. Type V subjects are unable to handle carbohydrate or fat challenges and may develop abdominal pain, pancreatitis and eruptive xanthomata on exposure to fat. In types I, IV, and V levels of the lipoprotein remnant form (LDL) and HDL are either low or normal.

Type III. Type III hyperlipoproteinemia is characterized by the appearance of unusual lipoprotein forms in the plasma. A beta migrating VLDL that may be identical to the lipoprotein intermediate form seen in normal VLDL metabolism accumulates (QUARFORDT et al., 1971). The defect in primary type III appears to reside in the second stage of glyceride particle removal from the plasma. Whereas lipoprotein lipase activity is normal in type III, and chylomicron and VLDL metabolism is initially brisk, remnant chylomicron forms, as well as VLDL-intermediate particles, accumulate. This defect in intravascular VLDL metabolism appears to be functional for it occurs in type III subjects challenged with normal or type III VLDL (BILHEIMER et al., 1971; HAZZARD and BIERMAN, 1971). The precise description of the defect awaits our gaining further insight into the enzymes involved in VLDL metabolism. Secondary forms of type III (myxedema, dysproteinemia) also seem to result from a block in VLDL catabolism. With this block in normal intravascular glyceride-rich particle clearance any load on the normal glyceride transport system usually results in severe hyperlipidemia. The accumulation of these intermediate forms in the plasma is associated with planar and tuboeruptive xanthomata and premature coronary and peripheral vessel disease.

Type II. In type II hyperlipoproteinemia LDL accumulates in the plasma in increased concentration. In the most common familial form of type II this appears to result from a decreased rate of clearance of LDL from the plasma. The cause of this delayed clearance is not known. Decreased LDL clearance also occurs secondary to myxedema and dysproteinemia. In porphyria and nephrosis, increased LDL production, presumably associated with increased VLDL synthesis and clearance, may cause the increased levels of LDL. Patients with type II develop coronary vessel disease prematurely and may have tendon and tuberous xanthomata. In obstructive liver disease, an unusual LDL form accumulates (Lpx), presumably secondary to the pile up of free cholesterol and phospholipids in the plasma (SEIDEL et al., 1969).

Hyperlipoproteinemia Summary

Abnormalities in lipoprotein metabolism will produce a heterogenous group of disorders dependent on the site of the basic defect. Overproduction of VLDL will result in a type IV or II pattern. Defective chylomicron hydrolysis results in tpye I. Delayed clearance of chylomicrons and VLDL will produce the type V or IV patterns. A block in VLDL conversion to LDL appears to result in type III hyperlipoproteinemia. Finally, delayed clearance of the LDL remnant appears to be the most common cause of type II. Thus, visualization of the processes involved in normal lipid transport enables us to explain the forms of hyperlipoproteinemia. The clinical value of translating hyperlipidemia to its equivalent form of hyperlipoproteinemia is discussed completely in a recent review (Levy et al., 1972)

V. Treatment of Hyperlipoproteinemia (Levy et al., 1972 a, b)

It is not the purpose of this chapter to review in depth available hypolipidemic diets and drugs. Rather, we would merely like to extend our recent understanding of normal and abnormal lipid transport to its logical therapeutic conclusions. If fat is removed from the diet chylomicrons will not be made. This obviously is beneficial in types I and V where chylomicrons accumulate. Decrease in total calories in the diet and/or dietary carbohydrates and alcohol will decrease available VLDL precursors and thus be useful in types II, IV, and V. Decreased consumption of cholesterol and increase in polyunsaturated fat intake will decrease LDL levels by increasing LDL removal from the plasma. This is obviously beneficial in type II.

Nicotinic acid, a drug that clearly works on VLDL production, is somewhat effective in all lipoprotein types involved in VLDL clearance (II to V), but most clearly effective in the disorders that represent derangements in the early stages of VLDL catabolism, types III, IV, and V. Clofibrate (Atromid-S) also appears to work on VLDL production and/or the earliest stages of VLDL clearance and is, therefore, useful in types III, IV, and V. Cholestyramine and the other bile acid sequestrants, D-Thyroxine, Beta-Sitosterol, Neomycin and PAS all seem to effect the last step of VLDL metabolism, the removal of LDL from the plasma. These drugs are thus very efficacious where LDL accumulates as in type II but are usually ineffective in disorders secondary to problems at earlier stages of VLDL metabolism types III to V. None of the presently available hypolipidemic drugs affect chylomicron formation, and hence there is no drug treatment available for type I.

It should be obvious from what has been said in this chapter that lipid transport in the plasma is a complex and highly ordered process. The lipoproteins, the units of lipid transport, can accumulate in the plasma for many different reasons. Since hyperlipoproteinemia is so heterogenous and secondary to so many different mechanisms, it is unlikely that there will ever be one drug or diet for all types of hyperlipoproteinemia. Understanding of the lipoproteins and their metabolism should enable us, however, to more rationally treat hyperlipoproteinemia in the future.

References

(Updated to January 1973)

Albers, J.J., Aladjem, F.: Precipitation of ^{125}I-labeled lipoproteins with specific polypeptide antisera. Evidence for two populations with differing polypeptide compositions in human high density lipoproteins. Biochemistry 10, 3436—3442 (1971).
Barter, P.J., Nestel, P.J.: Precursor-product relationship between pools of very low density lipoprotein triglyceride. J. clin. Invest. 51, 174—180 (1972).

BIERMAN, E. L.: Insulin and hypertriglyceridemia. Israel J. med. Sci. **8**, 303—307 (1972).

BILHEIMER, D., EISENBERG, S., LEVY, R. I.: Abnormal metabolism of very low density lipoproteins (VLDL) in type III hyperlipoproteinemia. Circulation Supp II, 56, 1971.

BILHEIMER, D. W., EISENBERG, S., LEVY, R. I.: The metabolism of very low density lipoproteins. I. Preliminary *in vitro* and *in vivo* observations. Biochim. biophys. Acta (Amst.) **260**, 212—221 (1972).

BREWER, H. B., SHULMAN, R., HERBERT, P., RONAN, R., WEHRLY, K.: The complete amino acid sequence of apoLP-Ala an apoprotein from very low density lipoproteins. Advanc. exp. Med. **26**, 280 (1972a).

BREWER, H. B., LUX, S. E., RONAN, R., JOHN, K. M.: Amino acid sequence of human apo LP-Gln II (apo-A II), an apolipoprotein isolated from the high density lipoprotein complex. Proc. nat. Acad. Sci. (Wash.) **69**, 1306—1308 (1972b).

BROWN, W. V., LEVY, R. I., FREDRICKSON, D. S.: Studies of the proteins in human plasma very low density lipoproteins. J. biol. Chem. **244**, 5687—5694 (1969).

BROWN, W. V., LEVY, R. I., FREDRICKSON, D. S.: Further separation of the apoproteins of the human plasma very low density lipoproteins. Biochim. biophys. Acta (Amst.) **200**, 573—575 (1970a).

BROWN, W. V., LEVY, R. I., FREDRICKSON, D. S.: Further characterization of apolipoproteins from the human plasma very low density lipoproteins. J. biol. Chem. **245**, 6588—6594 (1970b).

BUNGENBERG DE JONG, J.-J., MARSH, J. B.: Biosynthesis of plasma lipoproteins by rat liver microsomes. J. biol. Chem. **243**, 192—199 (1968).

DE LALLA, V. F., GOFMAN, J. W.: Ultracentrifugal analysis of serum lipoproteins. In: Methods of Biochemical Analysis, Vol. 1. New York: Interscience 1954.

EISENBERG, S., BILHEIMER, D. W., LEVY, R. I.: The metabolism of very low density lipoprotein proteins. II. Studies on the transfer of apoproteins between plasma lipoproteins. Biochim. biophys. Acta (Amst.) **280**, 94—104 (1972a).

EISENBERG, S., BILHEIMER, D. W., LINDGREN, F. T., LEVY, R. I.: On the apoprotein composition of human plasma very low density lipoprotein subfractions. Biochim. biophys. Acta (Amst.) **260**, 329—333 (1972b).

EISENBERG, S., BILHEIMER, D. W., LINDGREN, F. T., LEVY, R. I.: On the metabolic conversion of human plasma very low density lipoprotein to low density lipoprotein. Biochim. biophys. Acta (Amst.) **326**, 361—377 (1973a).

EISENBERG, S., WINDMUELLER, H. G., LEVY, R. I.: The metabolic fate of rat and human lipoprotein apoproteins in the rat. J. Lipid Res. **14**, 446—458 (1973b)

EISENBERG, S., RACHMILEWITZ, D.: Metabolism of rat plasma very low density lipoprotein. I. Fate in circulation of the whole lipoprotein. Biochim. Biophys. Acta **326**, 378—390 (1973c).

EISENBERG, S., RACHMILEWITZ, D.: Metabolism of rat plasma very low density lipoprotein II. Fate in circulation of lipoprotein subunits. Biochim. biophys. Acta **326**, 391—405 (1973d).

EWING, A. M., LINDGREN, F. T., ELLIOTT, H.: Analysis of human serum lipoprotein distribution. Advanc. Lipid Res. **3**, 25—61 (1965).

FIELDING, C. J., SHORE, V. G., FIELDING, P. E.: A protein cofactor of lecithin:cholesterol acyltransferase. Biochem. biophys. Res. Commun. **46**, 1493—1498 (1972).

FORTE, G. M., NICHOLS, A. V., GLAESER, R. M.: Electron microscopy of human serum lipoproteins using negative staining. Chem. Phys. Lipids **2**, 396—408 (1968).

FORTE, T., NORUM, K. R., GLOMSET, J. A., NICHOLS, A. V.: Plasma lipoproteins in familial lecithin:-cholesterol acyltransferase deficiency: Structure of low and high density lipoproteins as revealed by electron microscopy. J. clin. Invest. **50**, 1141—1148 (1971).

FREDRICKSON, D. S., MC COLLISTER, D. L., ONO, K.: The role of unesterified fatty acid transport in chylomicron metabolism. J. clin. Invest. **37**, 1335—1341 (1958).

FREDRICKSON, D. S., GOTTO, A. M., LEVY, R. I.: Familial lipoprotein deficiency. In Metabolic Basis of Inherited Disease, 3rd edition. New York: McGraw-Hill 1972a.

FREDRICKSON, D. S., LEVY, R. I.: Familial hyperlipoproteinemia. In Metabolic Basis of Inherited Disease, 3rd edition. New York: McGraw-Hill 1972b.

FREDRICKSON, D. S., LUX, S. E., HERBERT, P. N.: The apolipoproteins. Advanc. exp. Med. **26**, 25—56 (1972c).

Furman,R.H., Sanbar,S.S., Alaupovic,P., Bradford,R.H., Howard,R.P.: Studies of the metabolism of radioiodinated human serum alpha lipoprotein in normal and hyperlipidemic subjects. J. Lab. clin. Med. **63**, 193—204 (1964).

Gage,S.H.: The free granules (chylomicrons) of the blood as shown by the dark-field microscope. Cornell Vet. **10**, 154—155 (1920).

Gage,S.H., Fish,P.A.: Fat digestion and assimilation in man and animals as determined by dark-field microscope and fat-soluble dye. Amer. J. Anat. **34**, 1—85 (1924).

Ganesen,D., Bradford,R.H., Alaupovic,P., McConathy,W.J.: Differential activation of lipoprotein lipase from human post-heparin plasma, milk and adipose tissue by polypeptides of human serum apolipoprotein C. FEBS Letters **15**, 205—204 (1971).

Gitlin,D., Cornwell,D.G., Na'Casato,D., Oncley,J.L., Hughes,W.L., Janeway,C.A.: Studies on the metabolism of plasma proteins in the nephrotic syndrome. II. The lipoproteins. J. clin. Invest. **37**, 172—186 (1958).

Glomset,J.A.: The plasma lecithin: cholesterol acyltransferase reaction. J. Lipid Res. **9**, 155—167 (1968).

Gotto,A.M., Brown,W.V., Levy,R.I., Birnbaumer,M.E., Fredrickson,D.S.: Evidence for the identity of the major apoprotein in low density and very low density lipoproteins in normal subjects and patients with familial hyperlipoproteinemia. J. clin. Invest. **51**, 1486—1499 (1972).

Gotto,A.M., Levy,R.I., John,K., Fredrickson,D.S.: On the protein defect in abetalipoproteinemia. New Engl. J. Med. **284**, 813—818 (1971).

Greten,H., Levy,R.I., Fredrickson,D.S.: Evidence for separate monoglyceride hydrolase and triglyceride lipase in post-heparin human plasma. J. Lipid Res. **10**, 326—330 (1967).

Gustafson,A., Alaupovic,P., Furman,R.H.: Studies of the composition and structure of serum lipoproteins. Separation and characterization of phospholipid-protein residue obtained by partial delipidation of very low density lipoprotein of human serum. Biochemistry **5**, 632—640 (1966).

Haft,D.E., Roheim,P.S., White,A., Eder,H.A.: Plasma lipoprotein metabolism in perfused rat liver. I. Protein synthesis and entry into the plasma. J. clin. Invest. **41**, 842—849 (1962).

Hamilton,R.L.: Ultrastructural aspects of hepatic lipoprotein synthesis and secretion. In Proceedings of the Deuel Conference on Lipids, The Turnover of Lipids and Lipoproteins, pp. 3—28. U.S. Public Health Service Publication 1968.

Hamilton,R.L.: Synthesis and secretion of plasma lipoproteins. Advanc. exp. Med. Biol. **26**, 7—24 (1972).

Hammond,M.G., Fisher,W.: The characterization of a discrete series of low density lipoproteins in the disease hyper-pre-β-lipoproteinemia. Implications relating to the structure of plasma lipoproteins. J. biol. Chem. **246**, 5454—5465 (1971).

Hatch,F.T., Lees,R.S.: Practical methods for plasma lipoprotein analysis. Advanc. Lipid Res. **6**, 1—68 (1968).

Havel,R.J., Felts,J.M., Van Duyne,C.M.: Formation and fate of endogenous triglycerides in blood plasma of rabbits. J. Lipid Res. **3**, 297—308 (1962).

Hay,R.V., Pottenger,L.A., Reingold,A.L., Getz,G.S., Wissler,R.W.: Degradation of ^{125}I-labelled serum low density lipoprotein in normal and estrogen-treated male rats. Biochem. Biophys. Res. Commun. **44**, 1471—1477 (1971).

Hazzard,W.R., Bierman,E.L.: Impaired removal of very low density lipoprotein "remnants" in the pathogenesis of broad B disease (type III hyperlipoproteinemia). Clin. Res. **19**, 476 (1971).

Herbert,P., Levy,R.I., Fredrickson,D.S.: Correction of COOH-terminal amino acids of human plasma very low density apolipoproteins. J. biol. Chem. **246**, 7068—7069 (1971).

Hoffman,A.F.: Exchange of ^{131}I labeled chylomicron protein *in vitro*. Amer. J. Physiol. **199**, 433—436 (1960).

Jones,A.L., Ruderman,N.B., Herrera,M.G.: Electron microscopic and biochemical study of lipoprotein synthesis in the isolated perfused rat liver. J. Lipid Res. **8**, 429—446 (1967).

Kostner,G., Alaupovic,P.: Studies of the composition and structure of plasma lipoproteins. C- and N-terminal amino acids of the two nonidentical polypeptides of human plasma apolipoprotein A. FEBS Letters **15**, 320—324 (1971).

KOSTNER,G., HOLASEK,A.: Characterization and quantitation of the apolipoproteins from human chyle chylomicrons. Biochemistry 11, 1217—1223 (1972).

LANGER,T., FREDRICKSON,D.S., LEVY,R.I.: Dietary and pharmacologic pertubation of beta lipoprotein (BLP) turnover. Circulation Supp III, 14 (1969).

LANGER,T., STROBER,W., LEVY,R.I.: The metabolism of low density lipoprotein in familial type II hyperlipoproteinemia. J. clin. Invest. 51, 1528—1536 (1972).

LA ROSA,J.C., LEVY,R.I., HERBERT,P., LUX,S.E., FREDRICKSON,D.S.: A specific apoprotein activator for lipoprotein lipase. Biochem. Biophys. Res. Commun. 41, 57—62 (1970).

LA ROSA,J.C., LEVY,R.I., BROWN,W.V., FREDRICKSON,D.S.: Changes in high density lipoprotein protein composition after heparin-induced lipolysis. Amer. J. Physiol. 220, 785—791 (1971).

LA ROSA,J.C., LEVY,R.I., WINDMUELLER,H.G., FREDRICKSON,D.S.: Comparison of the triglyceride lipase of liver, adipose tissue, and post-heparin plasma. J. Lipid Res. 13, 356—363 (1972).

LEVY,R.I., BILHEIMER,D.W., EISENBERG,S.: The structure and metabolism of chylomicrons and very low density lipoproteins (VLDL). In Plasma Lipoproteins. London-New York: Academic Press 1971.

LEVY,R.I., LANGER,T.: Hypolipidemic drugs and lipoprotein metabolism. Advanc. exp. Med. Biol. 26, 155—163 (1972a).

LEVY,R.I., FREDRICKSON,D.S., SHULMAN,R., BILHEIMER,D.W., BRESLOW,J.L., STONE,N.J., LUX,S.E., SLOAN,H.R., KRAUSS,R.M., HERBERT,P.N.: Dietary and drug treatment of primary hyperlipoproteinemia. Ann. intern. Med. 77, 267—294 (1972b).

LEVY,R.I., LEES,R.S., FREDRICKSON,D.S.: On the nature of prebeta lipoproteins. J. clin. Invest. 45, 63—77 (1966).

LINDGREN,F.T., JENSEN,L.C., HATCH,F.T.: The isolation and quantitative analysis of serum lipoproteins. In Blood Lipids and Lipoproteins, pp.181—272. New York: Interscience 1972.

LO,C., MARSH,J.B.: Biosynthesis of plasma lipoproteins. Incorporation of ^{14}C-glucosamine by cells and subcellular fractions of rat liver. J. biol. Chem. 245, 5001—5006 (1970).

LOSSOW,W.J., LINDGREN,F.T., MURCHIO,J.C., STEVENS,G.R., JENSEN,J.C.: Particle size and protein content of six fractions of the $S_f > 20$ plasma lipoproteins isolated by density gradient centrifugation. J. Lipid Res. 10, 68—76 (1969).

LUX,S.E., LEVY,R.I., GOTTO,A.M., FREDRICKSON,D.S.: Studies on the protein defect in Tangier disease. Isolation and characterization of an abnormal high density lipoprotein. J. clin. Invest. 51, 2505—2519 (1972).

MACHEBOUF,M.M.A.: Recherches sur les phosphoaminolipides et les sterides du serum et du plasma sanguins. I. Entrainement des phospholipids, des sterols et des sterides par les diverses fractions au cours de fractionement des protudes du serum. Bull. Soc. chim. Biol. 11, 268—293 (1929).

MAHLEY,R.W., BENNETT,B:I., MORRE,D.J., GRAY,M.E., THISTLETHWAITE,W., LE QUIRE,V.S.: Lipoprotein associated with the Golgi apparatus isolated from epithelial cells of rat small intestine. Lab. Invest. 25, 435—444 (1971).

MAHLEY,R.W., BERSOT,T.P., LE QUIRE,V.S., LEVY,R.I., WINDMUELLER,H.G., BROWN,W.V.: Identity of very low density lipoprotein apoproteins of plasma and liver Golgi apparatus. Science 168, 380—382 (1970).

MARSH,J.B.: Biosynthesis of plasma lipoproteins. In Plasma Lipoproteins, pp.89—98. London-New York: Academic Press 1971.

MOLNAR,J.: Attachment of glucosamine to protein at the ribosomal site of rat liver. Biochemistry 6, 1941—1947 (1967).

NESTEL,P.J.: Relationship between plasma triglycerides and removal of chylomicrons. J. clin. Invest. 43, 943—949 (1964).

NICHOLS,A.V.: Human serum lipoproteins and their interrelationships. Advanc. Biol. Med. Phys. 11, 110—158 (1967).

NICHOLS,A.V., SMITH,L.: Effect of very low density lipoproteins on lipid transfer in incubated serum. J. Lipid Res. 6, 206—210 (1965).

NIKKILA,E.A.: Control of plasma and liver triglyceride kinetics by carbohydrate metabolism and insulin. Advan. Lipid Res. 7, 63—134 (1969).

NORUM,K.R., GJONE,E.: Familial plasma lecithin: cholesterol acyltransferase deficiency. Scand. J. clin. Lab. Invest. 20, 231—243 (1967).

Norum,K.R., Glomset,J.A., Gjone,E.: Familial lecithin: cholesterol acyltransferase deficiency. In: The Metabolic Basis of Inherited Disease. New York: McGraw-Hill 1972.

Norum,K.R., Glomset,J.A., Nichols,A.V., Forte,T.: Plasma lipoproteins in familial lecithin: - cholesterol acyltransferase deficiency: Physical and chemical studies of low and high density lipoproteins. J. clin. Invest. **50**, 1131—1140 (1971).

Olivecrona,T.: Metabolism of chylomicrons labeled with ^{14}C-glycerol-^{3}H-palmitic acid in the rat. J. Lipid Res. **3**, 439—444 (1962).

Olivecrona,T., Belfrage,P.: Mechanisms of removal of chyle triglyceride from the circulating blood as studied with (^{14}C) glycerol and (^{3}H) Palmitic acid labeled chyle. Biochim. biophys. Acta (Amst.) **98**, 81—93 (1965).

Pearlstein,E., Eggena,P., Aladjem,F.: The human serum high density lipoprotein peptides of very low density lipoproteins and chylomicrons. Immunochemistry **8**, 865—867 (1971).

Porter,H.P., Saunders,D.R., Tytgat,G., Branser,O., Rubin,C.E.: Fat absorption in bile fistula man. A morphological and biochemical study. Gastroenterology **60**, 1008—1019 (1971).

Quarfordt,S.H., Frank,A., Shames,D.M., Berman,M., Steinberg,D.: Very low density lipoprotein triglyceride transport in type IV hyperlipoproteinemia and the effects of carbohydrate rich diet. J. clin. Invest. **49**, 2281—2297 (1970).

Quarfordt,S.H., Goodman,D.S.: Metabolism of doubly labeled chylomicron cholesteryl esters in the rat. J. Lipid Res. **8**, 266—272 (1967).

Quarfordt,S., Levy,R.I., Fredrickson,D.S.: On the lipoprotein abnormality in type III hyperlipoproteinemia. J. clin. Invest. **50**, 754—761 (1971).

Rachmilewitz,D., Stein,O., Roheim,P.S., Stein,Y.: Metabolism of iodinated high density lipoproteins in the rat. II. Autoradiographic localization in the liver. Biochim. biophys. Acta (Amst.) **270**, 414—425 (1972).

Radding,C.M., Bragdon,J.H., Steinberg,D.: The synthesis of low and high density lipoproteins by rat liver *in vitro*. Biochim. biophys. Acta (Amst.) **30**, 443—444 (1958).

Redgrave,T.G.: Formation of cholesteryl ester-rich particulate lipid during metabolism of chylomicrons. J. clin. Invest. **49**, 465—471 (1970).

Robinson,D.S.: Removal of triglyceride fatty acids from the blood. In Comprehensive Biochemistry, Vol. 19, pp. 51—116. Amsterdam: Elsevier 1970.

Roheim,P.S., Gidez,L.I., Eder,H.A.: Extra-hepatic synthesis of lipoprotein of plasma and chyle: Role of the intestine. J. clin. Invest. **45**, 297—300 (1966).

Roheim,P.S., Hirsch,H., Edelstein,D., Rachmilewitz,D.: Metabolism of iodinated high density lipoprotein subunits in the rat. III. Comparison of the removal rate of different subunits from the circulation. Biochim. biophys. Acta (Amst.) **278**, 517—529 (1972).

Roheim,P.S., Rachmilewitz,D., Stein,O., Stein,Y.: Metabolism of iodinated high density lipoproteins in the rat. I. Half-life in the circulation and uptake by organs. Biochim. biophys. Acta (Amst.) **268**, 315—329 (1971).

Ruderman,H.B., Richards,K.C., Valles de Bourges,V., Jones,A.L.: Regulation of production and release of lipoproteins by the perfused rat liver. J. Lipid Res. **9**, 613—619 (1968).

Sabesin,S.M., Isselbacher,K.J.: Protein synthesis inhibition: Mechanism for the production of impaired fat absorption. Science **147**, 1149—1157 (1964).

Sardet,C., Hansma,H., Ostwald,R.: Characterization of guinea pig plasma lipoproteins: The appearance of new lipoproteins in response to dietary cholesterol. J. Lipid Res. **13**, 624—639 (1972).

Scanu,A., Hughes,W.L.: Further characterization of the human serum D 1.063—1.21, α_1-lipoproteins. J. clin. Invest. **41**, 1681—1689 (1962).

Scow,R.O.: Transport of triglyceride: Its removal from blood circulation and uptake by tissues. In Parenteral Nutrition, Chap. 24. Springfield, Ill.: Charles C. Thomas 1970.

Seidel,D., Alaupovic,P., Furman,R.H.: A lipoprotein characterizing obstructive jaundice. I. Methods of quantitative separation and identification of lipoproteins in jaundiced patients. J. clin. Invest. **48**, 1211—1223 (1969).

Shore,V., Shore,B.: Some physical and chemical studies on the polypeptide components of high density lipoproteins of human serum. Biochemistry **7**, 3396—3403 (1968).

Shore,B., Shore,V.: Isolation and characterization of polypeptides of human serum lipoproteins. Biochemistry **8**, 4510—4516 (1969).

SHORE, V. G., SHORE, B.: The apolipoproteins: their structure and functional roles in human serum lipoproteins. In: NELSON, G. J. (Ed.): Blood Lipids and Lipoproteins: Quantitation, Composition and Metabolism. New York: Wiley-Interscience 1972.

SHULMAN, R., HERBERT, P., WEHRLY, K., CHESEBRO, B., LEVY, R. I., FREDRICKSON, D. S.: The complete amino acid sequence of apoLP-ser: An apolipoprotein obtained from human very low density lipoprotein. Circulation **45—46**, Suppl. II, 246 (1972).

SKIPSKI, V. P.: Lipid composition of lipoproteins in normal and diseased states. In: Blood Lipids and Lipoproteins, pp. 471—583. New York: Interscience 1972.

SIMONS, K., EHNHOLM, C., RENKONEN, O., BLOTH, B.: Characterization of the LP(a) lipoprotein in human plasma. Acta Path. Microbiol. Scand. Sect. B **73**, 459—466 (1970).

STEIN, O., STEIN, Y.: Lipid synthesis, intracellular transport, storage and secretion. I. Electron microscopic radioautography study of liver after injection of tritiated palmitate or glycerol in fasted and ethanol treated rats. J. Cell. Biol. **33**, 319—339 (1967).

STEIN, O., STEIN, Y., FIDGE, A., GOODMAN, D. S.: The metabolism of chylomicron cholesteryl ester in rat liver. A combined radioautographic electron microscopic and biochemical study. J. Cell Biol. **43**, 410—431 (1969).

TYTGAT, G. N., RUBIN, C., SAUNDERS, D. P.: Synthesis and transport of lipoprotein particles by intestinal absorptive cells in man. J. clin. Invest. **50**, 2065—2078 (1971).

WAGNER, R. R., CYNKIN, M. A.: Glycoprotein biosynthesis. Incorporation of glucosyl groups into endogenous acceptors in a Golgi apparatus-rich fraction of liver. J. biol. Chem. **246**, 143—151 (1971).

WALDMAN, T. A., STROBER, W.: Metabolism of immunoglobulins. Prog. Allergy **13**, 1—110 (1969).

WINDMUELLER, H. G., HERBERT, P. N., LEVY, R. I.: Biosynthesis of lymph and plasma lipoprotein apoproteins by isolated perfused rat liver and intestine. J. Lipid Res. **14**, 215—223 (1973).

WINDMUELLER, H. G., SPAETH, A. E.: Fat transport and lymph and plasma lipoprotein biosynthesis by isolated intestine. J. Lipid Res. **13**, 92—105 (1972).

YOKOYAMA, A., ZILVERSMIT, D. B.: Particle size and composition of dog lymph chylomicrons. J. Lipid Res. **6**, 241—246 (1965).

ZILVERSMIT, D. B.: The surface coat of chylomicrons: lipid chemistry. J. Lipid Res. **9**, 180—192 (1968).

ZILVERSMIT, D. B.: The chylomicrons: In: Structural and Functional Aspects of Lipoproteins in Living Systems, p. 329. London-New York: Academic Press 1969.

CHAPTER 6

Animal Models for Atherosclerosis Research

D. KRITCHEVSKY*

Human atherosclerosis is a complex, progressive disease process of multiple etiology. There are a number of initiating factors, at least as many augmenting factors and the extent of their interaction is undoubtedly different for every individual. The extent of atherosclerotic involvement in any specific individual is not easily assessed and is essentially masked until it precipitates a clinical event. Thus, research in this field must be carried out using appropriate animal models.

There has been a continuing search for a suitable model in which to produce lesions similar in morphology to the human lesion. The lesion would have to be inducible with a minimum of trauma and in a relatively short time. This animal model could then be used for studies involving prevention, therapy or regression of the plaques.

Since IGNATOWSKI'S (1909) original experiments in rabbits, a number of animal models have been used. The animal studies in this field have been reviewed in books by ALTSCHUL (1950), ANITSCHKOW (1933), CONSTANTINIDES (1965), KATZ and STAMLER (1953) and ROBERTS and STRAUS (1965). There have also been a number of review chapters published on this subject (CLARKSON, 1963; HARTROFT and THOMAS, 1963; KRITCHEVSKY 1964a, 1974; WISSLER and VESSELINOVITCH, 1968). The mass of published work has understandingly increased our knowledge but has also demonstrated the complexity of the system being studied. Within any given species there are strains that are inordinately susceptible or resistant to the modalities being employed. Variations in diet, even relatively minor ones, can affect atherogenesis and, as with man, external factors may play a role. It is important for the investigator to maintain a sense of perspective vis-a-vis the relation of animal work to the human disease. However, animal experiments can, and do, provide important clues which can be used in diet and drug trials in man.

WISSLER and VESSELINOVITCH (1974) have recently reviewed some of the differences amongst experimental species and these are summarized in Table 1. Despite the differences, there is one thread of consistency-namely, it is virtually impossible to establish atherosclerosis in animals unless their serum β-lipoproteins are elevated. Hypercholesteremia without hyperbetalipoproteinemia will not result in atherosclerosis (KELLNER et al., 1951; HIRSCH and KELLNER, 1956). OLSON (1958) observed that while the dog and rat normally exhibited serum cholesterol levels 60 to 100% higher than that of the rabbit, they normally carried 2 to 6 times more cholesterol in the α

* Supported in part by USPHS grants HL 03299, HL 05209 and a Research Career Award HL 0734 from the National Heart and Lung Institute.

Table 1. Some characteristics of atherosclerosis in species commonly used in experimental atheroclerosis research[a] (0–4 Scale)

Species	Spontaneous disease	Sensitivity to diet	Distribution of lesions[b]	Small Artery involvement
Rabbit	0.5	4	1	4
Chicken	2	4	0.5	4
Rat	0	1	0.5	3
Pig	1	2	2.0	2
Squirrel Monkey	2	4	3.5	2
Rhesus Monkey	0	4	3.5	1

[a] After Wissler and Vesselinovitch (1974).
[b] Compared to Man.

lipoprotein fraction than did the rabbit. Thus the susceptibility of the rabbit may be more a function of his serum α/β lipoprotein cholesterol ratio than of his total serum cholesterol level.

The ensuing discussion will attempt to highlight those species more commonly used in atherosclerosis research.

I. Rabbit

To date, the animal most frequently used for induction of atherosclerosis has been the rabbit. The rabbit is readily available and easy to maintain. He is big enough to be amenable to most manipulative techniques and he develops lesions very quickly. Among the drawbacks attending use of the rabbit are the facts that since he is normally a herbivore, the distribution of his lesions does not resemble that found in man and his lesions rarely progress to the complicated plaque seen in the human. Nevertheless, since Anitschkow (1913) first showed that pure cholesterol was atherogenic for the rabbit, this species has been used in countless experiments.

It is important to know the characteristics of the particular rabbit strain being used. There are a number of reports indicating that normal cholesterol levels in rabbits vary by breed and sex (Wang et al., 1954; Fillios and Mann, 1956; Laird et al., 1970; Marquie and Agid, 1972; Roberts et al., 1974). Hyper- and hyporesponding (to cholesterol challenge) rabbits have been identified (Fillios and Mann, 1956) and the trait is suggested to be heritable (Roberts et al., 1974).

In general, rabbits become hypercholesteremic after only a few days on a high cholesterol diet. The extent of hypercholesteremia is a function of the dietary level of cholesterol (Scebat et al., 1961) but in time severe atherosclerosis will result. Thus, Scebat et al. (1961) found that when rabbits were fed 250 mg/day of cholesterol for 130 days, their serum cholesterol level was 545 mg/dl and average atherosclerosis 3.0. When the diet contained 1 gm/day of cholesterol that severity of atherosclerosis was achieved in 90 days with a serum cholesterol level of 1072 mg/dl. Most experiments involve cholesterol feeding for 6 to 8 weeks. It is possible to obtain severe lesions in a

shorter time but this usually requires extra-physiological treatment such as intravenous injections of allylamine and egg yolk emulsion (GIORDANO et al., 1970), injections of histamine, noradrenaline and thyroxine (PARWARESCH et al., 1973) or epinephrine and thyroxine (BROHON et al., 1974).

The type of dietary fat will make a difference in the level of atherosclerosis and
often in the cholesteremia. A diet containing cholesterol and no fat will give severe
atherosclerosis and relatively low cholesterol levels (KRITCHEVSKY et al., 1961a),
otherwise generally saturated fat is more atherogenic than unsaturated fat
(KRITCHEVSKY et al., 1954, 1956).

Table 2 summarizes one experiment showing the relationship of unsaturation of
dietary fat to severity of atherosclerosis. The presence of free fatty acid in the experimental diet will enhance its atherogenicity (KRITCHEVSKY et al., 1962). When rabbits
were fed diets containing 2% cholesterol and either no fat, 6% corn oil or 5.75%
corn oil plus 0.25% corn oil fatty acids—lesions appeared in the arteries of the no fat
and fatty acid groups within 2 weeks, and in the corn oil group within 4 weeks. At
5 weeks the average severity of lesions (arch plus thoracic/2) was: no fat—1.40; corn
oil plus fatty acid—1.50; and corn oil—0.65 (KRITCHEVSKY and TEPPER, 1973a).

One fat that has been found to be inordinately atherogenic (considering its iodine
value) is peanut oil. It has been shown (KRITCHEVSKY et al., 1971) that when fed with
2% cholesterol, the average atheromata observed with peanut oil is 1.60, with coconut oil, 1.81 and with corn oil 1.30.

It is possible to render rabbits hypercholesteremic and atheromatous by feeding a
semi-purified diet containing saturated fat (LAMBERT et al., 1958; MALMROS and
WIGAND, 1959). At first the atherogenicity of this diet was simply attributed to the
presence of saturated fat but collation of the literature (KRITCHEVSKY, 1964b)
showed that the nature of the dietary carbohydrate and nonnutritive fiber may also
play a role. It has been shown that the type of carbohydrate present in the diet does
indeed affect the atherogenicity of the diet, fructose and sucrose being more hypercholesteremic and atherogenic (KRITCHEVSKY et al., 1968a; 1973b) (Table 3). The
fiber present in the diet (KRITCHEVSKY and TEPPER, 1965, 1968b; MOORE, 1967) has a
profound effect on the atherogenicity of the diet. MOORE (1967) fed 20% butter and
found that the atherosis in rabbits fed 19% wheat straw was almost one-third of that
observed in rabbits fed 19% cellulose. The diet that is usually used does not promote
optimum weight gain, but WILSON et al. (1973) have devised a semi-purified diet
which is atherogenic but palatable and leads to normal weight gain.

One aim of atherosclerosis research is to find means of causing regression of
lesions: After removal of the dietary stimulus, serum cholesterol levels will decline,
but the lesions generally become more severe. Addition of unsaturated fat to the
post-cholesterol regimen will inhibit the exacerbation of the lesions (KRITCHEVSKY
and TEPPER, 1962; VLES et al., 1964; GUSKI and WEISS, 1972). GUPTA et al. (1971)
have confirmed these findings and found that if the rabbits are maintained on the
cholesterol-free diet for a sufficiently long time the plaques will regress to that point
at which they were when cholesterol feeding was suspended, but will not regress
further. Thus after eight weeks of cholesterol feeding 17% of the aortic intimal
surface was involved with lesions. Cholesterol feeding was halted at that point. Ten
weeks later intimal involvement was up to 58% of the surface but 10 weeks after that,
it was down to 18%. Recently VESSELINOVITCH et al. (1974a) have shown that admin-

Table 2. Effect of fat (6%) on atherosclerosis in rabbits fed 2% cholesterol for 8 weeks[a]

Fat	Iodine value	Serum cholesterol mg/dl	Average atherosclerosis (arch + thoracic/2)
None	—	1214	2.70
Coconut oil	10	2827	2.80
Lard	66	2245	2.35
Hydrogenated corn oil	79	1984	2.10
corn oil	134	1908	1.45

[a] After KRITCHEVSKY (1970).

Table 3. Influence of carbohydrates on atherosclerosis in rabbits fed semi-purified diets[a] (10 month feeding)

Carbohydrate[b]	Wt. gain (g)	Serum lipids, mg/dl		Average atherosis
		cholesterol	triglycerides	
Glucose	− 83	451 ± 102	92 ± 15	0.85
Fructose	− 22	922 ± 231	116 ± 51	1.50
Sucrose	+ 180	520 ± 119	248 ± 72	1.45
Lactose	+ 97	329 ± 144	107 ± 21	0.50
Starch	+ 95	532 ± 152	254 ± 102	1.35

[a] After KRITCHEVSKY et al. (1973b).
[b] Diet contains 25% casein, 14% hydrogenated coconut oil, 40% carbohydrate.

Table 4. Effects of various treatments (10 Weeks) on pre-established artheromatous lesions in rabbits[a]

Group	No.	Diet	100% O_2	Drug[b]	% Aortic intima involved ± SEM
I	12	Control atherogenic	−	−	65 ± 8.7
II	7	Atherogenic	−	−	75 ± 13.6
III	12	Stock	−	−	66 ± 7.5
IV	7	Stock	+	−	50 ± 11.0
V	7	Stock	−	a	37 ± 13.0
VI	7	Stock	+	a	29 ± 10.0
VII	7	Stock	−	b	37 ± 17.0
VIII	7	Stock	+	b	31 ± 11.4

[a] After VESSELINOVITCH et al. (1974a).
[b] a) 1% Cholestyramine b) 1.332 mg estradiol benzoate s.c.

istration of a combination of hypocholesteremic drug and oxygen administered after cessation of cholesterol feeding resulted in significant regression of lesions (Table 4). Earlier drug experiments (KRITCHEVSKY et al., 1961b, 1967, 1968c, 1973c) had shown only a modest effect on pre-established atheroma.

II. Rat

The availability and ease of handling would make the rat an ideal candidate for atherosclerosis research were he not resistant to simple dietary manipulation. Atherosclerosis can develop when the rat is fed cholesterol plus high levels of sodium cholate (WISSLER et al., 1954) or saturated fat, cholesterol, cholic acid and thiouracil (HARTROFT et al., 1952). Coronary atherosclerosis can be induced by feeding cholesterol to hypophysectomized rats (PATEK et al., 1963) or by feeding saturated fat to animals with essential fatty acid deficiency (MORIN et al., 1964). AUBERT et al. (1974) have reported rapid development of atherosclerosis in rats fed 0.5% cholesterol and high oral doses of Vitamin D_2. KOLETSKY (1973) has reported on an obese, hypertensive rat which may serve as a model for future work.

III. Chicken

The chicken, formerly in wide use in atherosclerosis research, has fallen into relative disfavor, although some investigators continue to work with this species. The book by KATZ and STAMLER (1953) summarized the means of induction of atherosclerosis in this species. Atherosclerosis could be induced or enhanced by dietary cholesterol, undernutrition, hypertension, pancreatectomy and stilbesterol. The chicken, like the rabbit, is very susceptible to cholesterol feeding. Saturation of the fat also plays a role in atherogenesis. Table 5 summarizes an experiment involving saturated and unsaturated fat and free fatty acids.

Table 5. Influence of 1% cholesterol and 10% fat on cholesteremia and atherosclerosis in chickens[a]

Fat	Plasma cholesterol mg/dl	Atherosclerosis		
		Grade	Incidence %	Index[b]
Coconut oil	832	1.0	100	100
Olive oil	704	1.6	78	125
Oleic acid	839	0.5	11	6
Cottonseed oil	1252	1.4	90	126
Safflower oil	650	1.0	70	70
Linoleic acid	1528	1.4	100	140

[a] After STAMLER et al. (1959).
[b] Grade × Incidence.

IV. Dog

The dog is another species considered to be resistant to cholesterol feeding *per se*. When thiouracil is added to a cholesterol-containing diet and when the diet is augmented with saturated fat, lesions can be induced (STEINER and KENDALL, 1946; STEINER et al., 1949; DiLUZIO and O'NEAL, 1962). Even the hypothyroid-cholesterol regimen does not affect dogs uniformly. Thus DePALMA et al. (1972) and MAHLEY et al. (1974) have observed hypo- and hyperresponding dogs. MAHLEY et al. (1974)

studied purebred foxhounds for 3 to 12 months on a 1% cholesterol diet. Hyporesponders showed no elevation in serum triglycerides and only modest cholesteremia.
All serum lipids were elevated in the hyperresponders and they exhibited atherosclerosis. DePalma et al. (1972) found 3 dogs hyporesponders (avg. serum cholesterol
362 mg/dl) as opposed to 5 dogs whose average cholesterol levels were 1511 mg/dl on
a 2% cholesterol, 200 mg/day propylthiouracil regimen. The former group exhibited
no atherosclerosis. In the latter group, mesenteric artery atherosclerosis fell from
+ 3.0 to 1.6 after they were returned to a normal diet and given 10 mg D-thyroxine/
day for 20 months. Aortic atherosclerosis at autopsy was + 2.8. Manning et al.
(1973) have observed familial hyperlipoproteinemia and thyroid dysfunction in beagles.

MALMROS and STERNBY (1968) have found that when dogs are fed a semi-purified
diet containing 5% cholesterol and 15 to 20% cocount oil they will become atherosclerotic. This regimen is physiologic in the sense that it does not require chemical
or surgical thyroidectomy.

V. Pigeons

The White Carneau pigeon develops spontaneous atherosclerosis of a type similar to
that seen in man (CLARKSON et al., 1959; LOFLAND and CLARKSON, 1959; PRICHARD
et al., 1962). In general, the serum cholesterol levels of these pigeons are similar to
those seen in other breeds of pigeons. The Silver King pigeon also shows spontaneous atherosclerosis. LINDSAY and NICHOLS (1971) have examined several breeds of
pigeons and their data compare well with those of LOFLAND and CLARKSON (1959).
LINDSAY and NICHOLS (1971) found the most severe lesions in White Carneau, White
King and Silver King pigeons. By selective breeding WAGNER et al. (1973) have
produced a strain of White Carneau pigeon with severe aortic atherosclerosis, a
strain of Show Racer with very little aortic atherosclerosis and Show Racer and F_2
strains which show a high frequency of myocardial infarction (43 and 60% respectively).

CLARKSON et al. (1973) have studied the "regression" of pre-established plaques in
White Carneau pigeons. Regression was studied over a 16 month period. Serum
cholesterol levels fell from an average of 1063 mg/dl to 298 mg/dl at 16 months. The
aortic index (% aortic intimal surface covered with fatty streaks and/or plaques) was
29 at the beginning of the regression. At 2, 4, 8, 12, and 16 months of regression the
aortic indices were 25, 18, 14, 34, and 15, respectively. The data resemble those seen
in rabbits and dogs.

VI. Swine

The pig is a useful animal for atherosclerosis because he is omnivorous, large, available in purebred lineage and has a coronary anatomy and cardiorespiratory physiology resembling that of man. On the other hand, the pig does get spontaneous lesions,
is hard to manipulate and thus requires special facilities, consumes large quantities of
expensive experimental diet and shows a limited capacity for development of progressive lesions.

Table 6. Spontaneous atherosclerosis in swine[a]

Age (yrs)	Number (M/F)	Percentage stained area[b]
1–2	8 (6/2)	6
2–3	7 (4/3)	22
3–4	6 (0/6)	14
4–5	7 (0/7)	19
5–6	2 (1/1)	28
6–7	5 (0/5)	14
7–8	5 (1/4)	38
8–9	5 (0/5)	31

[a] After SKOLD and GETTY (1961).
[b] (Abdominal + Thoracic + Iliac/3).

The pig develops atherosclerosis with age as has been shown by GOTTLIEB and LALICH (1954) and SKOLD and GETTY (1961) (Table 6). Saturated fat and cholesterol will enhance atherosclerosis in swine. DOWNIE et al. (1963) fed pigs a diet containing 25% egg yolk and observed a 37% increase in serum cholesterol levels and a 106% increase in aortic lesions. LEE et al. (1971) have found that a high cholesterol diet, if fed long enough, will produce atherosclerosis and myocardial infarction. They now find (NAM et al., 1973) that if the endothelium is injured before feeding the diet (2.75% cholesterol, 1.38% sodium cholate, 25% butter) severe atherosclerosis will result within 6 months. Thus in 7 pigs fed only the cholesterol diet for an average of 116 days the extent of surface involvement was 16%. In 9 pigs fed the diet after injury the surface involvement was 63% after an average of 97 days. Injury without diet yielded only 4% involvement. This same group has recently reported that returning the swine to stock diet for 14 months causes significant regression of plaques (DAOUD et al., 1974).

VII. Primates

Currently, the animal of choice for atherosclerosis research is some type of non-human primate. Primates are omnivorous, similar to man in many aspects of cardiovascular and pulmonary physiology and develop lesions resembling human lesions both in distribution and histology. The primary disadvantages presented by non-human primates are their expense and the requirement for special housing and handling.

The rhesus monkey (Macaca mulatta) can be rendered arteriosclerotic by pyridoxine deficiency (RINEHART and GREENBERG, 1951) and atherosclerotic by a high cholesterol diet (MANN and ANDRUS, 1956). The morphology and distribution of the lesions induced by diet resemble those seen in man (ARMSTRONG and WARNER, 1971). In general, the severity of the atherosclerotic lesions seen in rhesus monkeys is related to the degree of hypercholesteremia and one case of actual myocardial infarction has been observed (TAYLOR et al., 1962, 1963). Similar to the findings in rabbits (KRITCHEVSKY et al., 1971), peanut oil appears to be especially atherogenic for the

Table 7. Effect of various fats (25%) in rhesus monkeys fed 2% cholesterol for 50 weeks[a]

Fat	No.	Serum cholesterol mg/dl	Aortic lesions			Coronary lesions	
			Gross area (% ± SEM)	Microscopic		Frequency	Severity
				Frequency	Severity		
Corn oil	6	650	63 ± 6.3 ab	56	35	22	8
Butter fat	6	1100	82 ± 3.3 ac	62	57	53	18
Peanut oil	6	610	93 ± 1.3 bc	68	77	95	21

[a] After Vesselinovitch et al. (1974b).
[b] Values bearing same subscript are significantly different.

Table 8. Regression of fatty streaks in aortas of rhesus monkeys[a]

Group	Diet		Aorta Cholesterol, mg/g		Sudanophilia (%)	
	Atherogenic	Basal	Total	F/E	Thoracic	Abdominal
A	12 weeks	2 weeks	16.3	1.6	56.7	28.8
B	12 weeks	32 weeks	9.0	3.5	20.8	15.3
C	12 weeks	64 weeks	8.3	3.8	15.3	8.5
D	—	76 weeks	7.5	4.7	4.7	5.7

[a] After Eggen et al. (1974).

rhesus monkey (Vesselinovitch et al., 1974 b). Rhesus monkeys were fed diets containing 2% cholesterol and 25% corn oil, butter fat or peanut oil for 50 weeks. The gross lesions covered 63% of the aortic surface in the corn oil group, 82% in the butter group and 93% in the peanut oil group (Table 7).

Regression of induced lesions has been observed in the rhesus monkey (Armstrong et al., 1970). Armstrong and Megan (1972) fed rhesus monkeys a 40% egg yolk diet for 17 months. At this time one group of 10 was autopsied and the other animals, 20 in all, were returned for 40 months to a diet low in fat or to one containing 40% calories as corn oil. Arteries of control monkeys contained 6.8 mg/gm of total cholesterol and the ratio of free to esterified cholesterol (F/E) was 2.83. The atherosclerotic arteries had 51.2 mg/gm of total cholesterol with an F/E ratio of 0.36 and the regressed arteries contained 18.1 mg/gm total cholesterol and their F/E ratio was 0.53. The lipid spectrum of the arteries was normalizing on the regression regimen. Eggen et al. (1974) fed rhesus monkeys a diet containing cholesterol and saturated fat for 12 weeks and observed subgroups 2, 32, and 64 weeks after return to a basal diet. They found distinct reductions in total aortic cholesterol, F/E ratio and sudanophilia on the regression regimen (Table 8). Atherosclerotic lesions have been induced in *Cebus fatuella* by administration of a diet high in cholesterol and deficient in sulfur amino acids (Mann et al., 1953). *Cebus albifrons* were fed diets containing 0.5% cholesterol and 25% corn oil, butter or coconut oil for 45 weeks. All of the monkeys on coconut oil (4/4), three of four of the animals fed butter and none of the corn oil-fed group developed fatty intimal lesions. Their total serum cholesterol and F/E ratios were: corn oil—210 mg-%, 8.13; butter—185 mg-%, 6.71; and coconut oil—291 mg-%, 2.27 (Wissler et al., 1962). When young and adult *Cebus albifrons* were fed an atherogenic diet for two years, atherosclerosis was relatively light in the young monkeys (4/18) and severe in the adults (7/10) (BULLOCK et al., 1969).

The squirrel monkey *(Saimiri sciureus)* shows spontaneous atherosclerosis despite a relatively low serum cholesterol level (LOFLAND et al., 1967; McCOMBS et al., 1969) and experimental atherosclerosis can be induced easily in this species (MALINOW et al., 1966; MIDDLETON et al., 1967).

The spider monkey *(Ateles geoffroyi)* becomes hyperlipoproteinemic on a high cholesterol-high saturated fat diet (SRINIVASAN et al., 1972). When fed a diet containing 1 mg cholesterol/kcal the spider monkey *(Ateles sp.)* exhibits only slight hyper-cholesteremia and shows little exacerbation of spontaneous lesions (PUCAK et al., 1973). These findings emphasize the vast species differences in monkeys.

A high cholesterol (5%), high lard (23%) diet will induce atherosclerosis in marmosets (DREIZEN et al., 1973). This diet raises their serum cholesterol levels from 93 mg/dl to 1485 mg/dl after 73 weeks.

Atherosclerosis can be induced in baboons by feeding beef fat (GILLMAN and GILBERT, 1957) or butter plus cholesterol (GRESHAM et al., 1965). STRONG and McGILL (1967) fed baboons cholesterol (0.01 or 0.5%) in diets containing saturated or unsaturated fat and high or low levels of protein. On the low cholesterol diet the most severe atherosclerosis was observed in the high protein groups (saturated fat—3.2% of intimal surface with sudanophilia and unsaturated fat—4.8%). When high cholesterol diets were fed, the most severe sudanophilia was observed in the saturated fat, low protein groups (14.2%). KRITCHEVSKY et al. (1974a) have found that semi-purified diets containing 40% carbohydrate, 25% casein and 14% hydrogenated coconut oil were hyperlipemic when fed to baboons for one year. When the carbohydrate was fructose, serum cholesterol and triglyceride levels were 162 and 129 mg/dl, respectively. These levels represented increases of 25 and 72% above normal levels. The fructose diet caused the most severe aortic sudanophilia but aortic sudanophilia and lipemia were also observed when the diets contained sucrose, glucose or starch. This type of diet has been found to cause atherosclerosis in Vervet monkeys *(Cercopithecus aethiops)* (KRITCHEVSKY et al., 1974b).

The ideal laboratory model will be an animal that reacts as does man to all the major risk factors such as diet, hypertension and stress. Ideally the lesion produced should resemble the human lesion in chronology and in its pathology. Availability of such a model would permit integrated studies of the interaction of diet, drugs and environmental factors.

References

ALTSCHUL, R.: Selected Studies on Arteriosclerosis. Springfield, Illinois. C. C. Thomas 1950.

ANITSCHKOW, N.: Über die Veränderungen der Kaninchenaorta bei experimenteller Cholesterin-steatose. Beitr. Path. Anat. **56**, 379—404 (1913).

ANITSCHKOW, N.: Experimental arteriosclerosis in animals. In: COWDRY, E. V. (Ed.): Arteriosclerosis: A Survey of the Problem, pp. 271—322. New York: MacMillan Co. 1933.

ARMSTRONG, M. L., MEGAN, M. B.: Lipid depletion in atheromatous coronary arteries in rhesus monkeys after regression diets. Circulation Res. **30**, 675—680 (1972).

ARMSTRONG, M. L., WARNER, E. D.: Morphology and distribution of diet induced atherosclerosis in rhesus monkeys. Arch. Path. **92**, 395—401 (1971).

ARMSTRONG, M. L., WARNER, E. D., CONNOR, W. E.: Regression of coronary atheromatosis in rhesus monkeys. Circulation. Res. **27**, 59—67 (1970).

Aubert, D., Ferrand, J. C., Lacaze, B., Pepin, O., Panak, E., Podesta, M.: Athérogénèse expérimentale chez le rat Wistar. Atherosclerosis **20**, 263—280 (1974).

Brohon, J., Chomette, G., Sterne, J.: Technique accélérée de production d'une athérosclérose expérimentale chez la lapin. Paroi Arterielle **2**, 18—27 (1974).

Bullock, B. C., Clarkson, T. B., Lehner, N. D. M., Lofland, H. B., Jr., St. Clair, R. W.: Atherosclerosis in *Cebus albifrons* monkeys. III. Clinical and pathological studies. Exp. molec. Path. **10**, 39—62 (1969).

Clarkson, T. B.: Atherosclerosis—spontaneous and induced. Advanc. Lipid Res. **1**, 211—252 (1963).

Clarkson, T. B., King, J. S., Jr., Lofland, H. B., Feldner, M. A., Bullock, B. C.: Pathologic characteristics and composition of diet aggravated atherosclerotic plaques during "regression". Exp. molec. Path. **19**, 267—283 (1973).

Clarkson, T. B., Prichard, R. W., Netsky, M. G., Lofland, H. B.: Atherosclerosis in pigeons: Its spontaneous occurence and resemblance to human atherosclerosis. Arch. Path. **68**, 143—147 (1959).

Constantinides, P.: Experimental Atherosclerosis. Amsterdam: Elsevier Publ. Co. 1965.

Daoud, A. S., Jarmolych, J., Fritz, K., Augustyn, J.: Regression of advanced atherosclerosis in swine (morphologic studies). Circulation **49**, 92 (1974). (Abstract).

DePalma, R. G., Insull, W., Bellon, E. M., Roth, W. T., Robinson, A. V.: Animal models for the study of progression and regression of atherosclerosis. Surgery **72**, 268—278 (1972).

DiLuzio, N. R., O'Neal, R. M.: The rapid development of arterial lesions in dogs fed an "Infarct-producing" diet. Exp. molec. Path. **1**, 122—132 (1962).

Downie, H. G., Mustard, J. F., Rowsell, H. C.: Swine atherosclerosis: The relationship of lipids and blood coagulation to its development. Ann. N. Y. Acad. Sci. **104**, 539—562 (1963).

Dreizen, S., Levy, B. M., Bernick, S.: Diet-induced atherosclerosis in the marmoset. Proc. Soc. exp. Biol. (N.Y.) **143**, 1218—1223 (1973).

Eggen, D. A., Strong, J. P., Newman, W. P., III, Catsulis, C., Malcom, G. T., Kokatnur, M. G.: Regression of diet-induced fatty streaks in rhesus monkeys. Lab. Invest. **31**, 294—301 (1974).

Fillios, L. C., Mann, G. V.: The importance of sex in the variability of the cholesteremic response of rabbits fed cholesterol. Circulation Res. **4**, 406—412 (1956).

Gillman, J., Gilbert, C.: Atherosis in the baboon *(Papio ursinus)* its pathogenesis and etiology. Exp. Med. Surg. **15**, 181—221 (1957).

Giordano, A. R., Spraragen, S. C., Hamel, H.: A model for the rapid production of atheromatous lesions in rabbits. Lab. Invest. **22**, 94—99 (1970).

Gottlieb, H., Lalich, J. J.: The occurence of arteriosclerosis in the aorta of swine. Amer. J. Path. **30**, 851—855 (1954).

Gresham, G. A., Howard, A. N., McQueen, J., Bowyer, D. E.: Atherosclerosis in primates. Brit. J. exp. Path. **46**, 94—103 (1965).

Gupta, P. P., Tandon, H. D., Ramalingaswami, V.: Further observations on the reversibility of experimentally induced atherosclerosis in rabbits. J. Path. **105**, 229—238 (1971).

Guski, H., Weiss, P.: Zur Frage der spontanen Rückbildungsfähigkeit der experimentellen Atheromatose. Exp. Path. **6**, 214—224 (1972).

Hartroft, W. S., Ridout, J. H., Sellars, E. A., Best, C. H.: Atheromatous changes in aorta, carotid and coronary arteries of choline-deficient rats. Proc. Soc. exp. Biol. (N.Y.) **81**, 384—393 (1952).

Hartroft, W. S., Thomas, W. A.: Induction of experimental atherosclerosis in various animals. In: Sandler, M., Bourne, G. H.: (Eds.): Atherosclerosis and its Origin, pp. 439—457. New York: Academic Press, Inc. 1963.

Hirsch, R. L., Kellner, A.: The pathogenesis of hyperlipemia induced by means of surface-active agents. II. Failure of exchange of cholesterol between plasma and the liver in rabbits given Triton WR-1339. J. exp. Med. **104**, 15—24 (1956).

Ignatowski, A.: Über die Wirkung des tierschen Eiweißes auf die Aorta und die parenchymatosen Organe der Kaninchen. Arch. Path. Anat. Physiol. **198**, 248—270 (1909).

Katz, L. N., Stamler, J.: Experimental Atherosclerosis. Springfield, Ill.: C. C. Thomas 1953.

Kellner, A., Correll, J. W., Ladd, A. T.: Sustained hyperlipemia induced in rabbits by means of intravenously injected surface-active agents. J. exp. Med. **93**, 373—383 (1951).

KOLETSKY,S.: Obese spontaneously hypertensive rats.—A model for study of atherosclerosis. Exp. molec. Path. **19**, 53—60 (1973).

KRITCHEVSKY,D.: Experimental atherosclerosis in rabbits fed cholesterol-free diets. J. Atheroscler. Res. **4**, 103—105 (1964a).

KRITCHEVSKY,D.: Experimental Atherosclerosis. In: PAOLETTI,R. (Ed.) Lipid Pharmacology, pp.63—130. New York: Academic Press, Inc. 1964b.

KRITCHEVSKY,D.: Role of cholesterol vehicle in experimental atherosclerosis. Amer. J. clin. Nutr. **23**, 1105—1110 (1970).

KRITCHEVSKY,D.: Laboratory models for atherosclerosis. Advanc. Drug Res. **9**, 41—53 (1974).

KRITCHEVSKY,D., DAVIDSON,L.M., SHAPIRO,I.L., KIM,H.K., KITAGAWA,M., MALHOTRA,S., NAIR,P.P., CLARKSON,T.B., BERSOHN,I., WINTER,P.A.D.: Lipid metabolism and experimental atherosclerosis in baboons: Influence of cholesterol-free, semi-synthetic diets. Amer. J. clin. Nutr. **27**, 29—50 (1974a).

KRITCHEVSKY,D., DAVIDSON,L.M., VANDERWATT,J.J., WINTER,P.A.D., BERSOHN,I.: Hypercholesterolaemia and atherosclerosis induced in vervet monkeys by cholesterol-free, semisynthetic diets. S. Afr. Med. J. **48**, 2413—2414 (1974b).

KRITCHEVSKY,D., KIM,H.K., TEPPER,S.A.: Effect of colestipol (U-26, 597A) on experimental atherosclerosis in rabbits. Proc. Soc. exp. Biol. (N.Y.) **142**, 185—188 (1973c).

KRITCHEVSKY,D., LANGAN,J., MARKOWITZ,J., BERRY,J.F., TURNER,D.A.: Cholesterol vehicle in experimental atherosclerosis. III. Effects of absence or presence of fatty vehicle. J. Amer. Oil chem. Soc. **38**, 74—76 (1961a).

KRITCHEVSKY,D., MOYER,A.W., TESAR,W.C., LOGAN,J.B., BROWN,R.A., DAVIES,M.C., COX,H.R.: Effect of cholesterol vehicle in experimental atherosclerosis. Amer. J. Physiol. **178**, 30—32 (1954).

KRITCHEVSKY,D., MOYER,A.W., TESAR,W.C., MCCANDLESS,R.F.J., LOGAN,J.B., BROWN,R.A., ENGLERT,M.E.: Cholesterol vehicle in experimental atherosclerosis. II. Influence of unsaturation. Amer. J. Physiol. **185**, 279—280 (1956).

KRITCHEVSKY,D., MOYNIHAN,J.L., LANGAN,J., TEPPER,S.A., SACHS,M.L.: Effects of D- and L-thyroxine and of D- and L-3,5,3'-triiodothyronine on development and regression of experimental atherosclerosis in rabbits. J. Atheroscler. Res. **1**, 211—221 (1961b).

KRITCHEVSKY,D., SALLATA,P., TEPPER,S.A.: Experimental atherosclerosis in rabbits fed cholesterol-free diets. 2. Influence of various carbohydrates. J. Atheroscler. Res.**8**, 697—703 (1968a).

KRITCHEVSKY,D., SALLATA,P., TEPPER,S.A.: Influence of ethyl p-chlorophenoxy-isobutyrate (CPIB) upon establishment and progression of experimental atherosclerosis in rabbits. J. Atheroscler. Res. **8**, 755—761 (1968c).

KRITCHEVSKY,D., TEPPER,S.A.: Factors affecting atherosclerosis in rabbits fed cholesterol-free diets. Life Sci. **4**, 1467—1471 (1965).

KRITCHEVSKY,D., TEPPER,S.A.: Influence of D- and L-thyroxine on pre-established atheroma in rabbits: Effect of mode of administration. J. Atheroscler. Res. **7**, 103—110 (1967).

KRITCHEVSKY,D., TEPPER,S.A.: Experimental atherosclerosis in rabbits fed cholesterol-free diets: Influence of chow components. J. Atheroscler. Res.**8**, 357—369 (1968b).

KRITCHEVSKY,D., TEPPER,S.A.: Cholesterol vehicle in experimental atherosclerosis. 14. Diet and rate of appearance of atheromata. Nutrition Reports Int. **8**, 163—168 (1973a).

KRITCHEVSKY,D., TEPPER,S.A., KITAGAWA,M.: Experimental atherosclerosis in rabbits fed cholesterol-free diets. 3. Comparison of fructose and lactose with other carbohydrates. Nutrition Reports Int.**7**, 193—202 (1973b).

KRITCHEVSKY,D., TEPPER,S.A., LANGAN,J.: Cholesterol vehicle in experimental atherosclerosis. IV. Influence of heated fat and fatty acids. J. Atheroscler. Res. **2**, 115—122 (1962).

KRITCHEVSKY,D., TEPPER,S.A., VESSELINOVITCH,D., WISSLER,R.W.: Cholesterol vehicle in experimental atherosclerosis. 11. Peanut oil. Atherosclerosis **14**, 53—64 (1971).

LAIRD,C.W., FOX,R.R., SCHULTZ,H.S., MITCHELL,B.P., BLAU,E.M.: Strain variations in rabbits: biochemical indicators of thyroid functions. Life Sci. **9**, 203—214 (1970).

LAMBERT,G.F., MILLER,J.P., OLSEN,R.T., FROST,D.V.: Hypercholesteremia and atherosclerosis induced in rabbits by purified high fat rations devoid of cholesterol. Proc. Soc. exp. Biol. (N.Y.) **97**, 544—549 (1958).

226   D. Kritchevsky

LEE, K.T., JARMOLYCH, J., KIM, D.N., GRANT, C., KRASNEY, J.A., THOMAS, W.A., BRUNO, A.M.: Production of advanced atherosclerosis, myocardial infarction and "sudden death" in swine. Exp. molec. Path. **15**, 170—190 (1971).

LINDSAY, S., NICHOLS, C.W., JR.: Arteriosclerosis in the pigeon: Naturally occurring disease of the coronary arteries und aorta. Exp. Med. Surg. **29**, 42—60 (1971).

LOFLAND, H.B., CLARKSON, T.B.: Biochemical study of spontaneous atherosclerosis in pigeons. Circulation Res. **7**, 234—237 (1959).

LOFLAND, H.B., ST. CLAIR, R.W., MACNINTCH, J.E., PRICHARD, R.W.: Atherosclerosis in new world primates: Biochemical studies. Arch. Path. **83**, 211—214 (1967).

MAHLEY, R.W., WEISGRABER, K.H., INNERARITY, T.: Canine lipoproteins and atherosclerosis. II. Characterization of the plasma lipoproteins associated with atherogenic and non-atherogenic hyperlipidemia. Circulation Res. **35**, 722—733 (1974).

MALINOW, M.R., MARUFFO, C.A., PERLEY, A.M.: Experimental atherosclerosis in squirrel monkeys *(Saimiri sciurea)*. J. Path. Bact. **92**, 491—510 (1966).

MALMROS, H., STERNBY, N.H.: Induction of atherosclerosis in dogs by a thiouracil-free semisynthetic diet containing cholesterol and hydrogenated coconut oil. Prog. Biochem. Pharmacol. **4**, 482—487 (1968).

MALMROS, H., WIGAND, G.: Atherosclerosis and deficiency of essential fatty acids. Lancet 1959 II, 749—751.

MANN, G.V., ANDRUS, S.B.: Xanthomatosis and atherosclerosis produced by diet in an adult rhesus monkey. J. Lab. clin. Med. **48**, 533—550 (1956).

MANN, G.V., ANDRUS, S.B., McNALLY, A., STARE, F.J.: Experimental atherosclerosis in cebus monkeys. J. exp. Med. **98**, 195—218 (1953).

MANNING, P.J., CORWIN, L.A., JR., MIDDLETON, C.C.: Familial hyperlipoproteinemia and thyroid dysfunction in beagles. Exp. molec. Path. **19**, 378—388 (1973).

MARQUIE, G., AGID, R.: Influence de la race sur la sensibilité du Lapin à l'athérome expérimental. Experientia **28**, 1068—1069 (1972).

McCOMBS, H.L, ZOOK, B.C., McGANDY, R.B.: Fine structure of spontaneous atherosclerosis of the aorta in the squirrel monkey. Amer. J. Path. **55**, 235—252 (1969).

MIDDLETON, C.C., CLARKSON, T.B., LOFLAND, H.B., PRICHARD, R.W.: Diet and atherosclerosis of squirrel monkeys. Arch. Path. **83**, 145—153 (1967).

MOORE, J.H.: The effect of the type of roughage in the diet on plasma cholesterol levels and aortic atherosis in rabbits. Brit. J. Nutr. **21**, 207—215 (1967).

MORIN, R.J., BERNICK, S., ALFIN-SLATER, R.B.: Effects of essential fatty acid deficiency and supplementation on atheroma formation and regression. J. Atheroscler. Res. **4**, 387—396 (1964).

NAM, S.C., LEE, W.M., JARMOLYCH, J., LEE, K.T., THOMAS, W.A.: Rapid production of advanced atherosclerosis in swine by a combination of endothelial injury and cholesterol feeding. Exp. molec. Path. **18**, 369—379 (1973).

OLSON, R.E.: Atherosclerosis—a primary hepatic or vascular disorder? Perspect. Biol. Med. **2**, 84—121 (1958).

PARWARESCH, M.R., MADER, C., HILL, W., WISWEDEL, K.: Ein Kombiniertes Verfahren zur Erzeugung von Arteriosklerose bei Kaninchen in Kurzzeitversuchen. Res. exp. Med. **160**, 269—291 (1973).

PATEK, P.R., BERNICK, S., ERSHOFF, B.H., WELLS, A.: Introduction of atherosclerosis by cholesterol feeding in the hypophysectomnized rat. Amer. J. Path. **42**, 137—150 (1963).

PRICHARD, R.W., CLARKSON, T.B., LOFLAND, JR., H.B., GOODMAN, H.O., HERNDON, C.N., NETSKY, M.G.: Studies on the atherosclerotic pigeon. J. Amer. med. Ass. **179**, 49—52 (1962).

PUCAK, G.J., LEHNER, N.D.M., CLARKSON, T.B., BULLOCK, B.C., LOFLAND, H.B.: Spider monkeys (Ateles sp.) as animal models for atherosclerosis research. Exp. molec. Path. **18**, 32—49 (1973).

RINEHART, J.F., GREENBERG, L.D.: Pathogenesis of experimental arteriosclerosis in pyridoxine deficiency; with notes on similarities to human arteriosclerosis. Arch. Path. **51**, 12—18 (1951).

ROBERTS, D.C.K., WEST, C.E., REDGRAVE, T.G., SMITH, J.B.: Plasma cholesterol concentration in normal and cholesterol-fed rabbits. Its variation and heritability. Atherosclerosis **19**, 369—380 (1974).

ROBERTS, J.C.JR., STRAUS, R.: Comparative atherosclerosis. New York: Hoeber Medical Division, Harper and Row (1965).

SCEBAT, L., RENAIS, J., LENEGRE, J.: Athérosclérose expérimentale du lapin. Etude preliminaire. Rev. Atherosclerose **3**, 14—26 (1961).

SKOLD, B. H., GETTY, R.: Spontaneous atherosclerosis in swine. J. Amer. Vet. med. Ass. **139**, 655—660 (1961).

SRINIVASAN, S. R., DALFERES, E. R., JR., RUIZ, H., PARGAONKAR, P. S., RADHAKRISHNAMURTHY, B., BERENSON, G. S.: Rapid serum lipoprotein changes in spider monkeys on short-term feeding of high cholesterol-high saturated fat diet. Proc. Soc. exp. Biol. (N.Y.) **141**, 154—160 (1972).

STAMLER, J., PICK, R., KATZ, L. N.: Saturated and unsaturated fats. Effects on cholesterolemia and atherogenesis in chicks on high-cholesterol diets. Circulation Res. **7**, 398—402 (1959).

STEINER, A., KENDALL, F. E.: Atherosclerosis and arteriosclerosis in dogs following ingestion of cholesterol and thiouracil. Arch. Path. **42**, 433—444 (1946).

STEINER, A., KENDALL, F. E., BEVANS, M.: Production of arteriosclerosis in dogs by cholesterol and thiouracil feeding. Amer. Heart J. **38**, 34—42 (1949).

STRONG, J. P., MCGILL, H. C. JR.: Diet and experimental atherosclerosis in baboons. Amer. J. Path. **50**, 669—690 (1967).

TAYLOR, C. B., COX, G. E., MANALO-ESTRELLA, P., SOUTHWORTH, J., PATTON, D. E., CATHCART, C.: Atherosclerosis in rhesus monkeys. II. Arterial lesions associated with hypercholesteremia induced by dietary fat and cholesterol. Arch. Path. **74**, 16—34 (1962).

TAYLOR, C. B., MANALO-ESTRELLA, P., COX, G. E.: Atherosclerosis in rhesus monkeys. V. Marked diet-induced hypercholesteremia with xanthomatosis and severe atherosclerosis. Arch. Path. **76**, 239—249 (1963).

VESSELINOVITCH, D., WISSLER, R. W., FISHER-DZOGA, K., HUGHES, R., DUBIEN, L.: Regression of atherosclerosis in rabbits. 1. Treatment with low-fat diet, hyperoxia and hypolipidemic agents. Atherosclerosis **19**, 259—275 (1974 a).

VESSELINOVITCH, D., GETZ, G. S., HUGHES, R. H., WISSLER, R. W.: Atherosclerosis in the rhesus monkey fed three food fats. Atherosclerosis **20**, 303—321 (1974 b).

VLES, R. O., BULLER, J., GOTTENBOS, J. J., THOMASSON, H. J.: Influence of type of dietary fat on cholesterol-induced atherosclerosis in the rabbit. J. Atheroscler. Res. **4**, 170—183 (1964).

WAGNER, W. D., CLARKSON, T. B., FELDNER, M. A., PRICHARD, R. W.: The development of pigeon strains with selected atherosclerosis characteristics. Exp. molec. Path. **19**, 304—319 (1973).

WANG, C. J., SCHAEFER, L. E., DRACHMAN, S. R., ADLERSBERG, D.: Plasma lipid partition of the normal and cholesterol fed rabbit. J. Mt. Sinai Hosp. **21**, 19—25 (1954).

WILSON, R. B., NEWBERNE, P. M., CONNER, M. W.: An improved semisynthetic atherogenic diet for rabbits. Arch. Path. **96**, 355—359 (1973).

WISSLER, R. W., EILERT, M. L., SCHROEDER, M. A., COHEN, L.: Production of lipomatous and atheromatous arterial lesions in the albino rat. Arch. Path. **57**, 333—351 (1954).

WISSLER, R. W., FRAZIER, L. E., HUGHES, R. H., RASMUSSEN, R. A.: Atherogenesis in the cebus monkey. I. A comparison of three food fats under controlled dietary conditions. Arch. Path. **74**, 312—322 (1962).

WISSLER, R. W., VESSELINOVITCH, D.: Comparative pathogenic patterns in atherosclerosis. Advanc. Lipid Res. **6**, 181—206 (1968).

WISSLER, R. W., VESSELINOVITCH, D.: Differences between human and animal atherosclerosis. In: SCHETTLER, G., WEIZEL, A. (Eds.): Atherosclerosis III, pp. 319—325. Berlin-Heidelberg-New York: Springer 1974.

CHAPTER 7

Lipoprotein Formation in the Liver Cell Ultrastructural and Functional Aspects Relevant to Hypolipidemic Action

W. Stäubli and R. Hess

With 17 Figures

I. Introduction

The accumulation of lipids within the arterial wall is of fundamental importance in the development of atherosclerosis [58, 135, 508]. The constituent lipids of the mural deposits are presumably heterogeneous in origin: they may be synthesized in situ, or they may enter the arterial wall, probably by means of active or passive transport [1, 26, 141, 168, 315, 422]. The circulating lipoproteins, whether intact or modified, are considered likely candidates for vectorial transport [393, 407].

The evidence associating hyperlipidemia with the development of atherosclerosis is believed to be conclusive enough to warrant attempts to control hyperlipidemia by drug therapy [35].

The lipoproteins that are secreted into the blood originate mainly from the liver and, to some extent, from the intestine [202, 215, 257, 308, 309, 362, 489, 492, 493]. They are usually separated by ultracentrifugation and classified according to their density (d, measured in g per ml) into: very low-density lipoprotein (VLDL) $d < 1.006$; low-density lipoprotein (LDL) $d = 1.006—1.063$, and high-density lipoprotein (HDL) $d = 1.063—1.21$. The lipoprotein molecules of different density classes consist of one or several polypeptide chains ["apolipoprotein(s)"], polar and nonpolar lipids and carbohydrates. These chemical moieties are assembled into a composite particle [267] displaying class-specific compositional and physical properties [381]. Since the majority of serum lipoproteins are synthesized by the parenchymal cells of the liver, the secretory apparatus of the hepatocyte may be an important target for hypolipidemic drugs. In this article, various functional and structural aspects of hepatocellular lipoprotein secretion and potential sites of intervention by lipid-lowering agents will be discussed. The composite functions involved in the process of secretion may be considered within the scope of the membrane flow concept.

II. The Concept of Membrane Flow and Its Relevance to Secretion

A. The Model

The membrane flow concept, as it is known today, was elaborated by PALADE and his associates (reviewed in references [32, 193, 270, 318]) and the HOKINS (reviewed in reference [179]). The whole process of membrane flow may be imagined as a system

of mass transport of secretory products from within the cell where they are synthesized to the extracellular compartment.

Several aspects of the secretion cycle can be distinguished. One main feature was
brought to light by the observation that in the cells of the exocrine pancreas [194 to
196, 316] and in other secretory cells, such as antibody-producing cells [19, 43, 57,
83, 400] the bulk of the exportable proteins remains enclosed in cellular membranes
throughout the process. Secretion can therefore be regarded as an intracellular de-
vice for transporting secretory material enclosed in membranous containers. Secretion starts with the elaboration of the polypeptide chain(s) of the secretory proteins
on polysomes and ends in their extrusion through the plasma membrane into the
extracellular space.

Between these two events a succession of transfer steps takes place, involving
different membrane compartments, i.e. the endoplasmic reticulum, the Golgi complex, the secretory vesicles and the plasma membrane. It is thought that transcellular
transfer is at least partly made possible by the fusion of membrane material of
various types. Presumably, the translocation process enables the cell to collect, modify, package, concentrate and release affluent secretory materials. Its function depends
on an essentially irreversible [197] concentration gradient of membranous material
directed towards the cell periphery. In several tissues exhibiting a marked degree of
secretory activity, such as the exocrine pancreas [106, 190, 317], the parotid gland
[10] and the anterior pituitary [408], it was found that the discharge of proteins is
initiated by fusion of the boundary membrane of secretory granules with the plasmalemma and the subsequent release of the contents of the granules into the extracellular space. This process should accordingly increase the surface of the plasma membrane by the insertion of membrane stretches formerly located around the secretory
granule. In fact, there is a considerable increase in the surface of the apical portion of
the plasma membrane of secretagogue-stimulated cells of the exocrine pancreas [137,
196] and the parotid gland [10]. This transient enlargement of the luminal surface
my be taken as evidence of a membrane flow, which originates in the interior of the
cell and which is vectorially oriented towards its surface. At later stages, the excess
luminal plasma membrane is removed and the material is possibly reutilized. Several
mechanisms have been discussed in this regard. According to one hypothesis, the
membrane excess is degraded to smaller (molecular) components, which may be
reutilized as "building blocks" in the synthesis of new membrane material [119, 179];
other authors [10, 196] incline to the view that the excess membrane material is
removed in the form of intact vesicular structures that are eventually used in the
assembly of new secretory granules. A number of observations seem to favor this
latter concept. The stimulated discharge of secretory proteins *in vitro* by pancreas
slices is characterized by a concomitant increase of ^{32}P incorporation into the phospholipids of rough and smooth membranes [179, 271]; this stimulation is, however,
not paralleled by an increase in labeled amino acid incorporation into the membranes of microsomal subfractions [271]. Thus, the stimulated flux of secretion
products does not seem to be dependent on the *de novo* synthesis of complete
intracellular membranes. In addition, the extrusion of pancreatic secretory enzymes,
stimulated by secretogogues, is not impaired by protein synthesis inhibitors, such as
cycloheximide [197]. The same inhibitor also does not appear to interfere with
lipoprotein secretion by perfused rat livers [29]. It has even been shown that cycloheximide, when present at the time of pulse-labelling of pancreatic slices with a

radioactive amino acid, and throughout the whole secretion cycle, does not stop the release of pancreatic proenzymes into the incubation medium [197]. These and other observations [31] confirm that the intracellular movement of exportable proteins does not depend on any appreciable de novo synthesis of membranes that form the containers enclosing the secretion products. Certain morphological [137] and biochemical [85] evidence has been put forward, suggesting that redundant membrane stretches which had been inserted into the apical plasmalemma during discharge of secretory granules are internalized. Recently, however, it has been reported that the proteins of the limiting membranes of secretory granules of the parotid gland are labeled at the same rate as their contents, indicating that the synthesis of exportable proteins and of membranous envelopes is simultaneous and coordinated [11].

B. Individuality of Membrane Compartments

One of the intriguing aspects of secretion is the finding that, in spite of the postulated sequential transport of discrete and membrane-enveloped portions of material from one intracellular compartment to the other through membrane fusion, the different types of membrane obviously retain their characteristic composition [89, 95]. The membranes of secretion granules isolated from the exocrine pancreas [273]—the zymogen granules, which are thought to be structural derivatives of the endoplasmic reticulum—are clearly distinct from their presumed parent membranes with respect to their phospholipid composition, their cholesterol content [274], and their pattern of constitutive membrane proteins [272] and enzyme activities [275]. The lipid composition of secretion granules of several secretory cells, such as the zymogen granules of the exocrine pancreas [274], the hormone storage granules of the pituitary [448], and the chromaffin granules of the adrenal medulla [46], generally tends to be similar to that of the plasma membrane [459]. The Golgi membranes, which might be generated by fusion of elements of the smooth-surfaced endoplasmic reticulum, are also distinct from the other membranous compartments: several characteristic constitutive enzyme activities of the endoplasmic reticulum, for example, such as glucose-6-phosphatase, NADH- and NADPH-cytochrome c reductase, cytochrome b_5 and P-450 are partly or totally lacking [38, 80, 121, 122, 123, 139, 287].

In comparison with the endoplasmic reticulum membranes, the membranes of the Golgi complex are also deficient in enzymes involved in the biosynthesis of phospholipids, such as lecithin [458]. Conversely, there is ample biochemical [38, 78, 122, 132, 139, 186, 213, 232, 239, 287, 288, 383, 434, 458, 462, 463] and autoradiographic [101, 151, 293, 296, 433, 471, 479] evidence indicating that the Golgi apparatus functions as an important cellular site of attachment of carbohydrate components to secretory or sedentary proteins residing in this compartment during their intracellular transit. Thus, the Golgi membranes participate actively in the biosynthesis of glycoproteins[1] which may be distributed to various cellular sites including the lyso-

---

[1] Glycoproteins are defined as proteins to which carbohydrate units are covalently attached by a glycopeptide bond. In many glycoproteins, whether secretory or membrane-bound, the sugars are linked to specific amino acid residues (asparaginyl, seryl, threonyl) of the polypeptide backbone. The number of carbohydrate units per molecule, their size and their sugar sequence is extremely variable. In a number of glycoproteins the carbohydrate side chains are linked to the peptide through N-acetyl-D-glucosamine as a "bridge sugar", followed by mannose and additional N-acetylglucosamine residues, which form together the internal portion or "core" of the heteropolysaccharide unit. The non-reducing termini ot the carbohydrate chains may consist of sialyl-galactosyl-N-acetylglucosamine or fucosyl-galactosyl-N-acetylglucosamine sequences [410].

somes and the plasma membrane, or else may leave the cell as secretory products. In some types of cells, other enzyme activities, such as sulfotransferases [92, 121a, 218a, 503] and acid phosphatases [307] seem to be specifically confined to the Golgi membranes. The lipid and protein analyses of Golgi-membrane-rich fractions from different tissues reveal that this cytoplasmic component has an intermediary position between the endoplasmic reticulum and the plasma membrane [212, 214, 272, 274, 275, 287, 289, 459, 504]. This transitional character of the Golgi complex is further substantiated by the findings [38, 268a, 276a, 314a] that it apparently harbors, as indigenous constituents, some enzymes thought to be unequivocal markers for either the endoplasmic reticulum (e.g., the NADH-cytochrome c reductase-cytochrome b_5 electron transport system and glucose-6-phosphatase) or the plasma membrane (e.g., AMPase and adenylate cyclase).

Taken as a whole, these observations indicate that membrane flow does not entail the complete loss of the biochemical and structural individuality of a given membrane compartment. In a unitarian view [287, 289], all the membranes of eukaryotic cells are thought to form a functional and physical continuum (i.e., the "endomembrane system"). The structural and enzymatic individuality of the various membrane types is maintained by local differentiation processes. Since membrane flow would link the membrane compartments in different cellular locations, it follows that this compartment-specific remodeling process should be of a complex nature. It might involve selective modifications and dissections of the incoming membrane segments or insertion of new constituents into them [38, 271, 272, 275]. Furthermore, alterations in the intramembrane lipid environment could activate or inhibit constitutive enzymes already present in the transferred membrane [107]. Alternative explanations for the maintenance of compartmental individuality of cellular membranes have been suggested [38].

Further important aspects of the secretion process still remain to be elucidated. For example, it is not understood how the presumed fusion between membranes takes place. The fluidity of the plasma membrane [405], which appears to play an important part in several unrelated cell-surface phenomena [131, 297, 447], might favour membrane fusion. Recently experiments with spin-labeled phospholipid molecules have revealed that the sarcoplasmic reticulum also displays a considerable degree of fluidity [379]. Similarly, kinetic studies with cytochrome b_5 and cytochrome b_5 reductase revealed a high diffusional mobility of these proteins within the microsomal membranes of rat liver [360a]. More specifically, it has been speculated [330] that a local generation of lysolecithin, which is able to induce cell fusion [330], could equally well be responsible for membrane fusions. This hypothesis gains support from the fact that membrane-bound phospholipases are rather widely distributed [292, 458, 465]. The phospholipases could deacylate phospholipids and thus create favorable conditions for membrane interactions [250]. Although it is not known whether lysolecithin is reacylated, it has been mooted that a deacylation-reacylation cycle might be responsible for the modulation of fatty acid composition of membrane phospholipids [456]. It is assumed that by fulfilling certain regulatory functions such a cycle could influence the physico-chemical properties of membranes or of membrane segments.

C. Directional Flow of Membranes

The mechanisms responsible for directional flow of membranes are largely unknown. With some rare exceptions [244] the morphological analysis of many different kinds of cellular secretion has hitherto failed to demonstrate any striking topographical association between transporting "containers" and filamentous or tubular guiding structures. There is, however, indirect evidence that such cellular elements may indeed participate in the transport of secretory material. It is believed that cells contain a "cytoskeleton" built up of two components. One component is presumed to consist of microfilaments (about 50 to 70 Å in thickness), which are thought to be endowed with actin-like contractile properties. The microfilaments may play an important role in cell locomotion [411, 474]. The other component takes the form of microtubules, which are described as cylinders measuring about 240 Å in diameter. They are composed of proteinaceous subunits [472]. The function of the microtubules is not clearly understood. It has been suggested that they are elements providing the cell with a supporting framework. The experimental evidence in favor of the notion that these two cellular elements participate in the transport of exportable proteins is based on their capacity *in vitro* to bind certain secretion inhibitors. For example, cytochalasin B interacts with microfilaments, eventually causing their structural disruption [411]. Microtubular proteins display an affinity for the antimitotic alkaloids colchicine and vinblastin [52, 59]. The latter drug is capable of inducing an intracellular rearrangement of microtubular proteins followed by the formation of crystals [37, 259]. Cytochalasin B has been shown to interfere with thyroid [484] and pituitary [388] secretion, whereas it apparently facilitates insulin release by pancreatic beta-cells [312]. The mitotic spindle stabilizers, colchicine and vinblastin, have been reported to inhibit the discharge of secretory material upon stimulation by the thyroid gland [483] and by the pancreatic beta-cells [259]. Both drugs partially depress the release of zymogen by pancreatic tissue slices [197] and the secretion of procollagen by cultured embryonic chick cranial bone [104a]. In the beta-cells of the pancreas glucose seems to trigger an influx of calcium ions which, in turn, react with microtubular proteins to initiate insulin secretion [259]. This hypothesis is to some extent supported by recent experimental findings showing that bivalent cations participate in the aggregation of subunits isolated from brain microtubules [472]. Evidence has been presented that colchicine impairs the secretion of lipoproteins by perfused mouse liver [243a, 313], or by the intact rat [421, 422a], resulting, in both systems, in a hepatocellular accumulation of lipoprotein-containing secretory vesicles. Cytochalasin B and colchicine both interfere with the extrusion of α-amylase by stimulated parotid gland slices [69].

Neither of these agents seem to influence the release of immunoglobulins by plasmacytoma cells [319]. Since antibody-producing cells apparently do not package their exportable proteins into distinct secretory granules [57] this "refractory" behaviour of plasmacytoma cells has been interpreted as evidence of a modified secretion process allowing a continuous release of secretory proteins, as opposed to a more intermittent extrusion of secretory quanta by glandular cells [319].

These observations point to the possible participation of microfilaments and microtubules in the terminal steps of secretion which involve the migration of Golgi-derived secretory granules to the cell periphery and their interactions with the plasma membrane during extrusion of secretory material. The available evidence suggests that cytochalasin B and colchicine tend to interfere with the stimulated discharge of secretory material already formed. It should be mentioned, however, that cytochalasin B, for example, may also interfere with other cellular activities [325].

D. Energy Requirements of Secretion

The available information on the energetics of secretion is scanty. The release of amylase by slices of pancreas has been shown to be energy-dependent [179]. A detailed analysis of the whole secretion process in the exocrine pancreas suggested the existence of three functional segments with different energy requirements. The first segment, extending from the site of synthesis of exportable proteins in the rough-surfaced endoplasmic reticulum to the condensing vacuoles, is dependent on a supply of energy [197]; the second segment, which involves the transformation of condensing vacuoles into mature zymogen granules, is energy-independent [197]. Finally, the translocation of zymogen granules to the cell periphery and the release of their contents into the acinar lumen, again depends on the supply of respiration-chain-generated energy [197].

III. Formation and Secretion of Lipoproteins

A. Evidence of the Secretion of Lipoproteins by the Hepatocyte

The following section will be devoted specifically to the mechanisms of biosynthesis, transport and discharge of lipoproteins by the hepatic parenchymal cell. There is ample evidence [159, 268, 395] that these cells, by virtue of their capacity to esterify fatty acids, contribute largely to the lipoprotein contents of plasma in the post-absorptive state of the organism. Triglycerides are the main products that are transported into the circulation in the form of lipoproteins of very low density (VLDL) [44, 158, 160, 268, 297a, 435a]. Intestinal cells also contribute a considerable amount [309, 493] of endogenously synthesized lipoproteins to the pool of plasma lipoproteins [202, 257, 308, 362, 453, 489, 492]. Circulating lipoproteins thus originate from at least two different tissues, and it is not surprising that, in man at least, VLDL subpopulations exist [320].

B. Synthesis of Lipoproteins on Ribosomes

Human VLDL [7, 8, 61, 320] and rat VLDL [72, 104c, 219] contain several chemically and immunologically distinct polypeptides, although it is not known whether different molecules can coexist on the same lipoprotein particle, or are characteristic determinants of different VLDL subclasses. In spite of these uncertainties, it might be useful to remember that important proteins known to be composed of non-identical subunits such as hemoglobin and immunoglobulins are thought to be encoded by monocistronic messenger RNA [34, 96, 188, 211, 294, 391, 397, 485]. Although no information on the mode of coding of lipoproteins is available, it may be assumed, by analogy, that the primary structure of the different VLDL polypeptides is determined by individual messenger RNA molecules. Since actinomycin D

suppresses the normal [116] or fatty-acid stimulated [9] discharge of beta-lipoproteins by isolated perfused livers, the half-life of apoprotein-specific messenger RNAs
seems to be within the usual range.

Exportable proteins in general are believed to be synthesized on membrane-
bound polysomes, i.e., in the rough-surfaced endoplasmic reticulum [13, 73, 134,
355, 403, 460], although some remarkable exceptions to this rule have been described
[191, 446]. In the case of the liver this applies to serum proteins [133, 352] including
serum albumin [139, 323, 443 to 445] and transferrin [286]. Although experiments
to locate the site of synthesis of the apoprotein chains of lipoproteins in
intact hepatocytes have not been performed, it has been reported to take place in
isolated ribosome fractions from entire liver [65, 66] and in hepatic microsomes
[245, 264]. Indirect evidence for the participation of the endoplasmic reticulum in
lipoprotein synthesis may be derived from the fact that lipoproteins are glycoproteins [265, 266, 380] which, in various cell systems, are synthesized on membrane-
bound ribosomes [155, 233, 336, 399]. According to current views, the nascent
polypeptide chains of exportable proteins grow vectorially into the lumen of the
cisternae of the rough-surfaced endoplasmic reticulum, as they are sequentially
elongated by the protein synthesizing machinery, i.e. by the membrane-bound polyribosomes [47, 351, 354, 373]. Upon the release of the terminated polypeptide chain
it may either lie free in the cisternal lumen or be (transiently) bound to the inner
aspect of the endoplasmic reticulum membrane [223, 353, 377]. It was argued [353,
377] that this adhesion of the nascent polypeptide chain to the microsomal membrane may facilitate the contact between the growing acceptor protein and the
membrane-bound multi-glycosyltransferase system [383].

C. Stepwise Glycosylation of Exportable Proteins
by the Membrane-bound Multiglycosyl Transferase System

This multienzyme system catalyzes the stepwise glycosylation (cf. footnote on p. 231)
of exportable acceptor proteins, as they travel through the cavities of the cytoplasmic
membrane systems (e.g., rough-surfaced and smooth-surfaced endoplasmic reticulum,
Golgi apparatus, secretory granules, plasmalemma). As a corollary of this hypothesis
the sugars which are positioned adjacent to the polypeptide chain ("bridge" sugars)
would be added at an early stage in the glycoprotein synthesis, e.g., at the level of
the rough-surfaced endoplasmic reticulum. Subsequently, the carbohydrate residues
in internal positions ("core" sugars) would be attached as the acceptor protein moves
through the channels of the endoplasmic reticulum. In the region of the Golgi apparatus
(or possibly also at the level of the plasma membrane) the appropriate glycosyl
transferases would catalyze the attachment of the terminal sugar residues.

In fact, the early addition of sugar moieties, especially of the "bridge" sugar N-
acetyl-D-glucosamine, to the nascent, still ribosome-attached acceptor protein chain
has been reported to occur in immunoglobulin-secreting cells [384, 399] and in
hepatocytes [155, 233, 353]. Thus, the principal localisation of the N-acetylglucosa-
minyl transferase activity may be the membranes of the rough-surfaced endoplasmic
reticulum [56, 84, 233, 269, 281 to 284, 353, 383, 399, 455, 505]. During intracisternal
translocation the glycoprotein may reach the peripheral regions of the rough-sur-

faced endoplasmic reticulum where possibly the generation of smooth-surfaced membrane elements takes place. It is thought that in these locations the addition of the "core" sugars (e.g., mannose and additional N-acetylglucosamine) to the growing carbohydrate units of glycoproteins occurs [56, 84, 264, 353, 383]. It was claimed that in cells forming immunoglobulin glycoproteins [181, 298] the more terminal sugar residue galactose would be preferentially incorporated in smooth-surfaced membrane regions [176, 455]. There is an almost general agreement upon the fact that the Golgi membranes predominantly contain those glycosyltransferases that are responsible for the addition of terminal sugar residues to the polysaccharide units, namely galactose, fucose, and sialic acid [38, 78, 101, 121 a, 122, 139, 151, 166, 186, 213, 232, 239, 276 a, 287, 288, 293, 296, 314 a, 320 a, 383, 384, 433, 455, 458, 462 to 464, 471, 479, 505]. Thus during their residence within the channels of the Golgi complex the polysaccharide side chains of the exportable glycoproteins are eventually terminated, although the possibility remains that further glycosylations occur at the level of the secretory granules [276a, 314a]. Some observations on immunoglobulin M (IgM)-synthesizing lymphocytes indicate that the semiterminal and terminal sugar residues may be added somewhere distal to the Golgi apparatus, just before, or at the time of, exteriorization of the pentameric immunoglobulin molecule [12]; in this context, it should be remembered that the secretion cycle of antibody-forming cells could be regarded as an adaptive modification of the general cytological pattern as it occurs in secreting glandular cells [19, 57].

In the case of secretory proteins consisting of molecular complexes of two or more polypeptide protomers (e.g., hemoglobin, immunoglobulins, and possibly lipoproteins, etc.) the question arises how and where the interactions between the component polypeptide chains take place. Some insights into this problem were, for example, obtained through studies on the biosynthesis of antibodies. It should be mentioned, however, that a comparison between the assembly of lipoprotein-apoprotein protomers and immunoglobulin protomers might be of doubtful relevance since the subunits of immunoglobulins (IgG and IgM) are, as a rule, linked by disulfide bonds [276 b, 338], whereas corresponding information on lipoproteins is scarce. Nevertheless, it was reported that protomer polypeptides in particular apoprotein fractions of human serum HDL were linked by both noncovalent and disulfide bonds [103 a, 381 a]. Immunoglobulins (IgG) are composed of two light and two heavy polypeptide chains [338]. Since the two chain types are coded for in a monocistronic mode, light and heavy chains are synthesized and released by different size-classes of membrane-bound polyribosomes [34, 294, 391, 397, 485]. As light chains are synthesized much more rapidly than heavy chains [397], they tend to accumulate and establish an intracellular pool of free polypeptides. According to some authors [16, 425] two heavy chains react first to form a dimer linked by disulfide bonds; subsequently the light chains are linked to the heavy chain dimer. Apparently, these interactions between the component chains of immunoglobulins occur within the cisternae of the endoplasmic reticulum. Alternatively, light chains withdrawn from the pool may interact with nascent heavy chains on ribosomes to form mixed dimer precursors [70, 390, 391]. At a later stage, these dimers associate, possibly within the lumen of the cisternae, to form complete antibody molecules. It has recently been shown that the rate of synthesis of the heavy chains of immunoglobulins is controlled by a feed-back from the (intracisternally located) pool of fully assembled IgG molecules [425, 426]. A similar regulation mechanism could also be operative in the case of lipoprotein synthesis.

It should be stressed that, in addition to the foregoing regulation mechanism, the secretion cycle offers a great variety of potential post-transcriptional sites for other regulatory interventions. The most obvious ones are the following: the association of ribosomal particles with messenger RNA and the coupling of ribosomal subunits [25, 90, 128, 364, 367, 368], the attachment of ribosomal particles to the membrane of the endoplasmic reticulum [3, 47, 49 to 51, 68, 177, 191, 192, 206, 216, 217, 277, 311, 339, 354, 365, 366, 368, 373 to 375, 392, 398, 401, 402, 436, 437, 446, 482], the intraluminal translocation of the polypeptide chain [47, 351, 354, 373, 377], and the termination of a translational round by membrane-bound polyribosomes [117, 207, 209, 376].

The importance of the Golgi complex in the elaboration of secretory products should not obscure its possible participation in the biosynthesis and distribution of sedentary glycoproteins. Several observations point to the possibility that some glycoproteins ultimately inserted into the plasma membrane pass through the Golgi complex [54, 55, 154, 358a]. Recently, various plasma membrane-bound glycosyl transferase (ectoglycosyltransferase) activities have been described by several authors [38a, 53, 319a, 335, 467, 502a]. The metabolic relationship between these transferase enzymes and similar activities occurring at the level of the Golgi membranes [232, 268a, 383] is not known. Furthermore, the Golgi complex seems to play a role in the formation and in the disposal of lysosomal glycoproteins [36, 144]. In a recent review article these multiple activities of the Golgi apparatus were integrated into a scheme in which this organelle is supposed to exert important functions in the biosynthesis, disposal and catabolism of plasma membrane components [92].

Concerning the functional significance of glycoproteins, several hypotheses have been advanced. According to one of these, sedentary and secretory proteins are intracellularly sorted out by glycosylation [113]; there are, however, certain important exceptions that cannot be reconciled with this postulate [494]. According to other theories, the polysaccharide side chains contribute some "informational" capacities to the polypeptide backbone of glycoproteins, which enable them to participate in a multitude of specific recognition processes, such as intercellular recognition [92] and interactions with cell membrane-bound receptors [494]. An elaborate hypothesis suggests that intercellular recognition operates through a lock- and key-interaction between surface-bound glycosyl acceptors of one cell (the keys) and the corresponding glycosyltransferase of the other cell (the locks), resulting in an enzyme-substrate complex [368a]. Recent findings with a model system support some of the predictions evolving from this concept [502a].

D. Assembly of Protein and Lipid Moieties and Intracellular Transport

The general scheme of secretion postulates that the exportable products of cellular synthesis leave the rough-surfaced endoplasmic reticulum within smooth-surfaced vesicles [76, 194], i.e., within structures that are believed to be generated by a "pinching-off" process of terminal portions of the rough-surfaced membranes. On the basis of studies of the exocrine pancreas, the hypothesis was advanced that the vesicular structures of the smooth-surfaced endoplasmic reticulum might function as shuttle containers for secretory material. They might bridge the gap between rough-

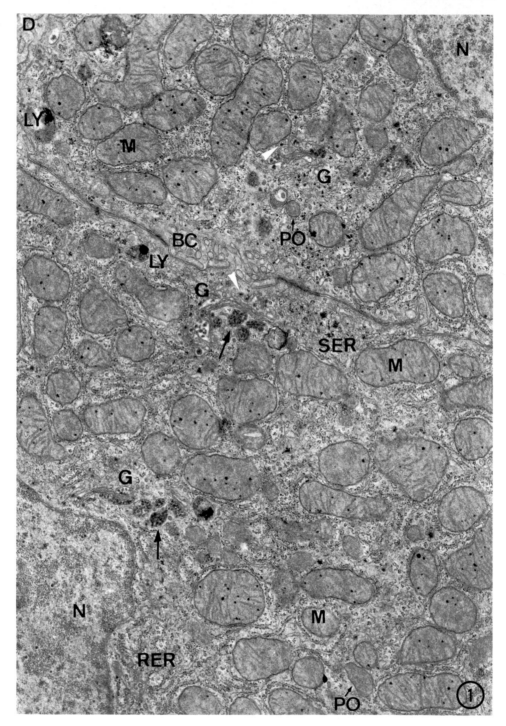

surfaced endoplasmic reticulum and the Golgi zone, the site of collection and concentration of pancreatic proenzymes [194 to 197]. This hypothesis is consistent with the apparent absence of any continuity between the elements of the rough-surfaced endoplasmic reticulum and of the Golgi complex. However, such continuities have been observed in other secretory cells [414, 499] as well as in hepatocytes [88, 287, 289, 314a].

In the case of lipoprotein secretion the process of translocation from rough membranes to smooth membranes is of particular interest. As visualized in the electron microscope, the lipoproteins appear in the form of more or less electron-opaque particles that lie within the cavities of various membrane compartments of the hepatocyte [14, 87, 88, 104, 156, 243a, 247, 255, 314a, 361, 419, 422a, 433, 450]. The lipoprotein nature of the intracellularly located spherules and their similarity to plasma lipoproteins have been unequivocally demonstrated. They have been isolated from Golgi-enriched fractions of rat and guinea-pig liver and characterized by structural, biochemical and immunological analysis [39, 78, 79, 254, 256, 258]. The lipoprotein particles emerge, in the form of spherical structures of variable diameter (300 to 1000 Å), in smooth-surfaced vesicles that may still be attached to terminal portions of the rough-surfaced membranes [88, 104, 205], or located between those membranes and the Golgi apparatus [88, 104] (Fig. 1). Since the lipoprotein granules are osmiophilic, it is reasonable to assume that they represent precursor particles of the plasma lipoproteins that contain at least part of the full lipid complement. The polypeptide determinants of Golgi-associated lipoprotein particles are very similar to those occurring in the plasma VLDL [78, 79, 104b, 104c, 258], including, therefore, apoproteins specific for the different plasma lipoprotein classes, e.g., VLDL, LDL (B protein) and HDL (A protein) (cf. [39]). These observations hence strongly support the notion that the lipoprotein particles present in Golgi-rich fractions of the liver are real precursors of the lipoproteins secreted by this organ.

With regard to the lipid components, it is known that the rate-limiting enzymes of the synthetic pathway of triglycerides [423, 481], phospholipids [82, 481] and cholesterol [97, 142, 200, 396] are localized preferentially in microsomes. At least in the case of triglycerides and phospholipids, this is borne out by autoradiographic studies indicating that the endoplasmic reticulum is the principal site of incorporation of the appropriate precursors [418 to 420]. In view of the fact that a small amount of free fatty acids is present in intrahepatocytic VLDL-particles [254, 256],

Fig. 1. Normal rat liver. Several Golgi complexes (G) are seen. More or less parallelized curved smooth-surfaced membranes are assembled to form the Golgi stacks (or dictyosomes). The functional polarity of this membrane system is visualized by the presence of small vesicles or tubules (arrow-heads) on one side, the forming face, of the stacked Golgi saccules. The profiles of these vesicles, which are considered to represent structural derivatives of the endoplasmic reticulum, may contain one or a limited number of lipoprotein (VLDL) particles (arrow-heads). The secreting face of the Golgi apparatus is characterized by an accumulation of secretory granules (arrows) containing many electron-dense VLDL particles and which are eventually translocated to the plasmalemma bordering the space of Disse (D). At this site the release of the VLDL particles into the extracellular space might occur. Other subcellular organelles of the hepatocytes are labeled as follows: N, nuclei; M, mitochondria; LY, lysosomes (peribiliar dense bodies); RER, rough-surfaced endoplasmic reticulum; SER, smooth-surfaced endoplasmic reticulum; PO (with arrow), peroxisomes. BC represents a bile canaliculus. × 16 300

the existence of a fatty acid-elongation system within microsomal membranes [100, 230] is noteworthy. The various systems for synthesizing complex lipids in rat liver seem to be about equally distributed between microsomal subfractions [458] with the exception of 3-hydroxy-3-methyl-glutaryl-coenzyme A reductase activity which was reported to be greatly enriched in smooth-surfaced endoplasmic reticulum membranes [142].

As judged by electron microscope autoradiography, precursors of triglycerides and phospholipids seem to become incorporated at the level of both rough and smooth membrane types [419, 420]. The body of available evidence suggests that the lipid components of lipoproteins are provided by the synthetic acitvities of the endoplasmic reticulum membranes and are coupled to the apoproteins that are transferred intracisternally. In fact, it has been observed that Golgi membranes isolated from guinea-pig liver contain lipoprotein particles belonging at least to two density classes which share common apoprotein determinants [78, 79]. The isolated Golgi particles could be separated into the LDL (density 1.007 to 1.063 g/ml) and VLDL (density <1.007 g/ml) density classes. The Golgi-associated VLDL particles differed from the LDL particles mainly in their higher content of triglyceride, as would be expected if the LDL particle represented the comparatively triglyceride-deficient precursor of the VLDL particles. The addition of triglycerides to the precursor LDL molecule would take place somewhere at the junction between the membranes of the endoplasmic reticulum and those of the Golgi apparatus [78, 79]. By investigating the incorporation of radioactive CMP-sialic acid into the various lipoproteins of Golgi-rich fractions of rat liver, the presence of a relatively lipid-deficient and sialic acid-containing lipoprotein-like product was noted [44a]. It was concluded that this particular molecular species may represent a Golgi-bound glyco-protein precursor of hepatic VLDL or HDL which had not already acquired its full lipid complement. This and the preceding observation both emphasize the concept of a stepwise biosynthesis of hepatic lipoproteins.

By simultaneous perfusion of isolated rat livers with differentially labeled leucine and palmitate it was shown that the lipid label appeared in the secreted lipoproteins earlier than the radioactivity due to the incorporated amino acid [64, 221]. It was concluded that this time-lag had occurred because of the existence of an intrahepatocytic pool containing preformed (non-radioactive) apoprotein molecules, to which the newly synthesized (radioactive) lipid moiety was attached. Similar conclusions have been drawn from observations made in kinetic studies in which cyclohex-imide was used as an inhibitor of protein synthesis [29]. A closer examination of the kinetics of radioacitve labeling of secreted lipoproteins revealed the possibility that the main apoproteins (e.g., A and B protein) are first individually loaded with their respective lipid complement and later on assembled to form the complete VLDL molecule [221, 222].

E. The Role of the Golgi Complex

According to the membrane-flow theory, the Golgi complex may be regarded as a turntable having the dual function of accepting and redistributing secretory products initially enclosed in membranes of the endoplasmic reticulum. Accordingly, the Golgi complexes of many cell types show a pronounced structural polarity [32, 74,

88, 92, 104, 287, 289, 435]. Stacked and parallelized plate-like membranes (cisternae, saccules, or lamellae) accept on their immature (forming, convex, proximal, or "cis") face the incoming, generally smooth-surfaced vesicles or tubules which are thought to contain the secretory materials. On the opposite side, at the mature (secreting, concave, distal, or "trans") face of the Golgi stacks, the exportable products are eventually released from the membrane complex, in most cases enclosed within secretory granules (cf. Figs. 1 to 6). The translocation of lipoprotein particles to the Golgi apparatus has been analysed extensively in rats by electron microscopy, following a dietary load with triglyceride [88]. The smooth-surfaced vesicles or tubules containing the lipoprotein particles accumulate at the accepting face of the Golgi complex (cf. Figs. 1 and 2). There, they are thought to fuse or coalesce to form essentially two-dimensional "fenestrated" plate-like structures (cf. Figs. 3 and 4). It is supposed that the plates resulting from this mass fusion are incorporated into the Golgi complex. Since the dilated terminal portions of the stacked Golgi lamellae also contain clustered lipoprotein particles (cf. Fig. 3) it was postulated that the "fenestrated" plates are gradually transformed into stacked lamellae, the bulb-like terminal distensions of which are finally pinched off to form secretory vesicles (cf. Figs. 3, 4, and 6).

An essentially similar sequence of events has been postulated by others [276a, 287, 289, 290, 314a] with the exception that solid continuities between the membranes of the endoplasmic reticulum and the secretory granules which form at the terminal portions of the stacking Golgi lamellae are assumed. Thus, the smooth-surfaced channels that link the rough-surfaced endoplasmic reticulum with the Golgi-associated secretory vesicles would provide a direct luminar continuity between the two membrane compartments. This connecting tubular system was designated as the "boulevard périphérique" [314a]. Nascent VLDL particles could then reach the Golgi-derived secretory vesicles without any migrational restriction. This detailed interpretation was partly based on morphological observations made with negatively stained preparations of Golgi-rich fractions in which the lipoprotein particles were seen to be located preferentially in distended tubules connected to the peripheral aspects of the cisternal plates (cf. Fig. 5). In addition, VLDL particles could not be observed to occur in the flat central segments of the Golgi cisternae, thus indicating that the packaging of incoming VLDL particles was limited to the periphery of the cisternal plates. In an attempt to subfractionate isolated rat liver Golgi complexes by means of enzymatic unstacking procedures combined with sucrose gradient centrifugation, three main fractions were obtained, which as judged by morphological criteria were enriched in secretory vesicles, boulevard périphérique, and plate-like cisternae, respectively [276a, 314a]. The determination of some enzyme activities (e.g., galactosyltransferase and glucose-6-phosphatase) of these fractions revealed an intermediary position of the boulevard périphérique-rich preparation in comparison with the fractions enriched either in secretory vesicles (highest galactosyltransferase activity) or Golgi cisternae (highest glucose-6-phosphatase activity). Although these results seem to favour the idea that the structural and functional heterogeneity of the Golgi membranes is paralleled by an enzymatic diversity, the relevance of some of the structural differentiations, as they regularly appear in negative stained Golgi-rich preparations (cf. Fig. 5), were called in question. Specifically, it was suggested that the appearance, after negative staining with phospho-

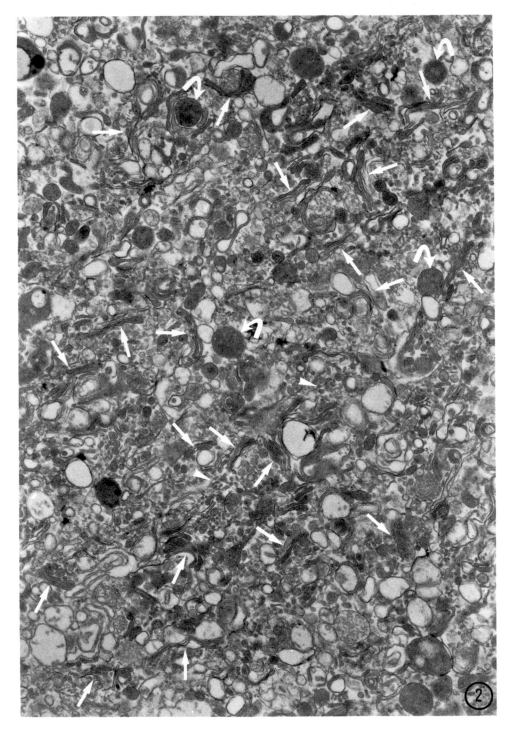

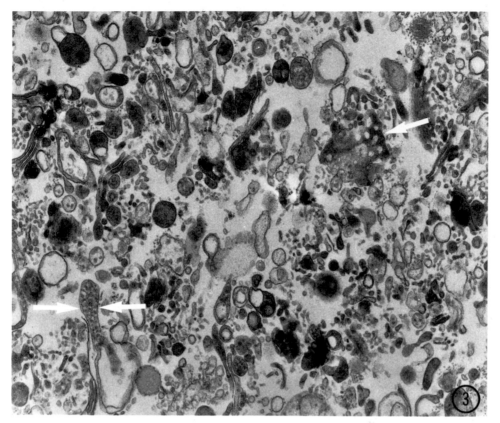

Fig. 3. Thin section of a fraction rich in Golgi membranes isolated from rat liver. This micrograph exemplifies some specific features related to the dynamic character of the Golgi apparatus. As discussed in the text "fenestrated" plates (single arrow) might be generated by multiple fusions of incoming vesicles. Dilated terminal portions of stacked Golgi saccules (double arrows) contain VLDL particles. Through a pinching-off process these portions of the saccules might form VLDL-containing secretory granules (cf. Figs. 1, 2, and 4). × 28000

tungstic acid, of isolated Golgi membranes in the form of fenestrated plates, tubules, and vesicles was the result of progressive alterations which occurred at the macromolecular level of the membranes as the consequence of their exposure to the degrading effect of enzymes and to the extractive capacity of phosphotungstate [90a]. Thus, the degree of structural complexity of isolated Golgi membranes may be determined essentially by the extent to which unfavourable factors can act on this membrane system during the isolation procedure. These observations [90a] may initiate a

Fig. 2. Thin section of a fraction rich in Golgi membranes isolated from rat liver. This preparation as well as the following ones were isolated in our laboratory by Mrs. Christiane Ody. The arrows point to stacked Golgi saccules. Note that the small vesicles (arrow-heads), as they occur on the forming face of the dictyosomes in situ (cf. Fig. 1), seem to co-sediment with the membrane stacks. The larger granules (curved arrows) are tentatively identified as secretory granules containing morphologically somewhat altered VLDL particles (cf. Fig. 1). × 28000

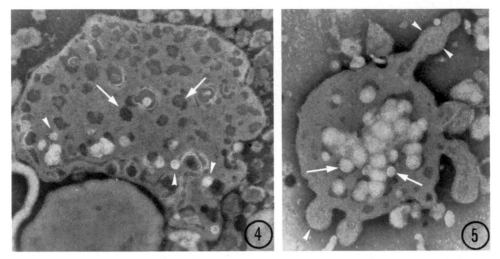

Fig. 4. Negatively stained fraction rich in Golgi membranes isolated from rat liver. As indicated in Fig. 3, "fenestrated" plates might be elaborated during the translocation of secretory material from the endoplasmic reticulum to the Golgi apparatus. The structure seen in this micrograph possibly represents such a fenestrated membrane, the "holes" (arrows) of which are penetrated by the negative stain (4% phosphotungstic acid). The arrow-heads point to structures which are tentatively interpreted as VLDL particles localized within the cavities of the fenestrated plate. × 56000

Fig. 5. Negatively stained fraction rich in Golgi membranes isolated from rat liver. This structure might represent an individual stacked Golgi lamella the central portion of which contains VLDL particles (arrows). Apparently, tubular protrusion (arrow-heads) emanate from the peripheral aspects of the lamella. They may either represent channels through which incoming VLDL particles reach the stacked saccules of the Golgi complex, or they may play a role in the morphogenesis of secretory granules. (cf. Fig. 3) × 56000

reinterpretation of the morphology of the Golgi system (and derived subfractions) as far as it was based on observations made on cell-free membrane preparations. However, it is conceivable that the Golgi membranes isolated from various cell types also display a different stability, and that this property has to be examined specifically for organelle fractions obtained from different cell sources. It was observed that two types of VLDL-containing secretory vacuoles can occur in the rat hepatocyte [276a]. One type of vesicles is preferentially located near the forming face of the Golgi complex and is characterized by an electron-translucent matrical space which surrounds relatively large VLDL particles. These structures were interpreted to represent immature secretory vesicles. In contrast, other vacuoles, occurring most frequently at the secreting face of the Golgi apparatus and in other cytoplasmic locations, had a darkly staining matrix which contained smaller VLDL particles than those observed in the "immature" species (and in the channels of the endoplasmic reticulum). This second kind of secretory granules are believed to represent a mature type of VLDL-carrying vacuoles. This interesting observation would imply that the VLDL particles are structurally altered during their migration and that the Golgi complex may represent the principal modifying site. It is, however, not clear

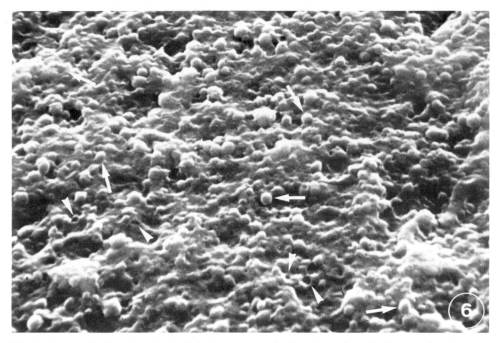

Fig. 6. Aspect of a fraction rich in Golgi membranes isolated from liver in the scanning electron microscope. Although the conventional preparation techniques used for scanning electron microscopy might introdue considerable artifacts into the preparations this (three-dimensional) micrograph nevertheless shows a number of bulb-like protrusions (arrows) which could possibly correspond to the tubular protrusions represented in Fig. 5. Arrow-heads indicate "holes" appearing in the more or less flat portions of the preparation. This micrograph was kindly supplied by Miss Christel Brücher. × 39600

whether the observed difference in size of VLDL particles is due to some changes pertaining the composition, mass, hydration, and/or conformation of the component molecules.

Thus, the morphological interpretation ascribes to the Golgi complex a collecting and packaging function which is possibly associated with a concomitant transformation or differentiation of the membranes within the stacks of Golgi lamellae [92, 287, 289]. In fact, many morphological [149], cytochemical [122, 130, 314, 341, 500], histochemical [81, 111] and autoradiographic observations [151] suggest that the Golgi membranes are heterogeneous in composition and enzymatic activity. It is conceivable that this heterogeneity could be a manifestation of chemical changes undergone by both the secretory products and the membranes themselves. The processes and the subcellular sites involved in the stepwise glycosylation of exportable acceptor proteins that were discussed in general terms in the previous sections, might also prove to be relevant to hepatocytic lipoprotein synthesis and release.

Some circumstantial evidence indicates that the final composition of circulating lipoproteins might be influenced by the synthetic activities of the Golgi apparatus. It has been shown that a particular polypeptide of human [62] and rat [39] serum apo-VLDL displays a chromatographic polymorphism likely to be due to variations in

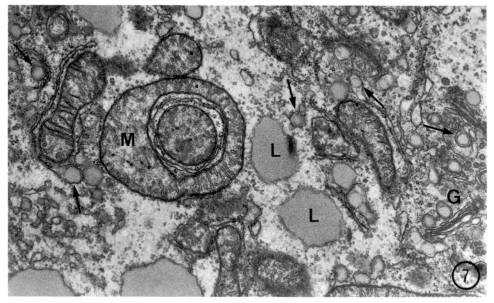

Fig. 7. Liver of rats fed a protein-deficient diet for 4 weeks. Apparently due to the dietary imbalance accumulations of lipid-rich particles or liposomes (arrows) occur within generally smooth-surfaced dilatations of the endoplasmic reticulum or near the Golgi apparatus (G). Note that the liposomes are, in contrast with the membrane-enclosed VLDL particles (cf. Fig. 1), electron-translucent and considerably larger. Large lipid droplets which possibly were generated by coalescence of liposomes are labeled by L. The deficiency in protein intake causes mitochondrial changes manifested by the occurence of ring-shaped organelles (M). × 20000

the sialic acid content of immunologically identical protein determinants. In addition, an extensive exchange *in vivo* and *in vitro* of low molecular apoprotein-polypeptides between VLDL and HDL was reported [104c, 105, 368b]. In human plasma at least one of these was shown to contain sialic acid [62, 62a]. It is thus conceivable that during this transfer the carbohydrate side chain of these apoproteins facilitates their mutual "recognition" [105]. Since the sugar components of plasma lipoprotein are thought to originate preferentially from the Golgi region of the hepatocyte, this organelle could therefore indirectly influence exchange processes between circulating lipoproteins.

It should be mentioned that some authors [126, 205] have proposed an alternative translocation scheme for lipoproteins, in which the Golgi apparatus is bypassed and the lipoprotein particles, possibly of a different quality [126], are directly transported by small smooth-surfaced vesicles from the rough-surfaced endoplasmic reticulum to the cell periphery facing the Disse space.

F. Release from the Cell

The lipoprotein particles may leave the Golgi region, clustered within smooth-surfaced secretory granules (Fig. 1), and eventually reach the plasma membrane facing the sinusoids [104, 156, 205, 420]. Since single lipoprotein particles have been observed to appear in the space of Disse [126, 156, 203 to 205, 243a, 422a] as well as in the perfusates during liver perfusion [29, 156, 204] it might be concluded that the membrane of secretory granules fuses with the plasma membrane [104, 156] in order to release, by a kind of "reversed pinocytosis", the VLDL particles into the extracellular space.

In the case of mammalian cells, the topographical details of this extrusion process are not known. During the exteriorization of secretory material by the protozoa tetrahymena, the membranes of the secretory granules were observed to interact with specific, structurally highly differentiated sites of the plasma membrane where the fusion of the two membrane types, prior to granule discharge, also occurred [376b]. Investigations on the phagocytosis by polymorphonuclear leukocytes indicated that the plasma membrane of these cells behaved like a functional mosaic in which membrane patches engaged in transmembrane transport were physically separated from those destinated to participate in phagocytosis [455a]. In the presence of antimitotic alkaloids (i.e., colchicine and vinblastine) the separation of these functionally different plasma membrane areas could no longer be observed, indicating that microtubules are possibly involved in the maintainance of important plasma membrane functions [455a]. By reasoning along these lines, the inhibitory effect of some antimitotic drugs on the secretion of lipoproteins by rat and mouse liver [243a, 313, 421, 422a] was tentatively interpreted in terms of an interaction of these compounds with microtubular elements which might lead to an impairment of contacts between VLDL-carrying secretory vacuoles and the hepatocytic plasma membrane [422a]. As a result of this inhibition, VLDL release into the circulation would be reduced, with a concomitant accumulation of secretory vacuoles in the cytoplasm of liver cells [243a, 422a]. By injecting radioactive fatty acids or glycerol into rats [27, 64, 140, 221], rabbits [160], or dogs [148], it was established that the first labeled triglycerides appear, presumably contained in secreted lipoproteins, after a lag of 7 to 20 min. A similar time schedule of phospholipid secretion was determined by means of autoradiography following the administration of choline-^{3}H to choline-deficient rats [420]. The "minimal transit time" of another hepatocytic secretory glycoprotein, transferrin, is roughly twice as long [286]. It seems, therefore, that the kinetics of the synthesis and secretion of lipoprotein by liver parenchymal cells are quite rapid [153] and comparable to those of albumin [322, 323], a non-glycosylated exportable protein which undergoes an apparently (cf. [136]) obligatory Golgi transit [139, 323].

G. Recapitulation

In summary, the biosynthesis and secretion of liver lipoproteins could be tentatively pictured as follows. It should be stressed, however, that only part of the proposed secretion scheme is based on work conducted in the field of lipoproteins, the other aspects having been imported from evidence collected in related areas of research. The component polypeptides of the VLDL molecule are synthesized on membrane-bound polyribosomes of the corresponding size. The nascent polypeptide chains grow vectorially into the channel system of the rough-surfaced endoplasmic reticulum. During this process of elongation of the ribosome-bound chain, the first sugar residues of the polysaccharide side chain are possibly added. The terminated protein chains are detached from the ribosome, and the majority of them now set out on their translocational path within the lumen of the endoplasmic reticulum. During the intracisternal displacement of the individual polypeptides, lipids (e.g., phospholipids, triglycerides, cholesterol, and cholesteryl esters) and sugar residues are added until, presumably at the junction between the rough- and smooth-surfaced endoplasmic reticulum, the component polypeptides are partially or fully charged with their respective lipid complement (cholesterol and its esters being added last). Their prosthetic carbohydrate groups now include all the "core" and semiterminal sugar residues. At this stage, a morphologically recognizable VLDL particle emerges.

Upon transfer to the Golgi complex, the growth of the polysaccharide chain is virtually completed by the addition of the terminal sugar residues. The VLDL particles are collected within Golgi-derived secretory vacuoles and transported to the plasmalemma which borders the space of Disse. At this site they are released into the extracellular space by a process resembling "reversed pinocytosis". It is clear that the above description is largely speculative; but it may reflect the obviously complex interplay between membrane-bound multienzyme systems which are progressively modifying moving macromolecules.

IV. Regulation of Lipoprotein Secretion

A. Compositional Variability of Lipoproteins

It is believed that the liver of normally fed animals secretes lipoprotein particles in which the various molecular components participate in more or less stoichiometric amounts [164, 165, 254, 256, 470]. Previously, it had been suggested that the compositional pattern of secreted VLDL was a rigid one, and that a metabolic deficiency in any one of its constituents would cause irregularities in lipoprotein secretion by the liver cell [165, 470]. Subsequent experiments, however, indicated that VLDL shows considerable compositional adaptability depending on various nutritional [79, 98, 163, 167, 180, 205, 220, 369, 370, 389, 404, 491] and hormonal [167, 253, 255] factors, as well as under certain experimental conditions such as experimental diabetes [164, 480]. Other experimental measures result in a more profound alteration of lipoprotein secretion.

There is ample evidence that choline-deficiency [248, 249, 285, 310] and treatment with ethionine [24, 44, 118, 189, 337], carbon tetrachloride [165, 189, 247], orotic acid [333, 363, 487, 488, 490], puromycin [203, 360], cycloheximide [199] and certain corticosteroids at high dosage [129, 341a] may interfere with lipoprotein metabolism at different levels of the biosynthetic pathways that converge to build up lipoproteins [247, 409]. As a result, triglycerides might accumulate in the liver, and its capacity to secrete lipoprotein is reduced or even abolished. During the establishment of a fatty liver these perturbations in lipoprotein biosynthesis possibly manifest themselves in the appearance of a particular kind of structures which are presumably rich in lipids, i.e., "liposomes".

B. The Nature of Cytoplasmic Lipid Particles

Characteristically, liposomal structures are spherical bodies of variable electron-density contained within smooth-surfaced cisternae or within smooth-surfaced vesicles in other cytoplasmic locations (Fig. 7). As a rule, their average diameter is greater

than that of typical VLDL particles [24, 247, 302, 385]. Eventually, individual liposomes may coalesce to form "giant liposomes" [24], which possess the morphological properties of typical cytoplasmic lipid droplets [24, 198, 302] and can be regarded as the structural expression of the fully developed fatty change. Liposomes
isolated from liver of rats treated with either ethionine [385] or orotic acid [333,
340] were shown to be rich in triglycerides and to contain considerable amounts of
proteins which may in part have electrophoretic and immunological properties in
common with apoproteins obtained from homologous plasma VLDL [333].

C. Effects of Lipid-lowering Agents

1. Actions of Aryloxyacetic acids

Regarding the formation of liposomes, the following sites of metabolic interference
have been considered [247, 310, 333]: a) fatty acid availability as influenced by the
influx, oxidation, synthesis *de novo*, and esterification of fatty acids; b) availability of
glycerophosphate; c) biosynthesis and utilization of triglycerides, including shifts
between the different intracellular pools; d) biosynthesis of phospholipids as constituents of lipoproteins and intracellular membranes; e) biosynthesis of proteins as
constituents of lipoproteins and intracellular membranes; f) biosynthesis of cholesterol and its esters as constituents of lipoproteins and intracellular membranes;
g) glycosylation of lipoproteins; h) generation of energy. There are obviously many
other possible sites of interference, and it is probable that the pharmacologic action
of any drug[2] effective in lowering the amount of circulating lipid will comprise
multiple metabolic effects. In fact, the following principal mechanisms of action have
been suggested to account for the lipid-lowering effect of CPIB and Su–13437:
a) displacement of hormones, especially of thyroxine, from binding sites on plasma
proteins, causing a hyperthyroid state in the liver [326, 327, 371]; b) stimulation of
peripheral removal of serum triglycerides [75, 77, 295, 372, 449, 466]; c) inhibition of
cholesterol biosynthesis [17, 23, 71, 228, 424, 477, 478]; d) decrease in hepatic fatty
acid synthesis [262, 263]; e) interference with the formation and secretion of lipoproteins by the liver [23, 41, 42, 71, 103, 145, 146, 169, 278, 321, 394, 430, 431, 473];
f) inhibition of hepatic biosynthesis of triglycerides [2, 229]; g) inhibitory or stimulating effects on mitochondria, possibly coupled with changes in the redox state of the
hepatocyte [208, 261, 321, 326, 502]; h) interference with the hepatic glycogen and
intermediary metabolism [382, 506]. Obviously, none of the presumptive mechanisms listed above would, by itself, explain the lipid-lowering effect of these drugs.
Wherever the decisive site or sites of interference of CPIB and Su–13437 may be, they
do not, according to the majority of authors, cause any appreciable accumulation of
triglycerides in liver [23, 91 a, 103, 146, 169, 278, 412]. These biochemical findings are
fully corroborated by morphological observations. In the livers of humans, monkeys
or rats, treated with either clofibrate or Su–13437 (Figs. 9, 14, 16), lipid-rich struc-

---

[2] In discussing drugs endowed with a hypolipidemic activity we shall confine ourselves mainly to
those belonging to the chemical group of α-aryloxyisobutyric acids, e.g. CPIB (Clofibrate,
Atromid S) and Su–13437 (nafenopin) [35]. Chemical, pharmacological and structural aspects of
other lipid-lowering agents have already been discussed in detail [35, 224, 439].

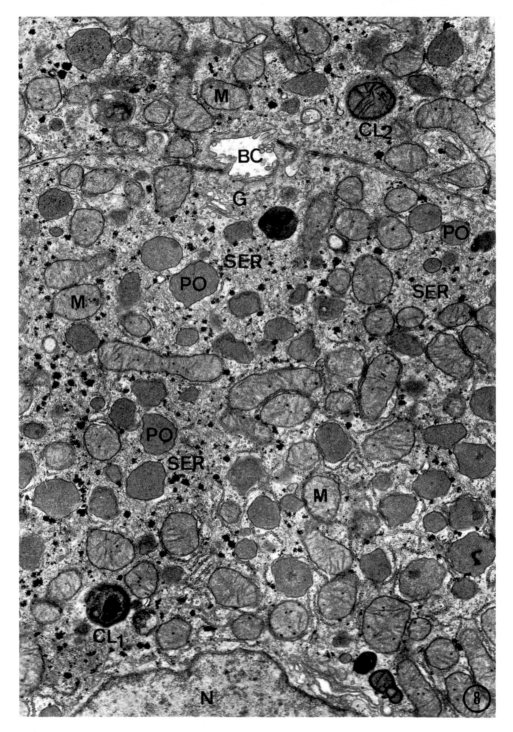

tures of the character and intracellular localization of liposomes (Fig. 7) have never been observed.

Obviously, the enumerations of conceivable mechanisms of action of fatty liver-inducing agents on the one hand and lipid-lowering compounds on the other have some items in common. In both cases a reduced release of lipoproteins by the liver is the most striking effect. Nevertheless, some specific metabolic events must intervene, in the case of the hypolipidemic drugs, which block the formation and accumulation of liposomal structures.

Since liposomes are known to be rich in triglycerides, it might be concluded that the metabolic handling and distribution of these lipids under the influence of the therapeutic agents is different from that observed when liposome-inducing "hepatotoxins" are administered. Morphological observations do indeed suggest that an essentially intact machinery for the synthesis, assembly, intracellular translocation and release of lipoproteins is slowed down by aryloxy acids. This conclusion is mainly based on the qualitative impression that in treated animals the occurrence of morphologically recognizable VLDL particles seems to be reduced (Fig. 8). Similar observations have been reported with respect to nicotinic acid [203]. The hypothesis that hepatic lipoprotein metabolism might be shifted to a lower steady state by the hypolipdemic drugs mentioned would, of course, not exclude the possibility that lipoproteins of an aberrant composition are secreted. In fact, some observations are in agreement with such an assumption [145, 174, 432]. Another experimental link between fatty-liver producing and hypolipidemic compounds was established when it was shown that CPIB and Su-13437 largely prevent the development of fatty livers after administration of orotic acid [108, 169, 475] or ethanol [60, 412]. More specifically, CPIB and Su-13437, along with other hypolipidemic drugs, restored the capacity of livers of orotic acid-treated rats to release beta-lipoproteins [108, 475]. Since isolated liposomes from orotic acid-induced fatty livers apparently contain the apoprotein determinants of all lipoprotein classes [333], it might be concluded that these drugs overcome or prevent the presumed lesions in the secretory apparatus of the hepatocyte caused by this steatogenic agent. The reasons why the lipid-lowering compounds stimulate the release of LDL rather than of VLDL by fatty livers is not understood; but it is conceivable that these drugs not only intervene at intracellular sites but also influence the metabolic interrelationships between circulating lipoproteins of different classes [104b, 104c, 105, 231, 368b, 486].

Fig. 8. Liver of rat treated with CPIB (100 mg/kg for 8 days). The most conspicuous change consists in a drug-induced expansion of the peroxisomal compartment. It is obvious that the numerical ratio mitochondria (M) to peroxisomes (PO) which in normal liver approximates 4 to 1 is shifted in favour of the peroxisomes (cf. Fig. 1). Characteristically, the smooth-surfaced endoplasmic reticulum (SER) is also expanded (cf. Fig. 1), indicating that the hepatocyte is in the induced state. The Golgi complexes (G) are, if anything, reduced in size and they often lack membrane-enclosed VLDL particles (cf. Fig. 1). The two structures labeled by CL represent cytolysosomes or autphagic vacuoles. They are thought to originate from a focal degradation event by means of which cytoplasmic constituents are segregated into a membrane-enclosed space. Affluent lysosomal particles would then participate in the breakdown of the segregated components. In fact, the autophagic vacuole labeled CL_1 contains an aggregate of glycogen particles, whereas the cytolysosome labeled CL_2 bears a structurally altered mitochondrion. N represents the nucleus and BC a bile canaliculus. × 16 300

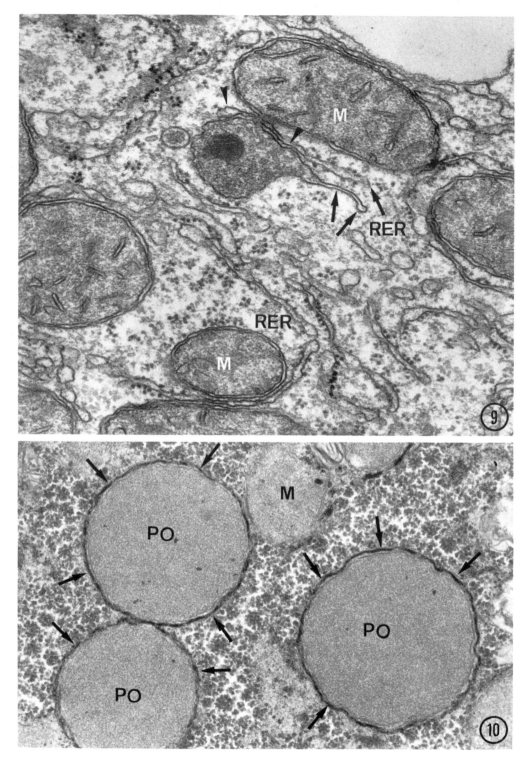

2. Liver Induction in the Rodent

Treatment of rodents with various α-aryloxyisobutyric acids elicits hepatomegaly [34a, 42, 91a, 169, 171, 184a, 244a, 327, 349a, 349b]. The question then arises whether the liver growth results from an increase in the number of hepatic cells or from enlargement of preexisting hepatic cells. It has been shown that CPIB treatment is followed by a slight increase in the total DNA content of the liver and a decrease per unit of weight, indicating a combined hypertrophic and hyperplastic effect [34a, 145]. This pattern of liver enlargement is reminiscent of that observed during phenobarbital induction of rat liver [416]. Following treatment with clofibrate or Su-13437 the enlarged liver contains, by comparison with untreated controls, more protein [23, 145, 327] and phospholipids [23, 145], whereas the estimations of the triglyceride contents are controversial [23, 42, 102, 145, 146, 169, 278, 321, 394]. These findings agree with the morphological aspect of livers of CPIB- or Su-13437-treated rats. They show a characteristic manifestation of the induced state of the hepatocyte [109, 138, 201, 356, 416] in the form of proliferation of the smooth-surfaced endoplasmic reticulum [21, 22, 171, 240, 241, 342, 438, 349b] (Fig. 8), increased amount of microsomal protein and phospholipid [91a], coupled with enhanced activity of a series of constitutive membrane enzymes belonging to the drug-metabolizing system of the endoplasmic reticulum [20, 91a, 169, 382]. It should be mentioned that some authors were unable to detect the biochemical manifestations of liver induction in treated animals [34a, 244a].

There is no published information available on the precise metabolic fate of aryloxyisobutyric acids. But it can be assumed that they are, possibly, chemically modified at the level of the hepatocytic endoplasmic reticulum. Subsequently, the drug or the metabolites are preferentially glucuronidized and excreted via bile or urine. It is known that part of this conjugation process takes place in the endoplasmic reticulum (cf. 147) and that its activity can be stimulated by some microso-

Fig. 9. Liver of rat treated with Su-13437 (10 mg/kg for 12 days). The peroxisome (or microbody) contains within its granular matrix an electron-dense tubular structure, the "core" or nucleoid. The nucleoid harbors exclusively the urate oxidase activity, whereas all of the other known peroxisomal enzymes are located in the matrix compartment. This particular peroxisome shows a tubular protrusion (double arrows) which is apparently devoid of matrix material and thus appears electron-translucent. Such finger-like smooth-surfaced structures have been interpreted to manifest an either permanent or intermittent membranous continuity between the smooth-surfaced endoplasmic reticulum and the peroxisomes. Note the close spatial relationship between the peroxisomal membrane and a smooth-surfaced profile (arrow-heads) which is continuous with the rough-surfaced endoplasmic reticulum (RER with arrow). Mitochondrial profiles and cisternae of rough-surfaced endoplasmic reticulum are labeled by M and RER, respectively. × 56000

Fig. 10. Liver of rat recovering from CPIB treatment (100 mg/kg for 14 days followed by withdrawal of the drug for 2 days). Individual peroxisomes (PO) are surrounded by membrane profiles (arrows) containing electron-dense reaction product (lead phosphate) which is deposited by the histochemical procedure revealing the activity of glucose-6-phosphatase. — This enzyme is regarded as a marker of the endoplasmic reticulum. This situation could be interpreted as representing an early stage in the formation of cytolysosomes (cf. Fig. 8). These particles may participate in the breakdown of the excess of peroxisomes which has formed under the stimulus of CPIB-treatment. A mitochondrial profile is labeled by M. × 42000

mal enzyme inducers [152, 218, 359, 507]. Thus, both drugs are endowed with the capacity to elicit the induced state of the hepatocyte.

3. The Peroxisome Problem

The hypolipidemic compounds clofibrate and Su-13437, like other aryloxyisobutyrates, share the rather uncommon ability to stimulate the volumetric and numerical expansion of the peroxisomal compartment [21, 171, 240, 241, 342, 343, 347, 348, 350, 413, 438, 441] (Fig. 8). Despite considerable experimental efforts, the metabolic significance of peroxisomes (microbodies) has not yet been fully elucidated [30, 93, 94, 182, 328]. According to the most comprehensive hypothesis, the peroxisomes of mammalian cells are particles containing a "primitive" (nonphosphorylating) respiratory chain [93, 94], which might, through a shuttling of various substrates of peroxisomal enzymes, be engaged in the reoxidation of cytosolic NADH [94, 457]. In addition, it has been suggested that some products of peroxisomal enzymes, such as α-keto acids, may be used as building blocks for gluconeogenesis [94]. Other theories ascribe to these particles a function in lipid metabolism [143, 301] or in the degradation of cholesterol [350]. Since the glycogen content of the livers of CPIB- and Su-13437-treated rats is generally reduced [506] and some key enzymes of gluconeogenesis are inhibited [382], increased generation of precursor for gluconeogenesis by peroxisomes seems to be an unlikely explanation. Although CPIB-treatment raises the hepatic $NAD/NADH_2$ ratio [326], the metabolic changes causing or motivating such a shift in the redox state of the hepatocyte are not understood. The peroxisomes of mammalian liver, unlike those of protozoa [178, 291], apparently lack the enzymes, e.g. isocitrate lyase, which are instrumental in linking lipid metabolism with gluconeogenesis [93]. The same difficulties are encountered in seeking a rational basis for a possible role of peroxisomes in the catabolism of cholesterol. It has been shown, for example, that the hypocholesterolemic effect of some drugs is not coupled with significant morphological or enzymatic changes in the peroxisomal compartment [185a].

Several observations indicate that the proliferating response of the peroxisomal compartment to CPIB treatment is not directly linked with the hypolipidemic effect of this drug. In hypothyroid rats, CPIB is ineffective in lowering serum lipids [40]. Nevertheless, it induces a rise in the number of peroxisomes and a corresponding increase in the specific activity of catalase in thyroidectomized animals [441]. Conversely, gonadectomy does not interfere with the hypolipidemic effect of CPIB [40], but this drug exerts its proliferating stimulus on peroxisomes in castrated rats only when supplemented with testosterone [441].

The peroxisomes of rat liver contain a set of hydrogen peroxide-producing oxidases [93] of which isocitrate dehydrogenase, urate oxidase, α-hydroxy acid oxidase and D-amino acid oxidase are of particular quantitative importance [243]. With the exception of urate oxidase, which is part of a highly ordered tubular core structure or nucleoid [183, 451], all these oxidative enzymes, along with the hydrogen peroxide-splitting catalase, are located within the more or less homogeneously structured peroxisomal matrix [94, 162]. Judging from the pattern of enzyme activity, the peroxisomes induced by CPIB or Su-13437 seem to be of a quality different from their normal counterparts. Although the specific activity of catalase in liver homogenates of treated rats is, at the most, doubled [21, 169, 171, 210, 343, 349 to 350, 441], the volumetric increase in the peroxisomal compartment is about 8-fold [413]. It follows that the proliferating peroxisomes should be deficient in catalase activity. A probably even more pronounced deficiency was also shown to occur in the case of some peroxisomal oxidases. It has been observed that the activity of α-hydroxy acid oxidase is greatly diminished [21], whereas conflicting data have been reported with regard to D-amino acid oxidase [21, 210]. The core-enzyme urate oxidase also showed reduced activity [171, 442], which was paralleled by a decrease in the frequency of core-containing particles among the expanding peroxisome population [210, 349b, 413, 438]. In addition, during purification experiments it was observed that the hepatic peroxisomes of clofibrate-treated rats seem to be more fragile than normal particles and to release a considerable amount of particle-bound catalase into the isolation medium [170]. Apparently the morphological aspect of proliferating peroxisomes is also changed: they become more polymorphic [210, 241, 349b, 438], the electron-density of their matrix possibly increases [184a, 241], new structural differentiations may occur in the matrical space [184a, 349b, 438], and they may show a greater frequency of membrane continuities with the smooth-surfaced endoplasmic reticulum [210, 349a, 438]. Taken as a whole, these observations point to the possibility that the administration of CPIB or Su-13437 to rats may provoke the emergence of a particular class of peroxisomes. The results of an analysis of particle diameters during Su-13437-stimulated proliferation and a successive recovery period could be interpreted in terms of the existence in hepatocytes of at least two populations, one representing the "normal" particles and the other comprising the expanding and recontracting pool of drug-induced peroxisomes [417].

Evidence based on inhibitor studies has been adduced indicating that drug-induced expansion of the peroxisomal compartment depends on the continuous formation of transcriptional and translational products [21, 350, 442]. But obviously, these conditions do not extend to the important peroxisomal enzyme catalase. Despite the presence of the effective inhibitor of catalase synthesis, allylisopropylacetamide [386], CPIB is still able to induce peroxisomal proliferation [241, 350]. Furthermore, CPIB exerts its stimulant effect on peroxisome formation in acatalasemic mice, which, owing to a genetic deficiency, are unable to produce a full complement of active catalase [342, 347, 348]. Thus, a continuous de novo synthesis of catalase is not essential to the peroxisome-inducing action of CPIB.

The question then arises as to the nature of the proteins contained within the proliferating peroxisomes. In normal peroxisomes, enzymes of known activity account for only about half of the total proteins of the particles [243]. Since, as already documented, the proliferating peroxisomes probably tend to be deficient in some particular enzymes, the proportion of proteins of obscure function should even be increased. With this argument in mind, experiments were performed with alkaline phosphatase-labeled anti-VLDL-antibodies [18] by means of established cytochemical techniques [187, 235, 236] to find out whether or not the expanding peroxisome population would contain proteins with the immunological properties of apo-VLDL [415].

Both direct and indirect procedures were unsuccessful, indicating either that hepatocytes of Su-13437-treated rats do not direct an excess of apoproteins, generated, for example, by a blockade of lipoprotein assembly, into the peroxisomal compart-

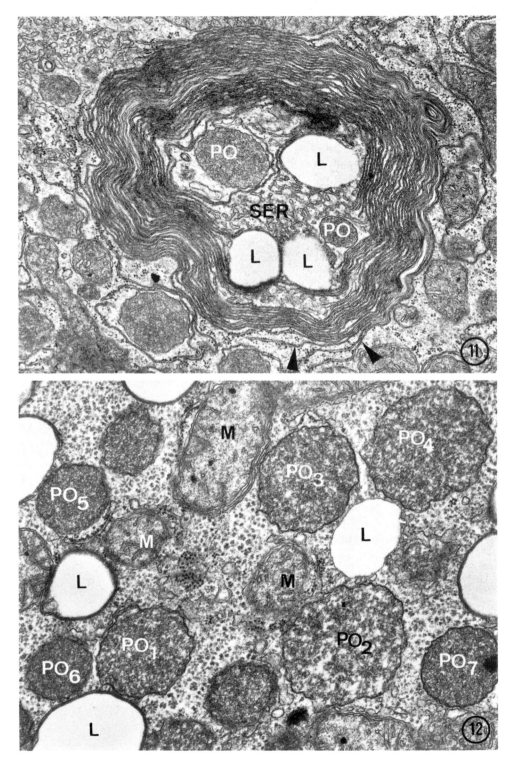

ment, or that the apoproteins at this subcellular locus are antigenically different from the serum VLDL of untreated animals used to provoke the antibody response. In this respect it should be mentioned that differences in the physico-chemical behaviour of lipoproteins of CPIB-treated rats, possibly due to aberrant properties of their protein moiety, have been demonstrated [175].

The uncertainty about the properties and functions of the majority of peroxisomal proteins also overshadows the problem of the morphogenesis of peroxisomes and their metabolic fate. Biochemical findings indicated that hepatic catalase is synthesized on a distinct class of polysomes [454], presumably (cf. [93a, 354a]) attached to the membranes of the endoplasmic reticulum [172, 173]. In an earlier study it was found that the catalase molecules subsequently appeared in the mitochondrial fraction [173] which most likely contained the peroxisomes also. Recent kinetic evidence, however, supports an alternative pathway for newly synthesized catalase [234, 234a, 234b, 354a]. The newly formed enzyme molecules are thought to be released by polysomes into the soluble fraction of the hepatocytes, most probably in the form of a aposubunit intermediate [234a]. These apoprotein monomers would then be transferred from the cytosol to the peroxisomal compartment, where the incorporation of the heme prosthetic group into the apoprotein would take place; in the same cellular location, the subunits would be assembled into the authentic tetrameric catalase molecule [234b]. It should be added that the biosynthetic pathway of other peroxisomal enzymes or components is unknown.

Morphological observations have disclosed an intimate spatial relationship between the peroxisomes and the endoplasmic reticulum [45, 110, 157, 210, 279, 300, 301, 303, 306, 342, 346, 438, 452]. Specifically, the occurence, within smooth-surfaced terminal dilatations of rough-surfaced cisternae, of deposits with similar optical properties to those of the peroxisomal matrix material and the presence of membranous continuities between the endoplasmic reticulum and the peroxisomes have been interpreted to reflect an involvement of the endoplasmic reticulum (Fig. 9) in the morphogenesis of peroxisomes. It has been postulated that these connections between the two compartments are maintained throughout the life-cycle of the peroxi-

Fig. 11. Liver of rats recovering from CPIB treatment (100 mg/kg for 14 days followed by withdrawal of the drug for 8 days). During recovery from drug treatment an extensive remodeling of the cell structure occurs. More specifically, the excess of peroxisomes and smooth-surfaced endoplasmic reticulum is disposed by means of different processes. In Figs. 8 and 9 the mode of autophagic disposal was depicted. This process possibly leads, by an exaggerated accretion of predominantly smooth-surfaced membranes, to large fingerprint-like membrane whorls. Peroxisomes *(PO)*, smooth-surfaced tubules *(SER)* and lipid droplets *(L)* may be enclosed within such structures. At some places (arrow-heads) the membranes leave the whorl and become rough-surfaced. It is not known how hydrolytic enzymes are introduced into these membrane complexes. × 22400

Fig. 12. Liver of rats recovering from CPIB-treatment (100 mg/kg for 14 days followed by withdrawal of the drug for 14 days). This micrograph illustrates the second pathway of destruction which is tentatively proposed for the removal of excess of peroxisomes. Some of the peroxisomal profiles $(PO_1$ to $PO_4)$ are distinguished from other ones $(PO_5$ to $PO_7)$ by a less electron-dense matrix. This loss in matrix density is interpreted as a sign of particle dissolution without the extensive participation of segregating membranes (cf. Figs. 8 and 9). Mitochondria *(M)* and lipid droplets *(L)* are present. × 28000

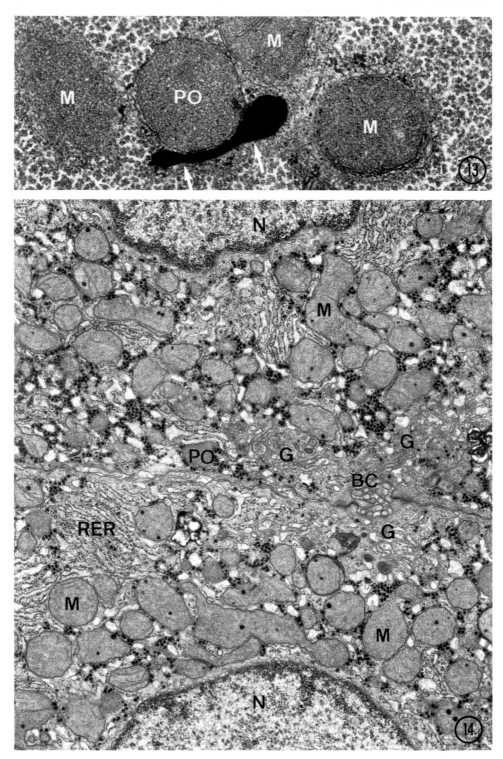

somes [300, 301]. According to this view, these two subcellular compartments would form a single pool in which peroxisomal material could flow unrestrictedly [342, 346]. The existence of such connections between endoplasmic reticulum membranes and catalase-bearing particles was also suggested by biochemical studies on the subcellular distribution of catalase in the normal liver and in hepatoma [468, 469]. Other authors have been unable to detect such patent continuities linking the peroxisomes to the endoplasmic reticulum [91, 114, 240]. In view of these contradictory findings and the observation that, following the histochemical demonstration of peroxidase activity, the reaction product occurs on free [114, 115] and membrane-bound ribosomes [114, 115, 242, 358, 501] in the neighbourhood of peroxisomes, alternative mechanisms of peroxisome formation have been postulated. According to one theory, peroxisomal proteins could be directly transferred from the site of their synthesis on ribosomes to pre-existing particles without an intracisternal passage [115, 240]; or possibly, during de novo biosynthesis of peroxisomes the catalase may focally accumulate within the cytoplasmic matrix and later on be enveloped by a limiting membrane [114]. Although this proposed sequence is compatible with many of the biochemical findings reported previously [234, 234a, 234b, 354a], some authors have expressed doubts concerning the relevance of the ribosomal location of the product generated by the histochemical peroxidase reaction [93a, 300, 305]. Indeed, recent experiments recognized the ribosomal location of peroxidase activity as a preparation artifact [114a]. In view of the still unsolved problem of peroxisome morphogenesis, recent morphological observations are of interest, describing the occurence of specialized structures of the endoplasmic reticulum which are claimed to participate in the formation of peroxisomes [184a]. These structures, by virtue of their particular organization, might be able to collect peroxisomal material from the soluble compartment of the hepatocyte and thus satisfy biochemical requirements [234, 234a, 234b, 354a].

There is a growing body of evidence in favor of the occurrence of fragmenting or fusioning peroxisomes during CPIB-induced proliferation [240, 342], liver regeneration [115, 358] and recovery from treatment with agents interfering with catalase activity or synthesis [241]. Since no peroxidase-deficient particles, as assayed by histochemical procedures, appeared under these experimental conditions, it has been suggested that the newly formed catalase may be extensively redistributed, possibly by multiple fission and fusion of particles, among the whole peroxisomal population.

Fig. 13. Liver of rats recovering from CPIB treatment (100 mg/kg for 14 days followed by withdrawal of the drug for 2 days). The histochemical demonstration of acid phosphatase activity (28) reveals the presence of a tubular structure (arrows) which is in close apposition to a peroxisome (PO). The electron-dense reaction product contained within the saccule is thought to be due to the presence of acid phosphatase activity which may participate in the dissolution process already refered to in the legend to Fig. 11. The structures labeled by M represent mitochondrial profiles. × 56000

Fig. 14. Liver biopsy of a female patient treated with Su-13437 (600 mg/day for 33 days). The treatment did not induce ultrastructural changes. Neither the peroxisomes (PO) nor the mitochondria (M) display numerical or structural alterations. N nucleus; RER rough-surfaced endoplasmic reticulum; G Golgi apparatus; BC bile canaliculus. The biopsy was obtained through the courtesy of Dr. M. SCHÖNBECK, Kantonsspital Zürich. × 16300

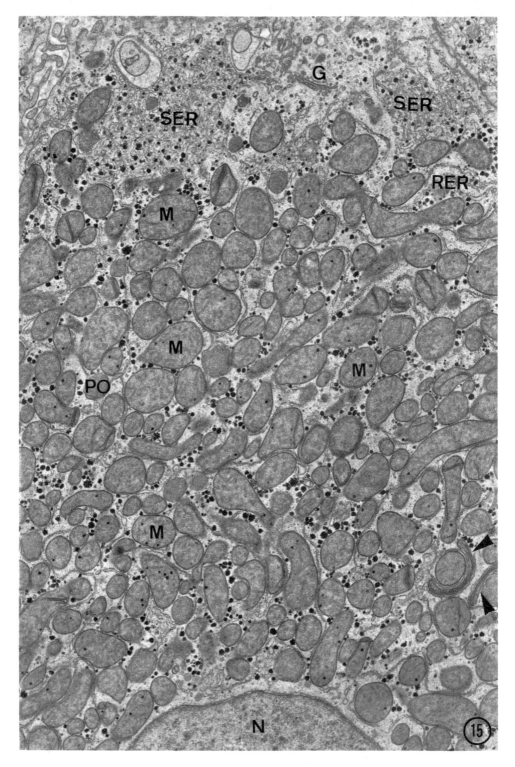

Irrespective of their actual volume, the peroxisomes incorporate labeled amino acids into their catalase to approximately the same extent [331]. Whether the peroxisome progressively enlarges during its morphogenesis is therefore unlikely to be of any relevance, and fragmentation and fusion of these particles have also been invoked to explain their uniform labeling [331].

The appearance of a large excess of peroxisomes in hepatocytes of α-aryloxyisobutyric acid-treated rats raises the question as to how the cell eliminates them upon withdrawal of the inducing drugs. Most of the biochemical data relating to the turnover of various peroxisomal proteins are in agreement with the notion that they all have a similar half-life and, consequently, the particles are destroyed as a unit [328, 332, 334]. It should be added, however, that the concept of peroxisomal proteins having identical half-lives has been in part revoked [329]. In most cases, comparatively large organelles, such as peroxisomes, would appear to be segregated as a whole into a space bounded by a membrane (Fig. 10)—the cytolysome or autophagic vacuole (Figs. 8 and 11)—where they are presumably destroyed by incoming hydrolytic enzymes [15, 99, 299].

In several instances, this concept of bulk destruction of peroxisomes has been questioned on the basis of histochemical and morphological observations. For example, during recovery from treatments interfering with the activity or biosynthesis of catalase, this enzyme showed a pattern of behavior apparently independent of the majority of peroxisomal proteins [241, 242]. The disposal of the excess of hepatic peroxisomes following the cessation of treatment with CPIB or Su-13437 was not necessarily coupled with the appearance of a large number of peroxisome-containing cytolysomes [442]. In fact, it seems that the destruction of microbodies involves two distinct pathways. The first follows the same pattern as cytolysosomal destruction, eventually culminating in the formation of whorl-like membranous structures (Fig. 11); the second is less dramatic and is suggestive of a progressive dissolution of peroxisomes within the cytoplasmic matrix, without the involvement of segregating membranes [241, 440, 442] (Fig. 12). It seems possible that this second process is assisted by vesicular structures of a rather uncommon intracellular location, which obviously contain acid hydrolases (Fig. 13). They may assumed tentatively to be related to the "reticulotubular structures" recently described [461]. It is not known whether the two mechanisms generate break-down products of a different quality that may be reutilized by the cell in separate metabolic pathways. It is noteworthy, however, that a similar dichotomy of peroxisomal destruction was observed during the developmental changes occurring in the fat body of an insect [246].

Fig. 15. Liver of monkey treated with Su-13437 (250 mg/kg for 90 days). Prolonged treatment of monkeys with a high dose of Su-13437 apparently causes, in contrast to the rodent, reversible changes in the mitochondrial compartment. The numer and structure of peroxisomes *(PO)* seems not to be altered. As compared to the controls the number of mitochondria *(M)* is considerably increased. In addition, the inner membranes of some of these organelles are redistributed and form parallelized or concentric arrays (arrow-heads). The rough-surfaced endoplasmic reticulum *(RER)* is scarce, whereas the smooth-surfaced membranes *(SER)* are extensively developed. The Golgi apparatus *(G)* appears to be reduced and somewhat fragmented. Part of the nucleus *(N)* appears on the bottom of the micrograph. The material was obtained through the courtesy of Drs. R.M. DIENER and S. THOMPSON, CIBA-GEIGY Corporation, Pharmaceuticals Division, Summit, N.J., USA. × 16250

Evidence is accumulating that in mammalian organisms peroxisomes are not mainly restricted to liver and kidney cells but are of rather widespread distribution [5, 6, 33, 86, 157, 166a, 184, 185, 251, 300, 304, 342, 344, 345, 387, 400a]. It has been speculated that the relatively large peroxisomes found in the liver and kidney may represent a class of particles distinct from the smaller peroxisomes ("microperoxisomes") occurring in most tissues [304], which are, as a rule, devoid of core-structures and connected by multiple continuities to the endoplasmic reticulum [300, 303, 304, 306]. Generally, CPIB and Su-13437 induce, in rodents, peroxisomal proliferation in the parenchymal cells of the liver and in the proximal tubular cells of the kidney [442]. It is not known what influence these drugs have on the fate of microperoxisomes, although it has been suggested that these may be morphogenetic precursors of the larger particles [300]. Little information is available as to whether or not treatment with CPIB or Su-13437 causes a volumetric or numerical increase in hepatic peroxisomes in higher mammals. Peroxisome counts made in a small number of liver biopsies from patients treated with clofibrate revealed a moderate decrease in the mitochondria:peroxisome ratio [439]. Electron microscopy of liver biopsies from a number of patients treated with Su-13437 did not disclose, except possibly in one single case, any notable increase in the number of microbodies present (Fig. 14). The same observations were made in livers obtained from rhesus monkeys given Su-13437 (Fig. 15).

4. Effects on Mitochondria

The lipid-lowering agents CPIB and Su-13437 may also affect various mitochondrial functions. They stimulate, for example, the activity of α-glycerophosphate dehydrogenase [169 to 171, 207a, 208, 321, 475, 476]. It has been suggested tentatively that this enzyme may be involved in a shuttle mechanism by means of which reducing equivalents are transported from the soluble compartment into the mitochondria, the net effect being a reoxidation of cytosolic NADH [63, 112]. The activity of α-glycerophosphate dehydrogenase is also increased by the administration of thyroxine [207a, 237, 238]. The metabolic reason for this apparent activation of the α-glycerophosphate shuttle is not fully understood. It has been interpreted as a means of controlling the availability of α-glycerophosphate for triglyceride synthesis [321]. It should be mentioned that the expanding peroxisomal compartment would probably also help to promote an accelerated NADH oxidation. Following the administration of a single dose of CPIB to rats, the subsequently isolated liver mitochondria showed, in contrast to other subcellular fractions, a greatly increased capacity to incorporate in vivo labeled amino acids; this stimulating effect was related to the enhanced activity of mitochondrial α-glycerophosphate dehydrogenase [321] which may be synthesized de novo [476]. The administration of these drugs in vivo enhanced the capacity of mitochondria to oxidize cholesterol [226] and deacylate acetoacetyl-CoA [67] in vitro, whereas some oxidative functions [210, 227] and the state of the respiratory chain [227] seemed not to be affected. Similarly, CPIB activated liver carnitine acetyltransferase [207a], an enzyme known to display a dual subcellular distribution, i.e. in mitochondria and peroxisomes [263a].

Neither of these hypolipidemic drugs apparently causes extensive quantitative or qualitative alterations in the mitochondrial compartment of rodent livers. CPIB has

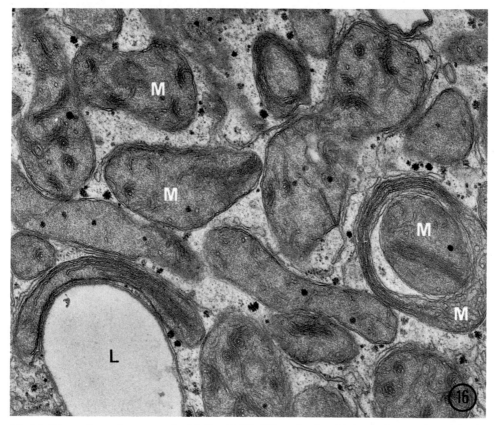

Fig. 16. Liver of monkey treated with Su-13437 (250 mg/kg for 90 days). As mentioned in the legend to Fig. 13, the main cytological changes by Su-13437 in monkeys affect the mitochondria. This micrograph shows a collection of structurally altered mitochondria *(M)*. The inner membranes are redistributed and may acquire a parallelized or concentric arrangement. Note the close spatial relationship between a lipid droplet *(L)* and a mitochondrium containing parallelized cristae. × 32500

been reported to increase the mitochondrial protein [91a, 227, 321] or to leave it unchanged [208]. Morphometric analysis of livers obtained from chronically CPIB-treated rats did not reveal any major fluctuations in the volumetric density of mitochondria, although a progressive decrease in their number was noted [413], indicating an increment in the volume of the individual organelle [357]. The structural organization of rat liver mitochondria remains relatively unchanged during drug treatment. They have been reported to be either unaltered [349b, 442] or to be more pleomorphic and to contain an increased number of matrix granules [241]. According to other observations, the mitochondria show transient swelling and deformation for a short time after the administration of CPIB [210].

In monkey liver, however, Su-13437 caused an increase in the number of mitochondria, concomitantly with an extensive rearrangement of inner membranes in some of them (Figs. 15 and 16). Human liver mitochondria from patients treated with Su-13437 did not manifest apparent morphological changes (cf. Fig. 14).

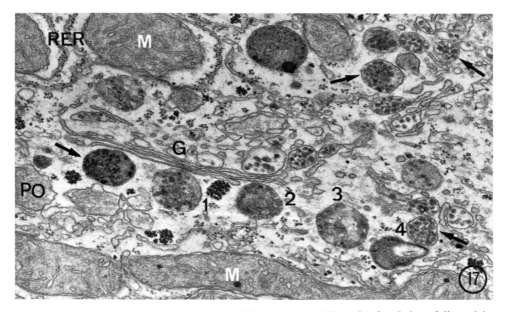

Fig. 17. Liver of rats recovering from Su-13437 treatment (100 mg/kg for 5 days followed by withdrawal of the drug for 7 days). This micrograph represents a Golgi zone *(G)* comprising stacked saccules and a series of secretory granules which contain VLDL particles (arrows). As mentioned in the text the possibility of a gradual transformation of VLDL-containing secretory granules into particles of a lysosomal aspect should be considered. The granules labeled by 1, 2, 3, and 4 might represent such a transformation sequence. Particle 1 bears clearly recognizable VLDL particles; within granule 2, the lipoprotein particles possibly have an altered appearance. Granule 3 contains clear (triglyceride-rich?) areas together with darker regions which might consist of confluent VLDL particles. Seemingly, these are no longer visible in granule 4, which, then, might represent a lysosome-like structure. Mitochondria *(M)*, peroxisomes *(PO)* and rough-surfaced endoplasmic reticulum *(RER)* are present. × 35000

5. Relationship between VLDL-Containing Secretion Granules and Lysosomes

During the physiological involution of mammotrophic hormone-producing cells of the rat anterior pituitary gland lysosomes have been shown to function in the regulation of the secretion process [408]. In the course of CPIB and Su-13437 treatment the activity of liver lysosomal enzymes remains relatively unchanged [22, 210, 226]. After the withdrawal of CPIB of Su-13437 the hepatomegaly is reversed. In addition to the disposal of the excess peroxisomes and endoplasmic reticulum membranes, this restoration involves the more frequent appearance in the Golgi zone of secretory vesicles containing lipoprotein particles (Fig. 17). Morphological observations suggest that a structural relationship between these VLDL-containing vesicles and lysosomal particles is established. The secretory granules seem to be progressively transformed into particles of a lysosomal character (Fig. 17), a process which has recently been reported to occur in the livers of ethanol-treated rats [104]. During this apparent transformation process, intermediary structures appear enclosing globular material displaying the optical characteristics of neutral lipids (Fig. 17). These particles bear some morphological resemblance to those found in the liver of cortisone-treated rabbits, which have also been interpreted as being lysosomes engaged in the catabolism of lipids [255]. In fact, lysosomes have been reported to display a spectrum of hydrolytic enzyme activities covering virtually all lipid classes [124, 127, 150, 252, 276, 292, 406, 427—429, 465]. The metabolic reasons underlying such transformation processes are not known, but they may reflect some imbalance in lipoprotein secretion, as has also been reported to occur in hepatocytes after administration of colchicine or vinblastine to rats [422a].

V. Concluding Remarks

The present review has emphasized the secretory aspect of the liver cell, and especially its capacity to synthesize, transport and release lipoproteins into the circulation. There are further aspects that have not been dealt with, for instance the important part played by the liver in the catabolism of serum lipoproteins [104b, 161, 422b].

The functional and structural framework within which the hepatocyte processes its exportable products has been described in detail, with special reference to the significant position occupied by the Golgi complex. In the context of the membrane flow concept, the correlative study of chemical, morphological and metabolic properties of purified fractions of Golgi membranes or of subfractions derived from them is considered to be of prime importance [104, 276a, 314a]. Investigations of the stability of Golgi membranes under different experimental conditions [280] and the analysis of their structural microenvironment [125] may lead to a better understanding of such phenomena as intermembrane cohesion and polarity.

The dual function of the Golgi apparatus as an accepting and delivering membrane system presupposes highly dynamic properties. These could possibly be assayed *in vitro* by means of transfer experiments between various purified subcellular fractions. Similar experiments already performed with artificial mixtures of microsomes and mitochondria [48, 378, 495 to 498] could serve as a model. Once established, such an *in vitro* transfer system could indicate dynamic deficiences of particular membrane compartments.

A further possibility might consist in testing the capacity of hypolipidemic drugs to interfere with specific steps in the secretion cycle of lipoproteins. Studies performed with a variety of agents have already shown that this approach can contribute valuable information [104, 132, 255, 421]. Finally, an example was given of the bewildering complexity of the biological effects exerted by two selected hypolipidemic drugs. The heterogeneous response pattern precluded a systematic and rational interpretation of the effects elicited by these compounds. One of their most interesting—though still in many respects obscure—properties is their ability to stimulate the reversible proliferation of peroxisomes in rodents.

Acknowledgement:

The assistance given by Mrs. A.M.KYBURZ, Mr. A.H.KIRKWOOD M.A., and by Mr. M.SCHLIENGER in the preparation of the manuscript is greatly acknowledged.

References

1. Adams, C. W. M.: Tissue changes and lipid entry in developing atheroma. In: Porter, R., Knight, J. (Eds.): Atherogenesis: Initiating Factors. CIBA Foundation Symposium, Vol. 12, pp. 5—30. Amsterdam: Elsevier 1973.

2. Adams, L, L., Webb, W. W., Fallon, H. J.: Inhibition of hepatic triglyceride formation by clofibrate. J. clin. Invest. **50**, 2339—2346 (1971).

3. Adelman, M. R., Sabatini, D. D., Blobel, G.: Ribosome-membrane interaction. Nondestructive diassembly of rat liver rough microsomes into ribosomal and membranous components. J. Cell Biol. **56**, 206—229 (1973).

4. Adelman, M. R., Borisy, G. G., Shelanski, M. L., Weisenberg, R. C., Taylor, E. W.: Cytoplasmic filaments and tubules. Fed. Proc. **27**, 1186—1193 (1968).

5. Ahlabo, I.: Observations on peroxisomes in the sustentocytus (sertoli cells) of the cat. J. Submicr. Cytol. **4**, 83—88 (1972).

6. Ahlabo, I., Barnard, T.: Observations on peroxisomes in brown adipose tissue of the rat. J. Histochem. Cytochem. **19**, 670—675 (1971).

7. Alaupovic, P., Lee, D. M., McConathy, W. J.: Studies on the composition and structure of plasma lipoproteins. Distribution of lipoprotein families in major density classes of normal human plasma lipoproteins. Biochim. biophys. Acta (Amst.) **260**, 689—707 (1972).

8. Albers, J. J., Scanu, A. M.: Isoelectric fractionation and characterization of polypeptides from human serum very low density lipoproteins. Biochim. biophys. Acta (Amst.) **236**, 29—37 (1971).

9. Alcindor, L. G., Infante, R., Soler-Argilaga, C., Raisonnier, A., Polonovski, J., Caroli, J.: Induction of the hepatic synthesis of β-lipoproteins by high concentrations of fatty acids. Effect of actinomycin D. Biochim. biophys. Acta (Amst.) **210**, 483—486 (1970).

10. Amsterdam, A., Ohad, I., Schramm, M.: Dynamic changes in the ultrastructure of the acinar cell of the rat parotid gland during the secretory cycle. J. Cell Biol. **41**, 753—773 (1969).

11. Amsterdam, A., Schramm, M., Ohad, I., Salomon, Y., Selinger, Z.: Concomitant synthesis of membrane protein and exportable protein of the secretory granule in rat parotid gland. J. Cell Biol. **50**, 187—200 (1971).

12. Andersson, J., Melchers, F.: Induction of immunoglobulin M synthesis and secretion in bone-marrow-derived lymphocytes by locally concentrated concanavalin A. Proc. nat. Acad. Sci. (Wash.) **70**, 416—420 (1973).

13. Andrews, T. M., Tata, J. R.: Protein synthesis by membrane-bound and free ribosomes of secretory and non-secretory tissues. Biochem. J. **121**, 683—694 (1971).

14. Arstila, A. U., Trump, B. F.: Ethionine induced alterations in the Golgi apparatus and in the endoplasmic reticulum. Virchows Arch. Abt. B Zellpath. **10**, 344—353 (1972).

15. Ashford, T. P., Porter, K. R.: Cytoplasmic components in hepatic cell lysosomes. J. Cell Biol. **12**, 198—202 (1962).

16. Askonas, B. A., Williamson, A. R.: Interchain disulfide-bond formation in the assembly of immunoglobulin G. Heavy chain dimer as an intermediate. Biochem. J. **109**, 637—643 (1968).

17. Avoy, D. R., Swyryd, E. A., Gould, R. G.: Effects of α-p-chlorophenoxyisobutyryl ethyl ester (CPIB) with and without androsterone on cholesterol biosynthesis in rat liver. J. Lipid Res. **6**, 369—376 (1965).

18. Avrameas, S.: Coupling of enzymes to proteins with glutaraldehyde. Use of the conjugates for the detection of antigens and antibodies. Immunochemistry **6**, 43—52 (1969).

19. Avrameas, S., Leduc, E. H.: Detection of simultaneous antibody synthesis in plasma cells and specialized lymphocytes in rabbit lymph nodes. J. exp. Med. **131**, 1137—1168 (1970).

20. Azarnoff, D. L.: Pharmacology of hypolipidemic drugs. Fed. Proc. **30**, 827—828 (1971).

21. Azarnoff, D. L., Svoboda, D.: Changes in microbodies in the rat induced by ethyl p-chlorophenoxyisobutyrate. J. Lab. clin. Med. **68**, 854 (1966).

22. Azarnoff, D. L., Tucker, D. R.: The effect of clofibrate on liver enzymes and substrates. Fed. Proc. **25**, 388 (1966).

23. Azarnoff, D. L., Tucker, D. R., Barr, G. A.: Studies with ethyl chlorophenoxyisobutyrate (clofibrate). Metabolism **14**, 959—965 (1965).

24. BAGLIO, C. M., FARBER, E.: Reversal by adenine of the ethionine-induced lipid accumulation in the endoplasmic reticulum of the rat liver. A preliminary report. J. Cell. Biol. **27**, 591—601 (1965).

25. BAGLIONI, C., BLEIBERG, I., ZAUDERER, M.: Assembly of membrane-bound polyribosomes. Nature (Lond.) New Biol. **232**, 8—12 (1971).

26. BAILEY, J. M.: Regulation of cell cholesterol content. In: PORTER, R., KNIGHT, J. (Eds.): Atherogenesis: Initiating Factors. CIBA Foundation Symposium, Vol. 12, pp. 63—88. Amsterdam: Elsevier 1973.

27. BAKER, N., SCHOTZ, M. C.: Use of multicompartmental models to measure rates of triglyceride metabolism in rats. J. Lipid Res. **5**, 188—197 (1964).

28. BARKA, T., ANDERSON, P. J.: Histochemical methods for acid phosphatase using hexazonium pararosanilin as coupler. J. Histochem. Cytochem. **10**, 741—753 (1962).

29. BAR-ON, H., KOOK, A. I., STEIN, O., STEIN, Y.: Assembly and secretion of very low density lipoproteins by rat liver following inhibition of protein synthesis with cycloheximide. Biochim. biophys. Acta (Amst.) **306**, 106—114 (1973).

30. BAUDHUIN, P.: Liver peroxisomes, cytology and function. Ann. N.Y. Acad. Sci. **168**, 214—228 (1969).

31. BAUDHUIN, H., REUSE, J., DUMONT, J. E.: Nondepence of secretion on protein synthesis. Life Sci. **6**, 1723—1731 (1967).

32. BEAMS, H. W., KESSEL, R. G.: The Golgi apparatus: structure and function Int. Rev. Cytol. **23**, 209—276 (1968).

33. BEARD, M. E.: Identification of peroxisomes in the rat adrenal cortex. J. Histochem. Cytochem. **20**, 173—179 (1972).

34. BECKER, M. J., RICH, A.: Polyribosomes of tissues producing antibodies Nature (Lond.) **212**, 142—146 (1966).

34 A. BECKETT, R. B., WEISS, R., STITZEL, R. E., CENEDELLA, R. J.: Studies on the hepatomegaly caused by the hypolipidemic drugs nafenopin and clofibrate. Toxicol. appl. Pharmacol. **23**, 42—53 (1972).

35. BENCZE, W. L., HESS, R., DE STEVENS, G.: Hypolipidemic agents. In: JUCKER, E. (Ed.): Progress in Drug Research, Vol. 13, pp. 217—292. Basel: Birkhäuser 1969.

36. BENNETT, G., LEBLOND, C. P.: Passage of fucose-^{3}H label from the Golgi apparatus into dense and multivesicular bodies in the duodenal columnar cells and hepatocytes of the rat. J. Cell Biol. **51**, 875—881 (1971).

37. BENSCH, K. G., MALAWISTA, S. E.: Microtubular crystals in mammalian cells. J. Cell Biol. **40**, 95—107 (1969).

38. BERGERON, J. J. M., EHRENREICH, J. H., SIEKEVITZ, P., PALADE, G. E.: Golgi fractions prepared from rat liver homogenates. II. Biochemical characterization. J. Cell Biol. **59**, 73—88 (1973).

38 a. BERNACKI, R. J.: Plasma membrane ectoglycosyltransferase activity of L 1210 murine leukemic cells. J. Cell Physiol. **83**, 457—466 (1974).

39. BERSOT, T. P., BROWN, W. V., LEVY, R. I., WINDMUELLER, H. G., FREDRICKSON, D. S., LEQUIRE, V. S.: Further characterization of the apolipoproteins of rat plasma lipoproteins. Biochemistry **9**, 3427—3433 (1970).

40. BEST, M. M., DUNCAN, C. H.: Hypolipemia and hepatomegaly from ethyl chlorophenoxyisobutyrate (CPIB) in the rat. J. Lab. clin. Med. **64**, 634—642 (1964).

41. BEST, M. M., DUNCAN, C. H.: Effects of clofibrate and dextrothyroxine singly and in combination on serum lipids. Arch. intern. Med. **118**, 97—102 (1966).

42. BEST, M. M., DUNCAN, C. H.: Lipid effects of a phenolic ether (Su-13437) in the rat: comparison with CPIB. Atherosclerosis **12**, 185—192 (1970).

43. BEVAN, M. J.: The vectorial release of nascent immunoglobulin peptides. Biochem. J. **122**, 5—11 (1971).

44. BEZMAN-TARCHER, A., NESTEL, P. J., FELTS, J. M., HAVEL, R. J.: Metabolism of hepatic and plasma triglycerides in rabbits given ethanol or ethionine. J. Lipid. Res. **7**, 248—257 (1966).

44 a. BIZZI, A., MARSH, J. B.: Further observations on the attachment of carbohydrate to lipoproteins by rat liver Golgi membranes. Proc. Soc. exp. Biol. Medicine **144**, 762—765 (1973).

45. BLACK, V. H., BOGART, B. I.: Peroxisomes in inner adrenocortical cells of fetal and adult guinea pigs. J. Cell Biol. **57**, 345—358 (1973).

46. BLASCHKO, H., FIREMARK, H., SMITH, A. D., WINKLER, H.: Lipids of the adrenal medulla. Lysolecithin, a characteristic constituent of chromaffin granules. Biochem. J. **104**, 545—549 (1967).
47. BLOBEL, G., SABATINI, D. D.: Controlled proteolysis of nascent polypeptides in rat liver cell fractions. I. Location of the polypeptides within ribosomes. J. Cell Biol. **45**, 130—145 (1970).
48. BLOK, M. C., WIRTZ, K. W. A., SCHERPHOF, G. L.: Exchange of phospholipids between microsomes and inner and outer mitochondrial membranes of rat liver. Biochim. biophys. Acta (Amst.) **233**, 61—75 (1971).
49. BLYTH, C. A., COOPER, M. B., ROBOOL, A., RABIN, B. R.: The binding of steroid hormones to degranulated microsomes from rat-liver endoplasmic reticulum. Europ. J. Biochem. **29**, 293—300 (1972).
50. BLYTH, C. A., FREEDMAN, R. B., RABIN, B. R.: Sex specific binding of steroid hormones to microsomal membranes. Nature (Lond.) New Biol. **230**, 137—139 (1971).
51. BORGESE, D., BLOBEL, G., SABATINI, D. D.: In vitro exchange of ribosomal subunits between free and membrane-bound ribosomes. J. molec. Biol. **74**, 415—438 (1973).
52. BORISY, G. G., TAYLOR, E. W.: The mechanism of action of colchicine. Binding of colchicine to cellular protein. J. Cell. Biol. **34**, 525—533 (1967).
53. BOSMANN, H. B.: Sialyl transferase activity in normal and RNA- and DNA-virus transformed cells utilizing desialyzed, trypsinized cell plasma membrane external surface glycoproteins as exogenous acceptors. Biochem. Biophys. Res. Commun. **49**, 1256—1262 (1972).
54. BOSMANN, H. B., HAGOPIAN, A., EYLAR, E. H.: Glycoprotein biosynthesis: the characterization of two glycoprotein: fucosyl transferases in Hela cells. Arch. Biochem. Biophys. **128**, 470—481 (1968).
55. BOSMANN, H. B., HAGOPIAN, A., EYLAR, E. H.: Cellular membranes: the biosynthesis of glycoprotein and glycolipid in Hela cell membranes. Arch. Biochem. Biophys. **130**, 573—583 (1969).
56. BOUCHILLOUX, S., CHABAUD, O., MICHEL-BÉCHET, M., FERRAND, M., ATHOUËL-HOAN, A. M.: Differential localization in thyroid microsomal subfractions of a mannosyltransferase, two N-acetylglucosaminyltransferase and a galactosyltransferase. Biochem. Biophys. Res. Commun. **40**, 314—320 (1970).
57. BOUTEILLE, M.: Protein renewal in anti-peroxidase antibody forming cells. I. In vivo incorporation of ^{3}H-leucine as studied by quantitative ultrastructure autoradiography. Exp. Cell Res. **66**, 465—477 (1971).
58. BOWYER, D. E., GRESHAM, G. A.: Arterial lipid accumulation. In: JONES, R. J. (Ed.): Atherosclerosis, Proc. Second Int. Symp., pp. 3—5. Berlin-Heidelberg-New York: Springer 1970.
59. BRIAN, J.: Definition of three classes of binding sites in isolated microtubule crystals. Biochemistry **11**, 2611—2616 (1972).
60. BROWN, D. F.: The effect of ethyl α-p-chlorophenoxybutyrate on ethanol-induced hepatic steatosis in the rat. Metabolism **15**, 868—873 (1966).
61. BROWN, W. V., LEVY, R. I., FREDRICKSON, D. S.: Studies of the proteins in human plasma very low density lipoprotein. J. biol. Chem. **244**, 5687—5694 (1969).
62. BROWN, W. V., LEVY, R. I., FREDRICKSON, D. S.: Further characterization of human very low density lipoprotein apoproteins (apo-VLDL). Fed. Proc. **29**, 327 (1970).
62a. BROWN, W. V., LEVY, R. I., FREDRICKSON, D. S.: Further characterization of apolipoproteins from the human plasma very low density lipoproteins. J. biol. Chem. **245**, 6588—6594 (1970).
63. BÜCHER, TH., KLINGENBERG, M.: Wege des Wasserstoffs in der lebendigen Organisation. Angew. Chem. **70**, 552—570 (1958).
64. BUCKLEY, J. T., DELAHUNTY, T. J., RUBINSTEIN, D.: The relationship of protein synthesis to the secretion of the lipid moiety of low density lipoprotein by the liver. Canad. J. Biochem. **46**, 341—349 (1968).
65. BUNGENBERG DE JONG, J. J., MARSH, J. B.: Synthesis of plasma lipoproteins. Fed. Proc. **25**, 581 (1966).
66. BUNGENBERG DE JONG, J. J., MARSH, J. B.: Biosynthesis of plasma lipoproteins by rat liver ribosomes. J. biol. Chem. **243**, 192—199 (1968).

67. BURCH, R. E., CURRAN, G. L.: Hepatic acetoacetyl-CoA deacylase activity in rats fed ethyl chlorophenoxyisobutyrate (CPIB). J. Lipid Res. **10**, 668—673 (1969).

68. BURKE, G. T., REDMAN, C. M.: The distribution of radioactive peptides synthesized by polysomes and ribosomal subunits combined *in vitro* with microsomal membranes. Biochim. biophys. Acta (Amst.) **299**, 312—324 (1973).

69. BUTCHER, F. R., GOLDMAN, R. H.: Effect of cytochalasin B and colchicine on the stimulation of α-amylase release from rat parotid tissue slices. Biochem. Biophys. Res. Commun. **48**, 23—29 (1972).

70. BUXBAUM, J., SCHARFF, M. D.: The synthesis, assembly, and secretion of γ-globulin by mouse myeloma cells. VI. Assembly of IgM proteins. J. exp. Med. **138**, 278—288 (1973).

71. BYERS, S. O., FRIEDMAN, M.: Effect of clofibrate on plasma lipids of rat and rabbit. Atherosclerosis **11**, 373—382 (1970).

72. CAMEJO, G.: Structural studies on rat plasma lipoproteins. Biochemistry **6**, 3228—3241 (1967).

73. CAMPBELL, P. N.: Functions of polyribosomes attached to membranes of animal cells. FEBS Letters **7**, 1—7 (1970).

74. CARASSO, N., OVTRACHT, L., FAVARD, M. P.: Observation, en microscopie électronique haute tension, de l'appareil de Golgi sur coupes de 0,5 à 5 μ d'épaisseur. C.R. Acad. Sci. (Paris) **273**, 876—879 (1971).

75. CARLSON, L. A.: Pharmacologic control of free fatty acid mobilization and plasma triglyceride transport. In: JONES, R. J. (Ed.): Atherosclerosis. Proc. Second Internat. Symp., pp. 516—521. Berlin-Heidelberg-New York: Springer 1970.

76. CARO, L. G., PALADE, G. E.: Protein synthesis, storage, and discharge in the pancreatic exocrine cell. An autoradiographic study. J. Cell Biol. **20**, 473—495 (1964).

77. CENEDELLA, R. J.: Preliminary studies of hypolipidemic drug effects upon plasma clearance and tissue distribution of chylomicron triglyceride in the dog. Pharmacologist **13**, 277 (1971).

78. CHAPMAN, M. J., MILLS, G. L., TAYLAUR, C. E.: Lipoprotein particles from the Golgi apparatus of guinea-pig liver. Biochem. J. **128**, 779—787 (1972).

79. CHAPMAN, M. J., MILLS, G. L., TAYLAUR, C. E.: The effect of a lipid-rich diet on the properties and composition of lipoprotein particles from the Golgi apparatus of guinea-pig liver. Biochem. J. **131**, 177—185 (1973).

80. CHEETHAM, R. D., MORRÉ, D. J., JUNGHANS, W. N.: Isolation of a Golgi apparatus-rich fraction from rat liver. II. Enzymatic characterization and comparison with other cell fractions. J. Cell Biol. **44**, 492—500 (1970).

81. CHEETHAM, R. D., MORRÉ, D. J., PANNEK, C., FRIEND, D. S.: Isolation of a Golgi apparatus-rich fraction from rat liver. IV. Thiamine pyrophosphatase. J. Cell Biol. **49**, 899—905 (1971).

82. CHESTERTON, C. J.: Distribution of cholesterol precursors and other lipids among rat liver intracellular structures. Evidence for the endoplasmic reticulum as the site of cholesterol and cholesterol ester synthesis. J. biol. Chem. **243**, 1147—1151 (1968).

83. CHOI, Y. S., KNOPF, P. M., LENNOX, E. S.: Subcellular fractionation of mouse myeloma cells. Biochemistry **10**, 659—667 (1971).

84. CHOI, Y. S., KNOPF, P. M., LENNOX, E. S.: Intracellular transport and secretion of an immunoglobulin light chain. Biochemistry **10**, 668—679 (1971).

85. CHRISTOPHE, J., VANDERMEERS, A., VANDERMEERS-PIRET, M. C., RATHÉ, J., CAMUS, J.: The relative turnover time *in vivo* of the intracellular transport of five hydrolases in the pancreas of the rat. Biochim. biophys. Acta (Amst.) **308**, 285—295 (1973).

86. CITKOWITZ, E., HOLTZMAN, E.: Peroxisomes in dorsal root ganglia. J. Histochem. Cytochem. **21**, 34—41 (1973).

87. CLAUDE, A.: Microsomes, endoplasmic reticulum and interactions of cytoplasmic membranes. In: GILETTE, J. R., CONNEY, A. H., COSMIDES, G. J., ESTABROOK, R. W., FOUTS, J. R., MANNERING, G. J. (Eds.): Microsomes and Drug Oxidations, pp. 3—39. New York: Academic Press, Inc. 1969.

88. CLAUDE, A.: Growth and differentiation of cytoplasmic membranes in the course of lipoprotein granule synthesis in the hepatic cell. I. Elaboration of elements of the Golgi complex. J. Cell Biol. **47**, 745—766 (1970).

89. Colbeau, A., Nachbaur, J., Vignais, P. M.: Enzymic characterization and lipid composition of rat liver subcellular membranes. Biochim. biophys. Acta (Amst.) **249**, 462—492 (1971).

90. Colombo, B., Vesco, C., Baglioni, C.: Role of ribosomal subunits in protein synthesis in mammalian cells. Proc. nat. Acad. Sci. (Wash.) **61**, 651—658 (1968).

90a. Cunningham, W. P., Staehelin, L. A., Rubin, R. W., Wilkins, R., Bonneville, M.: Effects of phosphotungstate negative staining on the morphology of the isolated Golgi apparatus. J. Cell Biol. **62**, 491—504 (1974).

91. Daems, W. Th.: The fine structure of mouse-liver microbodies. J. Microscopie **5**, 295—304 (1966).

91a. Dalton, C., Hope, W. C., Hope, H. R., Sheppard, H.: Relationship of serum triglyceride lowering to changes in hepatic composition induced by different classes of drugs. Biochem. Pharmacol. **23**, 685—696 (1974).

92. Dauwalder, M., Whaley, W. G., Kephart, J. E.: Functional aspects of the Golgi apparatus. Sub-Cell. Biochem. **1**, 225—275 (1972).

93. De Duve, C.: Evolution of the peroxisome. Ann. N.Y. Acad. Sci. **168**, 369—381 (1969).

93a. De Duve, C.: Biochemical studies on the occurence, biogenesis and life history of mammalian peroxisomes. J. Histochem. Cytochem. **21**, 941—948 (1973).

94. De Duve, C., Baudhuin, P.: Peroxisomes (microbodies and related particles). Physiol. Rev. **46**, 323—357 (1966).

95. Dehlinger, P. J., Schimke, R. T.: Size distribution of membrane proteins of rat liver and their relative rates of degradation. J. biol. Chem. **246**, 2574—2583 (1971).

96. Delovitch, T. L., Davis, B. K., Holme, G., Sehon, A. H.: Isolation of messenger-like RNA from immuno-chemically separated polyribosomes. J. molec. Biol. **69**, 373—386 (1972).

97. Dennis, E. A., Kennedy, E. P.: Intracellular sites of lipid synthesis and the biogenesis of mitochondria. J. Lipid Res. **13**, 263—267 (1972).

98. De Pury, G. G., Collins, F. D.: Composition and concentration of lipoproteins in the serum of normal rats and rats deficient in essential fatty acids. Lipids **7**, 225—228 (1972).

99. Deter, R. L.: Quantitative characterization of dense body, autophagic vacuole, and acid phosphatase-bearing particle populations during the early phases of glucagon-induced autophagy in rat liver. J. Cell Biol. **48**, 473—489 (1971).

100. Donaldson, W. E., Wit-Peeters, E. M., Scholte, H. R.: Fatty acid synthesis in rat liver: relative contributions of the mitochondrial, microsomal and non-particulate systems. Biochim. biophys. Acta (Amst.) **202**, 35—42 (1970).

101. Droz, B.: Elaboration de glycoprotéines dans l'appareil de Golgi des cellules hépatiques chez le rat; étude radioautographique en microscopie électronique après injection de galactose-^{3}H. C.R. Acad. Sci. (Paris) **262**, 1766—1768 (1966).

102. Duncan, C. H., Best, M. M.: Influence of a terminal period of fasting on the serum and tissue lipid effects of ethyl chlorophenoxyisobutyrate (CPIB). Metabolism **17**, 681—689 (1968).

103. Duncan, C. H., Best, M. M., Despopoulos, A.: Inhibition of hepatic secretion of triglyceride by chlorophenoxyisobutyrate (CPIB). Circulation **30** (Suppl. III), 7 (1964).

103a. Edelstein, C., Lim, C. T., Scanu, A. M.: On the subunit structure of the protein of human serum high density lipoprotein. I. A study of its major polypeptide components (Sephadex, fraction III). J. biol. Chem. **247**, 5842—5849 (1972).

104. Ehrenreich, J. H., Bergeron, J. J. M., Siekevitz, P., Palade, G. E.: Golgi fractions prepared from rat liver homogenates. I. Isolation procedure and morphological characterization. J. Cell Biol. **59**, 45—72 (1973).

104a. Ehrlich, H. P., Ross, R., Bornstein, P.: Effects of antimicrotubular agents on the secretion of collagen. A biochemical and morphological study. J. Cell. Biol. **62**, 390—405 (1974).

104b. Eisenberg, S., Rachmilewitz, D.: Metabolism of rat plasma very low density lipoprotein. I. Fate in circulation of the whole lipoprotein. Biochim. biophys. Acta (Amst.) **326**, 378—390 (1973).

104c. Eisenberg, S., Rachmilewitz, D.: Metabolism of rat plasma very low density lipoprotein. II. Fate in circulation of apoprotein subunits. Biochim. biophys. Acta (Amst.) **326**, 391—405 (1973).

105. EISENBERG, S., BILHEIMER, D. W., LEVY, R. I.: The metabolism of very low density lipoprotein proteins. II. Studies on the transfer of apoproteins between plasma lipoproteins. Biochim. biophys. Acta (Amst.) **280**, 94—104 (1972).
106. EKHOLM, R., ZELANDER, T., EDLUND, Y.: The ultrastructural organization of the rat exocrine pancreas. I. Acinar cells. J. Ultrastruct. Res. **7**, 61—72 (1962).
107. ELETR, S., ZAKIM, D., VESSEY, D. A.: A spin-label study of the role of phospholipids in the regulation of membrane-bound microsomal enzymes. J. molec. Biol. **78**, 351—362 (1973).
108. ELWOOD, J. C., RICHERT, D. A., WESTERFELD, W. W.: A comparison of hypolipidemic drugs in the prevention of an orotic acid fatty liver. Biochem. Pharmacol. **21**, 1127—1134 (1972).
109. ERNSTER, L., ORRENIUS, S.: Substrate-induced synthesis of the hydroxylating enzyme system of liver microsomes. Fed. Proc. **24**, 1190—1199 (1965).
110. ESSNER, E.: Endoplasmic reticulum and the origin of microbodies in fetal mouse liver. Lab. Invest. **17**, 71—87 (1967).
111. ESSNER, E., NOVIKOFF, A. B.: Cytological studies on two functional hepatomas. Interrelations of endoplasmic reticulum, Golgi apparatus, and lysosomes. J. Cell. Biol. **15**, 289—312 (1962).
112. ESTABROOK, R. W., SACKTOR, B.: α-Glycerophosphatase oxidase of flight muscle mitochondria. J. biol. Chem. **233**, 1014—1019 (1958).
113. EYLAR, E. H.: On the biological role of glycoproteins. J. theoret. Biol. **10**, 89—113 (1965).
114. FAHIMI, H. D.: Morphogenesis of peroxisomes in rat liver. Abstracts of the American Society of Cell. Biology, New Orleans, p. 87, 1971.
114a. FAHIMI, H. D.: Diffusion artifacts in cytochemistry of catalase. J. Histochem. Cytochem. **21**, 999—1009 (1973).
115. FAHIMI, H. D., VENKATACHALAM, M. A.: Microbody regeneration and catalase synthesis in rat liver. J. Cell Biol. **47**, 58 a (1970).
116. FALOONA, G. R., STEWART, B. N., FRIED, M.: The effect of actinomycin D on the biosynthesis of plasma lipoproteins. Biochemistry **7**, 720—725 (1968).
117. FALVEY, A. K., STAEHELIN, T.: Structure and function of mammalian ribosomes. II. Exchange of ribosomal subunits at various stages of *in vitro* polypeptide synthesis. J. molec. Biol. **53**, 21—34 (1970).
118. FARBER, E., SHULL, K. H., VILLA-TREVINO, S., LOMBARDI, B., THOMAS, M.: Biochemical pathology of acute hepatic ATP deficiency. Nature (Lond.) **203**, 34—40 (1964).
119. FAWCETT, D. W.: Physiologically significant specializations of the cell surface. Circulation **26**, 1105—1125 (1962).
120. FEINSTEIN, R. N.: Acatalasemia in the mouse and other species. Biochem. Genetics **4**, 135—155 (1970).
121. FLEISCHER, B., FLEISCHER, S.: Preparation and characterization of Golgi membranes from rat liver. Biochim. biophys. Acta (Amst.) **219**, 301—319 (1970).
121a. FLEISCHER, B., ZAMBRANO, F.: Localization of cerebroside—sulfotransferase activity in the Golgi apparatus of rat kidney. Biochem. Biophys. Res. Commun. **52**, 951—958 (1973).
122. FLEISCHER, B., FLEISCHER, S., OZAWA, H.: Isolation and characterization of Golgi membranes from bovine liver. J. Cell Biol. **43**, 59—79 (1969).
123. FLEISCHER, S., FLEISCHER, B., AZZI, A., CHANCE, B.: Cytochrome b$_5$ and P-450 in liver cell fractions. Biochim. biophys. Acta (Amst.) **225**, 194—200 (1971).
124. FOWLER, S., DE DUVE, C.: Digestive activity of lysosomes. III. The digestion of lipids by extracts of rat liver lysosomes. J. biol. Chem. **244**, 471—481 (1969).
125. FRANKE, W. W., KARTENBECK, J., KRIEN, S., VANDERWOUDE, W., SCHEER, U., MORRÉ, D. J.: Inter- and intracisternal elements of the Golgi apparatus. A system of membrane-to-membrane cross links. Z. Zellforsch. **132**, 365—380 (1972).
126. FRANKE, W. W., MORRÉ, D. J., DEUMLING, B., CHEETHAM, R. D., KARTENBECK, J., JARASCH, E.-D., ZENTGRAF, H.-W.: Synthesis and turnover of membrane proteins in rat liver: an examination of the membrane flow hypothesis. Z. Naturforsch. **26b**, 1031—1039 (1971).
127. FRANSON, R., WAITE, M., LA VIA, M.: Identification of phospholipase A$_1$ and A$_2$ in the soluble fraction of rat liver lysosomes. Biochemistry **10**, 1942—1946 (1971).
128. FRIDLENDER, B. R., WETTSTEIN, F. O.: Differences in the ribosomal protein of free and membrane bound polysomes of chick embryo cells. Biochem. Biophys. Res. Commun. **39**, 247—253 (1970).

129. Friedman, M., Van den Bosch, J., Byers, S. O., St. George, S.: Effects of cortisone on lipid and cholesterol metabolism in the rabbit and rat. Amer. J. Physiol. **208**, 94—105 (1965).

130. Friend, D. S., Murray, M. J.: Osmium impregnation of the Golgi apparatus. Amer. J. Anat. **117**, 135—150 (1965).

131. Frye, L. D., Edidin, M.: The rapid intermixing of cell surface antigen after formation of mouse-human heterokaryons. J. Cell Sci. **7**, 319—335 (1970).

132. Gang, H., Lieber, C. S., Rubin, E.: Ethanol increases glycosyl transferase activity in the hepatic Golgi apparatus. Nature (Lond.) New Biol. **243**, 123—125 (1973).

133. Ganoza, M. C., Williams, C. A.: In vitro synthesis of different categories of specific protein by membrane-bound and free ribosomes. Proc. nat. Acad. Sci. (Wash.) **63**, 1370—1376 (1969).

134. Gaye, P., Denamur, R.: Acides ribonucléiques et polyribosomes de la glande mammaire de la lapine au cours de la lactogénèse induite par la prolactine. Biochim. biophys. Acta (Amst.) **186**, 99—109 (1969).

135. Geer, J. C., Panganamala, R. V., Newman, H. A. I., Cornwell, D. G.: Mural metabolism. In: Jones, R. J. (Ed.): Atherosclerosis, Proc. Second Int. Symp., pp. 6—12. Berlin-Heidelberg-New York: Springer 1970.

136. Geller, D. M., Judah, J. D., Nicholls, M. R.: Intracellular distribution of serum albumin and its possible precursors in rat liver. Biochem. J. **127**, 865—874 (1972).

137. Geuze, J. J., Poort, C.: Cell membrane resorption in the rat exocrine pancreas cell after in vivo stimulation of the secretion, as studied by in vitro incubation with extracellular space markers. J. Cell Biol. **57**, 159—174 (1973).

138. Gillette, J. R.: Biochemistry of drug oxidation and reduction by enzymes in hepatic endoplasmic reticulum. Advanc. Pharmacol. **4**, 219—261 (1966).

139. Glaumann, H., Ericsson, J. L. E.: Evidence for the participation of the Golgi apparatus in the intracellular transport of nascent albuminum in the liver cell. J. Cell Biol. **47**, 555—567 (1970).

140. Göransson, G., Olivecrona, T.: The metabolism of fatty acid in the rat. I. Palmitic acid. Acta physiol. scand. **62**, 224—239 (1964).

141. Gofman, J. W., Young, W.: The filtration concept of atherosclerosis and serum lipids in the diagnosis of atherosclerosis. In: Sandler, M., Bourne, G. H. (Eds.): Atherosclerosis and Its Origin, pp. 197—229. New York: Academic Press Inc. 1963.

142. Goldfarb, S.: Submicrosomal localization of hepatic 3-hydroxy-3-methylglutaryl coenzyme A (HMG-CoA) reductase. FEBS Letters **24**, 153—155 (1972).

143. Goldfischer, S., Roheim, P. S., Edelstein, D., Essner, E.: Hypolipidemia in a mutant strain of "acatalasemic" mice. Science **173**, 65—66 (1971).

144. Goldstone, A., Koenig, H.: Biosynthesis of lysosomal glycoproteins in rat kidney. Life Sci. **11**, 511—523 (1972).

145. Gould, R. G., Swyryd, E. A., Avoy, D., Coan, B.: The effects of α-p-chlorophenoxyisobutyrate on the synthesis and release into plasma of lipoproteins in rats. In: Kritchevsky, D., Paoletti, R., Steinberg, D. (Eds.): Progress in Biochemical Pharmacology, Vol. 2, pp. 345—357. Basel: Karger 1967.

146. Gould, R. G., Swyryd, E. A., Coan, B. J., Avoy, D.: Effects of chlorophenoxyisobutyrate (CPIB) on liver composition and triglyceride synthesis in rats. J. Atheroscler. Res. **6**, 555—564 (1966).

147. Gram, T. E., Hansen, A. R., Fouts, J. R.: The submicrosomal distribution of hepatic uridine diphosphate glucuronyltransferases in the rabbit. Biochem. J. **106**, 587—591 (1968).

148. Gross, R. C., Eigenbrodt, E. H., Farquhar, J. W.: Endogeneous triglyceride turnover in liver and plasma of the dog. J. Lipid Res. **8**, 114—125 (1967).

149. Grove, S. N., Bracker, C. E., Morré, D. J.: Cytomembrane differentiation in the endoplasmic reticulum—Golgi apparatus vesicle complex. Science **161**, 171—173 (1968).

150. Guder, W., Weiss, L., Wieland, O.: Triglyceride breakdown in rat liver. The demonstration of three different lipases. Biochim. biophys. Acta (Amst.) **187**, 173—185 (1969).

151. Haddad, A., Smith, M. D., Herscovics, A., Nadler, N. J., Leblond, C. P.: Radioautographic study of in vivo and in vitro incorporation of fucose-³H into thyroglobulin by rat thyroid follicular cells. J. Cell Biol. **49**, 856—882 (1971).

152. HÄNNINEN, O., AITIO, A.: Enhanced glucuronide formation in different tissues following drug administration. Biochem. Pharmacol. **17**, 2307—2311 (1968).
153. HAFT, D. E., ROHEIM, P. S., WHITE, A., EDER, H. A.: Plasma lipoprotein metabolism in perfused rat livers. I. Protein synthesis and entry into the plasma. J. clin. Invest. **41**, 842—849 (1962).
154. HAGOPIAN, A., BOSMANN, H. B., EYLAR, E. H.: Glycoprotein biosynthesis: the localization of polypeptidyl: N-acetylgalactosaminyl collagen: glucosyl, and glycoprotein: galactosyl transferases in Hela cell membrane fractions. Arch. Biochem. Biophys. **128**, 387—396 (1968).
155. HALLINAN, T., MURTY, C. N., GRANT, J. H.: The exclusive function of reticulum bound ribosomes in glycoprotein biosynthesis. Life Sci. **7**, 225—232 (1968).
156. HAMILTON, R. L., REGEN, D. M., GRAY, M. E., LeQUIRE, V. S.: Lipid transport in liver. I. Electron microscopic identification of very low density lipoproteins in perfused rat liver. Lab. Invest. **16**, 305—319 (1967).
157. HAND, A. R.: Morphologic and cytochemical identification of peroxisomes in the rat parotid and other exocrine glands. J. Histochem. Cytochem. **21**, 131—141 (1973).
158. HAVEL, R. J.: Conversion of plasma free fatty acids into triglycerides of plasma lipoprotein fractions in man. Metabolism **10**, 1031—1034 (1961).
159. HAVEL, R. J.: Metabolism of plasma triglycerides. In: JONES, R. J. (Ed.): Atherosclerosis. Proc. Second Internat. Symp., pp. 210—220. Berlin-Heidelberg-New York: Springer 1970.
160. HAVEL, R. J., FELTS, J. M., VAN DUYNE, C. M.: Formation and fate of endogenous triglycerides in blood plasma of rabbits. J. Lipid Res. **3**, 297—308 (1962).
161. HAY, R. V., POTTENGER, L. A., REINGOLD, A. L., GETZ, G. S., WISSLER, R. W.: Degradation of I^{125}-labelled serum low density lipoprotein in normal and estrogen-treated male rats. Biochem. Biophys. Res. Commun. **44**, 1471—1477 (1971).
162. HAYASHI, H., SUGA, T., NIINOBE, S.: Studies on peroxisomes. I. Intraparticulate localization of peroxisomal enzymes in rat liver. Biochim. biophys. Acta (Amst.) **252**, 58—68 (1971).
163. HEIMBERG, M., WILCOX, H. G.: The effect of palmitic and oleic acids on the properties and composition of the very low density lipoprotein secreted by the liver. J. biol. Chem. **247**, 875—880 (1972).
164. HEIMBERG, M., VAN HARKEN, D. R., BROWN, T. O.: Hepatic lipid metabolism in experimental diabetes. II. Incorporation of $(1-^{14}C)$ palmitate into lipids of the liver and of the $d < 1.020$ perfusate lipoproteins. Biochim. biophys. Acta (Amst.) **137**, 435—445 (1967).
165. HEIMBERG, M., WEINSTEIN, I., DISHMAN, G., FRIED, M.: Lipoprotein lipid transport by livers from normal and CCL_4-poisoned animals. Amer. J. Physiol. **209**, 1053—1060 (1965).
166. HELGELAND, L., CHRISTENSEN, T. B., JANSON, T. L.: The distribution of protein-bound carbohydrates in submicrosomal fractions from rat liver. Biochim. biophys. Acta (Amst.) **286**, 62—71 (1972).
166a. HERZOG, V., FAHIMI, H. D.: Microbodies (peroxisomes) containing catalase in myocardium: morphological and biochemical evidence. Science **185**, 271—273 (1974).
167. HESS, R., DIETRICH, F. M.: Dietary and hormonal modifications of rat serum lipoproteins. In: PEETERS, H. (Ed.): Protides of the Biological Fluids. Proc. 19th Colloq., pp. 337—339. Oxford: Pergamon Press 1971.
168. HESS, R., STÄUBLI, W.: Ultrastructure of vascular changes. In: SCHETTLER, F. G., BOYD, G. S. (Eds.): Atherosclerosis, pp. 49—71. Amsterdam: Elsevier Publ. Comp. 1969.
169. HESS, R., MAIER, R., STÄUBLI, W.: Evaluation of phenolic ethers as hypolipidaemic agents effects of CIBA 13, 437-Su. In: HOLMES, W. L., CARLSON, L. A., PAOLETTI, R. (Eds.): Drugs Affecting Lipid Metabolism. Proc. 3rd Int. Symp., pp. 483—489. London: Plenum Press 1969.
170. HESS, R., RIESS, W., STÄUBLI, W.: Hepatic actions of hypolipidaemic drugs: effect of ethyl chlorophenoxy-isobutyrate (CPIB). In: KRITCHEVSKY, D., PAOLETTI, R., STEINBERG, D. (Eds.): Progress in Biochemical Pharmacology, Vol. 2, pp. 325—336. Basel: Karger 1967.
171. HESS, R., STÄUBLI, W., RIESS, W.: Nature of the hepatomegalic effect produced by ethylchlorophenoxy-isobutyrate in the rat. Nature (Lond.) **208**, 856—858 (1965).
172. HIGASHI, T., PETERS, T., JR.: Studies on rat liver catalase. I. Combined immunochemical and enzymatic determination of catalase in liver cell fractions. J. biol. Chem. **238**, 3945—3951 (1963).

173. Higashi,T., Peters,T., Jr.: Studies on rat liver catalase. II. Incorporation of ^{14}C-leucine nto catalase of liver cell fractions *in vivo*. J. biol. Chem. **238**, 3952—3954 (1963).

174. Hill,P., Dvornik,D.: Agents affecting lipid metabolism. XXXVII. Separation of rat serum lipoproteins with dextran sulfate. Canad. J. Biochem. **47**, 1043—1047 (1969).

175. Hill,P., Dvornik,D.: Agents affecting lipid metabolism. XL. Effect of ethyl chlorophenoxyisobutyrate on liver lipids and serum lipoproteins in rats. Can. J. Biochem. **49**, 903—910 (1971).

176. Hirano,H., Parkhouse,B., Nicolson,G.L., Lennox,E.S., Singer,S.J.: Distribution of saccharide residues on membrane fragments from a myeloma-cell homogenate: its implications for membrane biogenesis. Proc. nat. Acad. Sci. (Wash.) **69**, 2945—2949 (1972).

177. Hochberg,A.A., Stratman,F.W., Zahlten,R.N., Morris,H.P., Lardy,H.A.: Binding of rat liver and hepatoma polyribosomes to stripped rough endoplasmic reticulum *in vitro*. Biological or an artifact? Biochem. J. **130**, 19—25 (1972).

178. Hogg,J.F.: Peroxisomes in Tetrahymena and their relation to gluconeogenesis. Ann. N.Y. Acad. Sci. **168**, 281—290 (1969).

179. Hokin,L.E.: Dynamic aspects of phospholipids during protein secretion. Int. Rev. Cytol. **23**, 187—208 (1968).

180. Howard,A.N., Blaton,V., Vandamme,D., Van Landschoot,N., Peeters,H.: Lipid changes in the plasma lipoproteins of baboons given an atherogenic diet. Part 3. A comparison between lipid changes in the plasma of the baboon and chimpanzee given atherogenic diets and those in human plasma lipoproteins of type II hyperlipoproteinaemia. Atherosclerosis **16**, 257—272 (1972).

181. Howell,J.W., Hood,L., Sanders,B.G.: Comparative analysis of the IgG heavy chain carbohydrate peptide. J. molec. Biol. **30**, 555—558 (1967).

182. Hruban,Z., Rechcigl,M.,Jr.: Microbodies and related particles. Morphology, biochemistry and physiology. Int. Rev. Cytol. Suppl. 1 (1969).

183. Hruban,Z., Swift,H.: Uricase: localization in hepatic microbodies. Science **146**, 1316—1318 (1964).

184. Hruban,Z., Vigil,E.L., Martan,J.: Microbodies (peroxisomes) in sebaceous glands. 29th Ann. Proc. Electron Microscopy Soc. Amer., Boston, 1971.

184a. Hruban,Z., Gotoh,M., Slesers,A., Chou,S.: Structure of hepatic microbodies in rats treated with acetylsalicylic acid acid, clofibrate, and dimethrin. Lab. Invest. **30**, 64—75 (1974).

185. Hruban,Z., Vigil,E.L., Slesers,A., Hopkins,E.: Microbodies. Constituent organelles of animal cells. Lab. Invest. **27**, 184—191 (1972).

185a. Hruban,Z., Mochizuki,J., Gotoh,M., Slesers,A., Chou,S.: Effects of some hypocholesterolemic agents on hepatic ultrastructure and microbody enzymes. Lab. Invest. **30**, 474—485 (1974).

186. Hudgin,R.L., Murray,R.K., Pinteric,L., Morris,H.P., Schachter,H.: The use of nucleotide-sugar: glycoprotein glycosyltransferases to assess Golgi apparatus function in Morris hepatomas. Can. J. Biochem. **49**, 61—70 (1971).

187. Hugon,J., Borgers,M.: A direct lead method for the electron microscopic visualization of alkaline phosphatase activity. J. Histochem. Cytochem. **14**, 429—431 (1966).

188. Hunt,T., Hunter,T., Munro,A.: Control of haemoglobin synthesis: rate of translation of the messenger RNA for the α- and β-chains. J. molec. Biol. **43**, 123—133 (1969).

189. Hyams,D.E., Taft,E.B., Drummey,G.D., Isselbacher,K.J.: The prevention of fatty liver by administration of adenosine triphosphate. Lab. Invest. **16**, 604—615 (1967).

190. Ichikawa,A.: Fine structural changes in response to hormonal stimulation to hormonal stimulation of the perfused canine pancreas. J. Cell Biol. **24**, 369—385 (1965).

191. Ikehara,Y., Pitot,H.C.: Localization of polysome-bound albumin and serine dehydratase in rat liver cell fractions. J. Cell Biol. **59**, 28—44 (1973).

192. James,D.W., Rabin,B.R., Williams,D.J.: Role of steroid hormones in the interaction of polysomes with endoplasmic reticulum. Nature (Lond.) **224**, 371—372 (1969).

193. Jamieson,J.D.: Role of the Golgi complex in the intracellular transport of secretory proteins. In: Clementi,F., Ceccarelli,B. (Eds.): Advances in Cytopharmacology, Vol.1, pp.183—190. New York: Raven Press 1971.

194. JAMIESON, J. D., PALADE, G. E.: Intracellular transport of secretory proteins in the pancreatic exocrine cell, I. Role of the peripheral elements of the Golgi complex. J. Cell Biol. **34**, 577—596 (1967).

195. JAMIESON, J. D., PALADE, G. E.: Intracellular transport of secretory proteins in the pancreatic exocrine cell, II. Transport to condensing vacuoles and zymogen granules. J. Cell Biol. **34**, 597—615 (1967).

196. JAMIESON, J. D., PALADE, G. E.: Synthesis, intracellular transport, and discharge of secretory proteins in stimulated pancreatic exocrine cells. J. Cell Biol. **50**, 135—158 (1971).

197. JAMIESON, J. D., PALADE, G. E.: Condensing vacuole conversion and zymogen granule discharge in pancreatic exocrine cells: metabolic studies. J. Cell Biol. **48**, 503—522 (1971).

198. JATLOW, P., ADAMS, W. R., HANDSCHUMACHER, R. E.: Pathogenesis of orotic acid-induced fatty change in the rat liver. Amer. J. Path. **47**, 125—145 (1965).

199. JAZCILEVICH, S., VILLA-TREVIÑO, S.: Induction of fatty liver in the rat after cycloheximide administration. Lab. Invest. **23**, 590—594 (1970).

200. JONES, A. L., ARMSTRONG, D. T.: Increased cholesterol biosynthesis following phenobarbital induced hypertrophy of agranular endoplasmic reticulum in liver. Proc. Soc. exp. Biol. (N.Y.) **119**, 1136—1139 (1965).

201. JONES, A. L., FAWCETT, D. W.: Hypertrophy of the agranular endoplasmic reticulum in hamster liver induced by phenobarbital (with a review on the functions of this organelle in liver). J. Histochem. Cytochem. **14**, 215—232 (1966).

202. JONES, A. L., OCKNER, R. K.: An electron microscopic study of endogenous very low density lipoprotein production in the intestine of rat and man. J. Lipid Res. **12**, 580—589 (1971).

203. JONES, A. L., RUDERMAN, N. B., EMANS, J. B.: An electron microscopic study of hepatic lipoprotein synthesis in rat following antiinsulin serum, nicotinic acid and puromycin administration. Gastroenterology **56**, 402 (1969).

204. JONES, A. L., RUDERMAN, N. B., HERRERA, M. G.: An electron microscopic study of lipoprotein production and release by the isolated perfused rat liver. Proc. Soc. exp. Biol. (Wash.) **123**, 4—9 (1966).

205. JONES, A. L., RUDERMAN, N. B., HERRERA, M. G.: Electron microscopic and biochemical study of lipoprotein synthesis in the isolated perfused rat liver. J. Lipid Res. **8**, 429—466 (1967).

206. JOTHY, S., TAY, S., SIMPKINS, H.: The role of membrane phospholipids in the interaction of ribosomes with endoplasmic-reticulum membrane. Biochem. J. **132**, 637—640 (1973).

207. KABAT, D., RICH, A.: The ribosomal subunit-polyribosome cycle in protein synthesis of embryonic skeletal muscle. Biochemistry **8**, 3742—3749 (1969).

207a. KÄHÖNEN, M. T., YLIKAHRI, R. H.: Effect of clofibrate treatment on the activity of carnitine acetyltransferase in rat tissues. FEBS Letters **43**, 297—299 (1974).

208. KÄHÖNEN, M. T., YLIKAHRI, R. H., HASSINEN, I. E.: Ethanol metabolism in rats treated with ethyl-α-p-chlorophenoxyisobutyrate (clofibrate). Life Sci. **10**, 661—670 (1971).

209. KAEMPFER, R.: Ribosomal subunit exchange in the cytoplasm of a eukaryote. Nature (Lond.) **222**, 950—953 (1969).

210. KANEKO, A., SAKAMOTO, S., MORITA, M., ONOÉ, T.: Morphological and biochemical changes in rat liver during the early stages of ethyl chlorophenoxyisobutyrate administration. Tohoku J. exp. Med. **99**, 81—101 (1969).

211. KAZAZIAN, H. H., JR.: Separation of α- and β-globin messenger RNAs. Nature (Lond.) New Biol. **238**, 166—169 (1972).

212. KEENAN, T. W., MORRÉ, D. J.: Phospholipid class and fatty acid composition of Golgi apparatus isolated from rat liver and comparison with other cell fractions. Biochemistry **9**, 19—25 (1970).

213. KEENAN, T. W., MORRÉ, D. J., CHEETHAM, R. D.: Lactose synthesis by a Golgi apparatus fraction from rat mammary gland. Nature (Lond.) **228**, 1105—1106 (1970).

214. KEENAN, T. W., MORRÉ, D. J., HUANG, C. M.: Distribution of gangliosides among subcellular fractions from rat liver and bovine mammary gland. FEBS Letters **24**, 204—207 (1972).

215. KESSLER, J. I., STEIN, J., DANNACKER, D., NARCESSIAN, P.: Biosynthesis of low density lipoprotein by cellfree preparations of rat intestinal mucosa. J. biol. Chem. **245**, 5281—5288 (1970).

216. KHAWAJA, J. A.: Interaction of ribosomes and ribosomal subparticles with endoplasmic reticulum membranes *in vitro*: effect of spermine and magnesium. Biochim. Biophys. Acta **254**, 117—128 (1971).

217. KHAWAJA, J. A., RAINA, A.: Effect of spermine and magnesium on the attachment of free ribosomes to endoplasmic reticulum membranes *in vitro*. Biochem. Biophys. Res. Commun. **41**, 512—518 (1970).

218. KLAASEN, C. D.: Effects of phenobarbital on the plasma disappearance and biliary excretion of drugs in rats. J. Pharmacol. exp. Ther. **175**, 289—300 (1970).

218a. KNAPP, A., KORNBLATT, M. J., SCHACHTER, H., MURRAY, R. K.: Studies on the biosynthesis of testicular sulfoglycerogalactolipid: demonstration of a Golgi-associated sulfotransferase activity. Biochem. Biophys. Res. Commun. **55**, 179—186 (1974).

219. KOGA, S., HORWITZ, D. L., SCANU, A. M.: Isolation and properties of lipoproteins from normal rat serum. J. Lipid Res. **10**, 577—588 (1969).

220. KOHOUT, M., KOHOUTOVA, B., HEIMBERG, M.: The regulation of hepatic triglyceride metabolism by free fatty acids. J. biol. Chem. **246**, 5067—5074 (1971).

221. KOOK, A. I., RUBINSTEIN, D.: A comparison of the secretion of two components of very low density lipoproteins by perfused rat liver. Can. J. Biochem. **51**, 490—494 (1973).

222. KOOK, A. I., ECKHAUS, A. S., RUBINSTEIN, D.: The dissociation *in vitro* of the α- and β-lipoprotein components of human and rat very low density lipoproteins. Can. J. Biochem. **48**, 712—724 (1970).

223. KREIBICH, G., DEBEY, P., SABATINI, D. D.: Selective release of content from microsomal vesicles without membrane disassembly. I. Permeability changes induced by low detergent concentrations. J. Cell Biol. **58**, 436—462 (1973).

224. KRITCHEVSKY, D.: Newer hypolipidemic agents. Fed. Proc. **30**, 835—840 (1971).

225. KRITCHEVSKY, D.: Cholesterol metabolism in aorta and in tissue culture. Lipids **7**, 305—309 (1972).

226. KRITCHEVSKY, D., TEPPER, S. A.: Influence of 2-methyl-2-(p-1,2,3,4-tetrahydro-1-naphthylphenoxy) propionic acid on the oxidation of cholesterol by rat liver mitochondria. Experientia (Basel) **25**, 699—700 (1969).

227. KURUP, C. K. R., AITHAL, H. N., RAMASARMA, T.: Increase in hepatic mitochondria on administration of ethyl α-p-chlorophenoxy-isobutyrate to the rat. Biochem. J. **116**, 773—779 (1970).

228. LAKSHMANAN, M. R., PHILLIPS, W. E. J., BRIEN, R. L.: Effect of p-chlorophenoxyisobutyrate (CPIB) fed to rats on hepatic biosynthesis and catabolism of ubiquinone. J. Lipid Res. **9**, 353—356 (1968).

229. LAMB, R. G., FALLON, H. J.: Inhibition of monoacylglycerophosphate formation by chlorophenoxyisobutyrate and β-benzalbutyrate. J. biol. Chem. **247**, 1281—1287 (1972).

230. LANDRISCINA, C., GNONI, G. V., QUAGLIARIELLO, E.: Mechanisms of fatty acid synthesis in rat-liver microsomes. Biochim. biophys. Acta **202**, 405—414 (1970).

231. LANGER, T., BILHEIMER, D., LEVY, R. I.: Plasma low density lipoprotein (LDL): a remnant of very low density lipoprotein (VLDL) catabolism? Circulation **42**, (Suppl. III) 7 (1970).

232. LARSÉN, C., DALLNER, G., ERNSTER, L.: Association of sialic acid with microsomal membrane structures in rat liver. Biochem. Biophys. Res. Commun. **49**, 1300—1306 (1972).

233. LAWFORD, G. R., SCHACHTER, H.: Biosynthesis of glycoprotein by liver. The incorporation *in vivo* of ^{14}C-glucosamine into protein-bound hexosamine and sialic acid of rat liver subcellular fractions. J. biol. Chem. **241**, 5408—5418 (1966).

234. LAZAROW, P. B., DE DUVE, C.: Intermediates in the biosynthesis of peroxisomal catalase in rat liver. Biochem. Biophys. Res. Commun. **45**, 1198—1204 (1971).

234a. LAZAROW, P. B., DE DUVE, C.: The synthesis and turnover of rat liver peroxisomes. IV. Biochemical pathway of catalase synthesis. J. Cell Biol. **59**, 491—506 (1973).

234b. LAZAROW, P. B., DE DUVE, C.: The synthesis and turnover of rat liver peroxisomes. V. Intracellular pathway of catalase synthesis. J. Cell Biol. **59**, 507—524 (1973).

235. LEDUC, E. H., AVRAMEAS, S., BOUTEILLE, M.: Ultrastructural localization of antibody in differentiating plasma cells. J. exp. Med. **127**, 109—118 (1968).

236. LEDUC, E. H., SCOTT, G. B., AVRAMEAS, S.: Ultrastructural localization of intracellular immune globulins in plasma cells and lymphoblasts by enzyme-labeled antibodies. J. Histochem. Cytochem. **17**, 211—224 (1969).

237. LEE, Y. P., LARDY, H. A.: Influence of thyroid hormones on L-α-glycerophosphate dehydrogenases and other dehydrogenases in various organs of the rat. J. biol. Chem. **240**, 1427—1436 (1965).
238. LEE, Y. P., TAKEMORI, A. E., LARDY, H. A.: Enhanced oxidation of α-glycerophosphate by mitochondria of thyroid-fed rats. J. biol. Chem. **234**, 3051—3054 (1959).
239. LEELAVATHI, D. E., ESTES, L. W., FEINGOLD, D. S., LOMBARDI, B.: Isolation of a Golgi-rich fraction from rat liver. Biochim. biophys. Acta (Amst.) **211**, 124—138 (1970).
240. LEGG, P. G., WOOD, R. L.: New observations on microbodies. A cytochemical study on CPIB-treated rat liver. J. Cell Biol. **45**, 118—129 (1970).
241. LEGG, P. G., WOOD, R. L.: Effects of catalase inhibitors on the ultrastructure and peroxidase activity of proliferating microbodies. Histochemie **22**, 262—276 (1970).
242. LEGG, P. G., WOOD, R. L.: Effects of allylisopropylacetamide (AIA) on the fine structure and peroxidase activity of microbodies in rat hepatic cells. Z. Zellforsch. **128**, 19—30 (1972).
243. LEIGHTON, F., POOLE, B., LAZAROW, P. B., DE DUVE, C.: The synthesis and turnover of rat liver peroxisomes. I. Fractionation of peroxisome proteins. J. Cell Biol. **41**, 521—535 (1969).
243a. LE MARCHAND, J., SINGH, A., ASSIMACOPOULOS-JEANNET, F., ORCI, L., ROUILLER, CH., JEANRENAUD, B.: A role of the microtubular system in the release of very low density lipoproteins by perfused mouse livers. J. biol. Chem. **248**, 6862—6870 (1973).
244. LENTZ, T. L.: Rhabdite formation in planaria: the role of microtubules. J. Ultrastruct. Res. **17**, 114—126 (1967).
244a. LEVINE, W. G.: Effect of the hypolipidemic drug nafenopin {2-methyl-2-[p-(1, 2, 3, 4-tetrahydro-1-naphthyl) phenoxy] propionic acid; TPIA, Su-13,437}, on the hepatic disposition of foreign compounds in the rat. Drug Metab. Disp. **2**, 178—186 (1974).
245. LO, C., MARSH, J. B.: Biosynthesis of plasma lipoproteins. Incorporation of ^{14}C-glucosamine by cells and subcellular fractions of rat liver. J. biol. Chem. **245**, 5001—5006 (1970).
246. LOCKE, M., MCMAHON, J. T.: The origin and fate of microbodies in the fat body of an insect. J. Cell Biol. **48**, 61—78 (1971).
247. LOMBARDI, B.: Considerations on the pathogenesis of fatty liver. Lab. Invest. **15**, 1—15 (1966).
248. LOMBARDI, B., OLER, A.: Choline deficiency fatty liver. Protein synthesis and release. Lab. Invest. **17**, 308—321 (1967).
249. LOMBARDI, B., PANI, P., SCHLUNK, F. F.: Choline-deficiency fatty liver: impaired release of hepatic triglycerides. J. Lipid Res. **9**, 437—446 (1968).
250. LUCY, J. A.: Lysosomal membranes. In: DINGLE, J. T., FELL, H. B. (Eds.): Lysosomes in Biology and Pathology, Vol. 2, pp. 313—341. Amsterdam: North-Holland Publ. Comp. 1969.
251. MAGALHÃES, M. M., MAGALHÃES, M. C.: Microbodies (peroxisomes) in rat adrenal cortex. J. Ultrastruct. Res. **37**, 563—573 (1971).
252. MAHADEVAN, S., TAPPEL, A. L.: Lysosomal lipases of rat liver and kidney. J. biol. Chem. **243**, 2849—2854 (1968).
253. MAHLEY, R. W., GRAY, M. E., LEQUIRE, V. S.: Role of plasma lipoproteins in cortisone-induced fat embolism. Amer. J. Path. **66**, 43—62 (1972).
254. MAHLEY, R. W., HAMILTON, R. L., LEQUIRE, V. S.: Characterization of lipoprotein particles isolated from the Golgi apparatus of rat liver. J. Lipid Res. **10**, 433—439 (1969).
255. MAHLEY, R. W., GRAY, M. E., HAMILTON, R. L., LEQUIRE, V. S.: Lipid transport in liver. II. Electron microscopic and biochemical studies of alterations in lipoprotein transport induced by cortisone in the rabbit. Lab. Invest. **19**, 358—369 (1968).
256. MAHLEY, R. W., HAMILTON, R. L., GRAY, M. P., LEQUIRE, V. S.: Precursors of plasma very low density lipoproteins (VLDL) isolated from hepatocyte Golgi apparatus. Circulation **38** (Suppl. VI), 14 (1968).
257. MAHLEY, R. W., BENNETT, B. D., MORRÉ, D. J., GRAY, M. E., THISTLETHWAITE, W., LEQUIRE, V. S.: Lipoproteins associated with the Golgi apparatus isolated from epithelial cells of rat small intestine. Lab. Invest. **25**, 435—444 (1971).
258. MAHLEY, R. W., BERSOT, T. P., LEQUIRE, V. S., LEVY, R. I., WINDMUELLER, H. G., BROWN, W. V.: Identity of very low density lipoprotein apoproteins of plasma and liver Golgi apparatus. Science **168**, 380—382 (1970).

259. Malaisse-Lagae, F., Greider, M. H., Malaisse, W. J., Lacy, P. E.: The stimulus-secretion coupling of glucose-induced insulin release. IV. The effect of vincristine and deuterium oxide on the microtubular system of the pancreatic beta-cell. J. Cell Biol. **49**, 530—535 (1971).

260. Malaisse, W. J., Malaisse-Lagae, F., Walker, M. O., Lacy, P. E.: The stimulus-secretion coupling of glucose-induced insulin release. V. The participation of a microtubular-microfilamentous system. Diabetes **20**, 257—265 (1971).

261. Manyan, D. R., Fulton, J. E., Jr., Bradley, S., Hsia, S. L.: Atromid-S: an effective uncoupler of oxidative phosphorylation. 158th Meeting, American Chemical Society, Abstract no. 49, 1969.

262. Maragoudakis, M. E.: Inhibition of hepatic acetyl coenzyme A carboxylase by hypolipidemic agents. J. biol. Chem. **244**, 5005—5013 (1969).

263. Maragoudakis, M. E., Hankin, H.: On the mode of action of lipid-lowering agents. V. Kinetiks of the inhibition *in vitro* of rat acetyl coenzyme A carboxylase. J. biol. Chem. **246**, 348—358 (1971).

263 a. Markwell, M. A. K., McGroarty, E. J., Bieber, L. L., Tolbert, N. E.: The subcellular distribution of carnitine acyltransferases in mammalian liver and kidney. A new peroxisomal enzyme. J. biol. Chem. **248**, 3426—3432 (1973).

264. Marsh, J. B.: The incorporation of amino acids into soluble lipoproteins by cell-free preparations from rat liver. J. biol. Chem. **238**, 1752—1756 (1963).

265. Marsh, J. B., Fritz, R.: The carbohydrate components of rat serum lipoproteins. Proc. Soc. exp. Biol. (N.Y.) **133**, 9—10 (1970).

266. Marshall, W. E., Kummerow, F. A.: The carbohydrate constituents of human serum β-lipoprotein: galactose, mannose, glucosamine and sialic acid. Arch. Biochem. Biophys. **98**, 271—273 (1962).

267. Mateu, L., Tardieu, A., Luzzati, V., Aggerbeck, L., Scanu, A. M.: On the structure of human serum low density lipoprotein. J. molec. Biol. **70**, 105—116 (1972).

268. Mayes, P. A., Felts, J. M.: Regulation of fat metabolism in the liver. Nature (Lond.) **215**, 716—718 (1967).

268 a. McKeel, D. W., Jr., Jarett, L.: The enrichment of adenyle cyclase in the plasma membrane and Golgi subcellular fractions of porcine adenohypophysis. J. Cell Biol. **62**, 231—236 (1974).

269. Melchers, F.: Biosynthesis of the carbohydrate portion of immunoglobulins. Radiochemical and chemical analysis of the carbohydrate moieties of two myeloma proteins purified from different subcellular fractions of plasma cells. Biochemistry **10**, 653—659 (1971).

270. Meldolesi, J.: Studies on cytoplasmic membrane fractions from guinea pig pancreas. In: Clementi, F., Ceccarelli, B. (Eds.): Advances in Cytopharmacology, Vol. 1, pp. 145—157. New York: Raven Press 1971.

271. Meldolesi, J., Cova, D.: *In vitro* stimulation of enzyme secretion and the synthesis of microsomal membranes in the pancreas of the guinea pig. J. Cell Biol. **51**, 396—404 (1971).

272. Meldolesi, J., Cova, D.: Composition of cellular membranes in the pancreas of the guinea pig. IV. Polyacrylamid gel electrophoresis and amino acid composition of membrane proteins. J. Cell Biol. **55**, 1—18 (1972).

273. Meldolesi, J., Jamieson, J. D., Palade, G. E.: Composition of cellular membranes in the pancreas of the guinea pig. I. Isolation of membrane fractions. J. Cell Biol. **49**, 109—129 (1971).

274. Meldolesi, J., Jamieson, J. D., Palade, G. E.: Composition of cellular membranes in the pancreas of the guinea pig. II. Lipids. J. Cell Biol. **49**, 130—149 (1971).

275. Meldolesi, J., Jamieson, J. D., Palade, G. E.: Composition of cellular membranes in the pancreas of the guinea pig. III. Enzymatic activities. J. Cell Biol. **49**, 150—158 (1971).

276. Mellors, A., Tappel, A. L.: Hydrolysis of phospholipids by a lysosomal enzyme. J. Lipid Res. **8**, 479—485 (1967).

276 a. Merritt, W. D., Morré, J. D.: A glycosyl transferase of high specific activity in secretory vesicles from isolated Golgi apparatus of rat liver. Biochim. biophys. Acta (Amst.) **304**, 397—407 (1973).

276 b. Metzger, H.: Structure and function of γM macroglobulins. Advanc. Immunol. **12**, 57—116 (1970).

277. MILSTEIN, C., BROWNLEE, G. G., HARRISON, T. M., MATHEWS, M. B.: A possible precursor of immunoglobulin light chains. Nature (Lond.) New Biol. **239**, 117—120 (1972).
278. MISHKEL, M. A., WEBB, W. F.: The mechanisms underlying the hypolipidaemic effects of Atromid-S, nicotinic acid and benzmalecene. I. The metabolism of free fatty acid-albumin complex by the isolated perfused liver. Biochem. Pharmacol. **16**, 897—905 (1967).
279. MOCHIZUKI, Y.: An electron microscope study on hepatocyte microbodies of mice bearing Ehrlich ascites tumor. Tumor Res. **3**, 1—34 (1968).
280. MOLLENHAUER, H. H., MORRÉ, D. J., KOGUT, C.: Dietary modification of the stability of rat liver Golgi apparatus. Exp. molec. Path. **11**, 113—122 (1969).
281. MOLNAR, J.: Glycoproteins of Ehrlich ascites carcinoma cells. Incorporation of (^{14}C) glucosamine and (^{14}C) sialic acid into membrane proteins. Biochemistry **6**, 3064—3076 (1967).
282. MOLNAR, J., SHY, D.: Attachment of glucosamine to protein at the ribosomal site of rat liver. Biochemistry **6**, 1941—1947 (1967).
283. MOLNAR, J., CHAO, H., MARKOVIC, G.: Subcellular site of structural glycoprotein synthesis in Ehrlich ascites tumor. Arch. Biochem. Biophys. **134**, 533—538 (1969).
284. MOLNAR, J., ROBINSON, G. B., WINZLER, R. J.: Biosynthesis of glycoproteins. IV. The subcellular sites of incorporation of glucosamine-1-^{14}C into glycoprotein in rat liver. J. biol. Chem. **240**, 1882—1888 (1965).
285. MOOKERJEA, S.: Studies on the plasma glycolipoprotein synthesis by the isolated perfused liver: effect of early choline deficiency. Can. J. Biochem. **47**, 125—133 (1969).
286. MORGAN, E. H., PETERS, T., JR.: Intracellular aspects of transferrin synthesis and secretion in the rat. J. biol. Chem. **246**, 3508—3511 (1971).
287. MORRÉ, D. J., KEENAN, T. W., MOLLENHAUER, H. H.: Golgi apparatus function in membrane transformations and product compartmentalization: studies with cell fractions isolated from rat liver. In: CLEMENTI, F., CECCARELLI, B. (Eds.): Advances in Cytopharmacology, Vol. 1, pp. 159—182. New York: Raven Press 1971.
288. MORRÉ, D. J., MERLIN, L. M., KEENAN, T. W.: Localization of glycosyl transferase activities in a Golgi apparatus-rich fraction isolated from rat liver. Biochem. Biophys. Res. Commun. **37**, 813—819 (1969).
289. MORRÉ, D. J., MOLLENHAUER, H. H., BRACKER, C. E.: Origin and continuity of Golgi apparatus. In: REINERT, J., URSPRUNG, H. (Eds.): Origin and Continuity of Cell Organelles, pp. 82—126. Berlin-Heidelberg-New York: Springer 1971.
290. MORRÉ, D. J., HAMILTON, R. L., MOLLENHAUER, H. H., MAHLEY, R. W., CUNNINGHAM, W. P., CHEETHAM, R. D., LeQUIRE, V. S.: Isolation of a Golgi apparatus-rich fraction from rat liver. Method and morphology. J. Cell Biol. **44**, 484—491 (1970).
291. MÜLLER, M.: Peroxisomes of protozoa. Ann. N.Y. Acad. Sci. **168**, 292—301 (1969).
292. NACHBAUR, J., COLBEAU, A., VIGNAIS, P. M.: Distribution of membrane-confined phospholipases A in the rat hepatocyte. Biochim. biophys. Acta (Amst.) **274**, 426—446 (1972).
293. NAKAGAMI, K., WARSHAWSKY, H., LEBLOND, C. P.: The elaboration of protein and carbohydrate by rat parathyroid cells as revealed by electron microscope radioautography. J. Cell Biol. **51**, 596—610 (1971).
294. NAMBA, Y., HANAOKA, M.: Immunoglobulin synthesis by cultured myeloma cells. J. Immunol. **102**, 1486—1497 (1969).
295. NESTEL, P. J., AUSTIN, W.: The effect of ethyl chlorophenoxyisobutyrate (CPIB) on the uptake of triglyceride fatty acids, activity of lipoprotein lipase and lipogenesis from glucose in fat tissue of rats. J. Atheroscler. Res. **8**, 827—833 (1968).
296. NEUTRA, M., LEBLOND, C. P.: Radioautographic comparison of the uptake of galactose-^{3}H and glucose-^{3}H in the Golgi region of various cells secreting glycoproteins and mucopolysaccharides. J. Cell Biol. **30**, 137—150 (1966).
297. NICOLSON, G. L.: Topography of membrane concanavalin A sites modified by proteolysis. Nature (Lond.) New Biol. **239**, 193—197 (1972).
297a. NOEL, S.-P., RUBINSTERN, D.: Secretion of apolipoproteins in very low density and high density lipoproteins by perfused rat liver. J. Lipid Res. **15**, 301—308 (1974).
298. NOLAN, C., SMITH, E. L.: Glycopeptides. II. Isolation and properties of glycopeptides from rabbit γ-globulin. J. biol. Chem. **237**, 446—452 (1962).
299. NOVIKOFF, A. B., ESSNER, E.: Cytolysomes and mitochondrial degeneration. J. Cell Biol. **15**, 140—146 (1962).

300. Novikoff,P.M., Novikoff,A.B.: Peroxisomes in absorptive cells of mammalian small intestine. J. Cell Biol. **53**, 532—560 (1972).

301. Novikoff,A.B., Shin,W.-Y.: The endoplasmic reticulum in the Golgi zone and its relations to microbodies, Golgi apparatus and autophagic vacuoles in rat liver cells. J. Microscopie **3**, 187—206 (1964).

302. Novikoff,A.B., Roheim,P.S., Quintana,N.: Changes in rat liver cells induced by orotic acid feeding. Lab. Invest. **15**, 27—49 (1966).

303. Novikoff,A.B., Novikoff,P.M., Davis,C., Quintana,N.: Studies on microperoxisomes. II. A cytochemical method for light and electron microscopy. J. Histochem. Cytochem. **20**, 1006—1023 (1972).

304. Novikoff,A.B., Novikoff,P.M., Davis,C., Quintana,N.: Studies on microperoxisomes. V. Are microperoxisomes ubiquitous in mammalian cells? J. Histochem. Cytochem. **21**, 737—755 (1973).

305. Novikoff,A.B., Novikoff,P.M., Quintana,N., Davis,C.: Diffusion artifacts in 3,3'-diaminobenzidine cytochemistry. J. Histochem. Cytochem. **20**, 745—749 (1972).

306. Novikoff,P.M., Novikoff,A.B., Quintana,N., Davis,C.: Studies on microperoxisomes. III. Observations on human and rat hepatocytes. J. Histochem. Cytochem. **21**, 540—558 (1973).

307. Nyguist,S.E., Mollenhauer,H.H.: A Golgi apparatus acid phosphatase. Biochim. biophys. Acta (Amst.) **315**, 103—112 (1973).

308. Ockner,R.K., Bloch,K.J., Isselbacher,K.J.: Very-low-density lipoprotein in intestinal lymph: evidence for presence of the A protein. Science **162**, 1285—1286 (1968).

309. Ockner,R.K., Hughes,F.B., Isselbacher,K.J.: Very low density lipoproteins in intestinal lymph: origin, composition, and role in lipid transport in the fasting state. J. clin. Invest. **48**, 2079—2088 (1969).

310. Oler,A., Lombardi,B.: Further studies on a defect in the intracellular transport and secretion of proteins by the liver of choline-deficient rats. J. biol. Chem. **245**, 1282—1288 (1970).

311. Olsnes,S.: The isolation of polysomes from rat liver. Contamination by membrane proteins with high affinity to ribosomes. Biochim. biophys. Acta **232**, 705—716 (1971).

312. Orci,L., Gabbay,K.H., Malaisse,W.J.: Pancreatic beta-cell web: its possible role in insulin secretion. Science **175**, 1128—1130 (1972).

313. Orci,L., LeMarchand, Y., Singh,A., Assimacopoulos-Jeannet,F., Rouiller,Ch., Jean-renaud,B.: Role of microtubules in lipoprotein secretion by the liver. Nature (Lond.) **244**, 30—32 (1973).

314. Ovtracht,L., Thiéry,J.-P.: Mise en évidence par cytochimie ultrastructurale de compartiments physiologiquement différents dans un même saccule golgien. J. Microscopie **15**, 135—170 (1972).

314a. Ovtracht,L., Morré,D.J., Cheetham,R.D., Mollenhauer,H.H.: Subfractionation of Golgi apparatus from rat liver: method and morphology. J. Microscopie **18**, 87—102 (1973).

315. Page,I.H.: Atherosclerosis. An introduction. Metabolism **10**, 1—27 (1954).

316. Painter,R.G., Tokuyasu,K.T., Singer,S.J.: Immunoferritin localization of intracellular antigens: the use of ultracryotomy to obtain ultrathin sections suitable for direct immunoferritin staining. Proc. nat. Acad. Sci. (Wash.) **70**, 1649—1653 (1973).

317. Palade,G.E.: Functional changes in the structure of cell components. In: Hayashi,T. (Ed.): Subcellular Particles, pp.64—80. New York: Ronald Press Comp. 1959.

318. Palade,G.E., Siekevitz,P., Caro,L.G.: Structure, chemistry and function of the pancreatic exocrine cell. In: De Reuck,A.V.S., Cameron,M.P. (Eds.): The Exocrine Pancreas. CIBA Foundation Symposium, pp.23—49. London: Churchill 1962.

319. Parkhouse,R.M.E., Allison,A.C.: Failure of cytochalasin or colchicine to inhibit secretion of immunoglobulins. Nature (Lond.) New Biol. **235**, 220—222 (1972).

319a. Patt,L.M., Grimes,W.J.: Cell surface glycolipid and glycoprotein glycosyltransferases of normal and transformed cells. J. biol. Chem. **249**, 4157—4165 (1974).

320. Pearlstein,E., Aladjem,F.: Subpopulations of human serum very low density lipoproteins. Biochemistry **11**, 2553—2558 (1972).

320a. Pelletier,G.: Autoradiographic studies of synthesis and intracellular migration of glycoproteins in the rat anterior pituitary gland. J. Cell Biol. **62**, 185—197 (1974).

321. PEREIRA, J. N., HOLLAND, G. F.: Studies of the mechanism of action of p-chlorophenoxy-isobutyrate (CPIB). In: JONES, R. J. (Ed.): Atherosclerosis. Proc. Second Internat. Symp., pp. 549—554. Berlin-Heidelberg-New York: Springer 1970.

322. PETERS, T., JR.: The biosynthesis of rat serum albumin. II. Intracellular phenomena in the secretion of newly formed albumin. J. biol. Chem. **237**, 1186—1189 (1962).

323. PETERS, T., JR., FLEISCHER, B., FLEISCHER, S.: The biosynthesis of rat serum albumin. IV. Apparent passage of albumin through the Golgi apparatus during secretion. J. biol. Chem. **246**, 240—244 (1971).

324. PETRIK, P.: Fine structural identification of peroxisomes in mouse and rat bronchiolar and alveolar epithelium. J. Histochem. Cytochem. **19**, 339—348 (1971).

325. PLAGEMANN, P. G. W., ESTENSEN, R. D.: Cytochalasin B. VI. Competitive inhibition of nucleoside transport by cultured Novikoff rat hepatoma cells. J. Cell Biol. **55**, 179—185 (1972).

326. PLATT, D. S., COCKRILL, B. L.: Changes in the liver concentrations of the nicotinamide adenine dinucleotide coenzymes and in the activit,es of oxidoreductase enzymes following treatment of the rat with ethyl chlorophenoxyisobutyrate (Atromid-S). Biochem. Pharmacol. **15**, 927—935 (1966).

327. PLATT, D. S., THORP, J. M.: Changes in the weight and composition of the liver in the rat, dog and monkey treated with ethyl chlorophenoxyisobutyrate. Biochem. Pharmacol. **15**, 915—925 (1966).

328. POOLE, B.: Biogenesis and turnover of rat liver peroxisomes. Ann. N.Y. Acad. Sci. **168**, 229—243 (1969).

329. POOLE, B.: The kinetics of disappearance of labeled leucine from the free leucine pool of rat liver and its effect on the apparent turnover of catalase and other hepatic proteins. J. biol. Chem. **246**, 6587—6591 (1971).

330. POOLE, A. R., HOWELL, J. I., LUCY, J. A.: Lysolecithin and cell fusion. Nature (Lond.) **227**, 810—814 (1970).

331. POOLE, B., HIGASHI, T., DeDUVE, C.: The synthesis and turnover of rat liver peroxisomes. III. The size distribution of peroxisomes and the incorporation of new catalase. J. Cell Biol. **45**, 408—415 (1970).

332. POOLE, B., LEIGHTON, F., DE DUVE, C.: The synthesis and turnover of rat liver peroxisomes. II. Turnover of peroxisome proteins. J. Cell Biol. **41**, 536—546 (1969).

333. POTTENGER, L. A., GETZ, G. S.: Serum lipoprotein accumulation in the livers of orotic acid-fed rats. J. Lipid Res. **12**, 450—459 (1971).

334. PRICE, V. E., STERLING, W. R., TARANTOLA, V. A., HARTLEY, R. W., JR., RECHCIGL, M., JR.: The kinetics of catalase synthesis and destruction *in vivo*. J. biol. Chem. **237**, 3468—3475 (1962).

335. PRICER, W. E., JR., ASHWELL, G.: The binding of desialylated glycoproteins by plasma membranes of rat liver. J. biol. Chem. **246**, 4825—4833 (1971).

336. PRIESTLEY, G. C., PRUYN, M. L., MALT, R. A.: Glycoprotein synthesis by membrane-bound ribosomes and smooth membranes in kidney. Biochim. biophys. Acta (Amst.) **190**, 154—160 (1969).

337. PUDDU, P., CALDARERA, C. M., MARCHETTI, M.: Studies on ethionine-induced fatty liver. Biochem. J. **102**, 163—167 (1967).

338. PUTNAM, F. W.: Immunoglobulin structure: variability and homology. Science **163**, 633—644 (1969).

339. RAGLAND, W. L., SHIRES, T. K., PITOT, H. C.: Polyribosomal attachment to rat liver and hepatoma endoplasmic reticulum *in vitro*. A method for its study. Biochem. J. **121**, 271—278 (1971).

340. RAJALAKSHIMI, S., ADAMS, W. R., HANDSCHUMACHER, R. E.: Isolation and characterization of low density structures from orotic acid-induced fatty livers. J. Cell Biol. **41**, 625—636 (1969).

341. RAMBOURG, A., HERNANDEZ, W., LEBLOND, C. P.: Detection of complex carbohydrates in the Golgi apparatus of rat cells. J. Cell Biol. **40**, 395—414 (1969).

341a. REAVEN, E. P., KOLTERMAN, O. G., REAVEN, G. M.: Ultrastructural and physiological evidence for corticosteroid-induced alterations in hepatic production of very low density lipoprotein particles. J. Lipid Res. **15**, 74—83 (1974).

342. REDDY, J., SVOBODA, D.: Microbodies in experimentally altered cells. VIII. Continuities between microbodies and their possible biologic significance. Lab. Invest. **24**, 74—81 (1971).

343. Reddy,J., Svoboda,D.: Proliferation of microbodies and synthesis of catalase in rat liver. Induction in tumor-bearing host by CPIB. Amer. J. Path. **63**, 99—106 (1971).
344. Reddy,J., Svoboda,D.: Microbodies (peroxisomes). Identification in interstitial cells of the testis. J. Histochem. Cytochem. **20**, 140—142 (1972).
345. Reddy,J., Svoboda,D.: Microbodies in Leydig cell tumors of rat testis. J. Histochem. Cytochem. **20**, 793—803 (1972).
346. Reddy,J., Svoboda,D.: Further evidence to suggest that microbodies do not exist as individual entities. Amer. J. Path. **70**, 421—438 (1973).
346a. Reddy,J., Svoboda,D.: Microbody (peroxisome) matrix: transformation into tubular structures. Virchows Arch. Abt. B Zellpath. **14**, 83—92 (1973).
347. Reddy,J., Bunyaratvej,S., Svoboda,D.: Microbodies in experimentally altered cells. IV. Acatalasemic (Cs^b) mice treated with CPIB. J. Cell Biol. **42**, 587—596 (1969).
348. Reddy,J., Bunyaratvej,S., Svoboda,D.: Microbodies in experimentally altered cells. V. Histochemical and cytochemical studies on the livers of rats and acatalasemic (Cs^b) mice treated with CPIB. Amer. J. Path. **56**, 351—370 (1969).
349. Reddy,J., Chiga,M., Svoboda,D.: Stimulation of liver catalase synthesis in rats by ethyl-γ-p-chlorophenoxyisobutyrate. Biochem. Biophys. Res. Commun. **43**, 318—324 (1971).
349a. Reddy,J., Svoboda,D., Azarnoff,D.L.: Microbody proliferation in liver induced by nafenopin, a new hypolipidemic drug: comparison with CPIB. Biochem. Biophys. Res. Commun. **52**, 537—543 (1973).
349b. Reddy,J., Azarnoff,D.L., Svoboda,D., Prasad,J.D.: Nafenopin-induced hepatic microbody (peroxisome) proliferation and catalase synthesis in rats and mice. J. Cell Biol. **61**, 344—358 (1974).
350. Reddy,J., Chiga,M., Bunyaratvej,S., Svoboda,D.: Microbodies in experimentally altered cells. VII. CPIB-induced hepatic microbody proliferation in the absence of significant catalase synthesis. J. Cell Biol. **44**, 226—234 (1970).
351. Redman,C.M.: Studies on the transfer of incomplete polypeptide chains across rat liver microsomal membranes *in vitro*. J. biol. Chem. **242**, 761—768 (1967).
352. Redman,C.M.: The synthesis of serum proteins on attached rather than free ribosomes of rat liver. Biochem. Biophys. Res. Commun. **31**, 845—850 (1968).
353. Redman,C.M., Cherian,M.G.: The secretory pathways of rat serum glycoproteins and albumin. Localization of newly formed proteins within the endoplasmic reticulum. J. Cell Biol. **52**, 231—245 (1972).
354. Redman,C.M., Sabatini,D.D.: Vectorial discharge of peptides released by puromycin from attached ribosomes. Proc. nat. Acad. Sci. (Wash.) **56**, 608—615 (1966).
354a. Redman,C.M., Grab,D.J., Irukula,R.: The intracellular pathway of newly formed rat liver catalase. Arch. Biochem. Biophys. **152**, 496—501 (1972).
355. Redman,C.M., Siekevitz,P., Palade,G.E.: Synthesis and transfer of amylase in pigeon pancreatic microsomes. J. biol. Chem. **241**, 1150—1158 (1966).
356. Remmer,H., Merker,H.-J.: Drug-induced changes in the liver endoplasmic reticulum: association with drug-metabolizing enzymes. Science **142**, 1657—1658 (1963).
357. Riede,U.N., Ettlin,Ch., Von Allmen,R., Rohr,H.P.: Vergleichende ultrastrukturell-morphometrische Untersuchung zwischen der Leberparenchymzelle der Wistarratte (Rattus norvegicus) und der Wüstenratte (Meriones crassus) nach einer einmaligen CPIB (Clobifrat)-Verabreichung. Naunyn-Schmiedebergs Arch. Pharmak. **272**, 336—350 (1972).
358. Rigatuso,J.L., Legg,P.G., Wood,R.L.: Microbody formation in regenerating rat liver. J. Histochem. Cytochem. **18**, 893—900 (1970).
358a. Riordan,J.R., Mitchell,L., Slavik,M.: The binding of asialo-glycoprotein to isolated Golgi apparatus. Biochem. Biophys. Res. Commun. **59**, 1373—1379 (1974).
359. Roberts,R.J., Plaa,G.L.: Effect of phenobarbital on the excretion of an exogenous bilirubin load. Biochem. Pharmacol. **16**, 827—835 (1967).
360. Robinson,D.S., Seakins,A.: The development in the rat of fatty livers associated with reduced plasma-lipoprotein synthesis. Biochim. biophys. Acta (Amst.) **62**, 163—165 (1962).
360a. Rogers,M.J., Strittmatter,P.: Evidence for random distribution and translational movement of cytochrome b_5 in endoplasmic reticulum. J. biol. Chem. **249**, 895—900 (1974).

361. ROHEIM, P.S., BIEMPICA, L., EDELSTEIN, D., KOSOWER, N.S.: Mechanism of fatty liver development and hyperlipemia in rats treated with allylisopropylacetamide. J. Lipid Res. **12**, 76—83 (1971).

362. ROHEIM, P.S., GIDEZ, L.I., EDER, H.A.: Extrahepatic synthesis of lipoproteins of plasma and chyle: role of the intestine. J. clin. Invest. **45**, 297—300 (1966).

363. ROHEIM, P.S., SWITZER, S., GIRARD, A., EDER, H.A.: Alterations of lipoprotein metabolism in orotic acid-induced fatty liver. Lab. Invest. **15**, 21—23 (1966).

364. ROLLESTON, F.S.: The binding of ribosomal subunits to endoplasmic reticulum membranes. Biochem. J. **129**, 721—731 (1972).

365. ROLLESTON, F.S., MAK, D.: The binding of polyribosomes to smooth and rough endoplasmic-reticulum membranes. Biochem. J. **131**, 851—853 (1973).

366. ROOBOL, A., RABIN, B.R.: The binding of polysomes to smooth membranes of rat liver promoted by steroid hormones and extracts from either rough endoplasmic reticulum or from polysomes of the opposite sex. FEBS Letters **14**, 165—169 (1971).

367. ROSBASH, M.: Formation of membrane-bound polyribosomes. J. molec. Biol. **65**, 413—422 (1972).

368. ROSBASH, M., PENMAN, S.: Membrane-associated protein synthesis of mammalian cells. I. The two classes of membrane-associated ribosomes. J. molec. Biol. **59**, 227—241 (1971).

368a. ROTH, S., McGUIRE, E.J., ROSEMAN, S.: Evidence for cell-surface glycosyltransferases. Their potential role in cellular recognition. J. Cell Biol. **51**, 536—547 (1971).

368b. RUBENSTEIN, B., RUBINSTEIN, D.: Interrelationship between rat serum very low density and high density lipoproteins. J. Lipid Res. **13**, 317—324 (1972).

369. RUDERMAN, N.B., JONES, A.L., KRAUSS, R.M., SHAFIR, E.: A biochemical and morphologic study of very low density lipoproteins in carbohydrate-induced hypertriglyceridemia. J. clin. Invest. **50**, 1355—1368 (1971).

370. RUDERMAN, N.B., RICHARDS, K.C., VALLES DE BOURGES, V., JONES, A.L.: Regulation of production and release of lipoprotein by the perfused rat liver. J. Lipid Res. **9**, 613—619 (1968).

371. RUEGAMER, W.R., RYAN, N.T., RICHERT, D.A., WESTERFELD, W.W.: The effects of p-chlorophenoxyisobutyrate on the turnover rate and distribution of thyroid hormone in the rat. Biochem. Pharmacol. **18**, 613—624 (1969).

372. RYAN, W.G., SCHWARTZ, T.B.: The dynamics of triglyceride turnover: effect of Atromid-S. J. Lab. clin. Med. **64**, 1001 (1964).

373. SABATINI, D.D., BLOBEL, G.: Controlled proteolysis of nascent polypeptides in rat liver cell fractions. II. Location of the polypeptides in rough microsomes. J. Cell Biol. **45**, 146—157 (1970).

374. SABATINI, D.D., TASHIRO, Y., PALADE, G.E.: On the attachment of ribosomes to microsomal membranes. J. molec. Biol. **19**, 503—524 (1966).

375. SARMA, D.S.R., VERNEY, E., SIDRANSKY, H.: Studies on the nature of attachment of ribosomes to membranes in liver. II. Influence of monovalent cations on the detachment of membrane-bound ribosomes from membranes. Lab. Invest. **27**, 48—52 (1972).

376. SARMA, D.S.R., REID, I.M., VERNEY, E., SIDRANSKY, H.: Studies on the nature of attachment of ribosomes to membranes in liver. I. Influence of ethionine, sparsomycin, CCl_4, and puromycin on membrane-bound polyribosomal disaggregation and on detachment of membrane-bound ribosomes from membranes. Lab. Invest. **27**, 39—47 (1972).

376a. SATIR, B., SCHOOLEY, C., SATIR, P.: Membrane fusion in a model system. Mucocyst secretion in tetrahymena. J. Cell Biol. **56**, 153—176 (1973).

377. SAUER, L.A., BURROW, G.N.: The submicrosomal distribution of radioactive proteins released by puromycin from the bound ribosomes of rat liver microsomes labelled *in vitro*. Biochim. biophys. Acta **277**, 179—187 (1972).

378. SAUNER, M.-T., LÉVY, M.: Study of the transfer of phospholipids from the endoplasmic reticulum to the outer and inner mitochondrial membranes. J. Lipid Res. **12**, 71—75 (1971).

379. SCANDELLA, C.J., DEVAUX, P., McCONNELL, H.M.: Rapid lateral diffusion of phospholipids in rabbit sarcoplasmic reticulum. Proc. nat. Acad. Sci. (Wash.) **69**, 2056—2060 (1972).

380. SCANU, A.M.: Forms of human serum high density lipoprotein protein. J. Lipid Res. **7**, 295—306 (1966).

381. Scanu, A. M.: The structure of human serum low- and high-density lipoproteins. In Athero-genesis: Porter, R., Knight, J. (Eds.): Initiating Factors. CIBA Foundation Symposium, Vol. 12, pp. 223—246. Amsterdam: Elsevier 1973.

381a. Scanu, A. M., Lim, C. T., Edelstein, C.: On the subunit structure of the protein of human serum high density lipoprotein. II. A study of sephadex fraction, IV. J. Cell Biol. **247**, 5850—5855 (1972).

382. Schacht, U., Granzer, E.: On the effect of the hypolipidaemic phenyl ether CH 13437 on the liver metabolism of the rat. Biochem. Pharmacol. **19**, 2963—2971 (1970).

383. Schachter, H. I., Jabbal, R. L., Hudgin, R. L., Pinteric, L., McGuire, E. J., Roseman, S.: Intracellular localization of liver sugar nucleotide glycoprotein glycosyltransferases in a Golgi-rich fraction. J. biol. Chem. **245**, 1090—1100 (1970).

384. Schenkein, I., Uhr, J. W.: Immunoglobulin synthesis and secretion. I. Biosynthetic studies of the addition of the carbohydrate moieties. J. Cell Biol. **46**, 42—51 (1970).

385. Schlunk, F. F., Lombardi, B.: Liver liposomes. I. Isolation and chemical characterization. Lab. Invest. **17**, 30—38 (1967).

386. Schmid, R., Figen, J. F., Schwartz, S.: Experimental porphyria. IV. Studies of liver cata-lase and other heme enzymes in sedormid porphyria. J. biol. Chem. **217**, 263—274 (1955).

387. Schneeberger, E. E.: A comparative cytochemical study of microbodies (peroxisomes) in great alveolar cells of rodents, rabbit and monkey. J. Histochem. Cytochem. **20**, 180—191 (1972).

388. Schofield, J. G.: Cytochalasin B and release of growth hormone. Nature (Lond.) New Biol. **234**, 215—216 (1971).

389. Schonfeld, G.: Changes in the composition of very low density lipoprotein during carbo-hydrate induction in man. J. Lab. clin. Med. **75**, 206—211 (1970).

390. Schubert, D.: Immunoglobulin assembly in a mouse myeloma. Proc. nat. Acad. Sci. (Wash.) **60**, 683—690 (1968).

391. Schubert, D., Cohn, M.: Immunoglobulin biosynthesis. III. Blocks in defective synthesis. J. molec. Biol. **38**, 273—288 (1968).

392. Scott-Burden, T., Hawtrey, A. O.: Studies on the reattachment of ribosomes and riboso-mal subunits to ribosome-free membranes prepared from rat liver microsomes by means of lithium chloride. Hoppe-Seylers Z. physiol. Chem. **352**, 575—582 (1971).

393. Scott, P. J., Hurley, P. J.: The distribution of radio-iodinated serum albumin and low-density lipoprotein in tissues and the arterial wall. Atherosclerosis **11**, 77—103 (1970).

394. Segal, P., Roheim, P. S., Eder, H. A.: Mechanism of action of chlorophenoxyisobutyrate in hyperlipemic rats. Circulation **40** (Suppl. III), 182 (1969).

395. Shames, D. M., Frank, A., Steinberg, D., Berman, M.: Transport of plasma free fatty acids and triglycerides in man: a theoretical analysis. J. clin. Invest. **49**, 2298—2314 (1970).

396. Shapiro, D. J., Rodwell, V. W.: Regulation of hepatic 3-hydroxy-3-methylglutaryl coen-zyme A reductase and cholesterol synthesis. J. biol. Chem. **246**, 3210—3216 (1971).

397. Shapiro, A. L., Scharff, M. D., Maizel, J. V., Jr., Uhr, J. W.: Polyribosomal synthesis and assembly of the H and L chains of gamma-globulin. Proc. nat. Acad. Sci. (Wash.) **56**, 216—221 (1966).

398. Shelton, E., Kuff, E. L.: Substructure and configuration of ribosomes isolated from mam-malian cells. J. molec. Biol. **22**, 23—31 (1966).

399. Sherr, C. J., Uhr, J. W.: Immunoglobulin synthesis and secretion, V. Incorporation of leu-cine and glucosamine into immunoglobulin on free and bound polyribosomes. Proc. nat. Acad. Sci. (Wash.) **66**, 1183—1189 (1970).

400. Sherr, C. J., Uhr, J. W.: Immunoglobulin synthesis and secretion. VI. Synthesis and intra-cellular transport of immunoglobulin in nonsecretory lymphoma cells. J. exp. Med. **133**, 901—920 (1971).

400a. Shio, H., Farquhar, M. G., De Duve, C.: Lysosomes of the arterial wall, IV. Cytochemi-cal localization of acid phosphatase and catalase in smooth muscle cells and foam cells from rabbit atheromatous aorta. Amer. J. Path. **76**, 1—16 (1974).

401. Shires, T. K., Narurkar, L. M., Pitot, H. C.: Polysome interaction *in vitro* with smooth microsomal membranes from rat liver. Biochem. Biophys. Res. Commun. **45**, 1212—1218 (1971).

402. SHIRES, T. K., NARURKAR, L., PITOT, H. C.: The association *in vitro* of polyribosomes with ribonuclease-treated derivatives of hepatic rough endoplasmic reticulum. Characteristics of the membrane binding sites and factors influencing association. Biochem. J. **125**, 67—79 (1971).
403. SIEKEVITZ, P., PALADE, G. E.: Distribution of newly synthesized amylase in microsomal subfractions of guinea pig pancreas. J. Cell Biol. **30**, 519—530 (1966).
404. SINCLAIR, A. J., COLLINS, F. D.: Fatty livers in rats deficient in essential fatty acids. Biochim. biophys. Acta (Amst.) **152**, 498—510 (1968).
405. SINGER, S. J., NICOLSON, G. L.: The fluid mosaic model of the structure of cell membranes. Science **175**, 720—731 (1972).
406. SMITH, A. D., WINKLER, H.: Lysosomal phospholipases A_1 and A_2 of bovine adrenal medulla. Biochem. J. **108**, 867—874 (1968).
407. SMITH, E. P., SLATER, R. S.: The lipoproteins of the lesions. In: JONES, R. J. (Ed.): Atherosclerosis, Proc. Second Int. Symp., pp. 42—49. Berlin-Heidelberg-New York: Springer 1970.
408. SMITH, R. E., FARQUHAR, M. G.: Lysosome function in the regulation of the secretory process in cells of the anterior pituitary gland. J. Cell Biol. **31**, 319—347 (1966).
409. SMUCKLER, E. A., BENDITT, E. P.: Carbon tetrachloride poisoning in rats: alteration in ribosomes of the liver. Science **140**, 308—310 (1963).
410. SPIRO, R. G.: Glycoproteins. Ann. Rev. Biochem. **39**, 599—638 (1970).
411. SPOONER, B. S., YAMADA, K. M., WESSELS, N. K.: Microfilaments and cell locomotion. J. Cell Biol. **49**, 595—613 (1971).
412. SPRITZ, N., LIEBER, C. S.: Decrease of ethanol-induced fatty liver by ethyl-α-p-chlorophenoxyisobutyrate. Proc. Soc. exp. Biol. (N.Y.) **121**, 147—149 (1966).
413. STÄUBLI, W., HESS, R.: Quantitative aspects of heptomegaly induced by ethyl chlorophenoxyisobutyrate (CPIB). In: UYEDA, R. (Ed.): Proceedings of the 6th International Congress for Electron Microscopy, Kyoto, Vol. 2, pp. 625—626. Tokyo: Maruzen 1966.
414. STÄUBLI, W., FREYVOGEL, T. A., SUTER, J.: Structural modification of the endoplasmic reticulum of midgut epithelial cells of mosquitos in relation to blood intake. J. Microscopie **5**, 189—204 (1966).
415. STÄUBLI, W., HESS, R., DIETRICH, F. M.: Unpublished observations.
416. STÄUBLI, W., HESS, R., WEIBEL, E. R.: Correlated morphometric and biochemical studies on the liver cell. II. Effects of phenobarbital on rat hepatocytes. J. Cell Biol. **42**, 92—112 (1969).
417. STÄUBLI, W., WEIBEL, E. R., HESS, R.: In preparation.
418. STEIN, O., STEIN, Y.: Electronmicroscopic autoradiography of ^{3}H-glycerol labeled lipid in ethanol induced fatty liver. Exp. Cell Res. **42**, 198—201 (1966).
419. STEIN, O., STEIN, Y.: Lipid synthesis, intracellular transport, storage and secretion. I. Electron microscopic radioautographic study of liver after injection of tritiated palmitate or glycerol in fasted or ethanol-treated rats. J. Cell Biol. **33**, 319—339 (1967).
420. STEIN, O., STEIN, Y.: Lecithin synthesis, intracellular transport, and secretion in rat liver. IV. A radioautographic and biochemical study of choline-deficient rats injected with choline-^{3}H. J. Cell Biol. **40**, 461—483 (1969).
421. STEIN, O., STEIN, Y.: Colchicine-induced inhibition of very low density lipoprotein release by rat liver *in vivo*. Biochim. biophys. Acta (Amst.) **306**, 142—147 (1973).
422. STEIN, O., STEIN, Y., EISENBERG, S.: A radioautographic study of the transport of ^{125}I-labeled serum lipoprotein in rat aorta. Z. Zellforsch. **138**, 223—237 (1973).
422a. STEIN, O., SANGER, L., STEIN, Y.: Colchicine-induced inhibition of lipoprotein and protein secretion into the serum and lack of interference with secretion of biliary phospholipids and cholesterol by rat liver *in vivo*. J. Cell Biol. **62**, 90—103 (1974).
422b. STEIN, O., RACHMILEWITZ, D., SANGER, L., EISENBERG, S., STEIN, Y.: Metabolism of iodinated very low density lipoprotein in the rat. Autoradiographic localization in the liver. Biochim. biophys. Acta (Amst.) **360**, 205—216 (1974).
423. STEIN, Y., SHAPIRO, B.: Assimilation and dissimilation of fatty acids by the rat liver. Amer. J. Physiol. **196**, 1238—1241 (1959).
424. STEINBERG, D.: Drugs inhibiting cholesterol biosynthesis, with special reference to clofibrate. In: JONES, R. J. (Ed.): Atherosclerosis. Proc. Second Internat. Symp., pp. 500—508. Berlin-Heidelberg-New York: Springer 1970.

425. STEVENS, R. H., WILLIAMSON, A. R.: Translational control of immunoglobulin synthesis. I. Repression of heavy chain synthesis. J. molec. Biol. **78**, 505—516 (1973).

426. STEVENS, R. H., WILLIAMSON, A. R.: Translational control of immunoglobulin synthesis. II. Cell-free interaction of myeloma immunoglobulin with mRNA. J. molec. Biol. **78**, 517—528 (1973).

427. STOFFEL, W., GRETEN, H.: Studies on lipolytic activities of rat liver lysosomes. Hoppe-Seylers Z. physiol. Chem. **348**, 1145—1150 (1967).

428. STOFFEL, W., TRABERT, U.: Studies on the occurrence and properties of lysosomal phospholipases A_1 and A_2 and the degradation of phosphatidic acid in rat liver lysosomes. Hoppe-Seylers Z. physiol. Chem. **350**, 836—844 (1969).

429. STOKKE, K. J.: Subcellular distribution and kinetics of the acid cholesterol esterase in liver. Biochim. biophys. Acta (Amst.) **280**, 329—335 (1972).

430. STRISOWER, E. H.: The combined use of CPIB and thyroxine in treatment of hyperlipoproteinemias. Circulation **33**, 291—296 (1966).

431. STRISOWER, E. H., STRISOWER, B.: The separate hypolipoproteinemic effects of dextrothyroxine and ethyl chlorophenoxyisobutyrate. J. clin. Endocr. **24**, 139—144 (1964).

432. STRISOWER, E. H., NICHOLS, A. V., LINDGREN, F. T., SMITH, L.: The effect of Sf 20-10^5 concentration changes induced by ethyl chlorophenoxyisobutyrate on high-density lipoprotein lipid composition. J. Lab. clin. Med. **65**, 748—755 (1965).

433. STURGESS, J. M., KATONA, E., MOSCARELLO, M. A.: The Golgi complex. I. Isolation and ultrastructure in normal rat liver. J. Membrane Biol. **12**, 367—384 (1973).

434. STURGESS, J. M., MITRANIC, M., MOSCARELLO, M. A.: The incorporation of D-glucosamine-^{3}H into the Golgi complex from rat liver and into serum glycoproteins. Biochem. Biophys. Res. Commun. **46**, 1270—1277 (1972).

435. STURGESS, J. M., MINAKER, E., MITRANIC, M. M., MOSCARELLO, M. A.: The incorporation of L-fucose into glycoproteins in the Golgi apparatus of rat liver and in serum. Biochim. biophys. Acta (Amst.) **320**, 123—132 (1973).

435a. SUNDLER, R., ÅKESSON, B., NILSSON, Å.: Triacylglycerol secretion in very low density lipoproteins by isolated rat liver parenchymal cells. Biochem. Biophys. Res. Commun. **55**, 961—968 (1973).

436. SÜSS, R., BLOBEL, G., PITOT, H. C.: Rat liver and hepatoma polysome-membrane interaction *in vitro*. Biochem. Biophys. Res. Commun. **23**, 299—304 (1966).

437. SUNSHINE, G. H., WILLIAMS, D. J., RABIN, B. R.: Role for steroid hormones in the interaction of ribosomes with the endoplasmic membranes of rat liver. Nature (Lond.) New Biol. **230**, 133—136 (1971).

438. SVOBODA, D., AZARNOFF, D. L.: Response of hepatic microbodies to a hypolipidemic agent, ethyl chlorophenoxyisobutyrate (CPIB). J. Cell Biol. **30**, 442—450 (1966).

439. SVOBODA, D. J., AZARNOFF, D. L.: Effects of selected hypolipidemic drugs on cell ultrastructure. Fed Proc. **30**, 841—847 (1971).

440. SVOBODA, D., REDDY, J.: Microbodies in experimentally altered cells. IX. The fate of microbodies. Amer. J. Path. **67**, 541—554 (1972).

441. SVOBODA, D., AZARNOFF, D. L., REDDY, J.: Microbodies in experimentally altered cells. II. The relationship of microbody proliferation to endocrine glands. J. Cell Biol. **40**, 734—746 (1969).

442. SVOBODA, D., GRADY, H., AZARNOFF, D.: Microbodies in experimentally altered cells. J. Cell Biol. **35**, 127—152 (1967).

443. TAKAGI, M., OGATA, K.: Direct evidence for albumin biosynthesis by membrane bound polysomes in rat liver. Biochem. Biophys. Res. Commun. **33**, 55—60 (1968).

444. TAKAGI, M., OGATA, K.: Isolation of serum albumin-synthesizing polysomes from rat liver. Biochem. Biophys. Res. Commun. **42**, 125—131 (1971).

445. TAKAGI, M., TANAKA, T., OGATA, K.: Functional differences in protein synthesis between free and bound polysomes of rat liver. Biochim. biophys. Acta (Amst.) **217**, 148—158 (1970).

446. TATA, J. R.: Ribosomal segregation as a possible function for the attachment of ribosomes to membranes. Sub-Cell. Biochem. **1**, 83—89 (1972).

447. TAYLOR, R. B., DUFFUS, W. P. H., RAFF, M. C., DE PETRIS, S.: Redistribution and pinocytosis of lymphocyte surface immunoglobulin molecules induced by anti-immunoglobulin antibody. Nature (Lond.) New Biol. **233**, 225—229 (1971).

448. TESAR,J.T.: Hormone storage granules in beef pituitary. Isolation and composition. Fed. Proc. **26**, 534 (1967).
449. TOLMAN, E. L., TEPPERMAN, H. M., TEPPERMAN, J.: Effect of ethyl p-chlorophenoxyisobutyrate on rat adipose lipoprotein lipase activity. Amer. J. Physiol. **218**, 1313—1318 (1970).
450. TROTTER, N. L.: Electron-opaque bodies and fat droplets in mouse liver after fasting or glucose injection. J. Cell Biol. **34**, 703—711 (1967).
451. TSUKADA, H., MOCHIZUKI, Y., FUJIWARA, S.: The nucleoids of rat liver cell microbodies. Fine structure and enzymes. J. Cell Biol. **28**, 449—460 (1966).
452. TSUKADA, H., MOCHIZUKI, Y., KONISHI, T.: Morphogenesis and development of microbodies of hepatocytes of rats during pre- and postnatal growth. J. Cell Biol. **37**, 231—243 (1968).
453. TYTGAT, G. N., RUBIN, C. E., SAUNDERS, D. R.: Synthesis and transport of lipoprotein particles by intestinal absorptive cells in man. J. clin. Invest. **50**, 2065—2078 (1971).
454. UENOYAMA, K., ONO, T.: Nascent catalase and its messenger RNA on rat liver polyribosomes. J. molec. Biol. **65**, 75—89 (1972).
455. UHR, J. W., SCHENKEIN, I.: Immunoglobulin synthesis and secretion. IV. Sites of incorporation of sugars as determined by subcellular fractionation. Proc. nat. Acad. Sci. (Wash.) **66**, 952—958 (1970).
455a. UKENA, T. E., BERLIN, R. D.: Effect of colchicine and vinblastine on the topographical separation of membrane function. J. exp. Med. **136**, 1—7 (1972).
456. VAN DEENEN, L. L. M., VAN DEN BOSCH, H., VAN GOLDE, L. M. G., SCHERPHOF, G. L., WAITE, B. M.: Some structural and metabolic aspects of fatty acids in phosphoglycerides. Cellular Compartmentalization and Control of Fatty Acid Metabolism, pp. 89—109. Oslo: Universitetsforlaget, 1968.
457. VANDOR, S. L., TOLBERT, N. E.: Glyoxylate metabolism by isolated rat liver peroxisomes. Biochim. biophys. Acta (Amst.) **215**, 449—455 (1970).
458. VAN GOLDE, L. M. G., FLEISCHER, B., FLEISCHER, S.: Some studies on the metabolism of phospholipids in Golgi complex from bovine and rat liver in comparison to other subcellular fractions. Biochim. biophys. Acta (Amst.) **249**, 318—330 (1971).
459. VAN HOEVEN, R. P., EMMELOT, P.: Studies on plasma membranes. XVIII. Lipid class composition of plasma membranes isolated from rat and mouse liver and hepatomas. J. Membrane Biol. **9**, 105—126 (1972).
460. VASSART, G.: Specific synthesis of thyroglobulin on membrane bound thyroid ribosomes. FEBS Letters **22**, 53—56 (1972).
461. VORBRODT, A., GRUCA, S., KRZYZOWSKA-GRUCA, S.: Cytochemical studies on the participation of endoplasmic reticulum in the formation of lysosomes (dense bodies) in rat hepatocytes. J. Microscopie **12**, 73—82 (1971).
462. WAGNER, R. R., CYNKIN, M. A.: Enzymatic transfer of ^{14}C-glucosamine from UDP-N-acetyl-^{14}C-glucosamine to endogenous acceptors in a Golgi apparatus-rich fraction from liver. Biochem. Biophys. Res. Commun. **35**, 139—143 (1969).
463. WAGNER, R. R., CYNKIN, M. A.: Glycoprotein biosynthesis. Incorporation of glycosyl groups into endogenous acceptors in a Golgi apparatus-rich fraction of liver. J. biol. Chem. **246**, 143—151 (1971).
464. WAGNER, R. R., PETTERSSON, E., DALLNER, G.: Association of the two glycosyl transferase activities of glycoprotein synthesis with low equilibrium density smooth microsomes. J. Cell Sci. **12**, 603—615 (1973).
465. WAITE, M., VAN DEENEN, L. L. M.: Hydrolysis of phospholipids and glycerides by rat-liver preparations. Biochim. biophys. Acta (Amst.) **137**, 498—517 (1967).
466. WALTON, K. W., SCOTT, P. J., JONES, J. V., FLETCHER, R. F., WHITEHEAD, T.: Studies on low-density lipoprotein turnover in relation to atromid therapy. J. Atheroscler. Res. **3**, 396—414 (1963).
467. WARREN, L., FUHRER, J. P., BUCK, C. A.: Surface glycoproteins of normal and transformed cells: a difference determined by sialic acid and a growth-dependent sialyltransferase. Proc. nat. Acad. Sci. (Wash.) **69**, 1838—1842 (1972).
468. WATTIAUX, R., WATTIAUX-DE CONINCK, S.: Particules subcellulaires dans les tumeurs. I. Distribution intracellulaire de la glucose-6-phosphatase, la catalase et plusieurs hydrolases acides dans un hépatome chimique transplantable (hépatome HW). Europ. J. Cancer **4**, 193—200 (1968).

469. Wattiaux, R., Wattiaux-de Coninck, S.: Particules subcellulaires dans les tumeurs. II. A-nalyse de fractions mitochondriales et microsomiales de l'hépatome HW par centrifugation isopycnique. Europ. J. Cancer **4**, 201—209 (1968).

470. Weinstein, I., Dishmon, G., Heimberg, M.: Hepatic lipid metabolism in carbon tetrachloride poisoning. Incorporation of palmitate-1-^{14}C into lipids of the liver and of the d < 1.020 serum lipoprotein. Biochem. Pharmacol. **15**, 851—871 (1966).

471. Weinstock, A., Leblond, C. P.: Elaboration of the matrix glycoprotein of enamel by the secretory ameloblasts of the rat incisor as revealed by radioautography after galactose-^{3}H injection. J. Cell Biol. **51**, 26—51 (1971).

472. Weisenberg, R. C., Timasheff, S. N.: Aggregation of microtubule subunit protein. Effects of divalent cations, colchicine and vinblastine. Biochemistry **9**, 4110—4116 (1970).

473. Weiss, P., Dujovne, C. A., Margolis, S., Lasagna, L., Bianchine, J. R.: Effects of Su-13437 on serum lipids in hyperlipoproteinemic patients. Clin. Pharmacol. Ther. **11**, 90—96 (1970).

474. Wessels, N. K., Spooner, B. S., Ash, J. F., Bradley, M. O., Luduena, M. A., Taylor, E. L., Wrenn, J. T., Yamada, K. M.: Microfilaments in cellular and developmental processes. Science **171**, 135—143 (1971).

475. Westerfeld, W. W., Elwood, J. C., Richert, D. A.: Effect of clofibrate on the handling of dietary and liver fat. Biochem. Pharmacol. **21**, 1117—1125 (1972).

476. Westerfeld, W. W., Richert, D. A., Ruegamer, W. R.: The role of the thyroid hormone in the effect of p-chlorophenoxyisobutyrate in rats. Biochem. Pharmacol. **17**, 1003—1016 (1968).

477. White, L. W.: Mechanism of clofibrate inhibition of hepatic cholesterol biosynthesis. In: Jones, R. J. (Ed.): Atherosclerosis. Proc. Second Internat. Symp., pp. 545—549. Berlin-Heidelberg-New York: Springer 1970.

478. White, L. W.: Regulation of hepatic cholesterol biosynthesis by clofibrate administration. J. Pharmacol. exp. Ther. **178**, 361—370 (1971).

479. Whur, P., Herscovics, A., Leblond, C. P.: Radioautographic visualization of the incorporation of galactose-^{3}H and mannose-^{3}H by rat thyroids *in vitro* in relation to the stage of thyroglobulin synthesis. J. Cell Biol. **43**, 289—311 (1969).

480. Wilcox, H. G., Dishmon, G., Heimberg, M.: Hepatic lipid metabolism in experimental diabetes. IV. Incorporation of animo acid ^{14}C into lipoprotein-protein and triglyceride. J. biol. Chem. **243**, 666—675 (1968).

481. Wilgram, G. F., Kennedy, E. P.: Intracellular distribution of some enzymes catalyzing reactions in the biosynthesis of complex lipids. J. biol. Chem. **238**, 2615—2619 (1963).

482. Williams, D. J., Rabin, B. R.: The effects of aflatoxin B$_1$ and steroid hormones on polysome binding to microsomal membranes as measured by the activity of an enzyme catalyzing disulphide interchange. FEBS Letters **4**, 103—107 (1969).

483. Williams, J. A., Wolff, J.: Possible role of microtubules in thyroid secretion. Proc. nat. Acad. Sci. (Wash.) **67**, 1901—1908 (1970).

484. Williams, J. A., Wolff, J.: Cytochalasin B inhibits thyroid secretion. Biochem. Biophys. Res. Commun. **44**, 422—425 (1971).

485. Williamson, A. R., Askonas, B. A.: Biosynthesis of immunoglobulins: the separate classes of polyribosomes synthesizing heavy and light chains. J. molec. Biol. **23**, 201—216 (1967).

486. Wilson, D. E., Lees, R. S.: Metabolic relationships among the plasma lipoproteins. Reciprocal changes in the concentrations of very low and low density lipoproteins in man. J. clin. Invest. **51**, 1051—1057 (1972).

487. Windmueller, H. G.: An orotic acid induced, adenine-reversed inhibition of hepatic lipoprotein secretion in the rat. J. biol. Chem. **239**, 530—537 (1964).

488. Windmueller, H. G., Levy, R. I.: Total inhibition of hepatic β-lipoprotein production in the rat by orotic acid. J. biol. Chem. **242**, 2246—2254 (1967).

489. Windmueller, H. G., Levy, R. I.: Production of β-lipoprotein by intestine in the rat. J. biol. Chem. **243**, 4878—4884 (1968).

490. Windmueller, H. G., Spaeth, A. E.: Perfusion in situ with tritium oxide to measure hepatic lipogenesis and lipid secretion. Normal and orotic acid-fed rats. J. biol. Chem. **241**, 2891—2899 (1966).

491. WINDMUELLER, H. G., SPAETH, A. E.: De novo synthesis of fatty acid in perfused rat liver as a determinant of plasma lipoprotein production. Arch. Biochem. Biophys. **122**, 362—369 (1967).
492. WINDMUELLER, H. G., SPAETH, A. E.: Fat transport and lymph and plasma lipoprotein biosynthesis by isolated intestine. J. Lipid Res. **13**, 92—105 (1972).
493. WINDMUELLER, H. G., HERBERT, P. N., LEVY, R. I.: Biosynthesis of lymph and plasma lipoprotein apoproteins by isolated perfused rat liver and intestine. J. Lipid Res. **14**, 215—223 (1973).
494. WINTERBURN, P. J., PHELPS, C. F.: The significance of glycosylated proteins. Nature (Lond.) **236**, 147—151 (1972).
495. WIRTZ, K. W. A., ZILVERSMIT, D. B.: Exchange of phospholipids between liver mitochondria and microsomes *in vitro*. J. biol. Chem. **243**, 3596—3602 (1968).
496. WIRTZ, K. W. A., ZILVERSMIT, D. B.: Participation of soluble liver proteins in the exchange of membrane phospholipids. Biochim. biophys. Acta (Amst.) **193**, 105—116 (1969).
497. WIRTZ, K. W. A., ZILVERSMIT, D. B.: Partial purification of phospholipid exchange protein from beef heart. FEBS Letters **7**, 44—46 (1970).
498. WIRTZ, K. W. A., KAMP, H. H., VAN DEENEN, L. L. M.: Isolation of a protein from beef liver which specifically stimulates the exchange of phosphatidylcholine. Biochim. biophys. Acta (Amst.) **274**, 606—617 (1972).
499. WISE, G. E.: Connections between cisternae of the Golgi apparatus and the granular endoplasmic reticulum in Amoeba proteus. Z. Zellforsch. **126**, 431—436 (1972).
500. WISE, G. E., FLICKINGER, C. J.: Patterns of cytochemical staining in Golgi apparatus of amebae following enucleation. Exp. Cell Res. **67**, 323—328 (1971).
501. WOOD, R. L., LEGG, P. G.: Peroxidase activity in rat liver microbodies after aminotriazole inhibition. J. Cell Biol. **45**, 576—585 (1970).
502. YEH, R., KABARA, J. J.: Antagonistic effect of two forms of clofibrate on mitochondrial oxidation of succinate. Life Sci. **11**, 709—716 (1972).
502a. YOGEESWARAN, G., LAINE, R. A., HAKOMOTI, S.: Mechanism of cell contact-dependent glycolipid synthesis: further studies with glycolipid-glass complex. Biochem. Biophys. Res. Commun. **59**, 591—599 (1974).
503. YOUNG, R. W.: The role of the Golgi complex in sulfate metabolism. J. Cell Biol. **57**, 175—189 (1973).
504. YUNGHANS, W. N., KEENAN, T. W., MORRÉ, J. D.: Isolation of Golgi apparatus from rat liver. III. Lipid and protein composition. Exp. molec. Path. **12**, 36—45 (1970).
505. ZAGURY, D., UHR, J. W., JAMIESON, J. D., PALADE, G. E.: Immunoglobulin synthesis and secretion. II. Radioautographic studies of sites of addition of carbohydrate moieties and intracellular transport. J. Cell. Biol. **46**, 52—63 (1970).
506. ZAKIM, D., PARADINI, R. S., HERMAN, R. H.: Effect of clofibrate (ethyl-chlorophenoxy-isobutyrate) feeding on glycolytic and lipogenic enzymes and hepatic glycogen synthesis in the rat. Biochem. Pharmacol. **19**, 305—310 (1970).
507. ZEIDENBERG, P., ORRENIUS, S., ERNSTER, L.: Increase in levels of glucuronylating enzymes and associated rise in activities of mitochondrial oxidative enzymes upon phenobarbital administration in the rat. J. Cell Biol. **32**, 528—531 (1967).
508. ZILVERSMIT, D. B.: Metabolism of arterial lipids. In: JONES, R. J. (Ed.): Atherosclerosis, Proc. Second Int. Symp., pp. 35—41. Berlin-Heidelberg-New York: Springer 1970.

CHAPTER 8

Vascular Metabolism, Vascular Enzymes, and the Effect of Drugs

T. ZEMPLÉNYI

With 13 Figures

I. Notes on Vascular Metabolism

The aim of the study of vascular metabolism is to ascertain whether it plays an essential role in the pathogenesis of vascular disease, especially atherosclerosis; and if so, to find ways to influence vascular metabolism for the prevention and treatment of vascular disease.

Because of the specific properties of the arterial wall, it is very difficult to study the intermediary metabolism of this tissue by techniques that provide excellent results in the study of other organs, such as the liver or the heart. For example, until recently, the attempts to measure oxidative phosphorylation reliably failed because of the difficulties in preparing viable mitochondria from vascular tissue. Nevertheless, with the currently available sophisticated techniques, some basic properties of vascular biochemistry became evident. Although this review deals mainly with vascular enzymes—it will be edifying to summarize briefly some special aspects of vascular metabolism.

A. It is generally accepted that the arterial wall does not show any Pasteur effect and covers its energy needs by "aerobic glycolysis" (KIRK et al., 1954; PANTESCO et al., 1957). However, if the normal artery is kept at 37° C before glycolysis and tissue respiration are measured to avoid the "cold shock", as much as 60% af ATP is found to be derived from oxidative phosphorylation and only 40% from glycolysis (SCOTT et al., 1970a and b). This implies that the oxygen supply is important for the bioenergetics of the artery, and it is in agreement with other findings. ASTRUP and coworkers, and others, (ASTRUP et al., 1967; KJELDSEN et al., 1968, 1969, 1972; HELIN and LORENZEN, 1969) conclude, on the basis of studies involving the effect of carbon monoxide and hypoxia in man and cholesterol-fed rabbits, that tissue hypoxia is an essential factor in accelerating experimental as well as human atherosclerosis. It is suggested that the underlying mechanism consists of increased arterial permeability as a result of tissue hypoxia. Furthermore, changes in oxygen diffusivity, depending on plasmatic protein concentration, are claimed to produce hypoxia and increased cellular permeability of the artery (CHISOLM et al., 1972). In fact, it was demonstrated that the vascular permeability for albumin and other macromolecular substances increases in individuals exposed to hypoxic conditions (ASMUSSEN and KNUDSEN, 1943; SIGGAARD-ANDERSEN et al., 1968). In addition, studies using tissue cultures

* Supported by grant HL-14138, National Heart and Lung Institute and grant AMA-ERF-TKZ, American Medical Association Education and Research Foundation (Project for Research on Tobacco and Health).

from human and animal arterial intimal cells indicate that oxygen concentrations below five percent in the surrounding medium cause increased cell membrane permeability for lipoproteins (ROBERTSON, 1967).

Recently, MORRISON et al. (1972), using intima-media preparations from pig, rabbit, and rhesus monkey aortas, confirmed earlier reports of an increased oxygen uptake in atherosclerotic arteries as compared with the uptake of normal arteries (LOOMEIJER and OSTENDORF, 1959; MUNRO et al., 1961; WHEREAT, 1961; CHATTOPA-DHYAY, 1962; KRČÍLEK et al., 1962; WHEREAT, 1964; MAIER and HAIMOVICI, 1965; MANDEL et al., 1966; ROBERTSON, 1968; WEISS et al., 1971). However, measurements using $[1-^{14}C]$ and $[6-^{14}C]$ glucose demonstrated that most of the glucose had been degraded to lactic acid in both normal and atherosclerotic aortas, and only very little of it (approximately one percent) entered the Krebs cycle or the pentose phosphate pathway. This is unexpected, because the same authors reported previously that about 60% of ATP produced in the aorta is derived from oxidative phosphorylation (SCOTT et al., 1970a, b) and other investigators also reported higher involvement of the Krebs cycle (KRESSE et al., 1970). The question is whether other compounds, and especially free fatty acids, provide the substrate for utilization *via* the Krebs cycle for oxidative phosphorylation. HASHIMOTO and DAYTON (1971) observed that in incubation experiments of three hours duration normal rat aortas oxidized medium-chain fatty acids, octanoate through laurate, to the extent of 85 to 99% of the total uptake, while the longer chain fatty acids were only oxidized to the extent of 33 to 64%. The influence of carnitine on the oxidation of long-chain fatty acids was small as compared to heart and other tissues. MORRISON et al. (1971) showed that in atherosclerotic rabbit aortas a much larger percentage of energy production (29%) occurs *via* Krebs cycle degradation of free fatty acids than in normal aortas (3.3%).

It is probable that some of the inconsistencies may be caused by the fact that in incubation studies the perfusion of the vessel wall *via* the *vasa vasorum* is completely eliminated and the oxygenation by diffusion also is markedly impaired, so that tissue hypoxia necessarily results. It is interesting that studies with aortic mitochondrial preparations suggested that in atherosclerotic arteries mitochondrial damage and uncoupling of oxidative phosphorylation may be the cause of the rise in oxygen uptake (WHEREAT, 1966). However, MORRISON et al. (1973) were unable to find differences in oxygen uptake and oxidative phosphorylation between mitochondria from atherosclerotic or normal arteries in pigs and rabbits. On the other hand, HASHIMOTO and DAYTON (1974a) observed a reduced oxidation of $[1-^{14}C]$ palmityl CoA by mitochondria from atherosclerotic rabbit aortas. The authors postulate, as a consequence, an increase of the arterial acyl-CoA pool, thereby augmenting local synthesis of cholesterol ester and phospholipids. In all such experiments, where mitochondria are being used, a marked variability in the rate of oxidation is observed and one has to consider the possibility that differences in the severity of mitochondrial damage during sample preparation may account for the observed metabolic differences (HASHIMOTO and DAYTON, 1974a).

In spite of some uncertainty concerning the substrates used in addition to glucose by the arterial wall, there is no doubt that the tricarboxylic acid cycle plays an important role in the bioenergetics of the arterial wall and that the oxygen supply is an essential factor for the viability and biosynthetic activity of this tissue.

It has to be added that the pentose phosphate pathway may also play a certain role in arterial intermediary metabolism. This has been demonstrated not only by the presence of enzymes of this pathway in arterial tissue, but also by experiments using $[1-^{14}C]$ glucose and $[6-^{14}C]$ glucose (SBARRA et al., 1960; BEACONSFIELD, 1962; MANDEL and KEMPF, 1963). However, recent findings indicate that the importance of this pathway is in arterial tissue less than suggested previously (RITZ, 1968; LILLE and CHOBANIAN, 1969; MORRISON et al., 1972).

Pentoses (non-phosphorylated) are also involved in the glucuronic acid cycle. Here in a series of NADP and NAD-dependent enzymatic reactions (involving L-gulonic acid, 3-keto-L-gulonic acid, xylitol, and D-xylulose) glucuronic acid is decarboxylated and degraded to L-xylulose. RITZ and SANWALD (1970) demonstrated in human, rat, and guinea pig arteries the presence of all the enzymatic steps of this cycle. However, the relative contribution of the pathway to the overall arterial glucose metabolism is not known. It could perhaps play a role in the genesis of vascular abnormalities connected with diabetes mellitus.

B. Substantial evidence shows that serum lipids and lipoproteins, especially the low-density lipoproteins, enter the arterial wall (CHERNICK et al., 1949; GOULD et al., 1959; FIELD et al., 1960; CHRISTENSEN, 1962; 1964; NEWMAN and ZILVERSMIT, 1966, 1970; ADAMS and MORGAN, 1966; DAYTON and HASHIMOTO, 1970). The evidence summarized by ZILVERSMIT (1968) suggests that accumulation of cholesterol or cholesterol-containing lipoproteins proceeds in parallel with increased permeability of the arterial wall. However, there is also increasing data indicating that not all of the lipids (including cholesterol) in the normal and atherosclerotic lesions are derived from the serum and they can be synthesized in the artery (SHORE et al., 1955; ZILVERSMIT and McCANDLESS, 1959; BÖTTCHER, 1963; LOFLAND and CLARKSON, 1965; WHEREAT, 1966; CHOBANIAN and HOLLANDER, 1966; PARKER et al., 1966; DAY and WILKINSON, 1967; CHOBANIAN, 1967, 1968; NAKATAMI et al., 1967; LOFLAND et al., 1968; ST CLAIR et al., 1968a and b; HOWARD, 1968, 1971; KRESSE et al., 1969; PORTMAN and ALEXANDER, 1969; FELT and BENES, 1969; STEIN and STEIN, 1970; CHOBANIAN and MANZUR, 1972; KUPKE, 1972a, b and c). Ample evidence demonstrates that the arterial wall is able to synthesize phospholipids, and in the atherosclerotic artery more phospholipid is synthesized than in the normal vessel. This synthesis takes place predominantly in the foam cells of the lesion (DAY et al., 1966; DAY and WAHLQVIST, 1969; WAHLQVIST and DAY, 1969). More complicated lesions exhibit a higher proportion of sphingomyelin, but it is possible that the accumulation of this lipid is age-associated (ROUSER and SOLOMON, 1969). The local synthesis of phospholipids might exert a protective effect by facilitating the solubilization of hydrophobic high-surface tension lipids such as cholesterol and triglycerides (FRIEDMAN et al., 1957; DIXON, 1958; ADAMS and BAYLISS, 1963; DUNNIGAN, 1964). According to DIXON "micellar fat" stabilized by phospholipids appears to be the form in which fat is removed from the cell. Moreover, lecithin may be also involved in cholesterol esterification through the action of the "GLOMSET enzyme" (lecithin: cholesterol fatty acid transferase).

Since it has been shown that hypoxia increases the severity of experimental, as well as human atherosclerosis, the question arises as to what the effects of tissue hypoxia are on arterial lipogenesis.

Whereat et al. (1967) presented evidence that in rabbit heart mitochondia the driving force for the rate of fatty acid synthesis was the intramitochondrial ratio of the reduced to oxidized form of NAD. The synthetic system is stimulated by succinate because of the capacity of this Krebs cycle intermediate to reduce NAD by reversed electron flow (Chance and Hollunger, 1961). It was demonstrated (Hull and Whereat, 1967) that rotenone as well as hypoxia also enabled other Krebs cycle intermediates to maintain a high NADH/NAD ratio and to stimulate acetate-1-^{14}C incorporation into long chain fatty acids. Whereat (1965, 1966) also demonstrated the effect of succinate on fatty acid synthesis in rabbit aortic mitochondria as well as the requirement for NADH as a cofactor in incorporation of acetate into fatty acids in this tissue.

At this point it will be useful to recall that *de novo* synthesis of fatty acids is in most tissues accomplished by the malonyl Co A pathway and it takes place only in the soluble fraction of the cytoplasm (cytosol). In mitochondria medium chain length saturated fatty acids in the form of Co A esters are elongated by successive additions of acetyl Co A. This probably occurs by reversal of some enzymatic steps that are involved in fatty acid oxidation. Furthermore, both saturated and unsaturated fatty acyl Co A esters may be elongated by a microsomal elongation-desaturation pathway, but in this case, acetyl Co A is replaced by malonyl Co A. However, in the heart Whereat et al. (1969) isolated two mitochondrial systems. The outer mitochondrial membrane contains an elongation system and the inner membrane contains a *de novo* system. Both systems are regulated by NADH and the outer system is supposed to function as a shuttle for the intramitochondrial oxidation of extramitochondrial (cytoplasmic) NADH. The inner system operates only when intramitochondrial NADH cannot be oxidized and this initiates fatty-acid synthesis (Whereat, 1971). A similar mechanism could be operative in arterial mitochondria and explain some effects of hypoxia on arterial metabolism.

The studies by Kresse et al. (1969) revealed a five-fold increase of [1-^{14}C] acetate incorporation rate into the triglyceride fraction of total lipids in healthy calf aortas incubated in the absence of oxygen, and a concomitant rise of the NADH/NAD ratio was also observed. It is interesting that according to Kupke (1972b) nicotine exhibits in this respect similar metabolic effects as oxygen deficiency and the author suggests that nicotine impairs oxidative enzymes by damaging mitochondrial structures.

Further studies by Filipovic and Buddecke (1971) showed that under hypoxic conditions there is an increase of incorporation into aortic fatty acids which is accompanied by a rise of the NADH/NAD ratio. This agrees with the theory that the NADH/NAD ratio is the controlling factor of mitochondrial fatty acid synthesis. In these experiments separation by gas liquid chromatography and chemical decarboxylation indicated that the synthesis of fatty acids from acetate was preferentially accomplished by elongation of preformed acyl units, and that this biosynthetic system was active mainly with the shorter chain fatty acyl Co A derivatives. Elongation is, according to these authors, the predominant synthetic system both in the presence and absence of oxygen, but the rate of chain elongation rises up to 37-fold (in the case of lauric acid) under hypoxic incubation.

The above results, obtained with healthy calf aortic tissue, differ in several regards from results obtained recently by Howard (1972) in studies with atherosclerotic aortas; with [1-^{14}C] acetate as substrate it is found that synthesis by elongation is the only mechanism and limited to longer chain fatty acids. However, with $[2-{}^{14}C]$ glucose the mechanism is primarily by *de novo* synthesis for 14 and 16 carbon fatty-acids and by elongation for longer chain fatty acids. Furthermore, in contrast to findings with healthy calf aortas, the synthesis of fatty-acids, whether from $[2-{}^{14}C]$ glucose or from $[1-{}^{14}C]$ acetate, decreases during hypoxic conditions. In addition, there is a more than two-fold increase of $[2-{}^{14}C]$ glucose incorporation into total lipids under hypoxic conditions, but a similar rise is not found when $[1-{}^{14}C]$ acetate is used. The rise of incorporation in the glucose experiments results from a 3.5-fold increased radiosubstrate incorporation into the glycerol moiety of glycerides and a 1.5-fold increased incorporation into phospholipid glycerophosphate.

Further studies are necessary to clarify whether the contrasting biochemical events in healthy calf aortas and atherosclerotic rabbit aortas are due to the presence of excess exogenous lipid in the experimentally induced atherosclerotic lesions, or whether they are caused by species differences or other factors. It is, however, of considerable interest that FILIPOVIC and co-workers (1974), comparing atherosclerotic and healthy segments of human aortas and using labeled glucose and acetate, observed a diminished ${}^{14}CO_2$ production and an increased ${}^{14}C$-lactate formation in the atherosclerotic segments, accompanied by a decreased ATP/ADP ratio, a rise of NADH/NAD ratio and accelerated fatty acid synthesis. This metabolic rate closely resembles to the hypoxic incubation studies by the authors.

C. Accumulation of lipids in the arterial wall is one of the hallmarks of atherosclerosis. It is of great interest that serum β and pre-β lipoproteins *in vitro* form insoluble complexes with sulfated acid mucopolysaccharides in the presence of Ca^{++} ions (BURSTEIN and SAMAILLIE, 1960). It was demonstrated (GERÖ, 1964, 1968) that such complexes can be formed also with arterial mucopolysaccharides, and the mechanism of the binding has been studied thoroughly (KUMAR et al., 1967; BIHARI-VARGA et al., 1968; SRINIVASAN et al., 1970, 1972; BERENSON et al., 1971; DALFERES et al., 1971; and others). In the low density lipoprotein-mucopolysaccharide complexes from human atherosclerotic lesions chondroitin sulfates, heparitin sulfate (and possibly hyaluronic acid) were found. In fibrous plaques heparin was also detected (SRINIVASAN et al., 1972). It is suggested that Ca^{++} acts as a bridge between N-sulfate groups of the mucopolysaccharide and the phosphate groups of lipoprotein phospholipids (SRINIVASAN et al., 1970).

Reports are very controversial concerning whether atherosclerosis is preceeded or accompanied by qualitative or quantitative changes of arterial acid mucopolysaccharides. Results of histochemical studies, based on increased metachromasia, were interpreted as an increase in mucopolysaccharide content. Chemical measurements indicated conflicting results. A similar situation exists regarding radiosulfate uptake into arterial mucopolysaccharides of animal or human atherosclerotic aortas. It is possible that changes in the affinity of mucopolysaccharides to lipoproteins are more closely related to qualitative than quantitative alterations of mucopolysaccharides. The normal constituents are hyaluronic acid, chondroitin-4 and 6-sulfate, heparitin-sulfate and dermatan sulfate. Although the mucopolysaccharides are not necessarily changed in the atherosclerotic vessel, the concentration of the individual components changes independently in the aging or diseased artery (ROBERT, 1970). In addition, physicochemical changes, including depolymerization of mucopolysaccharides, may take place influencing not only the affinity to lipoproteins, but also the permeability of the arterial wall. For more details please refer to the recent publication by ROBERT and co-workers (1973) and the reviews in the volume on arterial mesenchyme and arteriosclerosis edited by WAGNER and CLARKSON (1973).

Recently, attention has again been directed to endothelial permeability. Electron microscopic studies clarified some uncertainties concerning the ultrastructural basis for the transport of macromolecules through the endothelium (ROBERTSON and KHAIRALLAH, 1973; SHIMAMOTO, 1973, 1975; STEIN and STEIN, 1973). The use of markers of different molecular size, namely horseradish peroxidase (50 Å), ferritin (110 Å) and India ink (200—700 Å) disclosed that the smaller macromolecules can pass through interendothelial junctions, whereas the larger macromolecules can be transported into the subendothelial space within the so called plasmalemmal versicles. Furthermore, it was demonstrated (ROBERTSON and KHAIRALLAH, 1973; SHIMA-MOTO, 1973) that under certain conditions the endothelial cells can contract, thus widen the interendothelial junctions and increase the permeability for the larger macromolecules. In fact, endothelial cells possess the machinery for contraction in the form of microfilaments. Angiotensin, epinephrine, bradykinin, serotonin, histamine, as well as hypoxia, changes in pH, hypertension and immunological reactions seem to increase endothelial permeability by this mechanism. According to SHIMA-MOTO (1975) cyclic AMP has an inhibitory effect on the contraction of endothelial cells and cAMP phosphodiesterase inhibitors were suggested to counteract endothelial „hyperreactivity".

We have seen before that platelets carry several vasoactive agents and platelet stickiness to the endothelium and degranulation is also accompanied by widening of inter-endothelial junctions as a result of contractions of endothelial cells (ROBERT-SON and KHAIRALLAH, 1973).

It is of considerable interest that macroscopically intact aortic areas—in which fatty streaks develop preferentially—manifest selective permeability to protein-bound dyes (Evans blue, trypan blue), colloidal India ink, and also labeled cholesterol (KLYNSTRA and BÖTTCHER, 1970; VERESS et al., 1970; SOMER and SCHWARTZ, 1971; FRY, 1973; BELL et al., 1974). Experiments in which human coronary vessels are perfused with labeled cholesterol and human plasma, also indicate the role of altered permeability in cholesterol uptake; cholesterol flux in the arteries is significantly increased by collagenase and carbon monoxide (SARMA et al., 1975). Cholesterol synthesis from ^{14}C-acetate is not observed as occurring in these perfusion experiments (MORITA and BING, 1972).

Altered endothelial permeability allows the plasma low density and very low density lipoproteins to permeate the endothelial barrier and appears to be one of the most important pathogenetic factors of atherosclerosis (BJÖRKERUD und BONDJERS, 1971; WALTON, 1975; ZILVERSMIT, 1975).

D. The difference in susceptibility of arteries and veins to sclerotic changes is well known. The question arises whether there are marked differences in the chemistry and metabolism of these vessels. The data that follow are based mainly on the comparison of aorta and vena cava in man and cattle. The elastin content of the aorta is markedly higher than in the vena cava, and the predominance of collagen as compared with elastin was reported in the human saphenous vein (ŠVEJCAR et al., 1962, 1963; LASZT, 1972a). The mucopolysaccharide concentration is lower in venous than arterial tissue and in the latter chondroitin sulfate is the main component. In contrast, human venous tissue is rich in dermatan sulfate, and in bovine vena cava

75% of mucopolysaccharides consist of hyaluronic acid. KRESSE et al. (1970) report that on *in vitro* incubation venous tissue metabolizes only about 33% of the added glucose in 12 hrs whereas glucose uptake by arterial tissue is almost 75%. However, most of the glucose (70%) is used for incorporation into glycogen and the production of lactate in arterial tissue, but only 25% of glucose is utilized in this way in the vein. Only three percent or less of glucose is in such incubation studies metabolized in arteries through the Krebs cycle (or other metabolic pathways except glycolysis—see previous sections) but 6.2% is used up in veins. Accordingly, the oxygen uptake is almost twice as high in veins as in arteries (KRESSE et al., 1970). The replacement of glucose by succinate caused a twenty-fold increase of oxygen uptake in similar incubation studies with bovine tibial veins (LASZT, 1972a and b). This stimulating effect of succinate is higher than in other tissue, including arterial tissue (MORRISON et al., 1972a).

E. The development and perfection of techniques for arterial explants and for cultivating arterial cells, particularly smooth muscle cells, opened new avenues for research (RUTSTEIN et al., 1958; POLLAK and KASAI, 1964; JARMOLYCH et al., 1968; POLLAK, 1969; ROSS, 1971; DAOUD et al., 1973; FISHER-DZOGA et al., 1973b). The formation of foam cells, which are the essential components of the early atherosclerotic lesion, is associated with proliferation of the smooth muscle cells of the arterial tunica intima. It was shown (FISHER-DZOGA, et al., 1973a, 1974; ROSS and GLOMSET, 1973) that exposure of arterial smooth muscle cell cultures to low density lipoproteins (LDL) induced proliferation and increased cell growth of these cells. Furthermore, the smooth muscle cells take up lipids when incubated with LDL (BIERMAN et al., 1973, 1974; FISHER-DZOGA, 1973b; STEIN and STEIN, 1975). Hypoxia is another factor causing proliferation and lipid accumulation in arterial smooth muscle cells (MAY et al., 1974, 1975).

Further studies by BIERMAN and co-workers (1974) and STEIN and STEIN (1975) demonstrated that although aortic smooth muscle cells can take up low density and also very low density lipoproteins rapidly, the cells have a limited ability to catabolize the ingested lipoproteins. Calculations based on perfusion studies and estimation of transport by plasmalemmal vesicles (STEIN and STEIN, 1973) suggest that such a process may account for the progressive accretion of cholesterol in the arterial smooth muscle cells. (See also later, notes on lysosomes.) Aortic cells in tissue culture also readily synthesize phospholipids from labeled precursors (DAY, 1973; STEIN and STEIN, 1975).

Lipoproteins are not the only plasmatic factors causing proliferation of arterial smooth muscle cells. STOUT et al. (1975) reported that insulin has an unequivocal stimulating effect, although this stimulation is much less than the effect of serum lipoproteins. It is inhibited by cyclic AMP in the medium. Platelets also have a significant stimulating effect on arterial smooth muscle cell proliferation (ROSS et al., 1974). In view of the effect of platelets on endothelial permeability, it is evident that these blood constituents play an essential role in initiating processes that have considerable importance in the pathogenesis of atherosclerosis.

Summary

1. In both normal and atherosclerotic aortas glucose is degraded primarily to lactate, and only a very small fraction enters the Krebs cycle. However, free fatty acids can provide the substrate for utilization *via* the Krebs cycle and in atherosclerotic

aortas a considerable percentage of energy production takes place by oxidation of this substrate. In spite of "aerobic glycolysis", oxidative phosphorylation is essential for the bioenergetics of vascular tissue and local hypoxia plays an important role in atherogenesis. It is accompanied by increased permeability of the vascular wall.

2. Not all the lipids in the normal and atherosclerotic artery are derived from serum. The artery can synthesize cholesterol, cholesterol esters and glycerides. Local synthesis of phospholipids might exert a protective effect by facilitating the solubilization and removal of hydrophobic lipids such as cholesterol and triglycerides. Hypoxia stimulates synthesis of some lipids probably by rising the NADH/NAD ratio in the mitochondria. Under hypoxic conditions there is a considerable increase of radiosubstrate incorporation from labeled glucose into the glycerol moiety of glycerides and into phospholipid glycerophosphate. In normal aortas oxygen deficiency stimulates synthesis of fatty acids from acetate, but there is no consensus that this also occurs in the atherosclerotic artery.

3. Serum lipoproteins form insoluble complexes with sulfated acid mucopolysaccharides in the presence of Ca^{++} ions. Qualitative and quantitative alterations of vascular mucopholysaccharides might influence their affinity to lipoproteins and enhance accumulation of lipids in the arterial wall.

4. The chemical composition and intermediary metabolism of arterial and venous tissue differs. For example, the mucopolysaccharide concentration is lower in venous than in arterial tissue. Veins synthesize less lactate from glucose than arteries and a higher proportion of glucose is metabolized in veins through the Krebs cycle. It is tempting to speculate that to some extent these differences mirror the well-known disparity in susceptibility of arteries and veins to sclerotic changes. However, one has to be cautious in the interpretation since cell content, structure, and intravascular pressure also differ in arteries and veins.

5. Proliferation of arterial smooth muscle cells, an essential event in early atherosclerosis, is stimulated by low density lipoproteins, hypoxia and a platelet factor. Platelets also increase endothelial permeability and appear to play a fundamental role in atherogenesis.

II. Vascular Enzyme Studies

The vascular wall is a metabolically-active living organ and it is reasonable to anticipate that most enzymes characteristic or all living matter will be found in this tissue. The most thoroughly investigated arterial enzymes are those of glycolysis and glycogen breakdown (Embden-Meyerhof pathway). Enzymes of the tricarboxylic acid cycle (Krebs cycle), of the pentose phosphate pathway, of the polyol pathway (CLEMENTS et al., 1969) and enzymes of the terminal respiratory chain also were studied in detail.

Other enzymes which were investigated either are difficult to fit into generally accepted metabolic pathways or have been studied only in the vessel wall independently from other related enzymatic reactions. Such enzymes are, for example, some enzymes of phosphorus metabolism, of connective tissue metabolism, of lipid synthesis and breakdown, of the glyoxalase system, and many oxidoreductases, aminotransferases, and hydrolases. Some of the latter enzymes (e.g. all enzymes of mucopolysaccharide catabolism, cathepsin and acid phosphomonoesterase) are lysosomal enzymes and their activity may be connected with cell injury, cell death and phago-cytosis. Recently, DNA and RNA polymerases also were studied in aortic nuclei (JANAKIDEVI, 1971). Enzyme cofactors, such as nicotinamide containing coenzymes, coenzyme A, flavin nucleotides, glutathione, carnitine, thiamine, lipoic acid, para-amino-benzoic acid, vitamin B_{12}, tocopherol, and metal ion activators have been also investigated in vascular tissue. (HOSODA and KIRK, 1969; KHEIM and KIRK, 1969, 1970; KIRK, 1969; ITO, 1969; SCHOFFENIELS, 1969; PALATY et al., 1971).

In this review results obtained mainly by biochemical methods will be summa-rized. For more complete information, especially on data published before 1968, please refer to monographs by ZEMPLÉNYI (1968) and KIRK (1969). No attempt will be made here to give a detailed report of data gathered by histochemical techniques. The histochemistry of vascular enzymes has been described in detail by LOJDA (1958, 1962), LOJDA and ZEMPLÉNYI (1961), SANDNER and BOURNE (1963), MAIER et al. (1969), STAVROU and DAHME (1971), HOFF (1972), and in great detail by ADAMS in his book on vascular histochemistry (ADAMS, 1967). Data on the coenzyme and vitamin contents of arterial tissue can be found in two recent monographs by KIRK (1973, 1974). Studies on arterial trace elements have been summarized by SCHROEDER (1974).

A. Enzymes in Venous Tissue

In Part I a few differences in the chemistry and the metabolism of arteries and veins have been mentioned. KIRK (1964, 1969) studied many enzymes in human venous tissue and Fig. 1 summarizes pertinent information about comparison of some en-zyme activities and cofactor levels in the aorta and vena cava. The data are calcu-lated on the wet-weight basis and some of the differences are very significant. Howev-er, one has to be cautious in the interpretation because the structure of both types of vessels and especially their cell content is different. Neither is the intravascular pressure the same in arteries and veins.

NIEBES and LASZT (1971) studied the activity of lysosomal enzymes involved in mucopolysaccharide catabolism in normal and varicose human saphenous veins. The activity of all of these enzymes, except cathepsin, were significantly increased in varicose veins. Furthermore, the activity of lactate dehydrogenase is also elevated in varicose veins, whereas the activity of the Krebs cycle enzyme succinate dehydrogen-ase exhibits an opposite pattern, being higher in the healthy veins.

MATAGNE and HAMOIR (1973) investigated the isoenzyme pattern of some glyco-lytic enzymes in the human saphenous vein. They did not detect differences between the human heart, psoas and vein in the multiple molecular forms of glyceraldehy-dephosphate dehydrogenase, aldolase, enolase, pyruvate kinase, or triosephosphate isomerase. However, venous creatine phosphokinase has a single BB form instead of the MM form present in skeletal muscle. Venous lactate dehydrogenase is character-ized by the predominance of more aerobic LDH forms than skeletal muscle. The isoenzymes of venous phosphoglucomutase also differ from those of skeletal muscle or heart. Although the LDH isoenzymes were not evaluated quantitatively their distribution agrees with the data obtained by ZEMPLÉNYI et al. (1970) in pig and dog veins.

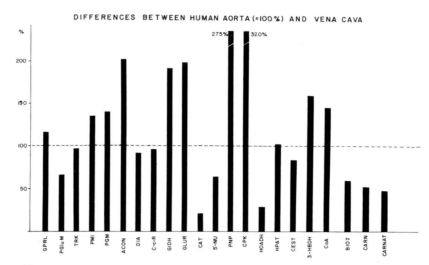

Fig. 1. Differences in enzyme activities and cofactor levels between the human aorta and inferior vena cava. The enzyme activities or cofactor levels of aortas, calculated on a wet weight basis equal 100 percent. (Constructed according to data from Kirk, Clin. Chem. **10**, 184 (1964), and some more recent publications by Kirk and co-workers.) For abbreviations see page 331

The same enzyme activity had been found in human veins and arteries by histochemical means (Stein et al., 1966). Comparison of normal and varicose human saphenous veins by Urbanová and Přerovský (1972) showed a marked increase in the activity of acid phosphomonoesterase, and a decreased activity of malate dehydrogenase, non-specific esterase (carboxylic esterase), AT Pase and 5'-nucleotidase in the varicose veins. The staining reaction for lactate dehydrogenase was increased in only 55% of the varicose veins. This corresponds with related biochemical data.

B. Interspecies and Intraspecies Differences

The varied susceptibility of different animal species to experimental and spontaneous atherosclerosis is an enigma in the study of the disease. For example, it is easy to induce atherosclerosis-like lesions by simple cholesterol feeding in the rabbit, chicken, or golden hamster; in the rat much more complicated procedures are required. Spontaneous as well as artificially aggravated arterial lesions occurring in primates or in the pig strongly resemble early human atherosclerotic lesions while in many other mammals and in avian species predominantly fibrous lesions or Mönckeberg-like medial calcifications only can be found, or no lesions can be detected.

Figure 2 shows that the rat aorta clearly has a higher lipolytic activity than the rabbit, guinea-pig, or chicken aorta. Mallov (1964) and Patelski et al. (1967) also observed much higher lipolytic activity in rat aortas than in the other species. Aortic esterolytic activity using β-napthol acetate as substrate is much higher in rat aorta than in the rabbit, chicken, or pig aorta (Zemplényi et al., 1963, 1965; Zemplényi, 1964). The activity of malate and succinate dehydrogenase, glutamate oxaloacetate transaminase, phosphomonoesterase I and II, and AT Pase also is higher in the rat than the rabbit or the chicken aorta (Zemplényi et al., 1966 a).

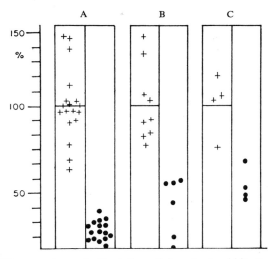

Fig. 2. Interspecies differences in aortic lipolytic activity. *A* rat-rabbit; *B* rat-guinea pig; *C* rat-chicken. The av. rat aorta activity equals 100%. [From ZEMPLÉNYI, LOJDA and GRAFNETTER, Circulation Res. **7**, 286 (1959)]

The high activity of all of the above enzymes in the rat aorta as compared to the other species reflects an overall higher level of metabolic activity, and it is reasonable to assume that the relative resistance of the rat to atherosclerosis may be connected to such metabolic characteristics.

Conspicuous differences can occur even among various strains of the same animal species. The White Carneau (WC) pigeon is susceptible to spontaneous and experimentally induced atherosclerosis in contrast to the resistant Show Racer (SR) strain. Blood lipid levels are essentially the same in both strains.

Recently it was shown that in old pigeons the activity of lipoamide dehydrogenase and malate dehydrogenase is lower in the WC than SR arteries (ZEMPLÉNYI and ROSENSTEIN, 1975a). The differences are not the result of ageing or atherosclerosis. In subsequent experiments they were also detected in arteries of very young preatherosclerotic pigeons (ZEMPLÉNYI et al., 1975; ZEMPLÉNYI and ROSENSTEIN, 1975a, b). Furthermore, the arteries of the young pigeons revealed a significantly higher activity of two glycolytic enzymes, namely phosphofructokinase (a regulatory enzyme of glycolysis) and aldolase, in the WC as compared with SR pigeons.

Moreover, in related studies, in which surviving arteries of young pigeons were incubated with [^{14}C] glucose, the steady-state level of lactate and the ratio of α-glycerol phosphate to dihydroxyacetone phosphate were significantly higher in the WC than they were in the SR pigeons (KALRA and BRODIE, 1974). It appears that the increased dependence of the White Carneau arteries on glycolysis may facilitate the development of atherosclerosis in this pigeon strain.

C. Effect of Age and Sex

Most enzyme activity tends to be less in the aortas or coronary arteries of children than in those of adults. However, over the age of 40 years the activity of most vascular enzymes and cofactors declines. In contrast, some enzymes, such as lactate

dehydrogenase, 5′-nucleotidase, acid phosphomonoesterase, ribosephosphate isomerase, all enzymes of mucopolysaccharide breakdown, and phospholipases are
exceptional because they exhibit a definite rise in activity (KIRK, 1966, 1969; KRESSE
and BUDECKE, 1968; ZEMPLÉNYI, 1968; EISENBERG et al., 1969).

The effect of hormones on vascular enzymes will be discussed in Part III. Here it
is sufficient to mention that some enzyme activity manifests clear-cut sex-linked
differences. The experiments by MALINOW et al. (1962) and MRHOVÁ and ZEM-
PLÉNYI (1965) indicated that gonadectomy also induces significant changes in the
activity of many aortic enzymes.

D. Enzyme Activities in Vascular Grafts

HAIMOVICI et al. (1958, 1959) studied the activity of several enzymes in segments of
aortic homografts implanted into dog abdominal or thoracic aortas. The activity of
cytochrome C oxidase, succinate oxidase and carboxylic esterase was significantly
lower in the implanted segment than in the recipient aortic tissue. KIRK (1969)
measured activity of several enzymes in the new tissue forming on the inner and
outer surface of synthetic prosthetic grafts implanted in pig thoracic aortas. The
activity of creatine phosphokinase and glutathione reductase was found to be lower
in the newly formed tissue than in the normal aortic tissue. In sharp contrast to the
findings with homografts, the tissue attached to the prosthetic graft exhibited greater
activity of carboxylic esterase, β-glucuronidase and thromboplastin. The newly
formed tissue which was attached to the pig and human prosthetic grafts showed
considerably higher cathepsin activity and proteolysis (with denatured hemoglobin
as substrate) than in the recipient artery. These results agree with the histochemical
findings of SZENDZIKOWSKI (1963) in the "neoadventitia" adjacent to prosthetic
grafts where the activity of hydrolytic enzymes (mainly lysosomal enzymes) was found
to be elevated. However, in the neointima the activity of hydrolases was low whereas
the activity of succinate, lactate and α-glycerophosphate dehydrogenases was relatively high.

Although it is difficult to conclude a logical synthesis from such scanty data,
further investigations using vascular grafts may reveal new aspects of vascular metabolism important for the pathogenesis and treatment of arterial disease.

E. Enzyme Activity in Atherosclerotic Vessels

Most enzymatic activities and cofactor levels tend to decline in human atherosclerotic arteries. As seen in Figs. 3, 4, and 5 almost all enzymes of the Krebs cycle,
glycolysis, the pentose phosphate pathway, and many other enzymes exhibit this
tendency in both human aorta and coronary artery. Other enzymes studied in human vessels (among them glutamic pyruvic transaminase, purine nucleotide phosphorylase, carboxylic esterase, acid phosphomonoesterase, cathepsin, and all enzymes of mucopolysaccharide breakdown) display increased activity either in the
atherosclerotic aorta, or coronary artery or both vessels (KRESSE and BUDDECKE,
1968; KIRK, 1969). It is not possible, however, to decide whether these changes in
enzymatic activity precede the development of atherosclerotic lesions or are secondary to the disease. This is, of course, a crucial problem in the search for the role of

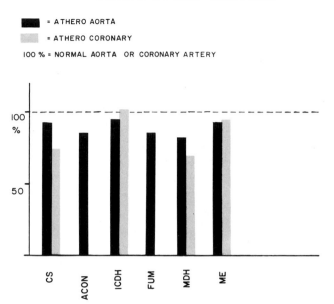

Fig. 3. Differences between atherosclerotic and normal human arteries in activities of the Krebs cycle. (Constructed according to data from KIRK, J.E., Enzymes of the Arterial Wall, New York: Academic Press, 1969.) For abbreviations see page 331

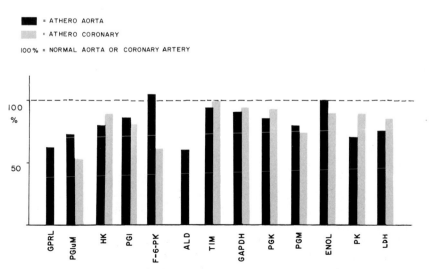

Fig. 4. Differences between atherosclerotic and normal human arteries in activities of enzymes of glycolysis and the glycogen pathway. (Constructed according to data from KIRK, J.E., Enzymes of the Arterial Wall, New York, Academic Press, 1969.) For abbreviations see page 331

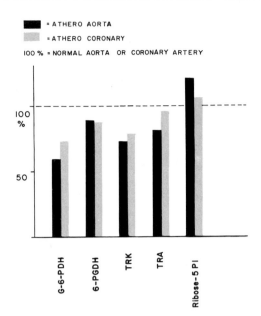

Fig. 5. Differences between atherosclerotic and normal human arteries in activities of enzymes of the pentose phosphate pathway. (Constructed according to data from KIRK, J. E., Enzymes of the Arterial Wall, New York, Academic Press, 1969.) For abbreviations see page 331

vascular metabolism in the pathogenesis of atherosclerosis, and other approaches had to be used.

First of all, different stages of experimental atherosclerosis had been studied. MAIER and HAIMOVICI (1958) have shown that aortic slices from rabbits and dogs subjected to an atherogenic diet exhibited decreased cytochrome oxidase activity prior to the development of atherosclerosis, whereas the succinoxidase system and the carboxyl esterase activity remained unchanged. In another series of experiments (ZEMPLÉNYI et al., 1963) it was demonstrated in experimental atherosclerosis in rabbits that the earliest changes of aortic enzyme activity consisted of increases in the activity of alkaline and acid phosphomonoesterase, β-glucuronidase, as well as declines in the activity of lactate dehydrogenase, succinate dehydrogenase and perhaps malate dehydrogenase (ZEMPLÉNYI, 1968). Data concerning glycerol 3-phosphate dehydrogenase are somewhat contradictory. While in canine atherosclerotic aortas the activity of the enzyme is stated to be increased (MAIER et al., 1969), in experimental rabbit atherosclerosis-and also in human atherosclerosis-it is lower than in normal arteries (MRHOVÁ et al., 1963; ZEMPLÉNYI et al., 1963; KIRK and RITZ, 1967; KIRK, 1969). It is interesting, that in the rabbit experiments increased lipolytic activity appeared only in later stages of atherosclerosis (ZEMPLÉNYI et al., 1959; ZEMPLÉNYI, 1964). No significant changes in the activities of AT Pase, 5'-nucleotidase and glucosephosphate isomerase were detected (ZEMPLÉNYI et al., 1963).

Another approach is based on the fact that different human arteries and even different segments of the same artery exhibit a considerable variation in suceptibility

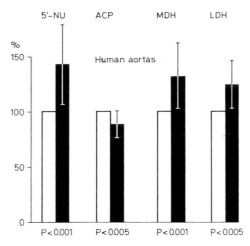

Fig.6. Enzyme activities in normal parts of human ascending aortas (black columns) as compared with normal parts of the abdominal aortas of the same persons (= 100 percent). Upright line with bars = S.D. (From ZEMPLÉNYI,T., Enzyme Biochemistry of the Arterial Wall as Related to Atherosclerosis, London: Lloyd-Luke, 1968.) For abbreviations see page 331

to atherosclerosis. For example, the severity of atherosclerosis is decidedly greater in the abdominal than ascending aorta; in the aorta than in the pulmonary artery; in the coronary artery than the abdominal organ arteries (e.g. splenic artery); in the femoral than brachial artery. Such disparities provide a useful basis for investigation of "local" factors in atherogenesis.

The following results were calculated either on the saline-extractable protein content basis or on the deoxyribonucleic acid content of the vessels investigated. In all cases, arteries or arterial segments from the same subjects were compared. Figure 6 shows that the activity of lactate, malate, and succinate dehydrogenases as well as of 5'-nucleotidase is higher in normal parts of the ascending than abdominal specimens of the same human aortas. In contrast, activity of acid phosphomonoesterase is higher in the abdominal than ascending aorta.

The same enzymes were studied while comparing activity in the femoral and brachial arteries or in the thoracic aortas and pulmonary arteries. The results were very similar, except that the activity ratio of 5'-nucleotidase was either reversed, or there was no difference among the specimens studied. The activity of Krebs cycle enzymes, especially malate and succinate dehydrogenase, was higher and the activity of acid phosphomonoesterase was lower in the relatively atherosclerosis-resistant (durable) arterial specimens (ZEMPLÉNYI et al., 1966; ZEMPLÉNYI, 1968).

When results are calculated on the wet-tissue basis the activity ratios of Krebs cycle enzymes in the pulmonary artery *versus* aorta are the same as in the above studies. KIRK et al. (1969) systematically compared not only enzymatic activities of the human aorta and pulmonary artery, but also the activity in the coronary arteries and vena cava. As can be seen in Fig.7a all Krebs cycle enzymes display a higher activity in the pulmonary artery and coronary artery than in the aorta. The phosphomonoesterase activity, on the other hand, is highest in the aorta. However, neither the enzymes of the glycolytic cycle (Fig.8), nor of the pentose phosphate shunt

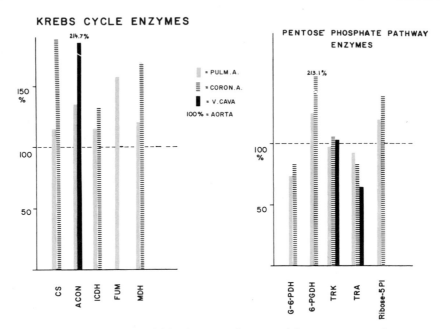

KREBS CYCLE ENZYMES

PENTOSE PHOSPHATE PATHWAY ENZYMES

Fig. 7. Differences in enzyme activities between the normal human aorta, pulmonary artery, coronary artery and vena cava. (Constructed according to data from Kirk, J.E., Enzymes of the Arterial Wall, New York: Academic Press, 1969.) For abbreviations see page 331

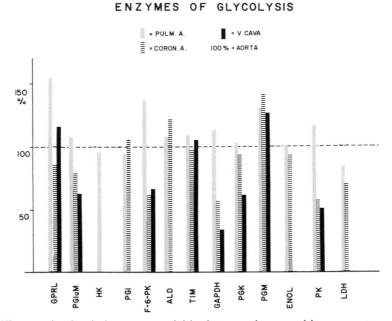

ENZYMES OF GLYCOLYSIS

Fig. 8. Differences in glycolytic enzyme activities between the normal human aorta, pulmonary artery, coronary artery, and vena cava. (Constructed according to data from Kirk, J.E., Enzymes of the Arterial Wall, New York: Academic Press, 1969.) For abbreviations see page 331

Table 1. Comparison of some enzyme patterns in human and animal arteries and arterial segments. (From ZEMPLÉNYI,T., Enzyme Biochemistry of the Arterial Wall as Related to Atherosclerosis, London: Lloyd-Luke, 1968)

	Tricarboxlic acid cycle enzymes	Ac. and/or alk. phosphomonoesterase
Abdominal as compared with asc. aorta in 30-day-old chickens	↗	↘
Abdominal as compared with asc. aorta in 50–60-day-old ducks	↗	→
Abdominal as compared with asc. aorta in 30-day-old calves	↗	→
Abdominal as compared with asc. aorta in young rhesus macaques	↗	→
Abdominal as compared with asc. aorta in young children	↗	→
Abdominal as compared with asc. aorta in older humans	↘	↗
Femoral as compared with brachial artery in older humans	↘	↗
Thoracic aorta as compared with pulmonary artery in older humans	↘	↗

(Fig. 7 b) show uniformity in enzyme activity ratio between the aorta and pulmonary artery, although in the coronary artery most glycolytic enzyme activities are lower than in the aorta. The activity of creatine phosphokinase and ATPase is greater in the pulmonary artery and coronary artery than in the aorta. This is probably due to lower actomyosin content of the aorta.

Actomyosin isolated from arteries reveals ATPase characteristics which are qualitatively similar to those of actomyosin prepared from skeletal muscle. The similarity also applies to the various ionic dependencies and increase of ATPase activity with lowered ionic strength (MAX-WELL et al., 1971). Nevertheless, some differences seem to exist. For example, whereas skeletal actomyosin can be extracted only by solutions of high ionic strength, vascular smooth muscle actomyosin can be extracted at low ionic strength and in the presence of traces of ATP (HAMOIR et al., 1965). Denaturating agents such as urea, ethanol and ethylenglycol, which at low concentration do not influence skeletal muscle myosin, considerably enhance Ca^{++}-ATPase activity of cow carotid myosin (GASPAR-GODFORD, 1970).

It is interesting that the actomyosin-bound ATPase can be separated easily from other ATPases by inhibition of the actomyosin ATPase by Salyrgan (KLIMESOVÁ and HEYEROVSKÝ, 1970). It was shown that there is a parallelism between the smooth muscle content and actomyosin-bound ATPase in various arteries. (For more details on ATPase see also the review by SOMLYO and SOMLYO, 1968.)

It must be emphasized that in most cases the above results were obtained from necropsied vessels of older persons and it is often very difficult, if not impossible, to decide whether "normal" vascular segments are really free of discrete atherosclerotic lesions. However, additional studies of the enzymatic pattern in arteries of children, young adults, and many young mammals and birds provided instructive data. They

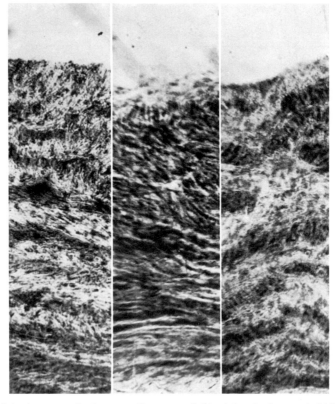

Fig. 9. Malate dehydrogenase in the ascending aorta (left), abdominal aorta (middle) and pulmonary artery (right) of a young duck (× 350). (From ZEMPLÉNYI, URBANOVÁ, and MRHOVÁ, Int. Symp. Biochemistry of the Vascular Wall, Basel and New York: Karger 1969)

are summarized in Table 1, and contrasted with the more important results obtained with arteries of older subjects.

In contrast to data obtained in studies of vessels of older persons, comparison of abdominal and ascending aortas of children (and young mammals and birds) reveals a ratio of Krebs cycle enzyme activity that is the reverse of that in older individuals. The activity of phosphomonoesterases is approximately the same in both segments. This is also true of the aortas of young ducks, calves, and monkeys, whereas in chickens the ratio of phosphomonoesterases is also reversed.

On the basis of these findings in human and animal vessels it can be inferred that the age-dependent changes in the enzymatic pattern are part of a general phenomenon, which may be an essential factor in determining the localization as well as the progression of atherosclerosis.

Simultaneous histochemical studies have revealed that enzyme activity in the smooth muscle cells is clearly the decisive factor that determines the overall activity in the arteries (LOJDA and ZEMPLÉNYI, 1961; ZEMPLÉNYI, 1968). All of the age-linked changes in susceptible arterial segments seem to depend on the quantity and conditions of the vascular smooth muscle cells. Figure 9 is an illustrative example of staining for malate dehydrogenase in the ascending aorta, abdominal aorta, and pulmonary artery of a young duck. The highest overall activity is confined to the abdominal and the lowest to the ascending aorta, the activity in the pulmonary artery being intermediate. The activity clearly corresponds to the localization of smooth muscle cells. Essentially the same histochemical pattern was observed in the staining for succinate dehydrogenase, ATPase and acid phosphomonoesterase.

F. The Role of Vascular Injury

What factors induce the age-dependent enzymatic alterations in the less durable arteries, especially in their smooth muscle cells? Many investigators believe that early atherosclerotic lesions in man and animals begin as a reparative response to injury caused by the wear-and-tear of daily life. To explore this, several experimental models of vascular injury were investigated (ZEMPLÉNYI and MRHOVÁ, 1965; ZEM-PLÉNYI et al., 1969a, b). The types of injuries that were chosen were also known in animals to facilitate the development of lesions similar to atherosclerosis if combined with induction of hyperlipidemia. Figure 10 is an example of the effects of such an injury induced in rats by injecting 7.5 mg of allylamine intravenously three times a week for 21 days (ZEMPLÉNYI et al., 1969b). Figures 11 and 12 illustrate some of the histochemical findings in rats fed 30000 units of vitamin D in oil for several days.

Table 2 summarizes some of the aortic enzyme activity changes resulting from different vascular injuries. In all five types of experiments acid phosphomonoesterase activity increased as compared with aortas of control animals. The activity of Krebs cycle enzymes (malate and succinate dehydrogenase) decreased in DOCA + NaCl hypertension, in allylamine intoxication, in thermal injury, and in the later stages of calciferol injury. The activity tends to decline in rats with hypertension induced by renal artery clamping. Other enzymatic alterations do not reveal such a uniformity.

From these results—assuming that vascular injury is a commom denominator in all of these experiments—it seems reasonable to conclude that decreased activity of Krebs cycle dehydrogenases, as well as increased phosphomonoesterase activity, constitute a common feature of vascular wall damage.

Experimental evidence from other tissues reveals that injury causes a decline in the concentration and activity of many cytoplasmic and mitochondrial enzymes, probably as a result of leakage accompanying permeability changes and damage to intracellular structures. On the other hand, the increased intracellular level and activity of other enzymes probably arises from damage and disruption of lysosomes (DEDUVE and WATTEAUX, 1966; MILLER and KOTHARI, 1969). It is likely that the same mechanism is responsible for the enzyme activity alterations observed in the arteries of animals subjected to selective vascular injury. Part of the elevated lysosomal enzyme activities accompanying arterial injury may sometimes also arise from monocytes and other cellular elements taking part in the repair of the arterial wall (GARBARSCH, 1973b).

One fact concerning the arterial wall emerges from the above studies: The enzymatic changes (in particular, the decrease in activity of Krebs cycle enzymes and the increase of phosphomonoesterase activity) which occur in experimental vascular injuries are the same as those which develop during life in susceptible human arterial segments. They are also similar to those observed in very early stages of experimental

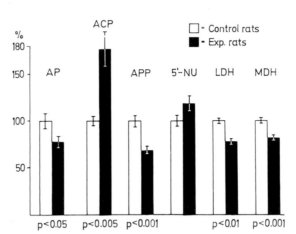

Fig. 10. Aortic enzyme activities in allylamine-treated rats. Results expressed as percentage differences. Upight line with bars = S.E.M. (From ZEMPLÉNYI, URBANOVÁ and MRHOVÁ, Int. Symposium Biochemistry of the Vascular Wall, Basel and New York: Karger 1969)

atherosclerosis. Such data justify an important conclusion: vascular segments which are more susceptible to atherosclerosis are also those that are preferentially exposed to damaging agents.

All of the physiological and pathological factors that may damage the arterial wall and thus contribute to the pathogenesis of atherosclerosis cannot be analyzed. There can be, for example, little doubt that hemodynamic and hemorrheologic factors such as lateral pressure, suction pressure, shearing strain, turbulence and other similar parameters play an essential role. Furthermore, immunologic injury seems to be important in certain cases (RENAIS et al., 1968; SCEBAT et al., 1968; SZIGETI et al., 1968; PAUTRIZEL et al., 1968; CROCKETT et al., 1968; ROBERT et al., 1970). The latter may also produce diffuse intimal thickening of the arterial wall which predisposes to development of atherosclerosis (HARDIN et al., 1972). There is also increasing evidence that platelet aggregates can release factors that increase vascular permeability and may produce focal injury of the vessel wall (ROBERT et al., 1969; MUSTARD, 1970).

Another factor contributing to vascular damage is arterial hypoxia (see Part I). Many investigators maintain that because of the anatomy of the arterial wall, in particular that of the aorta, the mid-zone layers of the arterial tunica media become poorly supplied with oxygen especially as a consequence of diffuse thickening of the intima (ADAMS, 1967).

Histochemical and biochemical studies (ADAMS, 1964; ZEMPLÉNYI, 1968; ZEMPLÉNYI et al., 1968) have demonstrated that in contrast to other enzymes, total lactate dehydrogenase activity is highest in the mid-zone of the tunica media. A study of isoenzymes of lactate dehydrogenase in multiple consecutive layers of human aortas (ZEMPLÉNYI, 1968; ZEMPLÉNYI et al., 1968) indicated that an adaptation to hypoxic

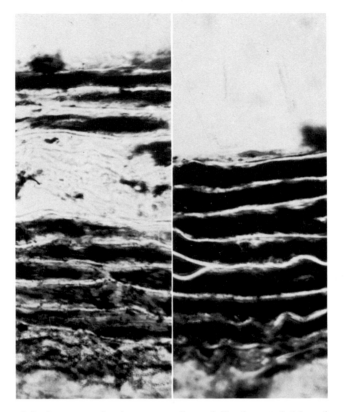

Fig. 11. Malate dehydrogenase in the aorta of a calciferol-treated (a) and normal (b) rat (× 500). (From ZEMPLÉNYI, URBANOVÁ, and MRHOVÁ, Int. Symp. Biochemistry of the Vascular Wall, Basel and New York: Karger 1969)

conditions in the middle zones of the human aorta may be brought about by increased activity of the anaerobic (muscle) forms of LDH isoenzymes, proportional to the increased total LDH activity. Furthermore, in human atherosclerotic arteries LOJDA and FRIČ (1966) demonstrated a high activity of the slow-moving (anaerobic) lactate dehydrogenase fractions, whereas the activity of the fast-moving (aerobic) fractions was negligibly low. However, in intact arteries of children, the activity of aerobic fractions prevailed. Figure 13 shows that in atherosclerotic human arteries the prevailing LDH isoenzyme fraction is the slow-moving anaerobic LDH_5. In contrast, in normal human or pig arteries the faster moving aerobic fractions dominate (ZEMPLÉNYI and BLANKENHORN, 1973).

Comparative investigations of arterial and venous tissue also yielded useful results (ZEMPLÉNYI et al., 1970). There is an unequivocal predominance of LDH_1 (the main aerobic fraction) and a lack of LDH_4 and LDH_5 (anaerobic fractions) in pig vena cava as compared with the aorta (Table 3). On the other hand, more than 40% of aortic LDH activity is confined to LDH_3 and only 15.6% to LDH_1. In dog vessels a similar pattern was detected.

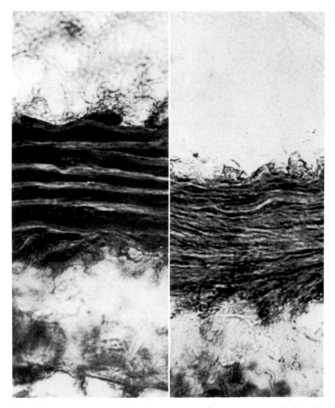

Fig. 12. Acid phosphomonoesterase in the aorta of a rat treated for 3 days by excess calciferol (a) as compared with the aorta of a normal (b) rat (× 500). (From Zempiényi, Urbanová, and Mrhová, Int. Symp. Biochemistry of the Vascular Wall, Basel and New York: Karger 1969)

According to current theory (Dawson et al., 1964) the slow moving cathodic LDH fractions are the principal isoenzymes in anaerobically metabolizing tissue while the fast-moving fractions are the most abundant isoenzymes in the heart and other tissue, where a steady supply of energy is maintained by complete oxidation in the presence of oxygen. Although some investigators have expressed doubt as to the general validity of this hypothesis, it appears to be the prevalent consensus that LDH isoenzyme patterns reflect long-term metabolic conditions of oxygen availability.

It was mentioned (Part I) that much recent evidence implicates hypoxic or anoxic damage of the arterial wall in the pathogenesis of atherosclerosis and results of LDH isoenzyme studies concur. It is also interesting that in the miniature pig subjected to high altitude hypoxia there is an increase in aortic lactate dehydrogenase and a decrease in succinate dehydrogenase activity (Frith et al., 1971; Will et al., 1972). Furthermore, in rats fed a cholesterol-rich diet a decrease of aerobic LDH fractions can be observed in the aorta (Seethanatan and Krup, 1970). Damage caused by pulling an inflated balloon catheter through the rabbit aorta also results in elevation of anaerobic lactate dehydrogenase isoenzymes (Lindy et al., 1972; Garbasch, 1973a) and severe hypertension has the same effect in miniature pigs (Will et al.,

Table 2. Some enzyme patterns in different types of experimental vascular injury. (Modified from ZEMPLÉNYI, URBANOVÁ and MRHOVÁ, Int. Symp. Biochemistry of the Vascular Wall, Basel and New York: Karger, 1969).

Vascular injury by	Acid Phosphomonoesterase	5'-Nucleotidase	ATPase	Carbesterase	Krebs cycle enzymes	
Allylamine intoxication	↗	→	↘	↘	↘	ZEMPLÉNYI et al., 1969
Excess vit. D feeding	↗	↗ (dashed)	↗ (dashed)	↘	↘	ZEMPLÉNYI and MRHOVÁ, 1965
DOCA + NaCl hypertension	↗	→	↘	↘	↘	ZEMPLÉNYI et al., 1968
Renovascular hypertension	↗	↗	→	↘	↘ (dashed)	ZEMPLÉNYI et al., 1968
Thermal lesion	↗	→	→	→	↘	JANDA et al., 1972

LDH Isoenzymes

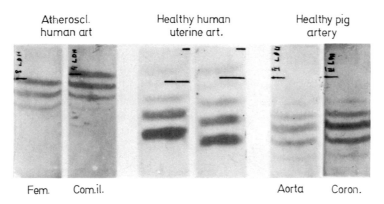

Fig. 13. Cellulose acetate electrophoresis of lactate dehydrogenase isoenzymes in normal human and pig artery and in atherosclerotic human artery. [From ZEMPLÉNYI and BLANKENHORN, Angiologica **9**, 429 (1972)]

1972). In experimental diabetes and in the femoral artery of diabetic patients the activity of the aerobic LDH fractions is decreased (WOHLRAB and GÖTZE, 1974; WOHLRAB and SCHMIDT, 1973).

The data so far noted seem to implicate age-dependent vascular injury as a cause of decreased durability of some parts of the arterial tree. However, it has to be pointed out that HAIMOVICI et al. (1964, 1966) demonstrated that canine arterial homografts, whether implanted into sites of maximum or minimum involvement, retained their original durability or susceptibility to atherosclerosis. Such findings suggest that susceptibility or durability is an inherent biologic local property of

Table 3. Comparison of distribution of lactate dehydrogenase isoenzymes in aorta and vena cava of pigs. (From ZEMPLÉNYI and BLANKENHORN, Angiologica, **9**, 429, 1972).

	LDH_1		LDH_2		LDH_3		LDH_4		LDH_5	
	A.	V.C.	A.	V.C.	A.	V.C.	A.	V.C.	A.	V.C.
Mean[a]	15.6	49.9	28.3	31.9	41.6	17.9	13.3	0	1.2	0
Range[a]	6–28	41–62	11–37	28–37	32–76	3–26	3–28	0–2[b]	0–6	0
S.E.M.	1.61	1.72	1.31	0.67	2.87	1.49	1.49	0	0.41	0
P	<0.001		<0.05		<0.001					

[a] Percents of total LDH activity.
[b] In most cases no band was found.

vascular tissue. It is, however, equally reasonable to expect that hemodynamic and hemorrheologic factors (the most likely damaging factors of daily wear-and-tear) have to exert their action for a long time before they provide a suitable "terrain" in the artery for the development of atherosclerosis. Therefore, the relatively short-term homograft experiments are not likely to either reject or confirm the role of "physiologic" damage in atherogenesis.

All the data which implicate vascular injury—including that caused by hypoxia—as a cause of altered susceptibility to atherosclerosis, also suggest that the ATP production of such a vessel is diminished; this results in lowering of all energy-requiring processes and failure of defense mechanisms of the arterial wall (ZEMPLÉNYI, 1967, 1968). Moreover, ATP deficiency may lead to decreased activity of ATP-dependent enzymes, such as the energy-linked nicotinamide nucleotide transhydrogenase (ERNSTER and LEE, 1964) or ATP-dependent cholesterol esterase. Instead, their action may be replaced by the increased and uncontrolled activity of the corresponding ATP-independent enzymes. The presence of the energy-linked transhydrogenase in arterial tissue has been reported by KALRA and BRODIE (1973). Both an ATP-dependent and ATP-independent aortic cholesterol esterase were detected by PROUDLOCK and DAY (1972) and the lecithin: cholesterol fatty-acid transferase found by ABDULLA et al. (1968) in arterial tissue, is also ATP-independent. According to JENSEN (1969) impairment of oxidation and stimulation of glycolysis is associated with increased cholesterol uptake by rabbit aorta.

G. Enzymes of Connective Tissue Metabolism

Local hypoxia is a stimulus for the activation of fibrogenic cell function, especially for the production of mucopolysaccharides and collagen (KROMPECHER, 1960; CHVAPIL, 1967). It may follow, therefore, that one of the stimuli leading to alterations in arterial connective tissue metabolism is hypoxia of this tissue. As a matter of fact, HELIN and co-workers (1969, 1970) observed an increase of aortic mucopolysaccharide and collagen in rabbits exposed to short-term hypoxia. Administration of small doses of monoiodoacetate seems to have a similar effect (SIDORENKOV, 1972). However, exposure to hypoxia for a longer period resulted in a reduction of the aortic content of mucopolysaccharides as well as collagen (HELIN et al., 1975).

Six enzymes of mucopolysaccharide breakdown have been identified and thoroughly studied in the vascular wall. In the first catabolic phase hyaluronidase and chondroitinsulfatase catalyze depolymerization and removal of ester sulfate. The resulting sulfate-free oligosaccharides subsequently are degraded by the alternating action of β-glucuronidase and β-acetyl-glucosaminidase. The protein component is degraded by cathepsin D and acid carboxypeptidase (HELD et al., 1968; BUDDECKE and KRESSE, 1969). The breakdown apparently is completed by such hydrolases as leucine aminopeptidase. The result is degradation into N-acetyl-agalactosamine, glucuronic acid, inorganic sulfate, oligosaccharides, glycopeptides, peptides, and amino acids (HELD et al., 1968). Chondroitinsulfatase has the least activity of these six enzymes, and the reaction catalyzed by it could represent a rate limiting step in the process of arterial mucopolysaccharide breakdown (HELD et al., 1968).

HAYASE et al. (1971) observed an identical activity of β-acetylglucosaminidase in human, chicken, and rat aortas but less activity in rabbit, pig, and dog aortas. In bovine aortas, (BUDDECKE and KRESSE, 1969) only cathepsin D and acid carboxypeptidase showed an increase of activity with age, whereas hyaluronidase activity decreased and the activities of β-acetylglucosaminidase and β-glucuronidase remained unchanged. Multiple forms of the enzyme also seem to be present in human aortas (HAYASE et al., 1971b). All of these activities were calculated on the DNA content basis of the arteries. In human arteries the data correlating age and enzyme activity, however, are conflicting (BUDDECKE and KRESSE, 1969; PLATT and LUBOENSKI, 1969).

More certainty exists concerning the activity in atherosclerotic vessels. In experimentally induced atherosclerosis in rabbits (MRHOVÁ et al., 1963) as well as in spontaneous atherosclerosis in rats (WEXLER and JUDD, 1966) there is an unequivocal increase in arterial β-glucuronidase activity. In human atherosclerosis an increased activity of β-glucuronidase, β-acetylglucosaminidase, cathepsin D, and acid carboxypeptidase was detected (DYRBYE and KIRK, 1956; BRANDWOOD and CARR, 1960; MILLER et al., 1966; BUDDECKE and KRESSE, 1969; KIRK, 1969; MILLER and KOTHARI, 1969). It is remarkable that normal segments of atherosclerosis-resistant vessels, such as the internal mammary artery, reveal a higher β-glucuronidase activity than the more susceptible abdominal aorta or coronary artery (MILLER et al., 1966). Perhaps the same is true for the pulmonary artery, but β-acetylglucosaminidase activity in the pulmonary artery and coronary artery is the same as in the aorta (KIRK, 1969). NIEBES and LASZT (1971a) studied the same enzymes in normal and varicose human saphenous veins. Except cathepsin, the activity of all enzymes is significantly increased in the diseased vein, especially the varix.

Only a few enzymes probably involved in mucopolysaccharide synthesis have been studied in arterial tissue. The activity of hexosephosphate aminotransferase ("hexosamine-synthesizing enzyme") is definitely lower in the pulmonary artery than in the aorta and there is a trend toward decreased activity in the atherosclerotic coronary artery (HARUKI and KIRK, 1965). RITZ and SANWALD (1970) demonstrated the transformation of ^{14}C-labeled D-glucose into D-glucuronic acid by rat aortas. This reaction is catalyzed by an NAD-dependent dehydrogenase. The activity was not changed in the aortas of alloxan-diabetic rats. Since the precursor of UDP glucuronic acid is UDP-glucose, it is relevant that KITTINGER et al. (1962) showed the presence of glucose-L-phosphate uridylyltransferase in arterial tissue. The activity of the enzyme significantly rises in the arteriosclerotic aortas of repeatedly-bred female rats. In aortas of rats fed an atherogenic diet VIJAYAKUMAR and KURUP (1975) observed a decrease in the activity of the hexosephosphate aminotransferase associated with an elevated activity of all mucopolysaccharide-degrading enzymes (see above).

Very little is known about enzymes of collagen and elastin metabolism in the arterial wall. Lysyl oxidase, an enzyme oxidizing peptidyl lysine to peptidyl α-aminoadipic-δ-semialdehyde, plays a key role in the synthesis of crosslinkings in elastin and collagen. It has been studied in chicken aortas (KAGAN and FRANZBLAU, 1971; KAGAN et al., 1974). The enzyme is in a catalytically functional insoluble complex form in the aorta and is inhibited by β-aminopropionitrile, copper chelators, carbonyl reagents and "deoxynation" with N_2. We will see later that some effects of flavonoids on arterial metabolism may be connected with their action on this enzyme. It is also possible that a soluble and particulate amino-oxidase recently, demonstrated in rabbit and bovine aortas (RUCKER and GOETTLICH-RIEMANN, 1972; HARRIS and O'DELL, 1972) is related to lysyl oxidase.

The activity of protocollagen proline hydroxylase (the enzyme considered to be a controlling factor in collagen synthesis) increases in rabbit aortas as early as four days after production of atherosclerosis-like plaques by simultaneous injection of epinephrine and thyroxine (FULLER and LANGER, 1970; FULLER et al., 1971). Mechanical injury has a similar effect (LINDY et al., 1972). An outstanding feature of this enzyme—as studied in other tissue—is that low oxygen pressure may influence its activity (CHVAPIL, personal communication). It was suggested that accumulation of lactate may enhance its activity (COMSTOCK and UDENFRIEND, 1970). This again brings to a focus hypoxia as an essential pathogenetic factor and emphasizes the desirability of further studies of the enzyme in relation to atherogenesis.

The last enzyme to be mentioned in respect to arterial connective tissue is elastase, a peptidase acting on elastin. There is also some evidence to indicate a possible relationship between enzymes of the elastase complex ("elastomucase") and lipoprotein lipase (BANGA and BALÓ, 1956; HALL, 1961; LOEVEN, 1967a, b). In human aortas GORE and LARKEY (1960) found only a weak elastase activity, but later CITTERIO and CUNEGO (1965) demonstrated a high activity in normal human cerebral arteries and a decline in activity in atherosclerotic vessels. PRETOLANI (1968) detected notable activity, but the method used is controversial (LOEVEN, 1969). Nevertheless, there is a small but consistently present amount of elastoproteinase and elastomucase both in calf and cow aortas. "Elastoliproteinase" could not be proved (LOEVEN, 1969).

In view of the recent findings of unequivocal arterial elastase activity, the possible pathogenetic significance of this enzyme should be taken into consideration. It is claimed that the elastoproteinase fraction of the elastase complex damages arterial elastic tissue primarily, whereas the elastomucase (or elastolipoproteinase?) fraction prevents secondary lipid infiltration (HALL and CZERKAWSKI, 1961; HALL, 1964). It is noteworthy that in the blood platelets there is also a protease attacking elastin, and the enzyme is liberated from platelets during their aggregation on collagen or by ADP (ROBERT et al., 1969). It is also of considerable interest that sodium salts of fatty acids manifest a very high stimulatory effect on the rate of elastolysis (JORDAN et al., 1974).

It has to be added that PLATT (1970) demonstrated in pig aortas a peptidyl-peptid hydrolase exhibiting similarity to collagenase. The subcellular localization of the enzyme is uncertain; probably it is not a typical lysosomal enzyme. Other peptidases (aminoacyloligopeptid hydrolases) have recently been studied by WAGNER and DUCK (1972) in normal and atherosclerotic rabbit aortas. Four isoenzymes were separated by column chromatography and no differences between normal and atherosclerotic aortas were observed.

H. Enzymes Related to Lipid Metabolism

The activity of carnitine transferase, an enzyme allowing the transfer of fatty-acids across the mitochondrial membrane and their oxidation by mitochondria, is very significantly lower in atherosclerotic human aortas and coronary arteries. The carnitine content of the atherosclerotic aorta is higher than that of the normal aorta, but the ratio is reversed in the coronary artery (KIRK, 1969).

Another enzyme of fatty acid turnover, 3-hydroxyacyl-CoA-dehydrogenase, has a high activity in human arteries and a tendency to decrease with age (SANWALD and KIRK, 1965). The activity in the vena cava is only about one-third of that in the arteries. In atherosclerotic aortas the activity decreases significantly.

It is evident that much more data on enzymes of fatty acid metabolism are needed before definite conclusions can be made on this important aspect of lipid metabolism in the arterial wall. However, a clearer picture seems to emerge from studies connected with other features of arterial lipid metabolism.

In 1955 KORN observed lipoprotein lipase activity in ammonia extracts of acetone-powders from several aortas, using chylomicrons as substrate (KORN, 1955). Independent of these observations, we subjected arterial lipolytic activity to detailed investigation. It was demonstrated, (using lipemic serum, rat chyle, or "activated" lipid emulsions as substrates and measuring the amount of free fatty acids liberated) that the degree of lipolytic activity of the aorta was significantly higher in the relatively atherosclerosis-resistant rat than in the rabbit, guinea pig, or chicken (ZEMPLÉNYI and GRAFNETTER, 1958; ZEMPLÉNYI et al., 1959). The lipolytic activity of the aorta significantly decreases in adult rats with increasing age (ZEMPLÉNYI and GRAFNETTER, 1959b), but rises in experimental rabbit atherosclerosis (ZEMPLÉNYI and GRAFNETTER, 1959a). The lipolytic activity in aortas of rats treated with high doses of calciferol significantly declines (GRAFNETTER and ZEMPLÉNYI, 1962). Others using basically the same or modified techniques, confirmed and extended the above findings (LEMPERT and LEITES, 1963; LEITES, 1964, 1965; MALLOV, 1964; CHMELAR and CHMELAROVÁ, 1968; ADAMS et al., 1969; CUPARENCU et al., 1970; SZABÓ et al., 1970). Human aortic mucopolysaccharide mixtures were also found to inhibit vascular lipolytic activity (GERÖ et al., 1962).

Experiments using various substrates and inhibitors indicated that besides lipoprotein lipase, other lipolytic enzymes were also involved in arterial lipolysis (GRAFNETTER and ZEMPLÉNYI, 1959; ZEMPLÉNYI, 1964; ZSOLDOS and HEINEMAN, 1964;

HAYASE and MILLER, 1970; JELINKOVÁ et al., 1972). However, lipoprotein lipase can be unequivocally demonstrated by increasing the specificity of the assay system using ^{14}C-triolein as substrate (VOST and POCOCK, 1974). NOMA and co-workers (1974) suggested that the intimal lipase might be lipoprotein lipase permeated from the serum while the medial lipase might be a "true" lipase acting on triglyceride molecules. It was also demonstrated that carboxylic (non-specific) esterase activity usually runs parallel with lipase activity, and the detection of the former by histochemical techniques is relatively simple. In experimentally induced atherosclerosis the early plaque constituents exhibit increased staining for non-specific exterase with all histochemical methods used for this enzyme (LOJDA and ZEMPLÉNYI, 1961; LOJDA, 1962; LEITES, 1963; TARARAK, 1968). In hypertensive animals there appears to be an increase in aortic lipolytic activity (MALLOV, 1964) although the esterase activity declines (ZEMPLÉNYI et al., 1969).

By actinomycin D treatment it is possible to prevent the increase of esterase activity in connective tissue cells (LEITES and FUKS, 1966). By analogy, one can assume that the elevated activity in atherosclerotic vessels is an adaptive change based on a substrate-linked induction of lipolytic enzymes (ZEMPLÉNYI, 1968).

The presence of lipoprotein lipase-like activity in human arteries was reported by several investigators. The activity in the normal thoracic aorta is approximately four times higher than in the abdominal aorta (PATELSKI et al., 1967). KIRK (1969) found a significantly higher activity in the pulmonary artery and vena cava than in the aorta. With aging, the activity in normal aortic tissue has a tendency to decrease (ADAMS et al., 1969). In atherosclerotic aortas from younger adults up to the fifth decade, there also is a tendency toward decreased activity (KIRK, 1969). The carboxylic esterase activity is, according to KIRK's findings, markedly higher in the atherosclerotic aorta and coronary artery segments than in normal portions of the same vessels. Fibrous lesions do not display such a change in activity. This concurs with previous histochemical data in human vessels (ZEMPLÉNYI, 1968).

It must be emphasized that not all arterial lipolytic activity is due to alkaline triglyceride lipase. HAYASE and MILLER (1970) demonstrated that normal human aortic tissue contains, beside the alkaline lipase (pH optimum 8.8), an acid lipase (pH optimum 5.4) differring in physicochemical characteristics. The acid lipase is more resistant to substrate inhibition so that the mechanism to dispose of excess triglycerides primarily may depend on the activity of acid lipase. By analogy with other tissues, the acid lipase may be lysosomal.

The evidence so far accumulated strongly suggests that the main function of arterial lipolytic activity consists in protecting the arterial wall against accumulation of potentially injurious lipids. In this regard the acid (and probably lysosomal) lipase may be more important than the alkaline lipoproteine lipase. However, even so it is very questionable whether one can accept the hypothesis recently proposed by ZILVERSMIT (1973). According to this hypothesis, high local concentrations of cholesterol-rich lipoproteins resulting from surface lipolysis by lipoprotein lipase and the release of potentially injurious fatty acids would enhance the uptake of cholesterol by the arterial intima.

The normal arterial wall possesses the ability to counterbalance an increased influx of not only triglycerides, but other lipids as well. In a series of very well documented papers STEIN and co-workers (STEIN and STEIN, 1962; STEIN et al., 1963,

1968, 1970; RACHMILEWITZ et al., 1967; EISENBERG et al., 1968, 1969a, b) reported on the presence and characteristics of phospholipases in animal and human arteries. The most interesting results deal with the activity of sphingomyelin choline phosphohydrolase, the enzyme that splits sphingomyelin into N-acylsphingosine ("ceramide") and phosphorylcholine. It can be shown that the activity of the enzyme, calculated on the DNA content basis, is much higher in the rat than rabbit aorta, and in animals as well as man the activity decidedly decreases with age. In contrast, the activity of phosphatide acyl-hydrolase, phospholipase, increases with age (up to five-fold) whether using lecthin or phosphatidyl ethanolamine as substrate. The activity of lysophosphatide hydrolase also increases.

Since the aortic sphingomyelin content rises with age and atherosclerosis (BÖTTCHER and VAN GENT, 1961; SMITH, 1965) the above facts throw some new light on the mechanism of regulation of the arterial phospholipid content. The accumulation of sphingomyelin with aging (70% of the total phospholipid increment) appears to result from an imbalance in the rate of its influx (synthesis *in situ* plus entry from the circulation) and the rate of removal (egress and degradation). The high activity of the other phosphohydrolases prevents a larger accumulation of the other phospholipids with age, and also most likely in atherosclerosis, in spite of the higher synthesis rate (EISENBERG et al., 1969b).

No data are available on the activity of these phosphohydrolases in human atherosclerosis; however, results have been assembled on the activity of phospholipase A in normal and atherosclerotic animal arteries (WALLIGÓRA, 1966; PATELSKI et al., 1967, 1968) and indicate that the aortas of rabbits fed on an atherogenic diet display a definite increase in the activity of this enzyme.

The last enzymes to be considered are connected with hydrolytic cleavage of cholesterol esters and/or with cholesterol esterification. PATELSKI and co-workers (1968, 1967, 1970) detected hydrolytic cholesterol esterase activity in pig, rat, and rabbit aortas. Feeding of an "atherogenic" diet to rats and rabbits caused a decline in the enzyme activity. Other investigators, using labeled cholesterol oleate as substrate, also were able to observe definite cholesterol esterase hydrolytic activity in rabbit (DAY and GOLD-HURST, 1966), rat, monkey (HOWARD and PORTMAN, 1966) as well as chicken aortas (SHYAMALA et al., 1966). No cholesterol esterase synthesizing activity was reported in these studies.

However, there is substantial evidence that arterial cholesterol esters do not originate only from deposition of the serum but also from local synthesis within the arterial wall (LOFLAND et al., 1965, 1968; NEWMAN et al., 1968; FELT and BENEŠ, 1969; ST. CLAIR et al., 1969, 1970, 1972; DAYTON and HASHIMOTO, 1970). Therefore, it is obvious that in addition to the cholesterol esterase hydrolytic activity an esterifying enzyme (or enzymes) must be active in the normal and atherosclerotic artery.

ST. CLAIR et al. (1970) detected in cell-free preparations from pigeon aortas an esterifying enzyme system which had an optimal pH of 7.4 to 7.8, and required ATP and coenzyme A as cofactors. Most of the activity was associated with the particulate fraction. PROUDLOCK and DAY (1972) demonstrated that there are at least two enzyme systems capable of incorporating labeled cholesterol and fatty-acid (oleic acid) into cholesterol ester in the atherosclerotic rabbit intima. The first had a pH optimum of 5.0 and did not require ATP and coenzyme A for activity. The other enzyme system, with a pH optimum in the region of 7.5 was found to be dependent on the presence of coenzyme A and ATP, and to require SH reagents for maximal activity. This enzyme appears to be similar to that described by St. CLAIR et al. (1970) in pigeon aortas and the enzyme activity observed by FELT and BENEŠ (1969) in normal rat aorta.

The failure to detect synthesizing activity in some of the previous studies seems to be clarified by recent data by KOTHARI et al. (1971, 1973). They demonstrated that the physicochemical state of the substrate greatly influences the possibility of detecting the synthesizing activity in acetone dry powder from normal rat and rabbit aorta. The synthetic activity is most effective with an emulsified substrate prepared from cholesterol, oleic acid, sodium taurocholate and NH_4Cl in phosphate buffer of pH 6.2. For the study of hydrolytic activity, a micellar substrate is used consisting of cholesterol oleate, sodium taurocholate and lecithin (or albumin) in phosphate buffer, pH 6.6 (with lecithin) or pH 7.4 (with albumin). With the micellar substrate hydrolysis is about three times more effective than with the emulsified substrate. The esterifying enzyme acts only on emulsified substrate, and this suggests a requirement for two phases or the presence of an interface. The enzyme requires sodium taurocholate for maximum activity.

It is interesting that the hydrolysis/synthesis ratio is much higher in the normal rat than rabbit aorta. Is there an innate inability in the rabbit to hydrolyze cholesterol esters which contributes to their susceptibility to cholesterol-induced atherosclerosis? In this respect, it is of additional interest that KRITCHEVSKY (1972) reported a similar difference in the hydrolysis/synthesis ratio in the aortas of two pigeon strains which differ in susceptibility to atherosclerosis. However, in rabbits fed for 5 months on a cholesterol diet FELT and BENEŠ (1971) observed in the aortas a 65% rise of cholesterol esterase hydrolyzing activity and only 40% rise of esterifying activity. This suggests an adaptation of the originally low hydrolysis/synthesis ratio to the high influx of cholesterol and cholesterol esters in the aortic wall. It is also noteworthy that increasing the atmospheric pressure during the incubation experiments causes a significant fall of both hydrolyzing and esterifying activity in rat aortas (FELT, 1971).

Besides cholesterol esterase, the existence of an alternate way for cholesterol esterification has been suggested in arterial tissue. ABDULLA et al. (1968, 1969) presented evidence indicating that in normal and atherosclerotic human and rabbit aortas esterification can be carried out by a lecithin: cholesterol fatty acid transferase. The activity tends to rise in aortas of older subjects and is definitely increased in human atherosclerotic lesions and aortas of cholesterol-fed rabbits. However, other investigators were unable to detect the transacylation reaction in the arterial wall (DAYTON and HASHIMOTO, 1970; St. CLAIR et al., 1970). Nevertheless, the transacylation reaction could represent an important link between cholesterol and phospholipid metabolism in the arterial wall. The reaction releases lysophosphatidylcholin (lysolecithin) from lecithin and, as a matter of fact, in the atherosclerotic aortas from squirrel monkeys the concentration of the latter compound is asserted to be nearly eight times higher than in comparable control tissue (PORTMAN and ALEXANDER, 1969). However, there is also evidence that lysolecithin is rapidly removed from plasma by arteries, and therefore, it may be a product of the lecithin: cholesterol fatty acid transferase reaction in plasma. The important aspect of arterial lysolecithin accumulation is the fact that this compound is of considerable importance in phospholipid and perhaps also triglyceride synthesis in aortic tissue (STEIN and STEIN, 1962; STEIN et al., 1963, 1968).

Lysosomal Enzymes

We have indicated in previous sections of this review that many of the arterial enzymes studied were lysosomal enzymes (e.g. acid phosphomonoesterase, β-glucuronidase and all enzymes of mucopolysaccharide catabolism). They manifested a conspicuous tendency toward increased activity associated with arterial injury and atherosclerosis. More recently this phenomenon has been investigated in particular by Dr. CHRISTIAN DE DUVE and co-workers. Rabbit aortic smooth muscle cells were fractionated by isopycnic centrifugation on sucrose density gradients. Several subcellular organelles, in particular lysosomes, could be characterized in the smooth muscle cells in this manner (PETERS et al., 1972). In rabbits with experimental atherosclerosis the specific activity of all lysosomal acid hydrolases (N-acetyl-β-galactosaminidase, α-mannosidase, N-acetyl-β-glucosaminidase, acid phosphomonesterase, cathepsin C, β-galactosidase and β-glucuronidase) increased progressively with increasing severity of arterial lesions. At the same time the lysosomes became more resistant to mechanical injury and their density decreased progressively, probably as a result of massive uptake of cholesterol in esterified form (BLACK et al., 1973; PETERS and DE DUVE, 1974). The typical lysosomal enzyme activities were also increased in the arteries of hypertensive rats and atherosclerotic or hypertensive rhesus monkeys (WOLINSKY et al., 1974, 1975); and the elevated activity in human atherosclerotic arteries has been mentioned before in relation to enzymes of connective tissue metabolism.

Moreover, aortic tissue contains an acid cholesterol ester hydrolase confined to lysosomes of the smooth muscle cells (TAKANO et al., 1974). Similarly, as the enzyme in peritoneal macrophages (WERB and COHN, 1972) this cholesterol esterase has an optimal activity at pH 4.25 and is several times more active on esters of unsaturated than saturated fatty acids. It appears to be similar to or identical with the cholesterol esterase detected by KOTHARI and co-workers (1971, 1973) whereas the enzyme studied by BRECHER and co-workers (1973) in subcellular fractions of rat and monkey aortic homogenates is associated with microsomes (similarly as the aortic cholesterol esterifying activity reported by HASHIMOTO and DAYTON, 1974, and HASHIMOTO et al., 1974) and apparently has no acid pH optimum.

A further finding of considerable interest is that the lipid-laden lysosomes from severely atherosclerotic rabbit smooth muscle cells possess much less cholesterol esterase activity (measured in relation to other lysosomal enzymes, especially to N-acetyl-β-glucosaminidase) than the activity exhibited by high density lysosomes which have a low lipid content (DE DUVE, 1974). This is in accord with observations of decreased cholesterol ester hydrolase activity reported by PATELSKI and co-workers (1970), and may explain the behavior of the hydrolysis/synthesis ratio changes as observed by KRITCHEVSKY (1972). It was also observed (SHIO et al., 1974) that the transformation of smooth muscle cells into foam cells is accompanied by increase in both size and in number of lysosomes.

On the basis of these findings DE DUVE suggested an attractive hypothetical "model" namely that the transformation of the arterial smooth muscle cell into the lipid-laden foam cell is the result of a relative deficiency of lysosomal cholesterol ester hydrolase, failing to deal with the increased influx of lipid into the cell. Implicit in this "model" is the identification of the lipid-laden vacuoles of the foam cells as being of lysosomal nature, resulting from fusion of pinocytic vacuoles with lysosomes and thus becoming secondary lysosomes or phagolysosomes (De Duve, 1974). It is not known whether the activity of the acid lipase, described by Hayase and Miller (1970) exhibits similar to the cholesterol ester hydrolase.

Summary

1. On *a priori* grounds one can anticipate that most enzymes characteristic of all living matter are present in arterial tissue. The evidence assembled shows conclusively that the arterial wall contains those enzymes which catalyze basic reactions of metabolic "mainstreams". Arterial tissue also contains enzymes catalyzing anabolic and catabolic reactions of connective tissue and lipid metabolism. The study of lipases, phospholipases and cholesterol esterases provided valuable data on the mechanism of lipid accumulation in arterial tissue and natural history of atherosclerosis.

2. Arterial enzyme activities manifest interspecies and intraspecies differences and some of those differences are in accordance with susceptibility to atherosclerosis. Arterial enzyme activity also changes with age and depends on hormonal factors, especially sex hormones.

3. Most enzymes display a marked alteration (mostly a decrease) in activity in atherosclerotic arteries. However, investigation of advanced lesions has not determined whether such changes in activity precede atherosclerosis or result from the disease. This is, of course, the crucial problem in the study of the relationship between vascular metabolism and atherosclerosis.

4. The study of very early stages of spontaneous and experimental animal atherosclerosis as well as the comparison of enzyme activity in various arteries indicates that "susceptible" vessels exhibit a lower activity of Krebs cycle enzymes and a higher activity of some glycolytic enzymes and phosphomonoesterases as compared to arteries resistant to atherosclerosis. Further experimental evidence shows that this pattern of enzyme activity develops during life, most likely as a result of damage by the wear-and-tear of the artery at hemodynamically vulnerable sites or as a result of increased intravascular pressure. However, some differences in enzyme activity appear to be of inherited (genetic) nature.

5. Evidence derived from studies of enzymes, particularly lactate dehydrogenase isoenzymes, supports the assumption that tissue hypoxia is an additional factor causing vascular damage. This agrees with data summarized in Part I and accentuates the role of arterial hypoxia in the pathogenesis of atherosclerosis.

6. Investigation of lysosomal enzyme activities in normal and diseased arteries indicates an essential role of lysosomal hydrolases in atherogenesis and particularly the role of acid cholesterol esterase in the transformation of the smooth muscle cell into the foam cell of the early atherosclerotic lesion.

III. The Effect of Drugs

On the basis of the data presented in Part I and II of this review, a working hypothesis can be formulated. A "favorable" metabolic drug effect on the arterial wall should fulfill at least one of these criteria:

a) Decrease the permeability of the inner layers of the arterial wall.

b) Decrease the ability of the arterial wall to synthesize hydrophobic lipids (cholesterol, triglycerides) and/or increase the synthesis of phospholipids.

c) Decrease the synthesis of abnormal vascular mucopolysaccharides and/or increase the catabolism of such mucopolysaccharides.

d) Decrease the possibility of vascular injury by hypertension or by such metabolic factors as local hypoxia or by damaging products released from platelet thrombi.

e) Increase the bioenergetics of vascular tissue by increasing the activity of the rate-limiting enzymatic steps in the Krebs cycle and in the mitochondrial electron transport system.

f) Decrease the lactate production in vascular tissue.

g) Increase the lipolytic (and esterolytic) activity and perhaps also change the cholesterol esterase activity of vascular tissue.

h) Decrease the uptake of lipoproteins.

Only a few drugs have been studied pertinent to these effects and the data are sometimes controversial and difficult to evaluate. However, some results are propitious for future research.

A. Bioflavonoids

Bioflavonoids are a group of substances which—according to many investigators—have the property of reducing the permeability and fragility of the vascular system, particularly capillaries. The commonly known and most studied flavonoids are rutin, various hydroxyethylrutosides, quercetin, naringin, the citrus complex (citrin), hesperidine, hesperidine methylchalcone, (+)cathechin, (+)epicathechin-2-sodium sulfonate and other derivatives of (+)catechin.

The mechanism by which the bioflavonoids exert their influence on permeability has been investigated extensively. It was found that they probably are capable of interacting with different metabolites and also enhance or inhibit various enzymatic activities. For example, it is maintained that some bioflavonoids are inhibitors of hyaluronidase and also inhibit epinephrine oxidation leading to a "tightening-up" of the vascular system. Some bioflavonoids are reported to be inhibitors of bovine pancreatic ribonuclease or liver tyrosine-aminotransferase. According to CARPENEDO et al. (1969) the membrane-bound sodium and potassium dependent ATPase (transport ATPase) is inhibited by quercetin. Copious data indicate that some flavonoids have an anthihistamine effect possibly involving a direct antihistaminic action, or interference with the formation of histamine, especially by inhibiting histidine decarboxylase or by preventing disruption of histamine- and serotonine-containing mast-cells (KATO and GOZSY, 1970). Endogenous histamine liberated from disrupted mast-cells may cause accumulation of macromolecular substances, including fat particles, in the vascular endothelium (ZEMPLÉNYI et al., 1960). HORN et al. (1970) found an increase of liver cytochrome oxidase activity in the presence of (+)catechin and its derivatives; and GAJDOS et al. (1969) reported an elevation of the hepatic ATP level in rats treated with (+)catechin.

Some effects of flavonoids on permeability and connective tissue may be connected with stabilization of the lysosomal membrane (VAN CANEGHEM, 1972) as well as inhibition of hyaluronidase, β-glucuronidase and other lysosomal enzymes (RODNEY et al., 1950). An interesting effect of flavonoids is their ability to impede blood cell and platelet aggregation (ROBBINS, 1966, 1967, 1971). The latter effect may be important in atherogenesis. (For further details concerning the physiologic and metabolic effects of flavonoids refer to reviews by MARTIN, 1954; BÖHM, 1968; GÁBOR, 1972 and others).

There is only a very limited number of publications dealing with flavonoid effects on the vascular wall. These studies are principally concerned with venous tissue, but some information on arterial metabolic effects is available.

LASZT (1972b) studied the oxygen consumption of human venous tissue incubated with hydroxyethylrutoside or (+)catechin. He observed that in the presence of the flavonoids there was a 50% rise of oxygen uptake and a concomitant fall in lactate production with glucose as the substrate. A similar effect was detected also in a few experiments with arterial tissue. NIEBES and LASZT (1971b) and NIEBES (1972) observed that in the bovine saphenous vein hydroxyethylrutin (1mg/ml) inhibited the activity of β-glucuronidase by 70% and arylsulfatase by 24%. The (+)catechin was a less potent inhibitor and the epicatechin sodium sulfonate inhibited only acid phosphomonoesterase by 51%.

The oxidation products of (+)catechin inhibited all the lysosomal enzymes investigated (except acid phosphomonoesterase) and inhibition of neuraminidase was also observed. No in vitro effect on lactate or succinate dehydrogenase activity could be detected. However, MATAGNE and HAMOIR (1972) observed a shift toward aerobic LDH isoenzyme fractions following pretreatment of human saphenous veins with 0.1 to 0.3% hydroxyethylrutoside. Under these experimental conditions, no effect of the flavonoid was observed on the activity and/or isoenzyme distribution of other enzymes, namely glyceraldehyde phosphate dehydrogenase, aldolase, enolase, pyruvate kinase, triosephosphate isomerase, phosphoglucomutase and creatine phosphokinase.

The effect of (+)cathechin on bovine arterial tissue (thoracic aorta) has been studied by FILIPOVIC et al. (1972). Using ^{14}C-labeled acetate and fatty-acids as substrates they observed a significant rise of cellular respiration, in particular fatty acid oxidation when the tissue was incubated with (+)catechin or hydroxyethylrutoside. Using [U-^{14}C] glucose instead of acetate, the main metabolic effect of (+)catechin was an unequivocally increased incorporation of ^{14}C-radioactivity into the glycerol component of phospholipids. Furthermore, labeling of the phospholipid fraction disclosed a more than 100% rise of ^{32}P-incorporation. The flavonoid also caused a slight decrease of lactate production and a 50% fall in ^{14}CO$_2$ production. However, contrary to what could be expected on the basis of similar studies in other tissue, no change in mucopolysaccharide metabolism was detected. The authors point out that this could be due to the fact that the incubations lasted only 15 hrs— not long enough to induce connective tissue changes.

In this regard it is of importance that in chronic experiments flavonoids exert a protective action on arterial collagen. In lathyric rats CETTA et al. (1971, 1972) observed that hydroxyethylrutoside and (+)catechin prevent the solubilization and reduction of crosslinkings in collagen. The enzyme lysyl oxidase, required for the formation of crosslinkings, is Cu^{++}-dependent and the lathyrogens (aminonitriles) appear to act by complexing the Cu^{++} ion. The favorable effect of flavonoids can be explained by competition for the Cu^{++} ion since their chelating capacity for metal ions seems to be established (BÖHM, 1968).

The question arises, of course, whether clinical studies confirm the "favorable" metabolic effects of flavonoids in the treatment of vascular disease. As far as chronic venous disorders are concerned several double-blind studies indicate a beneficial effect of some flavonoids on symptoms and signs caused by primary varicose veins (HALBORG-SØRENSEN and HANSEN, 1970; ROZTOČIL et al., 1971; PŘEROVSKÝ et al., 1972). Similar data on arterial disorders in man are not available.

A very significant effect of some flavonoids on the survival time of rats fed a thrombogenic or atherogenic regimen has been reported (ROBBINS, 1967). The alfalfa content of the experimental diet markedly reduces the degree of atherosclerotic lesions in cholesterol-fed rabbits (COOKSON et al., 1967; HOWARD, 1970) and extracts of alfalfa display the same effect (HORŇÁČEK et al., 1966). This may be due to the high flavonoid content of alfalfa. (Eight coumestan derivatives and several other phenolic compounds have been isolated from alfalfa—see BICKOFF et al., 1966).

B. Pyridinolcarbamate

This compound was synthesized in 1962 by SHIMAMOTO and ISHIKAWA. Chemically, it is 2,6-*bis* (hydroxymethyl) pyridine-*bis* (N-methylcarbamate). It was found by SHIMAMOTO et al. (1966a) to possess antibradykinin activity in some laboratory animals, but not in the guinea-pig. Subsequently, it was reported that pyridinolcarbamate is not a specific inhibitor of the kinins, but it has the capacity to counteract the increased permeability of vascular endothelium induced by bradykinin, kallidin, and kallikrein. Pyridinolcarbamate also impedes the permeability-increasing effect induced by the intradermal inoculation of the "lymph node permeability factor" (WILLOUGHBY et al., 1969). Diminution of exudation associated with some models of inflammation (e.g. in the anaphylactic reaction to egg albumin) also was reported when pyridinolcarbamate was applied. This compound is without effect, however, on the exudation evoked by serotonin or histamine (WILLOUGHBY et al., 1969) and does not prevent an edematous arterial reaction induced by the intravenous injection of horse serum to rabbits (DE OLIVIERA, 1969). In some animals as the rabbit and chicken (SHIMAMOTO et al., 1966b, 1969; DE OLIVIERA, 1969; PICK, 1969; NUMANO et al., 1971a) pyridinolcarbamate decreased the severity of experimentally-induced atherosclerosis; however, the results are conflicting (MÖTTONEN et al., 1972) and in nonprimate monkeys the compound was ineffective in altering the degree of aortic or coronary atherosclerosis (MALINOW et al., 1968, 1972).

Nevertheless—as permeability changes play an important role in the pathogenesis of vascular disease (see Part I)—it is of interest to investigate whether this compound has any effect on arterial wall metabolism.

MRHOVÁ et al. (1972a) observed that in rats fed a high-fat-cholesterol containing diet pyridinolcarbamate (30 mg/kg/day for eight weeks) increased the activity of aortic malate dehydrogenase and β-glucuronidase. In *in vitro* experiments pyridinolcarbamate (150 to 300 µg/ml) increased the activity of both aortic malate and lactate dehydrogenase.

In another experimental series MRHOVÁ et al. (1972b) studied the effect of pyridinolcarbamate on the aortas of calciferol-intoxicated rats. It was mentioned in Part II that vascular injury, including that induced by excess calciferol feeding, causes a rise of arterial acid phosphomonoesterase activity and fall of some Krebs cycle enzyme activities. In this experiment it was shown that the decreased activity of enzymes of the Krebs cycle did not occur if the rats have been treated with pyridinolcarbamate (25 mg/kg/day for three to nine weeks). However, the activity of acid phosphomon-oesterase was not affected by pyridinolcarbamate treatment.

In cholesterol-fed rabbits Numano et al. (1971b) observed in the aortas a decreased histochemical staining for glycogen phosphorylase, glucoes-6-phosphate dehydrogenase, aldolase, lactate dehydrogenase, succinate dehydrogenase and ATP-ase. Pyridinolcarbamate treatment was accompanied by a decrease of acid phosphomonoesterase, β-glucuronidase and carboxylic esterase activity.

C. Sex Hormones

It is a well established clinical experience (confirmed by most morphological studies) that premenopausal women have less coronary and peripheral atherosclerosis than men. The coronary arteries of elderly men, receiving prolonged stilbestrol treatment for prostatic carcinoma, reveal less atherosclerosis than matched control groups. On the other hand, bilateral ovariectomy in young women is followed by premature develpoment of atherosclerosis (see Zemplényi, 1968).

The sex differences and the effects of castration and sex hormones cannot be explained entirely as resulting from differences in circulating blood lipid levels; it is reasonable to assume direct action of sex hormones on arterial wall metabolism.

Most information in the literature concerns metabolic effects of sex hormones on tissue of reproductive organs (for details see e.g. Litwack and Kritchevsky, 1964). Interestingly enough, the studies of Chobanian et al. (1968a) demonstrate special affinity of sex hormones to arterial tissue. Both estrogen and testosterone enter the arterial wall rapidly, and here a chemical conversion of sex hormones may take place, probably requiring the presence of 17 β-dehydrogenase and a sulfatase. The artery can interconvert estrone and estradiol, and convert estrone sulfate to both estrone and estradiol. The metabolic effects of estrogenic hormones on the artery are similar to those reported for the uterus (Aizawa and Mueller, 1961) and suggest that the arterial intima is target tissue for estrogens (Chobanian, 1968b; Newmark et al., 1972).

This being the case, it is not surprising that the effects of sex, gonadectomy and sex hormones on arterial enzymes have been demonstrated. In the female rat the activity of aortic lactate dehydrogenase, malate dehydrogenase and 5'-nucleotidase is higher and the activity of β-glucuronidase and alkaline phosphomonoesterase lower than in the male (Mrhová and Zemplényi, 1965). Estradiol treatment (10000 I.U. daily for 14 days) causes a fall in the activity of acid and alkaline phosphomon-oesterase and carboxylic esterase in the male rat aorta, a rise of 5'-nucleotidase activity in both male and female aortas, and a trend toward increased malate dehy-drogenase activity in male aortas (Zemplényi and Mrhová, 1967). However, incubation of chicken aorta with estradiol is accompanied by enhancement of its alkaline phosphomonoesterase activity (Malinow, 1960).

In experiments dealing with the effect of gonadectomy on rat aortas Malinow et al. (1962) observed an increased activity of cytochrome oxidase and enhancement of α-ketoglutarate oxidation in the female aortas, a decreased oxidation of fumarate in the male aortas, and an increased succinate dehydrogenase activity in both male and female aortas. In another series of experiments (MRHOVÁ and ZEMPLÉNYI, 1965) it was shown that in the aortas of castrated male rats the activity of alkaline and acid phosphomonoesterase, malate dehydrogenase, and probably 5'-nucleotidase was higher than in the aortas of sham-operated animals. In ovariectomized female rats the activity of malate dehydrogenase and 5'-nucleotidase decreased significantly.

The results obtained by KIRK (1964, 1969) in work with human aortas indicate that male aortas, as compared with female aortas, display significantly higher activity of two NADP-dependent enzymes (glucose 6-phosphate dehydrogenase and decarboxylating malate dehydrogenase); the activity of two other "reduced NADP producing" enzymes (i.e., isocitrate dehydrogenase and decarboxylating phosphogluconate dehydrogenase) reveals a similar tendency. The same was observed for two of the above four enzymes in the male coronary arteries. Most interestingly, the activity of glycerol-3-phosphate dehydrogenase is also significantly higher in male than female aortas (KIRK and RITZ, 1967). Since reduced NADP is intimately involved in the synthesis of cholesterol and fatty-acids and since glycerol 3-phosphate ("active glycerol") is the common acceptor of fatty-acids in triglyceride and phospholipid synthesis, it is tempting to ascribe the above features of the male arteries to increased tendency toward synthesis of these lipids.

In addition to studies of arterial enzymes, useful information was obtained from studies of other metabolic parameters of arterial tissue influenced by sex hormones. MALINOW and MOGUILEVSKY (1961) observed in cockerels treated with estradiol or stilbestrol, a definite rise of arterial oxygen uptake. Unfortunately, experiments with gonadectomized rats (MALINOW et al., 1961) produced contradictory results and RIFKIND and MUNRO (1963) were unable to confirm the influence of either gonadectomy or sex hormones on aortic respiration. It would be desirable to repeat these experiments with the more sophisticated techniques presently available, including the measurement of oxidative phosphorylation.

Studies concerned with the effects of sex hormones on arterial phospholipid synthesis provided some important results (CHOBANIAN, 1968b). It was demonstrated that estrone sulfate and estradiol in vitro increased the incorporation of ^{32}P into phospholipid in human, canine, and rat arteries. The major augmentation was in the lecithin fraction. Testosterone produced no significant effect on incorporation of ^{32}P into phospholipid, but in combination with estrone sulfate, testosterone inhibited rise in incorporation induced by estrone sulfate. Estrone sulfate or estradiol had no significant effect on the incorporation of labeled acetate into total arterial lipids, although a slight incorporation into phospholipid was found. The estrogens had no in vitro effect on incorporation of labeled leucine into protein, and of ^{32}P into RNA. However, in the sexually immature rat intraperitoneal administration of 5.0 µg of estradiol four hours prior to killing was accompanied by a significant enhancement in incorporation of both ^{32}P and glycin into RNA and of glycin into protein. Contrary to the in vitro experiment, testosterone in vivo also exhibited an enhancing effect on incorporation of ^{32}P into RNA and of glycin into protein.

MORIN (1970) investigated the effect of estradiol on the in vitro incorporation of labeled acetate and choline into phospholipids of human peripheral arteries obtained immediately after surgery. Both choline-^{14}C and acetate-^{14}C incorporation in the presence of estradiol was significantly increased into phosphatidyl choline and slightly increased into sphingomyelin. Estradiol increased incorporation of acetate-

^{14}C into the palmitic acid component of phosphatidyl choline. Acetate-^{14}C incorporation into phosphatidyl ethanolamine was slightly reduced by estradiol.

It is also remarkable that estrogen influences vascular connective tissue (LOREN-ZEN and HEADINGS, 1966) and increases the turnover of collagen and elastin in arteries, resulting in lessening the stiffness and elasticity of the vascular wall (FISCHER, 1971; TSUKERSTEIN, 1971). Moreover, recently FISHER-DZOGA and co-workers (1974b) demonstrated that the addition of estradiol benzoate to the culture medium for rabbit aortic smooth muscle cells resulted in an inhibition of the proliferative effect of hyperlipemic serum.

In consideration of what has been outlined in the introduction to Part III of this review, some of the effects of estrogens, especially on phospholipid synthesis, can be undoubtedly considered "favorable"; they may contribute to the therapeutic effect of estrogens in the treatment of coronary heart disease and other forms of atherosclerosis (MARMORSTON et al., 1962; STAMLER et al., 1963, and others).

It will be appropriate to mention that recently the effects of other hormones on arterial metabolism were also investigated (NEWMARK et al., 1972). In rats hydrocortison reduces both the synthesis and breakdown of aortic glycogen and the synthesis of mucopolysaccharides from glucose. Similarly as in other tissues insulin stimulates in the aorta the synthesis of glycogen in diabetic rats and epinephrine enhances glucose utilization, lactate production and glycogen synthesis and breakdown.

D. Drugs Affecting Vascular Lipolytic and Esterolytic Activity

Interest in the relationship between atherosclerosis and hydrolytic splitting of fats originates from a fortuitous discovery by HAHN in 1943, who observed that intravenous injection of heparin to a highly lipemic dog led to rapid clearing of the plasma. Extensive investigations have shown that heparin releases a lipase—namely lipoprotein lipase—from the tissues, and the clearing of lipemic serum is caused by hydrolysis of triglycerides contained in chylomicrons and low-density lipoproteins. Heparin is an integral component of the system and enables the lipase to be bound to the lipoprotein substrate (KORN, 1958).

Lipoprotein lipase activity is confined principally to the capillary wall (HAVEL, 1958; ROBINSON and HARRIS, 1959), but arterial tissue also exhibits definite lipolytic and esterolytic activity. Relevant data have been described in Part II. The measurement of arterial lipolytic activity does not require the use of heparin in the assay system. However, SZABÓ and CSEH (1962) reported that addition of elastase to an acetone powder extract of blood vessels containing 5 μg/ml heparin significantly increased the lipoprotein lipase activity. PATELSKI et al. (1967) confirmed that in vitro the arterial lipase was activated by heparin in low concentration, but it was inhibited by higher concentration of heparin. This is in accord with KORN'S findings of the properties of the enzyme extracted from heart tissue. In vivo studies by DURY (1961) also indicate that heparin may enhance vascular lipolytic activity: heparin injections into young rats resulted in increased aortic lipolysis, but in old rats no such effect was observed. No comparable data are available in other animals or men.

PATELSKI et al. (1970) injected atherosclerotic rabbits with polyunsaturated lecithin (Lipostabil, Nattermann, Cologne), to change arterial lipolytic activity. The degree of atherosclerosis was lower in the injected animals, without significant effect on plasma cholesterol level and arterial lipase, phospholipase A or cholesterol esterase. However, serum and liver lipase activities were increased in the Lipostabil-treated animals.

CUPARENCU et al. (1970) report that the tranquilizer and muscle relaxant chlordiazepoxide in a daily dose of 10 mg/kg weight induces within a period of two months an elevation of aortic lipolytic activity in normal and cholesterol-fed rabbits. In the opinion of these authors the results may explain their previous findings showing an inhibitory effect of the drug on experimental rabbit atherosclerosis (CUPARENCU et al., 1969).

SZENDZIKOWSKI et al. (1961 to 1962) and LACUARA et al. (1962) reported sex differences in rat aorta lipolytic or esterolytic activity, but results of other studies were negative (ZEMPLÉNYI, 1964; MALLOV, 1964). Gonadectomy also resulted in questionable or conflicting changes of aortic esterolytic activity (LACUARA, 1962; MRHOVÁ and ZEMPLÉNYI, 1965). Although estradiol treatment of male rats is accompanied by a decline of aortic carboxylic esterase activity (ZEMPLÉNYI and MRHOVÁ, 1967), more studies are necessary to confirm the effect of sex hormones on lipolytic activity of the arterial wall.

While efforts to find a way to increase arterial lipolytic activity as a means of protecting the artery against accumulation of lipids produced only less than moderate results, several studies show adverse effects of some substances on vascular lipolytic or esterolytic activity. Some of them indicate, however, a possible link between lipolysis and atherogenesis. LEITES and CHOW-SU (1962, 1963) found that injection of noradrenaline (50 µg/100 gr. weight) to normal or adrenalectomized rats resulted in a significant fall in Tween-esterase activity. (This activity usually runs parallel with lipase activity in vascular tissue.) These investigators also observed a similar effect of "immobilization stress" on aortic esterolytic activity and they believe that this action is mediated through the sympathetic nervous system. In other experiments (LEITES, 1964, 1965a, b) it was demonstrated that alloxan diabetes and hypothyroidism are accompanied by a decrease in arterial lipolytic activity in rats and dogs. However, studies dealing with the direct effect of insulin, glucagon, or thyroid hormones have not been performed. According to PATELSKI and SZENDZIKOWSKI (1962), prolonged treatment with ACTH significantly reduces the aortic lipolytic activity in young male rats but not in older female rats. There are also indications that arterial lipoprotein lipase may be inhibited by nicotine by the formation of a nicotine-heparin complex (STEFANOVICH et al., 1969).

Summary

1. On the basis of data in Part I and II, a "favorable" drug effect on vascular metabolism should fulfill at least one of the following criteria: *decrease* permeability and activity of related lysosomal enzymes; *interfere* with synthesis of hydrophobic lipids, abnormal mucopolysaccharides or lactate; *enhance* synthesis of phospholipids; *increase* the activity of rate-limiting enzymatic steps in the Krebs cycle or mitochondrial electron transport system. Until now only a few drugs have been experimentally studied along these lines.

2. Bioflavonoids decrease tissue permeability. Furthermore the evidence assembled seems to indicate that some bioflavonoids decrease the activity of β-glucuroni-

dase, arylsulfatase and other lysosomal enzymes in venous and perhaps also arterial tissue. They increase cellular respiration, especially fatty acid oxidation, in arterial tissue and stimulate synthesis of phospholipids. Some bioflavonoids exert a protective action on arterial collagen.

3. It is claimed that pyridinolcarbamate increases the activity of the Krebs cycle enzyme malate dehydrogenase, of the glycolytic enzyme lactate dehydrogenase, and decreases the lysosomal acid phosphomonoesterase and carboxylic esterase. The effect on β-glucuronidase is controversial.

4. Estrogens stimulate the synthesis of arterial phospholipids, the opposite being true for testosterone. Estradiol causes a fall in some lysosomal arterial enzyme activity and a tendency toward an increase in malate dehydrogenase activity in male aortas. Sex differences in the enzyme activities of male and female arteries in man and animals also indicate the dependence of arterial metabolism on sex hormones. The difference in the arterial activity of "reduced NADP-producing" enzymes in males and females is of considerable interest. On the other hand, the effect of gonadectomy on arterial enzymes is a complex, controversial area, and no final conclusion can be made in this regard.

5. Vascular lipolytic activity has been studied primarily in regard to atherogenesis, and so far almost no attention has been paid to the effect of drugs on this property of vascular tissue. Heparin may increase arterial lipolysis, but very little data is available on this subject. In rats, polyunsaturated lecithin increases only serum and liver lipase activity without interfering with arterial lipase, phospholipase A, or cholesterol esterase activity. It is claimed that chlordiazepoxide elevates the lipolytic activity in normal and cholesterol-fed rabbits.

Concluding Remarks

The vascular wall is an organ with a distinctive metabolism associated with a particular form of nourishment and with specific functions in the transport and distribution of blood. The metabolic characteristics of this tissue, and particularly of its multifunctional smooth muscle cells (HAUST and MORE, 1963; CONSTANTINIDES, 1965; FRENCH, 1966; ZEMPLÉNYI, 1967; WISSLER, 1968; GETZ et al., 1969; SCOTT et al., 1970; GEER and HAUST, 1972) must be seriously considered in all studies of the pathogenesis, prevention, and treatment of vascular disease. For studying intermediary metabolism the artery is a difficult tissue to work with. This is why investigators interested in the pathogenesis and treatment of atherosclerosis preferred to pay attention to blood constituents most likely related to atherosclerosis, and metabolism of the artery remained a Cinderella of atherosclerosis research. The main purpose of this Chapter is to demonstrate that enough knowledge on arterial metabolism has been assembled to open the avenue for a rational prevention and treatment of vascular disease.

Acknowledgements

I wish to acknowledge the excellent assistance of Mrs. SYDNIE M. WASKEY, Mrs. MICHELLE T. WEST, and Mr. OTOKAR BREZINA in preparing the manuscript and illustrations of this chapter and Mrs. LEONA WEISS for "literary editing" of the manuscript. I would like to thank Dr. DAVID H. BLANKENHORN, Professor of Medicine for his continued interest in the topics contained in this chapter. I wish to record my gratitude to the editor of *Angiologica*, Professor L. LASZT, and the Karger Company for permission to reproduce Figs. 9, 11, and 12; to Lloyd-Luke-Medical Publishers, London, for permission to reproduce Fig. 6 and Table 1, and the American Heart Association and the editor of Circulation Research for permission to reproduce Fig. 2.

Abbreviations

ACP	Acid Phosphomonoesterase
ACON	Aconitase
ALD	Aldolase
AP	Alkaline phosphomonoesterase
APP	Adenosine-5′-triphosphatase
BIOT	Biotine
CAR	Carnitine
CARB. EST.	Carboxylic esterase
CARNAT	Carnitine acetyltransferase
CAT	Cathepsin
C-c-R	Cytochrome c reductase
CEST	Carboxylesterase
CoA	Coenzyme A
CPK	Creatine phosphokinase
CS	Citrate synthase
DIA	Diaphorase
ENOL	Enolase
F-6-PK	Fructose-6-phosphate kinase
FUM	Fumarase
GAPDH	Glyceraldehyde-3-phosphate dehydrogenase
GLUR	Glutathione reductase
G-6-PDH	Glucose-6-phosphate dehydrogenase
GPRL	Glycogen phosphorylase
3-HBDH	3-Hydroxybutyrate dehydrogenase
HK	Hexokinase
HOADH	3-Hydroxyacyl-CoA-dehydrogenase
HPAT	Hexose phosphate aminotransferase
ICDH	Isocitrate dehydrogenase
LDH	Lactate dehydrogenase
MDH	Malate dehydrogenase
ME	Malic enzyme

6-PGDH   6-Phosphogluconic dehydrogenase
PGI   Phosphoglucose isomerase
PGK   3-Phosphoglycerate kinase
PGluM   Phosphoglucomutase
PGM   Phosphoglycerate mutase
PK   Pyruvate kinase
PMI   Phosphomannose isomerase
PNP   Purine nucleoside phosphorylase

RIBOSE-5-PI   Ribose-5-phosphate isomerase

TIM   Triose phosphate isomerase
TRA   Transaldolase
TRK   Transketolase

References

ABDULLA, Y. H., ORTON, C. C., ADAMS, C. W. M.: Cholesterol esterification by transacylation in human and experimental atheromatous lesions. J. Atheroscler. Res. **8**, 967 (1968).

ABDULLA, Y. H., ADAMS, C. W. M., BAYLISS, O. B.: The location of lecithin-cholesterol transacylase activity in the atherosclerotic arterial wall. J. Atheroscler. Res. **10**, 229 (1969).

ADAMS, C. W. M.: Arteriosclerosis in man, other mammals and birds. Biol. Rev. **39**, 372 (1964).

ADAMS, C. W. M.: Vascular histochemistry. London: Lloyd-Luke 1967.

ADAMS, C. W. M., BAYLISS, O. B.: Phospholipids in atherosclerosis: The modification of the cholesterol granuloma by phospholipid. J. path. Bact. **86**, 431 (1963).

ADAMS, C. W. M., MORGAN, R. S.: Autoradiographic demonstration of cholesterol filtration and accumulation in atheromatous rabbit aorta. Nature (Lond.) **210**, 175 (1966).

ADAMS, C. W. M., ABDULLA, Y. H., MAHLER, R. F., ROOT, M. A.: Lipase, esterase and triglyceride in the ageing human aorta. J. Atheroscler. Res. **9**, 87 (1969).

AIZAWA, Y., MUELLER, G. C.: The effect *in vivo* and *in vitro* of estrogens on lipid synthesis in the rat uterus. J. biol. Chem. **236**, 381 (1961).

ASMUSSEN, E., KNUDSEN, E. O. E.: Studies in acute but moderate CO poisoning. Acta physiol. scand. **6**, 67 (1943).

ASTRUP, PL., KJELDSEN, K., WANSTRUP, J.: Enhancing influence of carbon monoxide on the development of atheromatosis in cholesterol-fed rabbits. J. Atheroscler. Res. **7**, 343 (1967).

BANGA, I., BALÓ, I.: Elastomucoproteinase and collagen-mucoproteinase, the mucolytic enzymes of the pancreas. Nature (Lond.) **178**, 310 (1965).

BEACONSFIELD, P.: Metabolism of the normal cardiovascular wall. 2. The pentose phosphate pathway. Experientia (Basel) **18**, 276 (1962).

BERENSON, G. S., SRINIVASAN, S. R., DOLAN, P. F., RADHAKRISHNAMURT, B.: Lipoprotein-acid mucopolysaccharide complexes from fatty streaks of human aorta. Circulation **43**, Suppl. II, 20 (1971).

BICKOFF, E. M., SPENCER, R. R., KNUCKLES, B. E., LUNDIN, R. E.: 3'-Methoxycoumestrol from alfalfa: isolation and caracterization. Agricult. Food Chem. **14**, 444 (1966).

BIHARI-VARGA, M., SIMON, J., GERÖ, S.: Identification of glycosaminoglycan-beta lipoprotein complexes in the atherosclerotic aorta intima by thermoanalytical methods. Acta Biochem. Biophys. Acad. Sci. Hung. **3**, 365 (1968).

BÖHM, K.: The flavonoids. A review of their physiology, pharmacodynamics and therapeutic uses. Aulendorf/Württ.: Cantor KG. 1968.

BÖTTCHER, C. J. F.: Phospholipids of atherosclerotic lesions in the human aorta. In: Evolution of the atherosclerotic plaque. Chicago: University of Chicago Press 1963.

BÖTTCHER, C. J. F., KLYNSTRA, F. B.: Acid mucopolysaccharides in human aortic tissue. Their distribution at different stages of atherosclerosis. **7**, 301 (1967).

BÖTTCHER, C. J. F., VAN GENT, C. M.: Changes in the composition of phospholipid fatty acids associated with altherosclerosis in the human aortic wall. J. Atheroscler. Res. **1**, 36 (1961).

BRANWOOD, A. W., CARR, J. A.: β-Glucuronidase activity of coronary atherosclerotic plaques. Lancet **1960** II, 1254.

BUDDECKE, E., KRESSE, H.: Mucopolysaccharide und Enzyme des Mucopolysaccharidstoffwechsels im Arterien- und Venengewebe. Angiologica **6**, 89 (1969).

BURSTEIN, M., SAMAILLE, J.: Sur un dosage rapide du cholesterol lie aux α- et β-lipoproteines du serum. Clin. chim. Acta **5**, 609 (1960).

CANEGHEM-VAN, V. P.: Influence of some hydrosoluble substances with vitamin B activity on the fragility of lysosomes *in vitro*. Biochem. Pharmacol. **21**, 1543 (1972).

CARPENEDO, F., BORTIGNON, C., BRUNI, A., SANTI, R.: Effect of quercetin on membrane-linked activities. Biochem. Pharmacol. **18**, 1495 (1969).

CAVALLERO, C., TUROLLA, E.: Istochimica enzimatica delle arterie in rapporto con l'aterosclerosi. Giorn. Gerontol. Suppl. **20**, 25 (1960).

CETTA, G., GERZELI, G., QUARTIERI, A., CASTELLANI, A. A.: Protective effect of flavonoids on the collagen of lathyritic rats. Experientia (Basel) **27**, 1046 (1971).

CETTA, G., GERZELI, G., CASTELLANI, A. A.: Effect des flavonoïdes sur le collagène dans le lathyrisme. Paper read at IV th International Angiologic Symposium, Nyon, Switzerland, September 4—6, 1972. Angiologica **9**, 235 (1972).

CHANCE, B., HOLLUNGER, G.: The interaction of energy and electron transfer reactions in mitochondria. J. biol. Chem. **236**, 1534 (1961).

CHATTOPADHYAY, D. P.: Influence of experimental atherosclerosis in rabbits on the rate of respiration and glycolysis by aortic tissue slices. Ann. Biochem. exp. Med. **22**, 77 (1962).

CHERNICK, S., SRERE, P. A., CHAIKOFF, I. L.: The metabolism of arterial tissue. II Lipid Synthesis: The formation *in vitro* of fatty acids and phospholipids by rat artery with ^{14}C and ^{32}P as indicators. J. biol. Chem. **179**, 113 (1949).

CHISOLM, G. M., GAINER, J., STONER, G. E., GAINER, J. V., JR.: Plasma proteins, oxygen transport and atherosclerosis. Atherosclerosis **15**, 327 (1972).

CHOBANIAN, A. V.: Sterol metabolism in the human arterial intima. Fed. Proc. **26**, 262 (1967).

CHOBANIAN, A. V.: Sterol synthesis in the human arterial intima. J. clin. Invest. **47**, 595 (1968 a).

CHOBANIAN, A. V.: Effects of sex hormones on phospholipid, RNA, and protein metabolism in the arterial intima. J. Atheroscler. Res. **8**, 763 (1968 b).

CHOBANIAN, A. V., HOLLANDER, W.: Phospholipid synthesis in the human arterial intima. J. clin. Invest. **45**, 932 (1966).

CHOBANIAN, A. V., BRECHER, P. I., LILLE, R. D., WOTIZ, H. H.: Metabolism of sex hormones in the aortic wall. J. Lipid Res. **9**, 701 (1968).

CHRISTENSEN, S.: Transfer of plasma phospholipid across the aortic intimal surface of cholesterol-fed cockerels. J. Atheroscler. Res. **2**, 131 (1962).

CHRISTENSEN, S.: Transfer with labeled cholesterol across the aortic intimal surface of normal and cholesterol-fed cockerels. J. Atheroscler. Res. **4**, 151 (1964).

CHVAPIL, M.: Physiology of connective tissue. London: Butterworths; Prague: Czechoslovak Medical Press 1967.

CHVAPIL, M.: Personal communication.

CITTERIO, C., CUNEGO, A.: Determinazione del principio elastolitico nelle arterie cerebrali umani. Giorn. Gerontol. **13**, 353 (1965).

CLEMENTS, R. S., JR., MORRISON, A. D., WINEGRAD, A. I.: Polyol pathway in aorta: regulation by hormones. Science **166**, 1007 (1969).

COMSTOCK, J. P., UDENFRIEND, S.: Effect of lactate on collagen proline hydroxylase activity in cultured L-929 fibroblasts. Proc. nat. Acad. Sci. (Wash.) **66**, 552 (1970).

CONSTANTINIDES, P.: Experimental atherosclerosis. Amsterdam: Elsevier 1965.

COOKSON, F. B., ALTSCHUL, R., FEDOROFF, S.: The effects of alfalfa on serum cholesterol and in modifying or preventing cholesterol-induced atherosclerosis in rabbits. J. Atheroscler. Res. **7**, 69 (1967).

CROCKETT, R., DALLOCCHIO, M., RAZAKA, G., BRICAUD, H., BROUSTET, P.: Etude biologique du serum chez le lapin au cours de l'immunisation par antigène aortique. In: Le Rôle De La Paroi Arterielle Dans L'Athérogenèse, p. 463. Paris: Center National De La Recherche Scientifique. 1968.

Cuparencu, B., Tisca, I., Safta, L., Rosenberg, A., Mocan, R., Brief, G. H.: Influence of some psychotropic drugs on the development of experimental atherosclerosis. Cor Vasa **11**, 112 (1969).

Cuparencu, B., Mocan, R., Safta, L.: The influence of chlordiazepoxide on the plasma lipoprotein lipase activity and on the lipolytic activity of the aorta in normal and cholesterol fed rabbits. Cor Vasa **12**, 248 (1970).

Dalferes, E. R., Jr., Ruiz, H., Kumar, B., Radhakrishnamurthy, B., Berenson, G. S.: Acid mucopolysaccharides of fatty streaks in young, human male aortas. Atherosclerosis **13**, 121 (1971).

Daly, M. M.: Effects of hypertension on the lipid composition of rat aortic intima-media. Circulation Res. **31**, 410 (1972).

Dawson, D. M., Goodfriend, T. L., Kaplan, N. O.: Lactic dehydrogenases: functions of the two types. Science **143**, 929 (1964).

Day, A. J., Gold-Hurst, P. R. S.: Cholesterol esterase activity of normal and atherosclerotic rabbit aorta. Biochem. biophys. Acta. **116**, 169 (1966).

Day, A. J., Wahlqvist, M. L.: Localization by autoradiography of phospholipid synthesis in rabbit atherosclerotic aorta. Exp. Mol. Path. **11**, 263 (1969).

Day, A. J., Wilkinson, G. K.: Incorporation of ^{14}C-labeled acetate into lipid by isolated foam cells and by atherosclerotic arterial intima. Circulation Res. **21**, 593 (1967).

Day, A. J., Newman, H. A. I., Zilversmit, D. B.: Synthesis of phospholipid by foam cells isolated from rabbit atherosclerotic lesions. Circulation Res. **19**, 122 (1966).

Dayton, S., Hashimoto, S.: Recent advances in molecular pathology: A review: Cholesterol flux and metabolism in arterial tissue and in atheromata. Exp. Mol. Path. **13**, 253 (1970).

Dayton, S., Hashimoto, S.: Origin of cholesteryl oleate and other esterified lipids of rabbit atheroma. Atherosclerosis **12**, 371 (1970).

Deduve, C., Wattiaux, R.: Function of lysosomes. Ann. Rev. Physiol. **28**, 435 (1966).

De Oliveira, J. M.: The effects of pyridinolcarbamate on experimental arteriosclerosis. In: Shimamoto, T., Numano, F. (Eds.): Atherogenesis. Tokyo: Excerpta Medica Foundation 1969.

Dixon, K. C.: Fatty deposition: A disorder of the cell. Quart. J. exp. Physiol. **43**, 139 (1958).

Dunnigan, M. G.: The distrubution of phospholipid within macrophages in human atheromatous plaques. J. Atheroscler. Res. **4**, 144 (1964).

Dury, A.: Lipolytic activity of aorta of young and old rats and influence of heparin *in vivo*. J. Gerontol. **16**, 114 (1961).

Dyrbye, M., Kirk, J. E.: The beta-glucuronidase activity of aortic and pulmonary artery tissue in individuals of various ages. J. Geront. **11**, 33 (1956).

Eisenberg, S., Stein, Y., Stein, O.: Phospholipases in arterial tissue. II Phosphotide acyl-hydrolase and lysophosphatide acylhydrolase activity in human and rat arteries. Biochim. biophys. Acta (Amst.) **164**, 205 (1968).

Eisenberg, S., Stein, Y., Stein, O.: Phospholipases in arterial tissue. III. Phosphatide acyl-hydrolase, lysophosphatide acyl-hydrolase and sphingomyelin choline phospohydrolase in rat and rabbit aorta in different age groups. Biochem. biophys. Acta **176**, 557 (1969).

Eisenberg, S., Stein, Y., Stein, O.: Phospholipases in arterial tissue. IV. The role of phosphatide acyl hydrolase, lysophosphatide acyl hydrolase, and sphingomyelin choline phosphohydrolase in the regulation of phospholipid composition in the normal human aorta with age. J. clin. Invest. **48**, 2320 (1969b).

Ernster, L., Lee, C. P.: Energy-linked pyridine nucleotide transhydrogenase. Ann. Rev. Biochem. **33**, 738 (1964).

Felt, V.: The effect of pressure changes on esterification of cholesterol and hydrolysis of cholesterol esters in rat aorta and serum. Experientia (Basel) **27**, 1412 (1971).

Felt, V., Beneš, P.: The incorporation of $[4 - ^{14}C]$ cholesterol into different cholesterol esters of rat aorta *in vitro*. Biochim. biophys. Acta (Amst.) **176**, 435 (1969).

Felt, V., Beneš, P.: Cholesterolesterase (veresternde und hydrolysierende) im Blutserum, in der Leber, den Nieren und Aorten bei Entwicklung der Kaninchen-Atherosklerose. Enzym. biol. clin. **11**, 511 (1970).

Field, H., Swell, L., Schools, P. E., Treadwell, C. R.: Dynamic aspects of cholesterol metabolism in different areas of the aorta and other tissues of men and their relationship to atherosclerosis. Circulation **22**, 547 (1960).

FILIPOVIC, I., BUDDECKE, E.: Increased fatty acid synthesis of arterial tissue in hypoxia. Europ. J. Biochem. **20**, 587 (1971).

FILIPOVIC, I., FIGURA, K. V., BUDDECKE, E.: Studies of the (+)-catechin action on the metabolism of bovine arterial tissue. Paper read at IVth International Angiologic Symposium, Nyon, Switzerland, September 4–6, 1972. Angiologica **9**, 204 (1972).

FRENCH, J. E.: Atherosclerosis in relation to the structure and function of the arterial intima. Int. Rev. exp. Pathol. **5**, 253 (1966).

FRIEDMAN, M., BYERS, S. O., ROSENMAN, R. H.: Resolution of aortic atherosclerosis infiltration in rabbit by phosphatide infusion. Proc. Soc. exp. Biol. (N. Y.) **95**, 586 (1957).

FRITH, C. H., ALEXANDER, A. F., WILL, D. H.: Influence of hypoxia on arterial enzymes. Fed. Proc. **30**, 481 (1971).

FULLER, G. C., LANGER, R. O.: Elevation of aortic proline hydroxylase: A biochemical defect in experimental arteriosclerosis. Science **168**, 987 (1970).

FULLER, G. C., MILLER, E., FARBER, T. M., VANLOON, E. J.: Elevation of aortic proline hydroxylase in miniature pigs fed a lipid-rich diet. Fed. Proc. **30**, 370 (1971).

GÁBOR, M.: The anti-inflammatory action of flavonoids. Budapest: Akademia Kiado 1972.

GAJDOS, A., GAJDOS-TOROK, M., HORN, R.: Augmentation du taux hepatique de l'ATP chez le Rat blanc par administration de (+)-catechine. C. R. Soc. Biol. **163**, 2089 (1969).

GASPAR-GODFROID, A.: Influence de differents agents denaturants et de la digestion tryptique sur l'activite adenosinetriphosphatasique de la myosine de carotide de bovide. Angiologica **7**, 273 (1970).

GEER, J. C., HAUST, M. D.: Smooth muscle cells in atherosclerosis. In: Monographs on Atherosclerosis. Vol. 2. Switzerland: S. Karger 1972.

GERÖ, S.: Investigations on the role of vascular mucopolysaccarides in the mechanism of lipid deposition. Zool. Soc. London Symp. **11**, 169 (1964).

GERÖ, S., GERGELY, J., DÉVÉNYI, T., VIRÁG, S., SZÉKELY, J., JAKOB, L.: Inhibitory effect of some mucopolysaccharides on the lipolytic activity of the aorta of animals. Nature (Lond.) **194**, 1181 (1962).

GERÖ, S., BIHARI-VARGA, M., VIRÁG, S., VÉGH, M.: Investigations on the role of mucopolysaccharides in atherosclerosis. In: Le Role De La Paroi Arterielle Dans L'Atherogenese, p. 789. Paris: Center National De La Recherche Scientifique 1968.

GETZ, G. S., VESSELINOVITCH, D., WISSLER, R. W.: A dynamic pathology of atherosclerosis. Amer. J. Med. **46**, 657 (1969).

GORE, I., LARKEY, B. J.: Functional activity of aortic mucopolysaccharides. J. Lab. clin. Med. **56**, 839 (1960).

GOULD, R. G., JONES, R. J., WISSLER, R. W.: Lability of labeled cholesterol in human atherosclerotic plaques. Circulation **20**, 967 (1959).

GRAFNETTER, D., ZEMPLÉNYI, T.: Vergleich der Eigenschaften von Gewebseigenen lipolytischen Enzymen und des »Klärungsfaktors« bei der Inkubation mit lipämischen Serum. Z. Physiol. Chem. **316**, 218 (1959).

GRAFNETTER, D., ZEMPLÉNYI, T.: Tissue lipolytic activity in calciferol intoxicated rats. Experientia (Basel) **18**, 85 (1962).

HADJIISKY, P., RENAIS, J., SCEBAT, L.: Histochimie et histoenzymologie de l'aorte de gallus gallus, jeunes et adultes. Comparaison avec conturnix conturnix. I. Metabolisme glucidique et energetique. Arch. Mal. Coeur, **63**, Suppl. 1, 40 (1970a).

HADJIISKY, P., RANAIS, J., SCEBAT, L.: Histochimie et histoenzymologie de l'aorte de gallus gallus, jeunes et adultes. Comparaison avec conturnix conturnix. II. Metabolisme lipidique et protidique. Arch. Mal. Coeur **63**, Suppl. 1, 53 (1970b).

HAHN, P. F.: Abolishment of alimentary lipemia following injection of heparin. Science **98**, 19 (1943).

HAIMOVICI, H., MAIER, H.: Fate of aortic homografts in canine atherosclerosis. Arch. Surgery **89**, 961 (1964).

HAIMOVICI, H., MAIER, N., STRAUSS, L.: Fate of aortic homografts in experimental canine atherosclerosis. Study of fresh thoracic implant into abdominal aorta. Arch. Surg. **76**, 282 (1958).

HAIMOVICI, H., MAIER, N., STRAUSS, L.: Role of arterial tissue susceptibility in experimental canine atherosclerosis. J. Atheroscler. Res. **6**, 62 (1966).

HALBORG,-SØRENSEN,A., HANSEN,A.: Chronic venous insufficiency treated with hydroxyethyl-rutosides (HR). Angiologia **7**, 192 (1970).

HALL,D.A.: The characterization of a new lipolytic enzyme in pancreatic extracts. Biochem. J. **78**, 491 (1961).

HALL,D.A.: Elastolysis and Aging. Springfield: Thomas 1964.

HALL,D.A., CZERKAWSKI,J.W.: The reaction between elastase and elastic tissue. 6. The mechanism of elastolysis. Biochem. J. **80**, 134 (1961).

HAMOIR,G., GASPAR-GODFROID,A., LASZT,L.: Changements d'etat d'agregation et de dissociation de la tonoactomyosine de carotides de bovide sous l'influence de la force ionique et de l'ATP. Angiologica **2**, 44 (1965).

HARRIS,E.D., O'DELL,B.L.: Comparison of soluble and particulate amine oxidases from bovine aorta. Biochem. Biophys. Res. Commun. **48**, 1173 (1972).

HARUKI,F., KIRK,J.E.: Hexosamine-synthesizing enzyme in human arterial tissue. Proc. Soc. exp. Biol. (N.Y.) **118**, 479 (1965).

HAUST,M.D., MORE,R.H.: Significance of the smooth muscle cell in atherogenesis. In: Evolution of the atherosclerotic plaque, p. 51. Chicago: Chicago University Press 1963.

HAVEL,R.J.: Transport and metabolism of chylomiera. Amer. J. clin. Nutr. **6**, 662 (1958).

HAYASE,K., MILLER,B.F.: Lipase activity in the human aorta. J. Lipid Res. **11**, 209 (1970).

HAYASE,K., REISHER,S., MILLER,F.B.: Partial purification and properties on N-acetyl-β-D-glucosaminidase from human human aortic wall. Fed. Proc. **30**, 481 (1971a).

HAYASE,K., REISHER,S.R., MILLER,B.F.: Evidence suggesting presence of at lease two forms of N-acetyl-B-D Hexosaminidase in human aorta. Circulation **44**, 17 (1971b).

HELD,E., BUDDECKE,E.: Nachweis, Reinigung und Eigenschaften einer Chondroitin-4-Sulfatase aus der Aorta des Rindes. Z. physiol. Chem. **348**, 1047 (1967).

HELD,E., HOEFELE,O., REICH,G., STEIN,U., WERRIER,E., BUDDECKE,E.: Wirtungssynergismus Chondroitin-4-Sulfat-protein abbauender Enzyme des Arteriengewebes. Z. Klin. Chem. Klin. Biochem. **6**, 244 (1968).

HELIN,P., LORENZEN,I.: Arteriosclerosis in rabbit aorta induced by systemic hypoxia; Biochemical and morphological studies. Angiology **20**, 1 (1969).

HELIN,P., LORENZEN,I., CARBASCH,C., MATTHIESSEN,M.E.: Arteriosclerosis and hypoxia, Part 2 (Biochemical changes in mucopolysaccharides and collagen or rabbit aorta induced by systemic hypoxia.) J. Atheroscler. Res. **9**, 295 (1969).

HELIN,G., HELIN,P., LORENZEN,I.: The aortic glycosaminoglycans in arteriosclerosis induced by systemic hypoxia. Atherosclerosis **12**, 235 (1970).

HOFF,H.F.: A histoenzymatic study of human intracranial atherosclerosis. Amer. J. Path. **67**, 583 (1972).

HORN,R., VONDERMUHLL,M., COMTE,M., GRANDROQUES,C.: Action de quelques catechines sur l'activité d'un enzyme (la cytochromeoxydase) de la chaine respiratoire. Experienta (Basel) **26**, 1081 (1970).

HORŇÁČEK,J., TRČKA,V., VEJDĚLEK,Z.: The effect of alfalfa extracts on experimental rabbit atherosclerosis. (In Czech.) Cs. fysiol. **15**, 33 (1966).

HOSODA,S., KIRK,J.E.: Vitamin B_{12} content of human vascular tissue in individuals of various ages. J. Gerontol. **24**, 298 (1969).

HOWARD,A.N.: Recent advances in nutrition and atherosclerosis. In: JONES,R.J. (Ed.): Atherosclerosis: Proceedings of the Second International Symposium. New York-Heidelberg-Berlin: Springer 1970.

HOWARD,C.F.,JR.: Lipogenesis from $[2-^{14}C]$ glucose and $[1-^{14}C]$ acetate in aorta. J. Lipid Res. **12**, 725 (1971).

HOWARD,C.F.,JR.: Aortic lipogenesis during aerobic and hypoxic incubation. Atherosclerosis **15**, 359 (1972).

HOWARD,C.F., PORTMAN,O.W.: Hydrolysis of cholesteryl linoleate by a high speed supernate preparation of rat and monkey aorta. Biochim. biophys. Acta (Amst.) **125**, 623 (1966).

HULL,F.E., WHEREAT,A.F.: The effect of rotenone on the regulation of fatty acid synthesis in heart mitochondria. J. biol. chem. **242**, 4023 (1967).

ITO,T.: Tocopherol, non-protein SH and metals in the human aorta. Jap. Circul. J. **33**, 25 (1969).

JANAKIDEVI,K.: Isolation and purification of aortic nuclei and characterization of the nuclear enzymes. Fed. Proc. **30**, 482 (1971).

JELINKOVÁ, M., STUCHLIKOVÁ, E., HRŮZA, Z., DEYL, Z., SMRŽ, M.: Hormonesensitive lipolytic activity of the aorta of different age groups of rats. Exp. Geront. **7**, 263 (1972).

JANDA, J., MRHOVÁ, O., URBANOVÁ, D.: Aortic thermal lesion. Cor Vasa **14**, 71 (1972).

KAGAN, H. M., FRANZBLAU, C.: Lysyl oxidase of chick aorta. Circulation **44**, No. 2, II–18 (1971).

KALRA, V. K., BRODIE, A. F.: α-Glycerol phosphate shuttle and energy-linked transhydrogenase in aortic mitochondria. Biochim. Biophys. Res. Commun. **51**, 414 (1973).

KATO, L., GOZSY, B.: Effets vasculaires des bioflavonoides chez le rat. Bordeaux Med. **No. 2**, 438 (1970).

KHEIM, T. F., KIRK, J. E.: Para-aminobenzoic acid and folic acid contents of human vascular tissue. J. Lab. clin. Med. **11**, 850 (1970).

KHEIM, T., KIRK, J. E.: Thiamine content of human arterial and venous tissue. Fed. Proc. **28**, 866 (1969).

KIRK, J. E.: Comparison of enzyme activities of arterial samples from sexually mature men and women. Clin. Chem. **10**, 184 (1964).

KIRK, J. E.: Aging in enzyme activities of human arterial tissue. In : SHOCK, N. W. (Ed.): Perspectives in experimental gerontology, p. 182. Springfield: Thomas 1966.

KIRK, J. E.: Enzymes of the arterial wall. New York-London: Academic Press 1969.

KIRK, J. E.: Free carnitine content and carnitine acetyltransferase activity of human vascular tissue. J. Lab. clin. Med. **11**, 892 (1969).

KIRK, J. E., RITZ, E.: The glyceraldehyde-3-phosphate and α-glycerophosphate dehydrogenase activities of arterial tissue in individuals of various ages. J. Gerontol. **22**, 427 (1967).

KIRK, J. E., EFFERSOE, P. G., CHIANG, S. P.: The rate of respiration and glycolysis by human and dog aortic tissue. J. Geront. **9**, 10 (1954).

KITTINGER, G. W., WEXLER, B. C., MILLER, B. F.: Enzymatic activities in aortas of normal and arteriosclerotic rats. In: PRUSIK, B., REINIS, Z., RIEDEL, O. (Eds.): Metabolismus Parietis Vasorum. Prague: State Medical Publ. House 1962.

KJELDSEN, K., WANSTRUP, J., ASTRUP, P.: Enhancing influence of arterial hypoxia on the development of atheromatosis in cholesterol-fed rabbits. J. Atheroscler. Res. **8**, 835 (1968).

KJELDSEN, K., ASTRUP, P., WANSTRUP, J.: Reversal of rabbit atheromatosis by hyperoxia. J. Atheroscler. Res. **10**, 173 (1969).

KJELDSEN, K., ASTRUP, P., WANSTRUP, J.: Ultrastructural intimal changes in the rabbit aorta after a moderate carbon monoxide exposure. Atherosclerosis **16**, 76 (1972).

KLIMEŠOVÁ, A., HEYROVSKY, A.: A note on the actomyosin content of the anterial wall. Atherosclerosis **11**, 27 (1970).

KORN, E. D.: Clearing factor, a heparin-activated lipoprotein lipase. I. Isolation and characterization of the enzyme from normal rat heart. J. biol. Chem. **215**, 1 (1955).

KORN, E. D.: In: PAGE, I. H. (Ed.): Chemistry of lipids as related to atherosclerosis, p. 169. A symposium. Springfield: C. C. Thomas 1958.

KOTHARI, H., MILLER, B. F., KRITCHEVSKY, D.: Properties of cholesterol ester hydrolase of rat and rabbit aorta. Circulation **43** and **44**, Suppl. II, II—5 (1971).

KOTHARI, H. V., MILLER, B. F., KRITCHEVSKY, D.: Aortic cholesterol esterase: Characteristics of normal rat and rabbit enzyme. Biochim. biophys. Acta (Amst.) **296**, 446 (1972).

KRESSE, H., BUDDECKE, E.: Veränderungen in der Aktivität Chondroitinsulfat-Protein abbauender Enzyme (Glykosaminoglykanohydrolasen und Peptidhydrolasen) des Arteriengewebes im Alter und bei Arteriosklerose. Z. klin. Chem. Klin. Biochem. **6**, 251 (1968).

KRESSE, H., WESSELS, G.: Methodische Untersuchungen zum In-Vitro-Stoffwechsel von Rinderarteriengewebe. Z. physiol. Chem. **350**, 1605 (1969).

KRESSE, H., FILIPOVIC, I., BUDDECKE, E.: Gesteigerte ^{14}C-Inkorporation in die Triacylglycerine (Triglyceride) des Arteriengewebes bei Sauerstoffmangel. Z. physiol. Chem. **350**, 1611 (1969).

KRESSE, H., FILIPOVIC, I., ISERLOH, A., BUDDECKE, E.: Comparative studies on the chemistry and the metabolism of arterial and venous tissue. Angiologica **7**, 321 (1970).

KRITCHEVSKY, S.: Cholesterol Metabolism in aorta and in tissue culture. Lipids **7**, 305 (1972).

KRČÍLEK, A., JANOUŠEK, V., ŠERÁK, L.: Respiratory activity of the vascular wall in experimental atherosclerosis measured by the polarographic method. In: PRUSIK, B., REINIS, Z., RIEDL, O. (Eds.): Metabolismus Parietis Vasorum. Prague: State Medical Publ. House 1962.

Krompecher, I.: Hypoxibiose und Mukopolysaccharide-Bildung in der Differenzierung und Pathologie der Gewebe sowie über den Zusammenhang zwischen Schilddrüsenfunktion und Mukopolysacchariden. Leipzig: Barth 1960.

Kumar, V., Berenson, G. S., Ruiz, H., Dalferes, E. R., Jr., Strong, T. P.: Acid mucopolysaccharides of human aorta. Part 2 (Variation with atherosclerotic involvement) J. Atheroscler. Res. 7, 583 (1967).

Kupke, I. R.: Biosynthesis of lipids in perfused dog aorta and coronary artery. I. Incorporation of $[2\text{-}^{14}C]$ acetate into the lipids of three aortic layers and of the coronary artery in normal and hyperlipemic dogs. J. Mol. Cell Cardiol. 4, 11 (1972a).

Kupke, I. R.: Biosynthesis of lipids in perfused dog aorta and coronary artery. II. Incorporation of $2\text{-}^{14}C$ Acetate into lipids of two aortic layers and of the coronary artery under the influence of nicotine. J. Mol. Cell. Cardiol. 4, 27 (1972b).

Kupke, I. R.: Biosynthesis of lipids in perfused dog aorta and coronary artery. III. Incorporation of $2\text{-}^{14}C$ Acetate into sterols and uptake of ^{3}H-cholesterol in three aortic layers and in coronary artery of normal and hyperlipemic dogs and under the influence of nicotine. J. Mol. Cell. Cardiol. 4, 255 (1972c).

Lacuara, J. L., Gerschenson, L., Moguilevsky, H. C., Malinow, M. R.: Sexual differences in the esterase activity of the aorta in rats. J. Atheroscler. Res. 3, 496 (1962).

Laszt, L.: Zur Biochemie der Venenwand. In: Die Venose Insuffizienz. Pathophysiologie, Klinik und Therapie. Herausgegeben von K. W. Schneider, p. 9. Baden-Baden-Brüssel: Gerhard Witzstrock 1972a.

Laszt, L.: Bases experimentales pour une pharmacologie des flavonoides. Paper read at IVth International Angiologic Symposium, Nyon, Switzerland, September 4—6, 1972b. Angiologica 9, 193 (1972).

Lazzarini-Robertson, A.: Respiration of human arterial intima and atherogenesis. Fed. Proc. 21, 101 (1962).

Leites, F. L.: Topography of lipolytic enzymes in various stages of evolution of the atherosclerotic plaques. (Russian) Dokl. Akad. Nauk. SSSR. 165(5), 1175 (1965a).

Leites, F. L.: Histochemical peculiarities of lipid metabolism and activity of lipolytic enzymes in alloxan diabetes. (Russian) Probl. Endokrinol. Gormonoterap. 11(3), 88 (1965b).

Leites, F. L., Golosvskaya, M. A.: Distribution of lipolytic enzymes in connection with age in man. (Russian) Arkh. Anat. Gistol. Embriol. 51(7), 61 (1966).

Leites, F. L., Fuks, B. B.: Mechanism of increasing the activity of lipolytic enzymes after introduction of lipids into tissues. (Russian) Byul. Exp. Biol. Med. 61(5), 46 (1966).

Leites, F. L., Lempert, B. L.: The histochemistry of lipoprotein lipase in the normal organism and in atherosclerosis. Cor et Vasa 10, 120 (1968).

Leites, S. M.: Lipolytic activity of organs and tissue in experimental alloxan diabetes. (Russian) Abhandl. dtsch. Akad. Wiss., Berlin, Kl. Med. 263, 267 (1964).

Leites, S. M., Chow-Su: On some features of lipid metabolism in stress. Vopr Med. Khim. 8, 289 (1962).

Leites, S. M., Chow-Su: Role of the sympathetic nervous system in mobilization of fats in a state of stress. (Russian) Kortikovisc. Vzaimootn. i Gorm. Regulatzia (Kharkov) 164 (1963).

Lempert, B. L., Leites, F. L.: The role of reduction of lipolytic activity of the wall of the aorta in the pathogenesis of its lipid infiltration. (Russian) Byul. Experim. Biol. Med. 56(10), 25 (1963).

Lillie, R. D., Chobanian, A. V.: Pathways of glucose metabolism in human and canine arteries. J. clin. Invest. 48, 52a (1968).

Lindy, S., Turto, H., Uitto, J., Helin, P., Lorenzen, I.: Injury and repair in arterial tissue in the rabbit. Circulation Res. 30, 123 (1972).

Litwack, G., Kritchevsky, D.: Actions of hormones on molecular process. New York: J. Wiley & Sons 1964.

Loeven, W. A.: Lypolytic activities of a partially purified enzyme of the elastase complex. Acta Physiol. Pharm. Neerl. 14, 475 (1967).

Loeven, W. A.: The effect of elastoproteinase on experimental atheromatosis in rabbits. Europ. J. Pharmacol. 1, 254 (1967).

Loeven, W. A.: Elastolytic enzymes in the vessel wall. J. Atheroscler. Res. 9, 35 (1969).

Lofland, H. B., Jr., Clarkson, T. B.: Certain metabolic patterns of atheromatous pigeon aortas. Arch. Path. 80, 291 (1965).

LOFLAND, H. B., ST. CLAIR, R. W., CLARKSON, T. B., BULLOCK, B. C., LEHNER, D. M.: Atherosclerosis in cebus monkeys. II. Arterial metabolism. Exp. Mol. Path. **9**, 57 (1968).

LOFLAND, H. B., JR., MOURY, D. M., HOFFMAN, C. W., CLARKSON, T. B.: Lipid metabolism in pigeon aorta during atherogenesis. J. Lipid. Res. **6**, 112 (1965).

LOJDA, Z.: Azocoupling reactions in histochemical detection of enzymes. Prague: State Medical Publ. House 1958.

LOJDA, Z.: Topochemistry of enzymes in the vascular wall. In: Metabolismus Parietis Vasorum, PRUSÍK, B., REINIŠ, K., RIEDL, O. (Eds.) Prague: State Medical Publ. House 1962, p. 232.

LOJDA, Z.: Histochemistry of the vascular wall. International Symposium, Morphology Histochemistry Vascular Wall, COMEL, M., LASZT, L. (Eds.), p. 364. Basel-New York: Karger 1966.

LOJDA, Z., FRIČ, P.: Lactic Dehydrogenase Isoenzymes in the aortic wall. J. Atheroscler. Res. **6**, 264 (1966).

LOJDA, Z., ZEMPLÉNYI, T.: Histochemistry of some enzymes of the vascular wall in experimental rabbit atheromatosis. J. Atheroscler. Res. **1**, 101 (1961).

LOOMEIYER, F. J., OSTENDORF, J. P.: Oxygen consumption of thoracic aorta of normal and hypercholesterolemic rats. Circulation Res. **7**, 466 (1959).

LORENZEN, I., HEADINGS, V.: Vascular connective tissue under the influence of estrogens. Part 2 (Reaction of the aortic wall to noradrenaline-induced injury in female and male rabbits). Acta endocr. (KbH.) **53**, 250 (1966).

MAIER, N., HAIMOVICI, H.: Oxidative activity of aortic tissue of man, the rabbit, and the dog with special reference to succinic dehydrogenase and cytochrome oxidase. Amer. J. Physiol. **195**, 476 (1958).

MAIER, N., HAIMOVICI, H.: Oxidative capacity of atherosclerotic tissue of rabbit and dog, with special reference to succinic dehydrogenase and cytochrome oxidase. Circulation Res. **41**, 65 (1965).

MAIER, N., RUBINSTEIN, L. J., HAIMOVICI, H.: Enzyme histochemistry of the normal and atherosclerotic canine aorta. J. Cardiovasc. Surgery **10**, 468 (1969).

MALINOW, M. R.: In vitro effects of estradiol on the aorta of chickens. Circulation Res. **8**, 506 (1960).

MALINOW, M. R., MOGUILEVSKY, J. A.: The effect of cholesterol feeding and of sex hormones on arterial oxygen uptake in chickens. J. Atheroscl. Res. **1**, 417 (1961).

MALINOW, M. R., MOGUILEVSKY, J. A., BUMASHNY, E.: Influence of the gonads and aortic oxygen uptake in rats. J. Atheroscler. Res. **1**, 128 (1961).

MALINOW, M. R., MOGUILEVSKY, J. A., LACUARA, J. L.: Modification of aortic oxidative enzymes in rats by gonadectomy and substitutive therapy. Circulation Res. **10**, 624 (1962).

MALINOW, M. R., PERLEY, A., McLAUGHLIN, P.: The effects of pyridinolcarbamate on induced atherosclerosis in monkeys. J. Atheroscler. Res. **8**, 455 (1968).

MALINOW, M. R., MacLAUGHLIN, P., PERLEY, A.: The effects of pyridinolcarbamate on induced atherosclerosis in cynomolgus monkeys (MACACA IRA). Atherosclerosis **15**, 31 (1972).

MALLOV, S.: Aortic lipoprotein lipase activity in relation to species, age, sex, and blood pressure. Circulation Res. **14**, 357 (1964).

MANDEL, P., KEMPF, E.: The pentose phosphate pathway in the degradation of glucose by aortic tissue. J. Atheroscler. Res. **3**, 233 (1963).

MANDEL, P., POIREL, G., SIMARD-DUQUESNE, N.: Oxygen uptake of normal and atherosclerotic rabbit aortae in mediums of normal and hyperlipaemic sera and plasmas. J. Atheroscler. Res. **6**, 463 (1966).

MARMORSTON, J., MOORE, F. J., HOPKINS, C. E., KUZMA, O. T., WEINER, J.: Clinical studies of long-term estrogen therapy in men with myocardial infarction. Proc. Soc. exp. Biol. (N. Y.) **110**, 400 (1962).

MARTIN, G. J.: Hesperidin and ascorbic acid: Naturally occurring Synergists. Exp. med. Surg. **12**, 535 (1954).

MATAGNE, D., HAMOIR, G.: Les enzymes glycolytiques de la veine saphène humaine saine et variqueuse. Action du Venoruton sur ces enzymes. Paper read at IVth International Angiologic Symposium, Nyon, Switzerland, September 4—6, 1972. Angiologica **9**, 213 (1972).

MAXWELL, L. C., BOHR, D. F., MURPHY, R. A.: Arterial actomyosin: effects of ionic strength on ATPase activity and solubility. Am. J. Physiol. **220**, 1871 (1971).

Miller, B. F., Aiba, T., Keyes, F. P., Curreri, P. W., Branwood, A. W.: Beta-glucuronidase-activity and its variation with pH in human atherosclerotic arteries. J. Atheroscler. Res. **6**, 352 (1966).

Miller, B. F., Kothari, H. V.: Increased activity of lysosomal enzymes in human atherosclerotic aortas. Exp. Mol. Path. **10**, 288 (1969).

Morin, R. J.: Effects of estradiol on the *in vitro* incorporation of Acetate-1-^{14}C into the phospholipids of human peripheral arteries. Experientia (Basel) **26**, 829 (1970).

Morrison, E. S., Scott, R. F., Kroms, M., Pastori, S. J.: A method for isolating aortic mitochondria exhibiting high respiratory control. Biochem. Med. **4**, 47 (1970).

Morrison, E. S., Scott, R. F., Frick, J., Kroms, M.: Changes in free fatty acid degradation by Krebs pathway in atherosclerotic aorta. Circulation **44**, II—7 (1971).

Morrison, E. S., Scott, R. F., Kroms, M., Frick, J.: Glucose degradation in normal and atherosclerotic aortic intima-media. Atherosclerosis **16**, 157 (1972).

Morrison, E. S., Scott, R. F., Kroms, M., Frick, J.: Aortic mitochondrial function in experimentally induced atherosclerosis in swine and rabbits. Biochem. Med. **7**, 308 (1973).

Möttönen, M., Pantio, M., Nieminen, L.: Enzyme histochemical observations on the effect of pyridinol carbamate on cholesterol-induced atheroslcerosis. Atherosclerosis **15**, 77 (1972).

Mrhová, O., Zemplényi, T.: The effect of sex and gonadectomy on some aortic enzymes of the rat. Quart. J. exp. Physiol. **50**, 289 (1965).

Mrhová, O., Zemplényi, T., Lojda, Z.: The effect of cholesterol-fat feeding on the activity of rabbit aorta dehydrogenase systems. Quart. J. exp. Physiol. **48**, 61 (1963a).

Mrhová, O., Zemplényi, T., Lojda, Z.: The beta-glucuronidase activity of the aorta in early stages of experimental rabbit atherosclerosis. J. Atheroscler. Res. **3**, 44 (1963b).

Mrhová, O., Shimamoto, T., Numano, F.: The metabolic effect of pyridinolcarbamate in rats. Acta Path. Jap. **22**(2), 353 (1972a).

Mrhová, O., Shimamoto, T., Numano, F.: Metabolic effect of pyridinolcarbamate on the vascular wall of rats with hypervitaminosis D. Atherosclerosis **16**, I—8 (1972b).

Mrhová, O., Grafnetter, D., Janda, J., Linhart, J.: Effect of Atromid-S on the activity of vascular enzymes in rats. Biochem. Pharm. **20**, 3069 (1971).

Munro, A. F., Rifkind, B. M., Leibescheutz, H. F., Campbell, R. S. F., Howard, B. R.: Effect of cholesterol feeding on the oxygen consumption of aortic tissue from the cockerel and the rat. J. Atheroscler. Res. **1**, 296 (1961).

Mustard, J. F.: Introduction to the platelet and the artery. In: Jones, R. J. (Ed.): Atherosclerosis, p. 76. New York-Heidelberg-Berlin: Springer 1970.

Murphy, R. A.: Contractile proteins of vascular smooth muscle: Effects of hydrogen and alkali metal actions on actomyosin adenosinetriphosphatase activity. Microvasc. Res. **1**, 344 (1969).

Nakatani, M., Sasaki, T., Miyazaki, T., Nakamura, M.: Synthesis of phospholipids in arterial walls. J. Atheroscler. Res. **7**, 747 (1967).

Newman, H. A. I., Zilversmit, D. B.: Uptake and release of cholesterol by rabbit atheromatous lesions. Circulation Res. **18**, 293 (1966).

Niebes, P.: Influence des flavonoïdes sur le métabolisme des mucopolysaccharides dans la paroi veineuse. Paper read at IVth International Angiologic Symposium, Nyon, Switzerland, September 4—6, 1972. Angiologica. **9**, 226 (1972).

Niebes, P., Laszt, L.: Recherches sur l'activite des enzymes dans le metabolisme des mucopolysaccharides des veines saphenes humaines saines ou variqueuses. Angiologica **8**, 7 (1971a).

Niebes, P., Laszt, L.: Influence *in vitro* d'une serie de flavonoides sur des enzymes du metabolisme des mucopolysaccharides de veines saphenes humaines et bovines. Angiologica **8**, 297 (1971b).

Newman, H. A. I., Gray, G. W., Zilversmit, D. B.: Cholesterol ester formation in aortas of cholesterol-fed rabbits. J. Atheroscler. Res. **8**, 745 (1968).

Newmark, M. Z.; Malfer, D. C., Wiese, C. D.: Regulation of arterial metabolism. I. The effects of age and hormonal status upon the utilization of glucose *in vitro* by rat aorta. Biochim. biophys. Acta (Amst.) **261**, 9 (1972).

Numano, F., Takenobu, K. K. M., Sagara, A., Shimamoto, T.: Comparative studies on the preventative effect of pyridinolcarbamate and estrogen against aortic and coronary atherosclerosis of cholesterol-fed rabbits. Part I: Topographic and pathological studies. Acta path. Jap. **21**, 177 (1971).

NUMANO, F., KATSU, K., TAKENOBU, M., SAGARA, A., SHIMAMOTO, T.: Comparative studies on the preventive effect of pyridinolcarbamate and estrogen against aortic and coronary atherosclerosis of cholesterol-fed rabbits. Part II: Histoenzymatic studies. Acta Path. Jap. **21**, 193 (1971b).

PANTESCO, V., VIAUD, J., FONTAINE, R., MANDEL, P.: Sur le mode de degradation du glucose par l'aorte de bovides. C. R. Soc. Biol. **151**, 1584 (1957).

PARKER, R., ORMSBY, J. W., PETERSON, N. F., ODLAND, G. F., WILLIAMS, R. H.: *In vitro* studies of phospholipid synthesis in experimental atherosclerosis: possible role of myointimal cells. Circulation Res. **19**, 700 (1966).

PATELSKI, J., SZENDZIKOWSKI, S.: Influence of cholinesterase inhibitor on lipolytic activity of rat aorta. Acta physiol. polon. **11**, 853 (1960).

PATELSKI, J., SZENDZIKOWSKI, S.: Lipolytic and esterolytic activity of aorta after prolonged ACTH treatment in rats. Bull. Soc. Amis. Sci. Lettres Poznan. C **11**, 37 (1962).

PATELSKI, J., WALIGÓRA, Z., SZULC, S., BOWYER, D. E., HOWARD, A. N., GRESHAM, G. A.: Lipolytic enzymes of the aortic wall. Progr. biochem. Pharmacol. Vol. 4, p. 287. Basel-New York: Karger 1968.

PATELSKI, J., BOWYER, D. E., HOWARD, A. N., GRESHAM, G. A.: Changes in phospholipase A, lipase and cholesterol esterase activity in aorta in experimental atherosclerosis in the rabbit and rat. J. Atheroscler. Res. **8**, 221 (1968).

PATELSKI, J., WALIGÓRA, Z., SZULC, S.: Demonstration and some properties of the phospholipase A, lipase and cholesterol esterase from the aortic wall. J. Atheroscler. Res. **7**, 453 (1967).

PATELSKI, J., BOWYER, D. E., HOWARD, A. N., JENNINGS, I. W., THORNE, C. J. R., GRESHAM, G. A.: Modification of enzyme activities in experimental atherosclerosis in the rabbit. Atherosclerosis **12**, 41 (1970).

PAUTRIZEL, R., DALLOCCHIO, M., GANDJI, F. A., RAZAKA, G., CROCKETT, R., BRICAUD, H., BROUSETET, P.: Une étude des reactions immunes provoqués par des antigènes aortiques. In: Le Rôle De La Paroi Arterielle Dans L'Atherogenèse, p. 353. Paris: Center National De La Recherche Scientifique 1968.

PICK, R.: The effect of pyridinolcarbamate on the induction and regression of aortic and coronary atherosclerosis in cholesterol-fed cockerls. In: SHIMAMOTO, T., NUMANO, F. (Eds.): Atherogenesis. Tokyo: Excerpta Medica Foundation 1969.

PLATT, D.: Nachweis einer Peptidyl-Peptid-Hydrolase (Kollagenase?) in der Aortenwand des Schweins. Klin. Wschr. **48**, 1420 (1970).

PLATT, D., LUBOEINSKI, H. P.: The activities of glycosaminoglycan hydrolases of normal and atherosclerotic human aorta. Angiologica **6**, 19 (1969).

PALATY, V., GUSTAFSON, B. K., FRIEDMANN, S. M.: Maintenance of the ionic composition of the incubated artery. Canad. J. Physiol. Pharmacol. **49**, 106 (1971).

PORTMAN, O. W., ALEXANDER, P.: Lysophosphatidylcholine concentrations and metabolism in aortic intima plus inner media: effect of nutritionally induced atherosclerosis. J. Lipid Res. **10**, 158 (1969).

PŘEROVSKÝ, I., ROZTOČIL, K., HLAVOVÁ, A., KOLEILAT, Z., RÁZGOVÁ, L., OLIVA, I.: The effect of hydroxyethylrutosides after acute and chronic oral administration in patients with venous diseases. (A double-blind study). Paper read at IVth International Angiologic Symposium, Nyon, Switzerland, September 4—6, 1972. Angiologica **9**, 408 (1972).

PRETOLANI, E.: Biochimica enzimatica delle arterie. Il "complesso" elastasi a livello parietale. Boll. Soc. ital. Biol. Sperm. **44**, 1 (1968).

PROUDLICK, J. W., DAY, A. J.: Cholesterol esterifying enzymes of atherosclerotic rabbit intima. Biochim. biophys. Acta (Amst.) **260**, 716 (1972).

RACHMILEWITZ, D., EISENBERG, S., STEIN, Y., STEIN, O.: Phospholipases in Arterial Tissue 1. Sphingomyelin Cholinephosphohydrolase activity in human, dog, guinea pig, rat and rabbit arteries. Biochim. biophys. Acta (Amst.) **144**, 624 (1967).

RENAIS, J., GROULT, N., SCEBAT, L., LENÈGRE, J.: Pouvoir antigénique et patho ène du tissue arteriel. In: Le Rôle De La Paroi Arterielle Dans L'Athérogenèse. VI, p. 323. Paris: Centre National De La Recherche Scientifique 1968.

RIFKIND, B. M., MUNRO, A. F.: Effect of sexual status on arterial respiration and glycolysis. J. Atheroscler. Res. **3**, 268 (1963).

RITZ, E.: The pentose cycle in arterial tissue. J. Atheroscler. Res. **8**, 445 (1968).

Ritz, E., Sanwald, R.: Glucuronic acid cycle in arterial tissue. Exp. Med. **153**, 237 (1970).

Robbins, R. C.: Effect of vitamin C and flavonoids on blood cell aggregation and capillary resistance. Int. Z. Vitaminforsch. **36**, 10 (1966).

Robbins, R. C.: Effect of flavonoids on survival time of rats fed thrombogenic or atherogenic regimens. J. Atheroscler. Res. **7**, 3 (1967).

Robbins, R. C.: Effects of phenyl benzo-pyrone derivatives (flavonoids) on blood cell aggregation: Basis for a concept of mode of action. Clin. Chem. **17**, No. 5, 433 (1971).

Robert, B., Legrand, Y., Pignaud, G., Caen, J., Robert, L.: Activité élastionlytique associée aux plaquettes sanguines. Path. Biol. **17**, 615 (1969).

Robert, L.: The micromolecular matrix of the arterial wall: Collagen, elastin, mucopolysaccharides. In: Jones, R. J. (Ed.): Atherosclerosis, p. 59. 1970.

Robert, L., Robert, B., Robert, A. M.: Molecular biology of elastin as related to aging and atherosclerosis. Exp. Gerontol. **5**, 339 (1970).

Robertson, A. L.: Transport of plasma lipoproteins and ultrastructure of human arterial intimacytes in culture. In: Rothblat, G. H., Kritchevsky, D. (Eds.): Lipid Metabolism in Tissue Culture Cells. The Wistar Institute Symposium Monograph, Number 6. Philadelphia: The Wistar Institute Press 1967.

Robertson, A. L.: Oxygen requirements of the human arterial intima in atherogenesis. Progr. Biochem. Pharmacol. **4**, 305 (1968).

Robinson D. S., Harris, P. M.: The production of lipolytic activity in the circulation of the hind limb in response to heparin. Quart. J. exp. Physiol. **44**, 80 (1959).

Rodney, G., Swanson, A. L., Wheeler, L. M., Smith, G. N., Worrel, C. S.: The effect of a series of flavonoids on hyaluronidase and some other related enzymes. J. biol. Chem. **183**, 739 (1950).

Rouser, G., Solomon, R. D.: Changes in phospholipid composition of human aorta with age. Lipids **4**, 232 (1969).

Roztočil, K., Fischer, A., Novák, P., Razgová, L.: The effect of 0-(β-hydroxyethyl)-rutosides (HR) on the peripheral circulation in patients with chronic venous insufficiency. Europ. J. clin. Pharmacol. **3**, 243 (1971).

Rucker, R. B., Goettlich-Riemann, W.: Properties of rabbit aorta amine oxidase Proc. Soc. exp. Biol. (N.Y.) **139**, 286 (1972).

Sandner, M., Bourne, G. F.: Histochemistry of atherosclerosis in the rat, dog and man. In: Sandner, M., Bourne, G. E. (Eds.): Atherosclerosis and its origin, p. 515. New York-London: Academic Press 1963.

Sandwald, R., Kirk, J. E.: Beta-hydroxyacyl dehydrogenase in human arterial tissue. Proc. Soc. exp. Biol. (N.Y.) **118**, 1088 (1965).

Sbarra, A. J., Gilfillan, R. F., Bardavil, W. A.: The hexose monophosphate pathway in arterial tissue. Biochem. Biophys. Res. Commun. **3**, 311 (1960).

Scebat, L., Renais, J., Iris, L., Groult, N., Lenègre, J.: Lésions arterielles generalisées declenchées chez le lapin par un traumatisme arteriel localise: Rôle possible d'autoanticorps antiaorte. In: Le Rôle De La Paroi Arterielle Dans L'Athérogenèse, p. 425. Paris: Center National De La Recherche Scientifique 1968.

Schoffeniels, E.: Ionic composition of the arterial wall. Angiologica **6**, 65 (1969).

Scott, R. F., Morrison, E. S., Kroms, M.: Effect of cold shock on respiration and glycolysis in swine arterial tissue. Amer. J. Physiol. **219**, 1363 (1970).

Scott, R. F., Jarmolych, J., Fritz, D. E., Imai, H., Kim, D. N., Morrison, E. S.: Reactions of endothelial and smooth muscle cells in the atherosclerotic lesion. In: Jones, R. J. (Ed.): Atherosclerosis, p. 50. New York-Heidelberg-Berlin: Springer 1970.

Seethanatan, P., Kurup, P. A.: Tissue lactate dehydrogenase isoenzyme patterns in rats fed a hypercholesterolemic diet. Atherosclerosis **12**, 393 (1970).

Shimamoto, T.: Experimental study of atherosclerosis. An attempt at its prevention and treatment. Acta path. jap. **19**, 15 (1969).

Shimamoto, T., Numano, F., Fujita, T.: Atherosclerosis-inhibiting effect antibradykinin agent, pyridinolcarbamate. Amer. Heart J. **71**, 216 (1966 a).

Shimamoto, T., Atsumi, T., Numano, F., Fujita, T.: Treatment of atherosclerosis with pyridinolcarbamate. Prog. Biochem. Pharmacol. **4**, 216 (1966 b).

Shore, M. L., Zilversmit, D. B., Ackerman, R. F.: Plasma phospholipid deposition and aortic phospholipid synthesis in atherosclerosis. Amer. J. Physiol. **181**, 527 (1955).

SHYAMALA, A. G., NICOLS, C. W., JR., CHAIKOFF, I. L.: The effect of aging on the hydrolysis of cho-
lesterol-7α-HS-oleate by homogenates of chicken aorta. Life Sci. **5**, 1191 (1966).

SIDORENKOV, I. V., SHARAEV, P. N.: The mechanism of disturbance of mucopolysaccharide and
collagen metabolism in experimental atherosclerosis. Cor Vasa **14**, 143 (1972).

SIGGAARD-ANDERSEN, J., BONDE-PETERSEN, F., HANSEN, T. I., MELLEMGAARD, K.: Plasma volume
and vascular permeability during hypoxia and carbon monoxide exposure. Scand. J. clin.
Lab. Invest. **22**, Suppl. 103, 39 (1968).

SMITH, E. B.: The influence of age and atherosclerosis on the chemistry of aortic intima. I. The
lipids. J. Atheroscler. Res. **5**, 224 (1965).

SOMLYO, A. P., SOMLYO, A. V.: Vascular smooth muscle. I. Normal structure, Pathology, biochemistry, and biophysics. Pharmacol. Rev. **20**, 197 (1968).

SRINIVASAN, S. R., LOPEZ, S., RADHAKRISHNAMURTHY, B., BERENSON, G. S.: Complexing of serum
pre-β and β-lipoproteins and acid mucopolysaccharides. Atherosclerosis **12**, 321 (1970).

SRINIVASAN, S., DOLAN, P., RADHAKRISHNAMURTHY, B., BERENSON, G.: Further studies on lipoprotein-acid mucopolysaccharide complexes from human atherosclerotic lesions. Circulation
46, No. 4, II—253 (1972).

STAVROU, D., DAHME, E.: Studie zur Arteriosklerosegenese beim Hanford-Miniatur-Schwein unter normalen und experimentellen Bedingungen, Teil 2 (Enzymtopochemische Befunde).
Atherosclerosis **14**, 169 (1971).

ST. CLAIR, R. W., LOFLAND, H. F., JR., PRICHARD, R. W., CLARKSON, T. B.: Synthesis of squalene
and sterols by isolated segments of human and pigeon arteries. Exp. Mol. Path. **8**, 201 (1968a).

ST. CLAIR, R. W., LOFLAND, H. B., JR., CLARKSON, T. B.: Composition and synthesis of fatty acids in
atherosclerotic aortas of the pigeon. J. Lipid. Res. **9**, 739 (1968b).

ST. CLAIR, R. W., LOFLAND, H. B., JR., CLARKSON, T. B.: Influence of atherosclerosis on the composition, synthesis and esterification of lipids in aortas of squirrel monkeys (*Saimiri sciurens*). J.
Atheroscler. Res. **10**, 193 (1969).

ST. CLAIR, R. W., LOFLAND, H. B., CLARKSON, T. B.: Influence of duration of cholesterol feeding on
esterification of fatty acids by cell-free preparation of pigeon aorta. Circulation Res. **27**, 213
(1970).

ST. CLAIR, CLARKSON, T. B., LOFLAND, H. B.: Effects of regression of atherosclerotic lesions on the
content and esterification of cholesterol by cell-free preparations of pigeon aorta. Circulation
Res. **31**, 664 (1972).

ST. CLAIR, R.: Esterification of fatty acids and cholesterol by pigeon aorta. Circulation **41**, Suppl.
III, p. III—3 (1970).

STAMLER, J., PICK, R., KATZ, L. N., PICK, A., KAPLAN, B. M., BERKSON, D. M., CENTURY, D.: Effectiveness of estrogens for therapy of myocardial infarction in middle-aged men. J. Amer. med.
Assn. **183**, 632 (1963).

STEFANOVICH, V., GORE, I., KAJIYAMA, G., IWANAGA, Y.: The effect of nicotine on dietary atherogenesis in rabbits. Exp. mol. Path. **11**, 71 (1969).

STEIN, A. A., ROSENBLUM, J., LEATHER, R.: Intimal sclerosis in human veins. Arch. Path. **81**, 548
(1966).

STEIN, O., STEIN, Y.: Lipid synthesis and transport in the normal and atherosclerotic aorta. Lab.
Invest. **23**, No. 5, 556 (1970).

STEIN, Y., STEIN, O.: Incorporation of fatty acids into lipids of aortic slices of rabbits, dogs, rats,
and baboons, J. Atheroscler. Res. **2**, 400 (1962).

STEIN, Y., STEIN, O., SHAPIRO, B.: Enzymic pathways of glyceride and phospholipid synthesis in
aortic homogenates. Biochim. biophys. Acta (Amst.) **70**, 33 (1963).

STEIN, Y., EISENBERG, S., STEIN, O.: Metabolism of lysolecithin by human umbilical and dog
carotid arteries. Progr. Biochem. Pharmacol. **4**, 253 (1968).

ŠVEJCAR, J., PŘEROVSKÝ, I., LINHART, J., KRUML, L.: Content of collagen elastin, and water in walls
of the internal saphenour vein in man. Circulation Res. **11**, 296 (1962).

ŠVEJCAR, J., PŘEROVSKÝ, I., LINHART, J., KRUML, J.: Content of collagen, elastin and hexosamine in
primary varicose veins. Clin. Sci. **24**, 325 (1963).

SZABÓ, I. K., CSEH, G.: Über die Wechselwirkung zwischen dem Elastase-Komplex und der Lipo-
proteidlipase der Blutgefäße. Naturwissenschaften **49**, 260 (1962).

SZABÓ, R., BENKÖ, S., SZARVAS, F., VARGA, L.: The lipolytic activity of the heart muscle and the
aorta in experimental cholesterol atherosclerosis. Cor Vasa **12**, 57 (1970).

Szendzikowski,S.: Histoenzymological investigation of the vascular channel developed after implantation of teritalprestheses into aorta. Folia Histochem. Cytochem. **1**, Suppl.I, 149 (1963).

Szendzikowski,S., Patelski,J., Pearse,A.G.E.: The influence of cholinesterase inhibitors on the lipolytic activity of rat aorta. Enzymol. Biol. Clin. **1**, 125 (1961—1962).

Szigeti,I., Piko,K., Doman,J.: The immunopathological importance of different structural protein antigens of human arterial vessel-wall in heterologous immunization of rabbits compared with immunoserological data of human coronary heart patients. In: Le Role De La Paroi Arterielle Dans L'Atherogenese, p.493. Paris: Center National De La Recherche Scientifique 1968.

Tararak,E.M.: Alterations in lipolytic enzymatic activity in rabbit aorta in the regressive phase of experimental atherosclerosis. Cor Vasa **10**, 135 (1968).

Tsukershtein,O.E.: The effect of sex hormones on the arterial elasticity. Cor Vasa **13**, 77 (1971).

Urbanová,D., Přerovský,I.: Enzymes in the wall of normal and varicose veins. Angiologica **9**, 53 (1972).

Wagner,J., Duck,H.: Säulenchromatographische Trennung von Aminoacyl-Oligo-Peptidhydrolasen normaler und arteriosklerotischer Kaninchenaorten. J. Chromatogr. **66**, 67 (1972).

Waligóra,Z.: Hydrolysis of lecithin by enzymes from the arterial wall. Poznan. Towarz. Prayjac. Nauk. **34**, 317 (1966).

Wahlqvist,M.L., Day,A.J.: Phospholipid synthesis by foam cells in human atheroma. Exp. Mol. Pathol. **11**, 275 (1969).

Weiss,H.S., Watson,N.J., Calhoon,T.B.: Respiration of the avian aorta in relation to spontaneous atherosclerosis. Comp. Biochem. Physiol. **38**, 675 (1971).

Wexler,B.C., Judd,J.T.: Increased aortic Beta-Glucuronidase activity with progressively severe arteriosclerosis in female breeder rats. Nature (Lond.) **209**, 383 (1966).

Whereat,A.F.: Oxygen consumption of normal and atherosclerotic intima. Circulation. Res. **9**, 571 (1961).

Whereat,A.F.: Lipid biosynthesis in aortic intima from normal and cholesterol-fed rabbits. J. Atheroscler. Res. **4**, 272 (1964).

Whereat,A.F.: Incorporation of tritium from succinate-2,3-^{2}H into long-chain fatty acids by aortic mitochondria. Proc. Soc. exp. Biol. (N.Y.) **118**, 888 (1965).

Whereat,A.F.: Fatty acid synthesis in cell-free system from rabbit aorta. J. Lipid Res. **7**, 671 (1966).

Whereat,A.F.: Fatty acid biosynthesis in aorta and heart. In: Paoletti,R., Kritchevsky,D. (Eds.): Advances in Lipid Research, Vol.9, p.119. New York-London: Academic Press 1971.

Whereat,A.F., Orishimo,M.W., Nelson,J., Phillips,S.: The location of different synthetic systems for fatty acids in inner and outer mitochondrial membranes from rabbit heart. J. biol. Chem. **244**, 6498 (1969).

Will,D.H., Frith,C.H., McMurtry,I.F.; MacCarter,D.J.: Effects of hypertension and hypoxemia on arterial metabolism and structure. Advanc. exp. Med. Biol. **22**, 185 (1972).

Willoughby,D.A., Lykke,A.W.J., Ryan,G.B.: A study of the antiinflammatory action of pyridinolcarbamate (anginin). In: Shimamoto,T., Numano,F. (Eds.): Atherogenesis. Tokyo: Excerpta Medica Foundation 1969.

Wissler,R.W.: The arterial medial cell, smooth muscle or multifunctional mesenchyme.[2] J. Atheroscler. Res. **8**, 201 (1968).

Wolinsky,H.: Effects of estrogen and progestrogen treatment on the response of the aorta of male rats to hypertension. Morphological and chemical studies. Circulation Res. **30**, 341 (1972).

Zemplényi,T.: Enzymes of the arterial wall. J. Atheroscler. Res. **2**, 2 (1962).

Zemplényi,T.: The lipolytic and esterolytic activity of blood and tissues and problems of atherosclerosis. In: Paoletti,R., Kritschevsky,D. (Eds.): Advances in Lipid Research, Vol.II, p.235. New York: Academic Press 1964.

Zemplényi,T.: Editorial: Vascular enzymes and atherosclerosis. J. Atheroscler. Res. **7**, 725 (1967).

Zemplényi,T.: Enzyme biochemistry of the arterial wall as related to atherosclerosis. London: Lloyd-Luke 1968.

Zemplényi,T.: Vascular enzymes and the relevance of their study to problems of atherogenesis. Med. Clin. N. Amer. **58**, 293 (1974).

ZEMPLÉNYI, T., BLANKENHORN, D. H.: Vascular permeability, hypoxia, and atherosclerosis. Paper read at IVth International Angiologic Symposium, Nyon, Switzerland, September 4—6 1972. Angiologica 9, 429 (1972).

ZEMPLÉNYI, T., GRAFNETTER, D.: Species and sex differences in fatty acid release on incubation of tissues and human lipaemic serum. Brit. J. exp. Pathol. 39, 99 (1958).

ZEMPLÉNYI, T., GRAFNETTER, D.: The lipolytic activity of heart and aorta in experimental atherosclerosis in rabbits. Brit. J. exp. Pathol. 40, 312 (1959a).

ZEMPLÉNYI, T., GRAFNETTER, D.: The lipolytic activity of the aorta, its relation to aging and to atherosclerosis. Gerontologia (Basel) 3, 55 (1959b).

ZEMPLÉNYI, T., MRHOVÁ, O.: Vascular enzyme activity changes accompanying the induction of experimental atherosclerosis. II. Rats fed excess vitamin D. J. Atheroscler. Res. 5, 548 (1965).

ZEMPLÉNYI, T., MRHOVÁ, O.: Activité enzymatique de la paroi arterielle et athérogenèse. Arch. Mal. Coeur, Suppl. 3, 59 (1966).

ZEMPLÉNYI, T., MRHOVÁ, O.: The effect of some drugs and hormones on the activity of vascular enzymes. Progr. Biochem. Pharmacol. 2, 141 (1967).

ZEMPLÉNYI, T., LOJDA, Z., GRAFNETTER, D.: The relationship of lipolytic and esterolytic activity of the aorta to susceptibility to experimental atherosclerosis. Circulation Res. 7, 286 (1959).

ZEMPLÉNYI, T., FODOR, J., LOJDA, Z.: Mast cell histamine and the accumulation of colloidal particles in the vascular endothelium. Quart. J. exp. Physiol. 45, 50 (1960).

ZEMPLÉNYI, T., LOJDA, Z., MRHOVÁ, O.: Enzymes of the vascular wall in experimental atherosclerosis in the rabbit. In: SANDLER, M., BOURNE, G. H. (Eds.): Atherosclerosis and its origin, p. 459. New York: Academic Press 1963.

ZEMPLÉNYI, T., KNÍŽKOVÁ, I., LOJDA, Z., MRHOVÁ, O.: The group-specific carboxylic esterase activity of aortic tissue. Cor Vasa 5, 107 (1963b).

ZEMPLÉNYI, T., MRHOVÁ, O., GRAFNETTER, D., LOJDA, Z.: Some enzymes of the arterial wall in physiological and pathological conditions. In: PRUSIK, B., REINIS, Z., RIEDL, O. (Eds.): Metabolismus Parietis Vasorum. Prague: State Medical Publ. House 1962.

ZEMPLÉNYI, T., HLADOVEC, J., MRHOVÁ, O.: Vascular enzyme activity changes accompanying the induction of experimental atherosclerosis. I. Rats fed Hartroft's diet. J. Atheroscler. Res. 5, 540 (1965a).

ZEMPLÉNYI, T., MRHOVÁ, O., URBANOVÁ, D., LOJDA, Z.: Comparative aspects of vascular enzymes. Acta Zool. Pathol. Atnverp. No. 39, 45 (1966a).

ZEMPLÉNYI, T., MRHOVÁ, O., URBANOVÁ, D., KRUML, J., SOPH, A.: Comparative studies of vascular enzymes in human and pig arteries. Il Giornale Del l'Arteriosclerosi. Anno IV, 12 (1966b).

ZEMPLÉNYI, T., MRHOVÁ, O., URBANOVÁ, D., KOHOUT, M.: Vascular enzyme activities and susceptibility of arteries to atherosclerosis. Ann. N.Y. Acad. Sci. 149, 585 (1968).

ZEMPLÉNYI, T., URBANOVÁ, D., MRHOVÁ, O.: Contributions of vascular enzyme studies to problems of atherogenesis. In: LASZT, L. (Ed.): International Symposium of Biochemistry of the Vascular Wall, Part II, p. 162. Basel-New York: Karger 1969a.

ZEMPLÉNYI, T., MRHOVÁ, O., URBANOVÁ, D.: Allylamine-induced arterial enzyme changes and the role of injury in atherogenesis. Circulation 39, Suppl. III, III—27 (1969b).

ZEMPLÉNYI, T., CHIN, H. P., BLANKENHORN, D. H.: Isoenzymes of creatine phosphokinase, malate, and lactate dehydrogenase in arterial and venous tissue. Clin. Res. 18, 1591 (1970).

ZILVERSMIT, D. B.: Cholesterol flux in the atherosclerotic plaque. N.Y. Acad. Sci. 149, 710 (1968).

ZILVERSMIT, D. B.: Metabolism of arterial lipids. In: JONES, R. J. (Ed.): Atherosclerosis. Proceedings of the second international symposium, p. 35. New York-Heidelberg-Berlin: Springer 1970.

ZILVERSMIDT, D. B., McCANDLESS, E. L.: Independence of arterial phospholipid synthesis from alterations in blood lipids. J. Lipid Res. 1, 118 (1959).

ZSOLDOS, S. F., HEINEMAN, H. O.: Lipolytic activity of rabbit aorta in vitro. Amer. J. Physiol. 206, 615 (1964).

Additional References

BELL, F. P., ADAMSON, I. L., GALLUS, A. S., SCHWARTZ, C. J.: Endothelial permeability: Focal and regional patterns of ^{131}I-albumin and ^{131}I-fibrinogen uptake and transmural distribution in the pig aorta. In: SCHETTLER, G., WEIZEL, A. (Eds.): Atherosclerosis III, p. 235. New York-Heidelberg-Berlin: Springer 1974.

BIERMAN, E. L., EISENBERG, S., STEIN, O., STEIN, Y.: Very low density lipoprotein "remnant" particles: uptake by aortic smooth muscle cells in culture. Biochem. biophys. Acta **329**, 163 (1973).

BIERMAN, E. L., STEIN, O., STEIN, Y.: Lipoprotein uptake and metabolism by rat aortic smooth muscle cells in tissue culture. Circulation Res. **35**, 136 (1974).

BJÖRKERUD, S., BONDJERS, G.: Arterial repair and atherosclerosis after mechanical injury. Part 1: Permeability and light microscopic characteristics of endothelium in non-atherosclerotic and atherosclerotic lesions. Atherosclerosis **13**, 355 (1971).

BLACK, W. J., TAKANO, T., PETERS, T. J.: Subcellular distribution of cholesteryl esterase in rabbit aortic smooth muscle cells. J. Cell Biol. **59**, 26a (1973).

BRECHER, P., KESSLER, M., CLIFFORD, C., CHOBANIAN, A. V.: Cholesterol ester hydrolysis in aortic tissue. Biochem. biophys. Acta **316**, 386 (1973).

CHMELAR, M., CHMELAROVÁ, M.: Lipolytic effect of insulin and other hormones *in vitro* in aortic tissue of experimental animals. Experientia (Basel) **24**, 1118 (1968).

CHOBANIAN, A. V., MANZUR, F.: Metabolism of lipid in the human fatty streak lesion. J. Lipid Res. **13**, 201 (1972).

DE DUVE, C.: The participation of lysosomes in the transformation of smooth muscle cells to foamy cells in the aorta of cholesterol-fed rabbits. Acta Cardiol. Suppl. **XX**, 9 (1974).

DAOUD, A. S., FRITZ, K. E., JARMOLYCH, J., AUGUSTYN, J. M.: Use of aortic medial explants in the study of atherosclerosis. Exp. molec. Path. **18**, 177 (1973).

DAY, A. J.: Lipid metabolism by rabbit aortic intimal and medical cells in tissue culture. Virchows Arch. A Path. Anat. Histol. **362**, 2 (1973).

FILIPOVIC, I., VON FIGURA, K., BUDDECKE, E.: Glucose and lipid metabolism in the human arteriosclerotic aorta. In: SCHETTLER, G., WEIZEL, A. (Eds.): Atherosclerosis III, p. 107. New York-Heidelberg-Berlin: Springer 1974.

FISHER-DZOGA, K. JONES, R. M., VESSELINOVITCH, D., WISSLER, R. W.: Ultrastructural and immunohistochemical studies of primary cultures of aortic medial cells. Exp. molec. Path. **18**(2), 162 (1973a).

FISHER-DZOGA, K., CHEN, R., WISSLER, R. W.: Effects of serum lipoproteins on the morphology, growth, and metabolism of arterial smooth muscle cells. In: WAGNER, W. D., CLARKSON, T. B. (Eds.): Arterial Mesenchyme and Arteriosclerosis, p. 299. New York-London: Plenum Press 1973b.

FISHER-DZOGA, K., JONES, R. M., VESSELINOVITCH, D., WISSLER, R. W.: Increased mitotic activity in primary cultures of aortic medial smooth muscle cells after exposure to hyperlipemic serum. In: SCHETTLER, G., WEIZEL, A. (Eds.): Atherosclerosis III, p. 193. New York-Heidelberg-Berlin: Springer 1974a.

FISHER-DZOGA, K., VESSELINOVITCH, D., WISSLER, R. W.: The effect of estrogen on the rabbit aortic medial tissue culture cells. Amer. J. Path. **74**, 52a (1974b).

FRY, D. L.: Responses of the arterial wall to certain physical factors. In: Atherogenesis, Initiating Factors, p. 93. CIBA Foundation Symposium 12, New York: Elsevier 1973.

GARBARSCH, C.: I. Distribution of urea-stable and urea-labile lactate dehydrogenease activity in rabbit aorta following a single mechanical dilatation injury. Acta Histochem. **46**, 288 (1973a).

GARBARSCH, C.: II. Enzyme histochemistry of rabbit thoracic aorta following a single mechanical dilatation injury. Acta Histochem. **46**, 300 (1973b).

HASHIMOTO, S., DAYTON, S.: Oxidation of palmityl-Co-A to CO_2 by normal and atherosclerotic aortic mitochondria. Life Sci. **14**, 945 (1974a).

HASHIMOTO, S., DAYTON, S.: Cholesterol-esterifying activity of aortas from atherosclerosis-resistant and atherosclerosis-susceptible species. Proc. Soc. exp. Biol. **145**, 89 (1974b).

HASHIMOTO, S., DAYTON, S., ALFIN-SLATER, R. B., BUI, P. T., BAKER, N., WILSON, L.: Characteristics of the cholesterol-esterifying activity in normal and atherosclerotic rabbit aortas. Circulation Res. **34**, 176 (1974).

HELIN, P., GARBARSCH, C., LORENZEN, I.: Effects of intermittent and continuous hypoxia on the aortic wall in rabbits. Analysis of glycosaminoglycans, hydroxyproline and vascular histochemistry. Atherosclerosis **21**, 325 (1975).

JARMOLYCH, J., DAOUD, A. S., LANDAU, J., FRITZ, K. E., McELVENE, E.: Aortic medial explants. Cell proliferation and production of mucopolysaccharides, collagen and elastic tissue. Exp. molec. Path. **9**, 171 (1968).

JENSEN,J.: On the relationship between metabolic activity and cholesterol uptake by intima-media of the rabbit aorta. Biochem. biophys. Acta **183**, 204 (1969).

JORDAN,R.E., HEWITT,N., LEWIS,W., KAGAN,H., FRANZBLAU,C.: Regulation of elastase-catalyzed hydrolysis of insoluble elastin by synthetic and naturally occurring hydrophobic ligands. Biochemistry **13**, 3497 (1974).

KALRA,V.K., BRODIE,A.F.: Metabolic differences between the arteries of atherosclerosis susceptible and resistant pigeons. Biochem. Biophys. Res. Commun. **61**, 1372 (1974).

KIRK,J.E.: Vitamin contents of arterial tissue. Monographs on Atherosclerosis, Vol. 3. Basel: S. Karger 1973.

KIRK,J.E.: Coenzyme contents of arterial tissue. Monographs on Atherosclerosis, Vol. 4. Basel: S. Karger 1974.

KLYNSTRA,F.B., BÖTTCHER,C.J.F.: Permeability patterns in pig aorta. Atherosclerosis **11**, 451 (1970).

MAY,J.F., ZEMPLÉNYI,T., PAULE,W.J., KALRA,V.K., BLANKENHORN,D.H., BRODIE,A.F.: Studies on the effect of hypoxia on arterial smooth muscle cell cultures. In: WOLF,S., WERTHESSEN,N.T. (Eds.): The Smooth Muscle of the Arterial Wall, p. 144. New York: Plenum Press 1975.

MAY,J.F., PAULE,W.J., ZEMPLENYI,T., KALRA,V.K., BRODIE,A.F., BLANKENHORN,D.H.: Effect of hypoxia on cultured arterial smooth muscle cells. Clin. Res. **22**, 110A (1974).

MORITA,T., BING,R.J.: Lipid metabolism in perfused human coronary arteries. Proc. Soc. exp. Biol. **140**, 617 (1972).

NOMA,A., OKABE,H., SAKURADA,T., ORIMO,H., MURAKAMI,M.: Properties and positional specificity of lipases in the human aorta. In: SCHETTLER,G., WEIZEL,A. (Eds.): Atherosclerosis III, p.143. New York-Heidelberg-Berlin: Springer 1974.

PETERS,T.J., MÜLLER,M., DE DUVE,C.: Lysosomes of the arterial wall. J. Exp. Med. **136**, 1117 (1972).

PETERS,T.J., DE DUVE,C.: Lysosomes of the arterial wall. Exp. molec. Path. **20**, 228 (1974).

POLLAK,O.J.: Tissue cultures. Monographs on Atherosclerosis, Vol. 1. Basel: S. Karger 1969.

POLLAK,O.J., KASAI,T.: Appearance and behavior of aortic cells *in vitro*. Amer. J. Med. Sci. **248**, 71 (1964).

ROBERT,L., KADAR,A., ROBERT,B.: The macromolecules of the intercellular matrix of the arterial wall: Collagen, elastin, proteoglycans, and glycoproteins. Advanc. exp. Med. Biol. **43**, 85 (1974).

ROBERTSON,A.L., JR., KHAIRALLAH,P.A.: Arterial endothelial permeability and vascular disease. Exp. molec. Path. **18**, 241 (1973).

ROSS,R.: The smooth muscle cell. J. Cell Biol. **50**, 172 (1971).

ROSS,R., GLOMSET,J.A.: Atherosclerosis and the arterial smooth muscle cell. Science **180**, 1332 (1973).

ROSS,R., GLOMSET,J., KARIYA,B., HARKER,L.: A platelet-dependent serum factor that stimulates the proliferation of arterial smooth muscle cells *in vitro*. Proc. nat. Acad. Sci. (Wash.) **71**, 1207 (1974).

RUTSTEIN,D.D., INGENITO,E.F., CRAIG,J.M., MARTINELLI,M.: Effects of linolenic and stearic acids on cholesterol induced lipoid deposition in human aortic cells in tissue culture. Lancet **1958I**, 7020.

SARMA,J.S.M., TILLMANNS,H., IKEDA,S., GRENIER,A., COLBY,E., BING,R.J.: Lipid metabolism in perfused human and dog coronary arteries. Amer. J. Cardiol. **35**, 579 (1975).

SHIMAMOTO,T.: Contraction of endothelial cells as a key mechanism in atherogenesis and treatment of atherosclerosis with endothelial cell relaxants. In: SCHETTLER,G., WEIZEL,A. (Eds.): Atherosclerosis III, p.64. New York-Heidelberg-Berlin: Springer 1974.

SHIMAMOTO,T.: Hyperreactive arterial endothelial cells in atherogenesis and cyclic AMP phosphodiesterase inhibitor in prevention and treatment of atherosclerotic disorders. Jap. Heart J. **16**, 76 (1975).

SHIMAMOTO,T., NUMANO,F.: Beta-lipoprotein entry into the arterial wall and its prevention. In: SCHETTLER,G., WEIZEL,A. (Eds.): Atherosclerosis III, p.89. New York-Heidelberg-Berlin: Springer 1974.

SHIO,H., FARQUHAR,M.G., DEDUVE,C.: Lysosomes of the arterial wall. Amer. J. Path. **76**, 1 (1974).

SOMER, J. B., SCHWARTZ, C. J.: Focal ^{3}H-cholesterol uptake in the pig aorta. Atherosclerosis **13**, 293 (1971).

SCHROEDER, H. A.: The role of trace elements in cardiovascular diseases. Med. Clin. N. Amer. **58**, 381 (1974).

STEIN, Y., STEIN, O.: Lipid synthesis and degradation and lipoprotein transport in mammalian aorta. In: Atherogenesis, Initiating Factors, p. 165. CIBA Foundation Symposium 12, New York: Elsevier 1973.

STEIN, O., STEIN, Y.: Comparative uptake of rat and human serum low density and high density lipoproteins by rat aortic smooth muscle cells in culture. Circulation Res. **36**, 436 (1975 a).

STEIN, Y., STEIN, O.: Turnover of phospholipids in rat aortic smooth muscle cells in culture. Amer. J. Cardiol. **35**, 572 (1975 b).

STOUT, R. W., BIERMAN, E. L., ROSS, R.: Effect of insulin on the proliferation of cultured primate arterial smooth muscle cells. Circulation Res. **36**, 319 (1975).

TAKANO, T., BLACK, W. J., PETERS, T. J., DE DUVE, C.: Assay, kinetics, and lysosomal localization of an acid cholesteryl esterase in rabbit aortic smooth muscle cells. J. biol. Chem. **249**, 6732 (1974).

VERESS, B., BÁLINT, A., KÓCZÉ, A.: Increasing aortic permeability by atherogenic diet. Atherosclerosis **11**, 369 (1970).

VIJAYAKUMAR, S. T., KURUP, P. A.: Metabolism of glucoaminoglycans in atheromatous rats. Enzymes concerned with synthesis, degradation and sulphation of glycosaminoglycans. Atherosclerosis **21**, 245 (1975).

VOST, A., POCOCK, D. E.: Aortic uptake of chylomicron triglyceride in vivo and aortic lipoprotein triglyceride lipase in rat. In: SCHETTLER, G., WEIZEL, A. (Eds.): Atherosclerosis III, p. 150. New York-Heidelberg-Berlin: Springer 1974.

WAGNER, W. D., CLARKSON, T. B. (Eds.): Arterial Mesenchyme and Arteriosclerosis. New York and London: Plenum Press 1974.

WALTON, K. W.: Pathogenetic mechanisms in atherosclerosis. Amer. J. Cardiol. **35**, 542 (1975).

WERB, Z., COHN, Z. A.: Cholesterol metabolism in the macrophage. J. exp. Med. **135**, 21 (1972).

WOHLRAB, V. F., SCHMIDT, S.: Zur Verteilung der Isoenzyme der Laktatdehydrogenase in der Wand der Arteria Femoralis diabetischer und nichtdiabetischer Patienten. Dtsch. Gesundh.-Wes. **28**, 1350 (1973).

WOHLRAB, V. F., GÖTZE, J.: Laktat-Dehydrogenase-Isoenzyme in der Wand der Rattenaorta beim experimentellen Streptozotocin-Diabetes. Dtsch. Z. Verdau.- u. Stoffwechselkr. **34**, 53 (1974).

WOLINSKY, H., GOLDFISCHER, S., SCHILLER, B., KASAK, L. E.: Modification of the effects of hypertension on lysosomes and connective tissue in the rat aorta. Circulation Res. **34**, 233 (1974).

WOLINSKY, H., GOLDFISCHER, S., DALY, M. M., KASAK, L. E., COLTOFF-SCHILLER, B.: Arterial lysosomes and connective tissue in primate atherosclerosis and hypertension. Circulation Res. **36**, 553 (1975).

ZEMPLÉNYI, T., ROSENSTEIN, A. J.: Arterial enzymes and their relation to atherosclerosis in pigeons. Exp. molec. Path. **22**, 225 (1975 a).

ZEMPLÉNYI, T., ROSENSTEIN, A. J.: Elevation of arterial phosphofructokinase activity associated with susceptibility to atherosclerosis in pigeons. Atherosclerosis **21**, 167 (1975 b).

ZEMPLÉNYI, T., BLANKENHORN, D. H., ROSENSTEIN, A. J.: Inherited depression of arterial lipoamide dehydrogenase activity associated with susceptibility to atherosclerosis in pigeons. Circulation Res. **36**, 640 (1975).

ZILVERSMIT, D. B.: A proposal linking atherogenesis to the interaction of endothelial lipoprotein lipase with triglyceride-rich lipoproteins. Circulation Res. **33**, 633 (1973).

ZILVERSMIT, D. B.: Mechanisms of cholesterol accumulation in the arterial wall. Amer. J. Cardiol. **35**, 559 (1975).

CHAPTER 9

Hypolipidemic Agents

W. L. BENCZE

I. Introduction

Epidemiological studies have repeatedly shown that coronary heart disease tends to be associated with hyperlipemia. The typing of hyperlipemic states by FREDRICKSON et al. (1967) has been adopted, with a slight modification, by the World Health Organisation (cf. BEAUMONT et al., 1970). According to this classification, hyperlipoproteinemia may be characterized by abnormally high levels of plasma cholesterol or triglycerides, or both.

Hyperlipemic states concomitant with vascular atherosclerotic lesions can be produced in several species of experimental animals by the addition of cholesterol, saturated fats, or even certain plant fats to the diet.

From the clinical point of view KHACHADURIAN (1968) sketched the dramatic sequence of events that determine the fate of his young Lebanese patients with familial type II hyperlipoproteinemia. These unfortunate children exhibit marked hypercholesterolemia with xanthomas in their first decade of life. Angina pectoris becomes manifest in their teens followed by myocardial infarctions. The average life expectancy of these patients is 25 years.

It was therefore not surprising that the correction or normalization of the hyperlipemic state of patients with atherosclerosis was advocated as a reasonable approach toward arresting atherogenesis. Consequently, controlled long-term clinical studies have been planned, in which patients with ischemic heart disease in relatively early stages or survivors of one or more myocardial infarctions are being treated with hypolipidemic drugs.

Preliminary results of a few of these preventive trials suggest that hyperlipemia can be modified or corrected by the administration of hypolipidemic drugs. However, these clinical trials have hitherto failed to furnish any data that would be of use in devising effective therapeutic measures against coronary heart disease. Moreover, it appears that normalization of hyperlipidemia will not suffice to halt the spread of atherosclerotic lesions in the affected arteries. Nevertheless, partial success has been achieved: treatment with clofibrate has, in some patients at least, resulted in amelioration of angina pectoris, an accepted corollary of ischemic heart disease.

A thorough historical survey of about 200 hypolipidemic agents has been compiled by BENCZE et al. (1969). It is felt that for the purposes of the present volume a discussion of pharmacological and clinical studies undertaken during the past four years with a variety of hypolipidemic agents will be more fruitful than a long parade of old and new drugs.

Considering that both pharmacological and clinical studies have raised more questions than they have been able to answer, a survey of such reports can hardly be expected to dispel the obscurity surrounding the new epidemic called coronary heart disease, to which more and more young men are falling victim. However, this review may provide a few faint glimmers that eventually become just bright enough to disclose the paths toward an effective antiatherosclerotic therapy to those who are not discouraged by the present state of research into coronary heart disease.

II. The Coronary Drug Project

In 1967 a national collaborative study was launched in the United States to determine the efficacy of four hypolipidemic drugs in the long-term treatment of men with a history of one or more myocardial infarctions. It was planned that the study should include 8000 or more patients to afford statistically significant results. The primary end-point is survival. Clinical and laboratory data are analyzed during the projected five-year period. From 1965 to 1969 the 53 clinical centers participating recruited 8341 patients, who were randomly assigned to six groups.

Group 1.	Nicotinic acid	3.0 g/day
2.	Conjugated estrogens	2.5 mg/day
3.	Conjugated estrogens	5.0 mg/day
4.	Dextrothyroxine	6.0 mg/day
5.	Clofibrate	1.8 g/day
6.	Placebo	

A safety-monitoring committee systematically reviews the data bimonthly. By early 1970 this committee of the CORONARY DRUG PROJECT RESEARCH GROUP (1970) had noted that in the group receiving 5.0 mg/day of conjugated estrogens an excessive number of nonfatal myocardial infarctions, pulmonary embolisms, and instances of thrombophlebetis had occurred compared with that recorded in the placebo group. This regimen has therefore been discontinued. In a small group of patients with frequent ectopic heart beats in the resting EEG receiving treatment with dextrothyroxine, mortality has been somewhat higher than among similar patients on placebo. In this subgroup medication has been discontinued.

By the fall of 1971, with an average follow-up of 36 months, the accumulated data reviewed quarterly by the safety monitoring committee of the CORONARY DRUG PROJECT RESEARCH GROUP (1972) showed that 14.8% of the patients in the group receiving dextrothyroxine had died, compared with 12.5% in the placebo group. The absolute difference in the mortality rate between the two groups increased progressively with the duration of the medication. No significant sustained reduction in mortality was recorded in any of the subgroups receiving the dextrothyroxine medication. Therefore, dextrothyroxine administration has been discontinued for all patients.

As of 1 February 1973, with an average follow-up of 56 months, data on the low-dose (2.5 mg/day) estrogen group indicated no evidence of a beneficial therapeutic effect in terms of mortality from all causes. Rather there were adverse trends with this estrogen regimen, in the form of excess incidence of venous thromboembolism and excess mortality from cancer. The mean cholesterol level of the low-dose estrogen group was reduced slightly from the base line levels. However, serum triglyceride content increased with low-estrogen medication. Based on these findings the CORONARY DRUG PROJECT RESEARCH GROUP (1973) announced the discontinuation of the low-dose estrogen regimen.

Administration of the two remaining hypolipidemic drugs, nicotinic acid and clofibrate led to the completion of the Coronary Drug Project. The initial report on the findings of the therapeutic effect of these two drugs has been published by the CORONARY DRUG PROJECT RESEARCH GROUP (1975). In short, the staff members of the Project, most of them experienced and well-known cardiologists, concluded that there was no evidence on which to recommend the use of nicotinic acid, or clofibrate in the treatment of survivors of myocardial infarction or of persons with coronary heart disease, respectively. Comments on this issue will be made in the section concluding remarks.

The further aspect of this review will address itself to a survey of the status of research on hypolipidemic agents and their therapeutic effects.

III. Nicotinic Acid and Analogs

The trivial name of 3-pyridine-carboxylic acid is nicotinic acid. The compound is often called niacin in biology. Another designation is P-P (pellagra-preventive) factor. Nicotinic acid (1) has been listed among the water-soluble vitamins with a recommended daily dietary allowance of 15 and 18 mg for the adult human female and male, respectively. The daily requirement is influenced by the dietary intake of the essential amino acid tryptophan, 60 mg of which is considered to give rise to 1 mg of nicotinic acid.

The relative innocuousness of the nicotinoyl residue and its presence in the vital coenzymes nicotinamide adenine dinucleotide and nicotinamide adenine dinucleotide phosphate stimulated considerable pharmacological experimentation with nicotinic acid. Almost two decades ago ALTSCHUL et al. (1955) observed that the administration of large oral doses (3 g/day) of nicotinic acid resulted in a significant reduction of serum cholesterol level in man. Shortly thereafter an extensive clinical study of the hypolipidemic, antiatherosclerotic and hepatic effects of substance 1 was initiated at the Mayo Clinic. As a result, PARSONS JR. (1961) accumulated a great amount of clinical data which was influential in the selection of nicotinic acid as one of the four drugs currently under trial in the Coronary Drug Project.

CARLSON (1965) has shown that compound (1) is a powerful inhibitor of lipolysis. As a consequence of the inhibition of lipid mobilization from adipose tissue, the reduced hepatic inflow of free fatty acids diminishes the biosynthesis of lipoproteins. The decreased assembly of lipoproteins, in turn, affords an unused pool cholesterol in the liver, which is then excreted via the biliary tract. Sterol balance studies reported by MIETTINEN (1970) indicated that nicotinic acid increased cholesterol elimination in more than three-fourths of the patients with familial hypercholesterolemia. Serum cholesterol reduction and increased fecal neutral steroid excretion occurred even during a total fast, when the biosynthesis of cholesterol is suppressed. In the fed state the increment of elimination appeared to be partly compensated by stimulation of cholesterol synthesis. This view was supported by studies with ^{14}C-acetate-^{3}H-mevalonate mixture in man. According to Kritchevsky (1968) opinions as to whether nicotinic acid increases or decreases cholesterogenesis are almost equally divided.

It was suggested by Lassers et al. (1971) that plasma free fatty acids (FFA) can suppress the myocardial uptake of glucose, lactate, and pyruvate in man. This conclusion was supported by the observation that a reduction of arterial FFA concentration, such as can be achieved by the administration of nicotinic acid, caused increased myocardial extraction of glucose, pyruvate, and lactate. Suppression of blood FFA levels, as induced by nicotinic acid administration, may not be a simple, straightforward effect. Thus, Pereira and Mears (1971) reported that nicotinic acid given at a dose of 10 mg/kg i.v. to rats, caused an initial decrease in plasma FFA concentration, followed by a rise to markedly elevated levels. At a low dose of 1 mg/kg only the increase in FFA was observed. The authors reasoned that the biphasic effects were due to two separate and opposing effects on the rate of adipose tissue lipolysis. Nicotinic acid may stimulate ACTH secretion, which may be involved in the secondary rise of FFA levels. If ACTH is involved, a similar rebound effect of plasma FFA would not occur in man, because ACTH does not induce lipolysis in human adipose tissue.

The Scandinavian authors Nordoey and Roedset (1971) suggested that platelets in patients with hyperbetalipoproteinemia are adversely affected by their plasma lipoproteins. This interaction could increase the tendency to thrombosis and would be counteracted by nicotinic acid administration.

A long-term study of treatment of hypercholesterolemia with nicotinic acid has been reported by Charman et al. (1972). Some of the 160 patients have been followed up for more than a decade. The mean percentage decrease of serum cholesterol was 26%. Side effects were a definite deterrent to some users of nicotinic acid. Nevertheless, the authors considered that this drug is still of major importance in the therapy of hypercholesterolemia. Mosher (1970) reviewed the side effects and toxicity of large doses of nicotinic acid given to man. Gaut et al. (1971) reported that during administration of hypolipidemic doses of nicotinic acid to hyperlipemic patients, all subjects sustained increases in plasma uric acid levels, as well as in carbohydrate intolerance. Since plasma insulin levels increased along with glucose in nondiabetics,

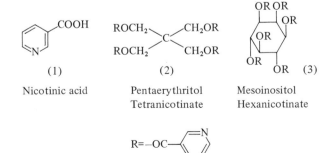

(1)	(2)	(3)
Nicotinic acid	Pentaerythritol Tetranicotinate	Mesoinositol Hexanicotinate

the data suggested that inhibition of insulin release was not the mechanism by which carbohydrate intolerance was produced or intensified. Renal clearance of plasma uric acid decreased by 50 to 75%. Hence, increases in plasma uric acid levels may be due to diminished renal clearance.

Nicotinic acid has been esterified with the purpose of prolonging its hypolipidemic activity. Moreover, the alcohol component may contribute its own share to the activity. Thus, BRATTSAND and LUNDHOLM (1971) reported that pentaerythritol tetranicotinate (2) tended to be more active than nicotinic acid (1) in reducing the lipid infiltrated area of the aorta in the cholesterol-fed rabbit. Serum cholesterol and triglyceride levels were also decreased. OLSSON et al. (1974) observed that administration of compound 2 in a daily dose of 3 g lowered serum cholesterol and triglyceride levels in patients with different types of hyperlipidemia. In contrast to nicotinic acid, substance 2 did cause an elevation of plasma uric acid concentration, but is was more effective than plain nicotinic acid in reducing elevated cholesterol levels. Sorbitol and myoinositol (mesoinositol) hexanicotinate (3) polyesters have been employed in the treatment of patients with atherosclerosis obliterans. BRATTGARD et al. (1966) reported that a considerable part of mesoinositol hexanicotinate (3) ciruculated unhydrolyzed in the blood of the cat. It should be noted here that esters of primary alcohols are generally rapidly hydrolyzed by intestinal lipases. However, the sterically hindered polyesters may escape enzymatic cleavage for a considerable length of time. Indeed, MATTSON and VOLPENHEIN (1972) observed that rat pancreatic lipase did not hydrolyze acylated polyols containing more than three ester groups, e.g. sorbitol hexaoleate.

Not only do some alcohols forming esters with niacin (1) impart novel features to the spectrum of biological properties of nicotinic acid, but even some bases merely associated as cations with the nicotinate anion may also alter the activity of nicotinic acid. BRENNER and BRENNER (1972) reported that the passage of glucose through the blood-brain barrier increased by 22% upon pretreatment of the rat with xanthinol nicotinate (4). Equimolar doses of the xanthinol base and nicotinic acid administered separately to the rat, showed only an insignificant influence on glucose transfer. Xanthinol nicotinate markedly increased the biosynthesis of adenosine nucleotides in the liver, myocardium, and brain of the rat.

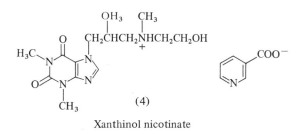

(4)

Xanthinol nicotinate

In another instance, SCHRAVEN et al. (1972) observed that resorption of ^{28}Magnesium from the alimentary tract of the rat was poor when ^{28}MgCl$_2$ was fed, but resorption of this important cation was considerably enhanced when ^{28}Mg nicotinate was given.

Chemical modifications of the structure of nicotinic acid have also been carried out in the search for analogs with enhanced activity and less toxicity. Some of these efforts are illustrated by the following examples.

The homologue of nicotinic acid, 3-pyridineacetic acid (5) has been evaluated as a hypolipidemic agent by Bizzi and Grossi (1961), who showed that compound 5 prevented triton-induced hypercholesterolemia in the rat more effectively than nicotinic acid. Two other Italian research groups, Preziosi et al. (1961), as well as Ratti and Defina (1959) found that substance 5 was comparable or superior to nicotinic acid as a hypolipidemic agent in experimental animals and man. Skidmore et al. (1971) observed that 3-pyridineacetic acid (5) and nicotinic acid (1) decreased lipolysis, adenylcyclase activity and cyclic AMP synthesis in a similar fashion. Compound 5 was introduced in Italy as a hypolipidemic drug in 1960 by Lepetit Co.

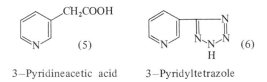

3−Pyridineacetic acid   3−Pyridyltetrazole

A prolongation of the duration of the hypolipidemic activity of nicotinic acid was achieved by the exchange of the carboxyl group for the tetrazole moiety. The single proton on a 5-substituted tetrazole ring and the proton of the carboxyl group exhibit comparable acidity. In several instances, e.g. plant growth regulators, anti-inflammatory compounds, etc., the biological activity was preserved by the exchange of the carboxyl substituent for the tetrazole group. Among 24 compounds containing the tetrazole function Holland and Pereira (1967) found that 5-(3-pyridyl)-tetrazole (6) depressed plasma FFA levels in the fasted dog most effectively, although compound 6 was a much weaker inhibitor of lipolysis *in vitro* than nicotinic acid. In addition, the activity persisted longer than that induced by compound 1. Pereira et al. (1968) reported that administration of substance 6 to man resulted in decreased levels of plasma cholesterol within 7 to 10 days of treatment. The close relationship between compounds 6 and 1 is also evident from the action of substance 6 on sugar metabolism. Thus, Gagliardino et al. (1972) demonstrated that the tetrazole derivative 6 stimulated glycogen synthesis in muscle *in vitro*.

Another way of masking a carboxyl group is its reduction to the primary alcohol function, which can then be oxidized to the carboxyl moiety in the living organism. Raaflaub (1966) was able to show, by way of a perfusion technique, that rat liver readily oxidized 3-pyridylcarbinol (7) to nicotinic acid. Moreover, the metabolic oxidation resulted in the prolongation of the hypocholesterolemic activity. Lengsfeld and Gey (1971) reported that oral administration of compound 7 to fasted rats resulted in a biphasic lowering of plasma cholesterol levels. There was a slight decrease of blood cholesterol concentration 5 hrs after administration and a second, more pronounced decrease 14 to 18 hrs thereafter. Both nicotinic acid and 3-pyridylcarbinol are able to extract cholesterol even from the slow-turnover pool. Zoellner and Wolfram (1970) reported that the size of xanthoma diminished in all patients during treatment with compounds 1 or 7.

The primary hydroxyl group of substance 7 lends itself to acylation to form esters. The acid component of the ester may also be a hypolipidemic agent in its own right. MARMO et al. (1971) found that the hypolipidemic effect of ester 8 was superior to that of 3-pyridylcarbinol or p-chlorophenoxyisobutyric acid (CPIB) in the rat, the dog, the cat, and the chicken.

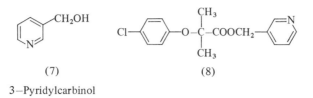

(7)   (8)

3–Pyridylcarbinol

Yet another way of masking the carboxyl group of nicotinic acid is its conversion to an amide function. HOLLAND and PEREIRA (1967) demonstrated that nicotinamide was about 10^{-4} times less active than nicotinic acid as an inhibitor of lipolysis. DALTON et al. (1970) confirmed this finding; however, they also observed hypolipidemic activity *in vivo* in the rat in response to a dose of nicotinamide only three times greater than the active dose of nicotinic acid. The *in vivo* activity of nicotinamide was considered to be due to metabolic deamination to nicotinic acid. Following this line of thought, BAILEY et al. (1972) prepared a number of compounds structurally related to nicotinic acid. These substances were designed to afford nicotinic acid upon metabolic deamination, oxidation, or hydrolysis. Three representative compounds 9 to 11, are recorded here. All three substances reduced serum levels of free fatty acids in the rat and were practically as active as nicotinic acid. The data obtained in this study suggests that the hypocholesterolemic and hypotriglyceridemic activity of these compounds depended on their metabolic conversion to nicotinic acid. It was concluded that such chemical modifications of nicotinic acid would probably offer no clinical advantage over the parent drug.

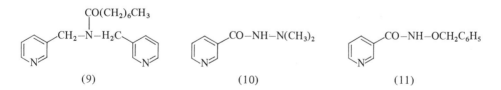

(9)   (10)   (11)

The positional isomers of nicotinic acid, 4-pyridine-carboxylic (isonicotinic) acid and 2-pyridine-carboxylic (picolinic) acid, are known to be very weak inhibitors of lipolysis. Hexahydro-2-pyridine-carboxylic (pipecolic) acid (12) has been reported by FREYSS-BEGUIN et al. (1970) to cause a rise in serum free fatty acids (FFA). Substitution of the heterocyclic ring of compounds 1 and 7 preserved the antilipolytic activity. CARLSON et al. (1969) and (1972) reported that esters derived from 5-fluoronicotinic acid (13) and the corresponding carbinol (14) inhibited mobilization of serum FFA in the dog. ROWE et al. (1973) studied the effect of 5-fluoro-3-hydroxymethylpyridine (14) on the raised plasma FFA levels in patients after myocardial infarction. The compound was given orally to the patients in doses of 200 mg every two hrs and found to maintain a sustained reduction of the elevated plasma FFA levels. Unlike nicotinic acid substance 14 rarely produced flushing and showed no significant hemodynamic effects. HAMILTON et al. (1971) found that 2-hydroxy-nicotinic acid (15) was about ten times more active than nicotinic acid in inhibiting both fatty acid and cholesterol biosynthesis in rat liver. 2-Chloro-6-hydroxynicotinic acid (16) was found to be the most active inhibitor of fatty acid biosynthesis among 30 derivatives of nicotinic acids tested. However, compound 16 was less active than nicotinic acid in blocking the biosynthesis of cholesterol.

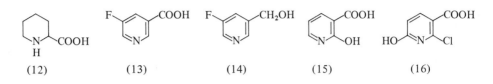

(12)   (13)   (14)   (15)   (16)

IV. Pyrazoles and Isoxazoles

The heterocyclic carboxylic acids 17 to 19 resemble nicotinic acid in their capacity to inhibit lipolysis. The prospects of these acids proving suitable for clinical use are poor. PEREIRA and HOLLAND (1967) found that repeated administration of acid 17 to dogs and rats for several days resulted in a loss of effect on plasma FFA. This resistance took 2 days to develop in the rat. The resistant animals regained the ability to respond to compound 17 after a 3-day rest period. Nicotinic acid did not induce resistance, but was ineffective in reducing plasma FFA levels in rats rendered resistant to substance 17. Development of similar tachyphylaxis to the antilipolytic activity of acid 19 has been observed by GERRITSEN and DULIN (1967). An intact pituitary adrenal system is required in the induction of the resistance.

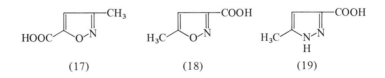

(17)   (18)   (19)

TAMASI et al. (1968) reported that nicotinic acid reduced serum cholesterol concentration in normal rats, but compound 19 had an effect in alloxan-treated rats only. HOLLOBAUGH et al. (1967) suggested that the mechanism of the lipolytic action of acid 19 was similar to that of nicotinic acid. Interesting aspects of the mechanism of action of the heterocyclic acids 1, as well as 17 to 19 were discussed by SCHWABE and EBERT (1969), who observed that these acids did not increase the activity of purified phosphodiesterase unless adipose tissue homogenate was also present in the incubation medium. Phosphodiesterase inhibited by theophylline could be fully reactivated by the addition of acid 18. Another feature of acid 18 was emphasized by KUPIECKI (1970), who observed that lipolysis in adipose tissue obtained from rats treated orally with acid 18 was increased in relation to lipolysis in tissue from untreated rats. This paradoxical stimulation of lipolysis depends upon an intact pituitary adrenal system.

The carboxylic acids 17 to 19 display a more pronounced hypoglycemic activity than nicotinic acid. LOTTI and VEZZOSI (1972) found that several analogs of acid 19 were more active hypoglycemic agents than tolbutamide. The antilipolytic and anti-diabetic action of compounds 17 and 19 has been reviewed by HOLCOMB (1969).

V. Diethyl Chelidonate

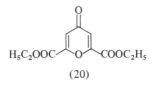

$$H_5C_2OOC \quad \quad COOC_2H_5$$

(20)

A novel inhibitor of lipolysis has been announced by ZAMPAGLIONE et al. (1970), who noted that lipolysis in rat epididymal fat pads induced by ACTH, norepinephrine, isoproterenol, theophylline or dibutyryl cyclic AMP, was inhibited by diethyl chelidonate 20. Chelidonic acid is a natural compound that has been obtained from the herb celandine (Chelidonium majus). A simple synthesis of chelidonic acid has been described by RIEGEL and ZWILGMEYER (1943).

It seems appropriate at this stage to discuss the mode of action of several natural and synthetic substances capable of altering the hormonal regulation of lipolysis. The following section is devoted to this aspect of lipid metabolism.

VI. The Role of the Second Messenger in Lipolysis

Whenever hormones elicit a fast reaction at their target tissues, it is considered that the rapidity of the response generally involves equally fast changes in the levels of intracellular cyclic AMP. Thus, in the case of lipolysis in adipose tissue, catecholamines, ACTH, TSH, LH and glucagon can all act as first messengers. Upon arrival at the outer surface of the adipocyte, these first messengers stimulate the membrane-bound enzyme system, known as adenyl cyclase. This enzyme system converts ATP to cyclic AMP and releases it at the inner side of the cell membrane. Cyclic AMP, also called the second messenger, in turn sets the internal cellular machinery into motion. In the case of the adipocyte the intracellular enzymes activated by cyclic AMP consist of a triglyceride lipase interlinked with a complex phosphorylase system. Experiments done by CORBIN and KREBS (1969), CORBIN et al. (1970), and HUTTUNEN et al. (1970) suggest that the activation of lipase in the adipose tissue involves a cascade of enzymatic reactions of protein kinases, illustrating the selectivity and amplification that is an essential part of the second messenger concept. It appears that similar systems govern the release of metabolic fuel from glycogen deposited in liver or muscle, and from the fat stores in adipose tissue.

Having served its purpose, cyclic AMP is inactivated by intracellular phosphodiesterase, whereupon the actions of both the first and second messengers are brought to a halt. Consequently, inhibitors of phosphodiesterase capable of penetrating the cell will prolong the life of cyclic AMP and thus act as stimulators of lipolysis in adipose tissue.

SUTHERLAND (1972) emphasized in his Nobel lecture, that the discovery of cyclic AMP made it possible to study hormonal activity at the molecular level experimentally. Thus, KLAINER et al. (1962) have shown that epinephrine-induced lipolysis generates cyclic AMP even in a cell-free preparation of adipose tissue. In a similar fashion, VAUGHAN and MURAD (1968) demonstrated that the polypeptide lipolytic hormones did the same. While there seems to be a direct relationship between the action of the first and second messengers in the stimulation of lipolysis, the sequence of events taking place during the inhibition of lipolysis is very complex. Although there seems to be little doubt that the antilipolytic effect of insulin is mediated by a decrease of cyclic AMP levels, this could only be demonstrated in intact adipose tissue. Insulin has not lowered adenyl cyclase activity in cell-free preparations under varied experimental conditions tried by BUTCHER (1971). Unraveling the chain of events taking place in the cyclic AMP mediated antilipolytic action of insulin remains an urgent task, essential in the design of new therapeutic measures for the treatment of hyperlipidemia, obesity, and atherosclerosis.

The most prominent effect of insulin, the stimulation of glucose entry into peripheral cells, appears to be independent of cyclic AMP mediation, as was asserted by SNEYD et al. (1968).

An intriguing feature of cyclic AMP mediated stimulation of lipolysis in adipose tissue is its species specificity. BRAUN and HECHTER (1970) provided evidence that ACTH induced lipolysis in adipose tissue from adult rabbits, but catecholamines failed to do so. In rat adipose tissue both ACTH and epinephrine are active stimulators, while in human and canine adipose tissue the catecholamines are effective and ACTH is not, as was reported by CARLSON et al. (1970).

VII. Catecholamines, Adrenergic Blocking Agents

It has been known for many years that the sympathetic nervous system plays an important role in the regulation of lipid mobilization, transport, deposition, and oxidation. Injection of epinephrine causes a prompt rise in plasma free fatty acid (FFA) concentrations in the dog, the rat, the sheep, the monkey, and man. Continuous infusion of epinephrine, however, merely produces a temporary rise in plasma FFA, most probably due to the concomitant hyperglycemia also produced by this hormone. Hyperglycemia results in the release of insulin which in turn decreases the plasma FFA levels. Norepinephrine, on the other hand, produces a sustained increase in plasma FFA upon infusion, because it exerts only a slight effect on hepatic glycogenolysis, as was reported by HAVEL (1964).

Isoproterenol (21), a synthetic sympathomimetic agent also has a potent effect in elevating plasma FFA values in man, as was demonstrated by BRUCE et al. (1961). It was AHLQUIST (1948) who suggested that the sympathetic effector cells that showed the greatest sensitivity to isoproterenol (21) possessed beta receptors. In contrast, the effector cells most sensitive to epinephrine were said to possess alpha receptors. Subsequently, isoproterenol became known as the eminently pure beta-adrenergic stimulant. Upon administration of 25 mg/kg of isoproterenol (21) to rats for two days, LEON et al. (1971) found that this beta adrenergic agent caused infarct-like myocardial lesions at the apex of the heart. Prolonged infusion of norepinephrine also produced such lesions. It appears that cardiac damage and an excessive concentrations of catecholamines in the heart go hand in hand. Nevertheless, short-term use of inotropic agents is still being practised clinically in cardiac shock. MUELLER et al. (1972) studied the action of isoproterenol (21) and norepinephrine in 21 patients who were in shock due to acute myocardial infarction. Isoproterenol improved coronary blood flow. However, after an initial improvement, the hemodynamics tended to deteriorate. Norepinephrine improved the cardiac index, though oxygen extraction from coronary blood remained high. With respect to myocardial lactate metabolism, the two catecholamines caused opposite effects. Isoproterenol induced myocardial lactate production, while norepinephrine induced the heart to extract lactate from the blood. The authors stressed that the normal heart extracts lactate from the blood and functions as an aerobic oxidative organ. In severe hypoxia, however, the heart resorts to the additional utilization of the small amount of anaerobic energy it gains from the oxidation of NADH to NAD by the linked reduction of pyruvate to lactate. Consequently, norepinephrine normalizes lactate metabolism in the heart and isoproterenol (21) deteriorates it.

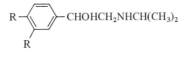

$$R-C_6H_3(R)-CHOHCH_2NHCH(CH_3)_2$$

R=OH, Isoproterenol   (21)
R=Cl, Dichloroisoproterenol (22)

    The normal heart responds promptly and forcefully to adrenergic stimulation, as is evidenced by exertional or emotional tachycardia. The ischemic heart, however, experiences difficulty in coping with the work load imposed upon it by exertion. Hence, there was reason to suppose that benefit might accrue from selective cardiac beta receptor blockade, especially in patients with angina pectoris. Indeed, cervical sympathectomy afforded a marked to moderate improvement in exercise tolerance in about half of the anginal subjects. LINDGREN (1950) has reviewed the results of this surgical procedure.
    The medicinal chemist responded to the challenge. The aim was to replace the surgeon's scalpel by drugs which would selectively inhibit cardiac catecholamine activity. Many of the early problems and pitfalls associated with the predictive value of tests of such drugs in the animal in relation to their clinical usefulness were discussed in an informal fashion at a symposium at the CIBA Foundation by BLACK (1967). In the laboratories of the I.C.I. a great number of β-adrenergic blocking agents have been developed. Four of these substances may be regarded as milestones in the advancement of our knowledge about adrenergic mechanisms. Dichloroisoproterenol (22) almost completely abolished the increase in plasma FFA produced by isoproterenol in the dog. MAYER et al. (1961) also observed that in small doses this agent caused a rise in plasma FFA, due to its residual adrenergic agonist activity. The first effective agent discovered was pronethalol (23). It was introduced into clinical trial specifically for the study of the prevention of catecholamine effects on the heart. Later, it was found to cause lymphomata in mice and was replaced by propranolol (24). The next step was the development of a cardioselective agent that

would antagonize the effect of catecholamines in the heart only. The screening procedures employed in the search for such an agent have been discussed by Fitz-Gerald (1971), and the result of the search was practolol (25). Another widely used β adrenergic blocking agent, oxprenolol (26), was developed by Wilhelm et al. (1967). The profile of the biological activity of compound 26, as well as of several analogs, has been evaluated by Brunner et al. (1971).

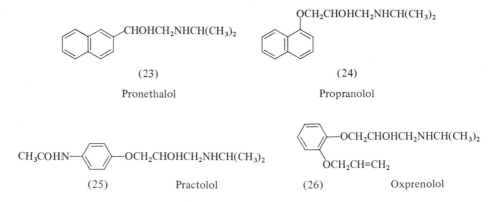

(23)

Pronethalol

(24)

Propranolol

(25)   Practolol

(26)   Oxprenolol

The further discussion of the β-adrenergic blocking agents will be restricted to the effects of the three compounds 24 to 26. Maroko et al. (1971) demonstrated that in experimental myocardial infarction the infarcted area was increased by the administration of isoproterenol (21) and decreased by the administration of propranolol (24). The negative chronotropic effect of the β-adrenergic blocking agents may be most beneficial in the treatment of patients with coronary heart disease. Berkson et al. (1970) found that in a cohort of 1329 men, resting heart rates over 80 appeared to be a risk factor, independent of the other major risk factors of ischemic heart disease, such as age, hyperlipidemia, hypertension, etc. Angina pectoris, a generally recognized warning sign of atherosclerotic coronary arteries, is the main indication for the use of β blocking agents. In a double-blind assessment and comparison with placebo, Sharma et al. (1971) noted that both compounds 24 and 26 produced an amelioration of symptoms in patients with angina pectoris. Prichard and Gillam (1971) reported that maximum benefit was obtained with an average dose of 417 mg/day of propranolol (24) in the treatment of angina pectoris. It was hoped that the new agents 25 and 26 would show activity at lower doses.

The effectiveness of oxprenolol (26) in angina pectoris was clearly established in a well-controlled study by Wilson et al. (1969). Forrest (1972) observed that oxprenolol reduced the number of anginal attacks even in patients who failed to respond to treatment with propranolol (24). The cardioselective agent, practolol (25) has been found to be a valuable drug in patients with angina pectoris by Areskog and Adolfson (1969) and by Nestel (1972). Lambert (1972) noted that there seemed to be a lower incidence of both fatal and nonfatal myocardial infarction in groups of patients taking the drugs 24 to 26.

Opinions about the hypolipidemic activity of the β-adrenergic blocking agents are divided. Lloyd-Mostyn et al. (1971) reported that the oral administration of 40/ mg/day of compounds 24 to 26 for 14-day periods to patients with hyperlipidemia had no significant effect on serum triglyceride and cholesterol levels. WEGENER et al. (1969), however, found that the long-term administration of compound 24 caused a sustained reduction of serum lipids, which was especially marked with respect to triglycerides in patients with hyperkinetic cardiac syndrome. Interruption of the administration of the drug regularly led to a marked rise in serum lipid levels. PALONKANGAS and VIHKO (1971) gave propranolol in a dose of 12.5 mg/kg i.p. to titmice and observed a rise in the plasma concentrations of palmitic acid and C_{18}-unsaturated fatty acids. There is no doubt, however, that catecholamine-induced elevations of plasma FFA are consistently inhibited by β-adrenergic blockers. TAGGART and CARRUTHERS (1972) showed that an oral dose of 40 mg of oxprenolol (26), given 1 hr before a racing car drive, suppressed the usual stress-induced rise in plasma FFA, blood glucose, and tachycardia, previously demonstrated in the same racing drivers in the absence of β blockade.

Other metabolic effects of the β-adrenergic blocking agents may also contribute to their beneficial action in patients with atherosclerotic heart disease. MANCHESTER and SHELBURNE (1972) assume that the efficacy of propranolol (24) in angina pectoris may be due, in part, to an increase in myocardial oxygen supply resulting from the decrease in hemoglobin–oxygen affinity caused by the drug. PONARI et al. (1972) observed that oxprenolol (26) markedly activated plasma fibrinolysis in man, while both antipodes of propranolol (24) were inactive in this respect.

Although the β-adrenergic blocking agents are the most selective inhibitors of lipolysis in adipose tissue, they are considerably less active than the non-specific inhibitors of cyclic AMP-mediated lipolysis. BUTCHER (1971) indicated the following order of potencies: insulin and the prostaglandins lower cyclic AMP levels at a concentration of 10^{-10} to 10^{-9}, nicotinic acid at 10^{-7} and the β-blocking agent 24 at 10^{-6} to 10^{-5} in rat adipose tissue. This order of activity may not be the same in man, because WENKE (1970) asserted that the affinity of propranolol (24) for human adipose tissue was one hundred times greater than its affinity for the adipose tissue of the rat.

A thorough study of the metabolic interactions of catecholamines, lipids, and carbohydrates in the heart is a prerequisite for the design of drugs causing inhibition or reversal of the damaging action of accumulated catecholamines in the myocardium. ARNOLD (1972) has reviewed the pharmacological data obtained from the study of the adrenergic blocking agents. It has been suggested that lipolysis and calorigenesis is regulated by β^1 receptors and lactacidemia by the β^2 receptors. RODBELL (1970) discusses the complex nature of the receptor sites and suggests that there are six differently structured discriminators on the cell membrane. These discriminators, which are proteins, selectively attract the first messengers. Between the discriminator and the enzyme system, adenyl cyclase, there is a coupling unit, the transducer, which contains lipids. Removal of these lipids results in a loss of the action induced by the first messenger. LEFKOWITZ and LEVEY (1972) assert that such a coupling unit isolated from a solubilized preparation of cat ventricular myocardium consists of a distinct phospholipid.

The presence of both α- and β-adrenergic receptors in human coronary vessels has been demonstrated by ANDERSSON et al. (1972). These authors argue that β blockade will increase the vasoconstricting action of the α receptors in the coronary vessels. This indirect stimulation of the alpha receptors may be the cause of the increased lactate/pyruvate ratio and the lowered oxygen content in the coronary venous blood. Therefore, a combination of α- and β-adrenergic blockade may be desirable. In order to avoid excessive reduction of the blood pressure a selective α-blocking agent acting on the coronary vessels only would have to be used.

Another challenging idea was put forward by GILLIS and MELVILLE (1972), who presented evidence that in experimental coronary atherosclerosis in the rabbit the response of the myocardium to norepinephrine-induced stimulation of heart rate and coronary flow is greatly diminished. The epinephrine content of the atherosclerotic hearts was greater than that of normal hearts. The authors concluded that the problem in the atherosclerotic heart was not one of inhibition, but of resensitization to catecholamines. Such a sensitization of the myocardium to catecholamines can be achieved by drugs. BLACK (1967) described experimentally induced sudden death of dogs in a lecture delivered at a CIBA symposium. He gave an oral dose of 200 mg/kg of a guanidine derivative to dogs. The animals bounded about friskily, tails wagging, for 90 to 150 min and then literally dropped dead. After considerable work, the author found out that death had been due to ventricular fibrillation and a "tremendous" sensitization of the myocardium to catecholamines. Unfortunately, he did not mention the possibility of less dramatic sensitization occurring in response to lower doses of the drug.

Investigations over the years 1968 to 1974 have gone far to confirm the original expectations of BLACK (1967) that β-adrenergic blockade would reduce the consumption of oxygen by the ischemic myocardium. Reduction of oxygen consumption has a similar net effect as an increment in oxygen supply of the heart. Thus, MUELLER et al. (1974) presented evidence that myocardial oxygenation and metabolic abnormalities associated with acute transmural myocardial infarction improved in 20 patients following administration of propranolol (24), 0.1 mg/kg i.v. Patients exhibiting signs of left ventricular failure were excluded from the study.

Incorporation of the β-blocking agents into the realm of the hypolipidemic agents is still a controversial issue. However, there is no doubt about the interference of these agents with the metabolism of lipids. Startling observations are often recorded. FABIAN et al. (1973) reported that a 2 mg/kg dose of propranolol lowered the plasma FFA levels in mice after an electric foot shock, but a dose of 10 mg/kg did not. TAGGART et al. (1973) studied the hypolipidemic activity of oxprenolol (26) in 8 normal and 7 coronary subjects. Under the stress of speaking before an audience increases in plasma FFA levels were found. A single oral dose of 40 mg oxprenolol abolished or decreased this stress-induced increments of FFA. Blood cholesterol concentrations remained unchanged, while there were variable increases in plasma triglyceride levels. WHITTINGTON-COLEMAN et al. (1973) observed that administration of propranolol (24), 5 mg/kg/day in the diet of cholesterol-fed rabbits profoundly reduced the fat deposition along the intimal layer and inside the endothelial cells of the aortae, while increasing the serum cholesterol levels twofold. This finding suggests that some factor other than serum cholesterol concentration may be responsible for the intimal development of the atheromatous plaques. WEXLER (1973) induced massive myocardial infarction in rats by subcutaneous injections of high doses of isoproterenol (21). Animals pretreated with 10 mg/kg of propranolol manifested significantly less cardiac necrosis, less excursion of serum triglycerides, FFA, and total cholesterol than animals that received isoproterenol only. However, the necrosis-protecting effects of propranolol were marred by an increase in blood urea nitrogen (BUN), persistance of fatty liver, and a shift in the output of less glucocorticoids and more mineralocorticoids from the adrenal cortex.

Propranolol treatment of 8 patients with high fasting plasma triglyceride levels and type IV hyperlipoproteinemia and of 6 normal subjects disclosed an unusual derangement in the lipid metabolism of the type IV hyperlipidemic patients. BARBORIAK and FRIEDBERG (1973) showed that a meal containing 60 g of fat caused an equal rise in plasma triglyceride levels 6 hr postprandially in both the normolipemic and hyperlipemic (type IV) subjects. Pretreatment with propranolol for two weeks resulted in a cut of the postprandial rise of triglycerides into half in the normolipemic subjects. In contrast, the 8 patients with elevated fasting triglyceride levels and type IV hyperlipoproteinemia exhibited a twofold enhancement of the alimentary lipemic response after the 2-week treatment with propranolol.

Next the study of the activity of the combination of a β-adrenergic blocking agent with hypolipidemic agents commenced. LIPSON et al. (1971) were able to show that the combined administration of propranolol (24) and nicotinic acid (1) to dogs resulted in an effective depression of serum triglyceride and FFA levels, at doses sufficiently low to reduce the risks of side effects materially. Treatment of type IV hyperlipemic patients with a combination of niacin and propranolol in very low doses has been usefully employed by AVOGARO et al. (1974).

VIII. Miscellaneous Inhibitors of Lipolysis

A novel and powerful inhibitor of lipolysis, phenylisopropyl adenosine (27) has been announced by BIECK et al. (1969). When injected intraperitoneally in a dose of 4 µg/kg, compound 27 was found to be 20 times more active than adenosine and 500 times more active than nicotinic acid, as an inhibitor off lipid mobilization in fasting rats. The L-form was 70 times more active than the D-form. MAY and LEINWEBER (1971) observed that serum FFA levels in human volunteers were reduced by 40 to 50% after the administration of substance 27. Total lipids, however, were only lowered in hyperlipidemic patients. WESTERMANN and STOCK (1970) suggested that phenylisopropyl adenosine (27) inhibited lipolysis by hindering the binding of ATP to the adenyl cyclase enzyme system.

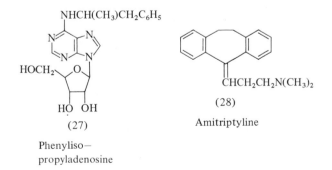

(27)

Phenyliso—
propyladenosine

(28)

Amitriptyline

The complex nature of adipose tissue lipolysis is demonstrated by the action of the tricyclic antidepressant drug amitriptyline (28). Despite increasing the intracellular concentration of cyclic AMP in the isolated fat cell, amitriptyline markedly inhibited lipolysis caused by DL-norepinephrine and theophylline, as has been reported by LOVRIEN et al. (1972).

IX. The Prostaglandins

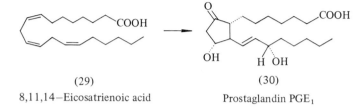

(29)
8,11,14–Eicosatrienoic acid

(30)
Prostaglandin PGE$_1$

Very potent antilipolytic agents are the prostaglandins. They are C_{20} carboxylic acids derived from essential fatty acids. Thus 8,11,14-eicosatrienoic acid (29) is converted by a series of enzymic reactions to the prostaglandin PGE$_1$ (30). The most typical step of this biogenetic synthesis is the formation of a new carbon–carbon bond between carbon atoms 8 and 12 of arachidonic acid which furnishes the characteristic skeleton of the prostaglandins. In most of the tissues where prostaglandins are active they cause an increase in cyclic AMP levels, most probably by activating adenyl cyclase. SHIO et al. (1971) noted that prostaglandins can also be identified with decreased intracellular cyclic AMP levels, inhibition of lipolysis, or inhibition of pancreatic secretion. Even at high concentrations, PGE$_1$ (30) inhibits hormone stimulated lipolysis only to the extent of about 50%. In contrast, the β blocking agents can cause complete inhibition. PGE$_1$ does not inhibit basal lipolysis in rabbits, but does so in rats. WEEKS (1971) has reviewed the metabolic actions of the prostaglandins.

CARLSON et al. (1968) showed that PGE$_1$ (30) increased arterial plasma levels of FFA in fasting human subjects. This effect of PGE$_1$ is intriguing because *in vitro* it exhibits a potent inhibitory action on lipolysis. A possible explanation of the opposite effects of PGE$_1$ on lipolysis *in vitro* and *in vivo* was offered by EFENDIC (1970), who suggested that in man PGE$_1$ blocks the α adrenergic receptors more effectively *in vivo*. Inhibition of the α receptors in human adipose tissue induces lipolysis.

ILLIANO and CUATRECASAS (1971) regard endogenous prostaglandins as modulators of lipolytic processes in adipose tissue. A specific stimulus initiates prostaglandin synthesis and release in the adipocyte following exposure to lipolytic agents. It appears that the rise in the endogenous levels of prostaglandins mediates a negative feedback control of cyclic AMP concentration in the adipose tissue.

Although most of the research into prostaglandins is directed toward the development of drugs for fertility control, the treatment of respiratory ailments, etc., it is certain that these studies will also result in a greater understanding of lipid metabolism.

X. Thyroid Hormones

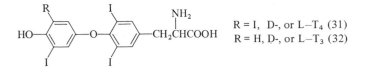

$$R = I, \quad D\text{-, or } L\text{-}T_4 \ (31)$$
$$R = H, \quad D\text{-, or } L\text{-}T_3 \ (32)$$

Clinical observations have established that in myxedema, a hypothyroid state, there is usually a rise in plasma cholesterol level, which is then rapidly reduced after administration of thyroxine (31). The converse condition, thyrotoxicosis may be attended by a plasma concentration of cholesterol that is lower than normal. It has been suggested that thyroid deficiency impairs the catabolism of cholesterol to a greater extent than its biosynthesis, so that hypercholesterolemia is the necessary consequence.

Synthetic thyroxine has been available since 1949. The synthetic racemate has been resolved to afford the natural levorotatory antipode (L-T_4), and the unnatural dextrorotatory form (D-T_4).

The COUNCIL ON DRUGS of the American Medical Association (1969) noted that D-T_4 tended to concentrate more in the liver and kidneys of the rat, while the natural antipode L-T_4, in the same dose, was more evenly distributed in various organs. This may be the reason, why the hepatic accumulation of D-T_4 enhances oxidative elimination of cholesterol in relation to its calorigenic effect. The hypocholesterolemic activity of D-T_4 is about 20% of that of L-T_4, whereas its calorigenic activity is only 5 to 10% as great. Because of this favorable ratio of the hypocholesterolemic to the calorigenic dose, the dextrorotatory isomer has been selected as the drug of choice by several clinical groups for the treatment of hypercholesterolemia associated with coronary heart disease.

BECHTOL and WARNER (1969) analyzed the clinical data relating to more than 6000 patients treated with dextrothyroxine foe an average pariod of 12 months. The authors observed a significant reduction of plasma cholesterol levels in response to a daily dose of 2 to 6 mg of D-T_4. The mortality rate among the treated patients was considered not to be higher than anticipated. PARSONS (1965), however, questioned the usefulness of thyroxine administration in the treatment of hyperlipidemia. He stressed that D-T_4 increased the frequency of angina and sudden death among the treated patients. The CORONARY DRUG PROJECT Research Group (1972) arrived at the same conclusion and instituted the discontinuance of dextrothyroxine administration to all patients in the D-T_4 group.

Several industrial sponsors have planned clinical trials with dextrotriiodothyronine, D-T_3 (32). Since L-T_3 is 5 times as active as L-T_4 in the goiter prevention test in rats, it appeared that the hypocholesterolemic potency of D-T_3 was also greater than that of D-T_4. However, in consideration of the fate of dextrothyroxine in the Coronary Drug Project, convincing experimental data may now be necessary to prove that D-T_3 is free of the inherent cardiotoxic effects of D-T_4.

In the course of the past decade, the direct action of thyroxine (41) upon the heart has been the concern of a number of research groups. VAUGHAN (1967) came to the conclusion that thyroxine alone seemed to have little or no effect on lipolysis, but enhanced epinephrine induced lipolysis in the intact fat pads of rats. The situation in the myocardium, however, may be quite different from that in the adipocyte. LEVEY and EPSTEIN (1969) furnished evidence that there may be at least two separate adenyl cyclase systems in the heart, one responsive to norepinephrine and the other to thyroid hormone. The β-adrenergic blocking agent propranolol (24) abolished the norepinephrine induced activation of myocardial adenyl cyclase, but failed to alter the activation caused by L-T$_4$. A similar conclusion was recorded by McDEWITT et al. (1968), who studied the differences in heart rate between hyperthyroid and hypothyroid patients. They stressed that thyroxine is acting directly on the heart and not via potentiation of the action of catecholamines. In an electronmicroscopical study KOBAYASHI (1969) described and illustrated the arteriosclerotic lesions in the rabbit aorta induced by simultaneous intravenous injection of L-T$_4$ and epinephrine. SIMONS and MYANT (1974) suggested that the deleterious cardiac effects of D-T$_4$ can be eliminated when propranolol (24) is administered in combination with D-T$_4$. They reported that mobilization of cholesterol from the tissues and increased faecal excretion of endogenous steroids resulted in type II patients during treatment with D-T$_4$ combined with propranolol (24).

The last word about the value of thyroxine therapy in atheroslcerosis may not yet have been said. BARNESS (1972) claimed that in a 20-year study among more than 1500 patients maintained with physiological doses of thyroid hormone, new cases of coronary disease were rare when compared to the incidence found in the Framingham study. The maximum safe dose of levothyroxine was estimated to be 0.2 mg. He cautioned that the use of 6 mg D-T$_4$ in the Coronary Drug Project may have been dangerously high for patients with coronary disease.

Studies on experimental animals tendend to suggest that both L-T$_4$ and D-T$_4$ may be capable of arresting atherogenesis. KRITCHEVSKY et al. (1968) reported that administration of thyroxine to cholesterol-fed rabbits inhibited development of atherosclerosis.

The number of the advocators of thyroxine therapy in hyperlipemia associated with coronary heart disease appears to be dwindling. Those who persist will have to furnish evidence that low doses of thyroid hormones are free of cardiotoxicity and still elicit hypolipidemic or antiatherogenic response.

XI. Estrogens, Progestagens, Anabolic and Androgenic Compounds

For a long time it was believed that there was an inverse correlation between ovarian activity and atherogenesis. This view was supported by the repeated observations that estrogens lowered serum cholesterol levels in experimental animals, as well as in patients with hypercholesterolemia.

FURMAN (1969) analyzed clinical statistical data and found that the ratio of male/ female death rates from coronary artery disease in the United States is about 8/1 for whites at the age of 40. After this age the acceleration of coronary artery disease mortality in men diminishes. Inspection of the semilogarithmic plot of the mortality rate against age for men suggests that there may be two subgroups within the male population, one of them being highly vulnerable to death from coronary heart disease at an early age. In coincidence with the shrinking of this sizeable pool of heart attack candidates, the male and female death rates approach each other. On the other hand, the semilogarithmic plot of mortality rate against age for females is a straight line with no inflection at the age of the onset of the menopause. TRACY (1966) derived an equation from statistical data describing the death rates from atherosclerotic heart disease in the U.S. white female. The conclusion from this mathematical study was that estrogens have no protective influence whatsoever on coronary heart disease.

The statistical studies point to the presence of serious derangements in the enzymatic and hormonal regulation of the vascular system in the vulnerable white male subgroup, rather than to the existence of an estrogen-mediated protective effect in the female.

The following three long-term studies, which were completed a decade ago, may illustrate the influence of estrogen treatment on the course of ischemic heart disease.

OLIVER and BOYD (1961) selected 100 men with a history of myocardial infarction. Half of the men received 0.2 mg ethynyl estradiol (33) daily for five years. The remaining 50 patients constituted the control group. In the treatment group, there was a 33% fall in serum cholesterol levels but also 10 fatal myocardial infarctions, 9 episodes of thrombophlebetis, and 5 episodes of cerebral thrombosis, compared with 10, 4, and 1, respectively, in the control group.

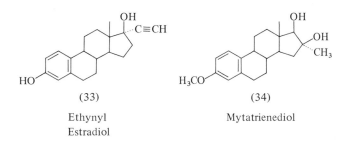

(33)   (34)

Ethynyl   Mytatrienediol
Estradiol

MARMORSTON et al. (1962) studied the effects of three estrogen preparations: a) premarin, a mixture of conjugated equine estrogens, b) ethynyl estradiol (33) and c) mytatrienediol (34) on the survival rate of male patients with a history of myocardial infarction. Premarin administration improved survival, particularly in the first two years of treatment. The other two estrogens had no effect on survival. There was no correlation between alteration of the serum lipids and survival.

STAMLER et al. (1963) administered premarin to patients with coronary heart disease. It appeared that the poor-risk patients benefited most from the treatment. An unexpected number of deaths occurred in the first two months of the study among those men who started at the high dose of 10 mg of premarin within three months of their most recent infarction.

In none of these three studies were the triglycerides measured. In the meantime it has been established that estrogen administration results in an elevation of the serum triglyceride levels. GLUECK et al. (1972) reviewed the hypertriglyceridemic effect of estrogens an oral contraceptive regimens.

OLIVER (1969) concluded that in view of the inevitable feminizing side effects and the triglyceride elevating effect, the prospects of estrogen treatment of patients with

atherosclerosis appeared to be poor. The Safety Monitoring Committee of the COR-
ONARY DRUG PROJECT Research Group (1970) requested discontinuation of
the regimen 5 mg/day of conjugated estrogens because of toxic side effects. The
2.5 mg/day regimen was still continuing in 1972.

The worldwide acceptance of the estrogen–progestogen oral contraceptive regimen induced numerous investigators to study the influence of the synthetic anovulatory hormones on lipid metabolism. In general, increases in plasma triglyceride
levels have been reported in healthy women taking a variety of oral contraceptives.

HAZZARD et al. (1969) demonstrated that the estrogen component alone appears
sufficient to cause hypertriglyceridemia. GLUECK et al. (1972a) noted that previously
covert familial type V hyperlipoproteinemia became overt in patients following estrogen administration. The increase in plasma triglyceride concentration in women
taking oral contraceptives was measured by KEKKI and NIKKILAE (1971) and found to
be 1.5-fold. There was an increased rate of triglyceride formation that was only
partially compensated by a simultaneous acceleration of triglyceride efflux. Changes
in lipoprotein distribution and ratio in women receiving the anovulatory regimen
was attributed mainly to the estrogen component in a study conducted by ALFIN-
SLATER and AFTERGOOD (1971). STOKES and WYNN (1971) observed that the most
estrogenic pills gave the highest triglyceride values, while the most progestational
gave the highest cholesterol values. In a similar fashion, ROESSNER et al. (1971) have
also shown that it was mainly the estrogenic component that caused an increase of
200% in the fasting levels of plasma triglycerides. GLUECK et al. (1972), as well as
OSMAN et al. (1972) suggested several mechanisms that may be responsible for the
alterations in lipid metabolism elicited by the contraceptive regimen such as: a) depressed postheparin lipolytic activity, b) estrogen-induced apolipoprotein and triglyceride synthesis, c) increased basal immunoreactive insulin levels, d) defective peripheral triglyceride removal, e) impaired hepatic excretory function, f) reduced glucose tolerance and the diabetogenic action of estrogens.

GLUECK et al. (1970) claimed that in direct contrast to estrogens, progestational
compounds lower triglyceride levels in normals and hypertriglyceridemic patients. It
should be noted, however, that most of the oral progestagens used in the contraceptive regimen are closely related in structure to the androgens and anabolic agents.
These synthetic steroids possess very dissimilar endocrine properties. Upon close
scrutiny their effects on lipid metabolism may also be found to vary to a considerable
degree. Only three substances will be discussed here with respect to their hypolipidemic properties.

Norethindrone acetate (35) is a typical oral progestogen. EDGREN et al. (1967)
classified this agent as an androgen with progestational effect. GLUECK et al. (1972)

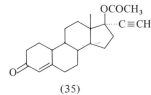

(35)

Norethindrone acetate

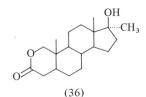

(36)

Oxandrolone

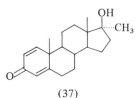

(37)

Methandrostenolone

studied the hypolipidemic effect of compound 35 most intensively and found that it effectively lowered triglycerides in patients with types III and IV hyperlipoproteinemia. Whereas abdominal pain in patients with type V hyperlipoproteinemia intensified and plasma triglyceride levels increased during estrogen administration, abdominal pain and pancreatitis ameliorated and plasma triglycerides decreased abruptly in the same patients when they received oxandrolone, an anabolic agent (36). GLUECK (1971) suggested that the two dissimilar steroid hormones 35 and 36 exhibited a potential similarity in their mode of hypotriglyceridemic action in patients with familial types III, IV, and V hyperlipoproteinemia. SACHS and WOLFMAN (1968) found that oxandrolone (36) elicited a highly selective response in each patient with carbohydrate-induced hypertriglyceridemia. One patient with the rare hyperchylomicronemia, type I, showed further elevations in plasma triglyceride levels upon administration of oxandrolone (36). Another anabolic agent, methandrostenolone (37) has been given to normal adult males. The data obtained by SRIKANTIA et al. (1967) showed that compound 37 lowered serum triglyceride and cholesterol levels in normal men, even in subjects whose triglyceride levels were in the lower part of the normal range.

GLUECK et al. (1972) expressed their hope that compounds 35 and 36, coupled with diet, may well be the treatment of choice in patients with familial type V hyperlipoproteinemia.

The data collected during long-term administration of the hormonal anovulatory regimen greatly diminished the prospects of estrogenic substances being employed for the prevention of atherosclerosis and coronary heart disease. OLIVER (1970) noted that oral contraceptives by themselves do not appear to increase the risk of developing myocardial infarction. However, they may accelerate atherogenesis in women prone to ischemic heart disease. He made some suggestions for the identification of these women.

Expectations about the potential protective action of estrogens in hyperlipidemia associated with coronary atherosclerosis are fading. It may then be worthwhile to search for the villains among the androgens and their metabolites. Such a search might reveal pathologic states in lipid metabolism which could perhaps be corrected by chemical means.

The C_{19} steroids 40 to 44 are not merely the inactive end-products of the spent hormone testosterone (39) ready for elimination; they are in fact effective hormonal modulators of a set of crucial metabolic functions.

The two androgens dehydroepiandrosterone (38) and testosterone (39) are converted to the central C_{19} steroid metabolite androstenedione (40). Enzymatic reduction of the double bond and the carbonyl function in ring A of androstenedione gives rise to the four possible metabolites 41 to 44. Reduction of the 3,4-unsaturated bond affords a new asymmetric carbon atom at position 5. Introduction of a hydrogen atom at position 5 can occur either in the α configuration, resulting in a trans junction of rings A and B of the steroid skeleton, or in the 5-β position, representing an A:B cis ring structure. Consequently, the 5-α and 5-β steroid reductases furnish profoundly different metabolites. Their pertinent stereochemical forms are illustrated in the partial structures 45 and 46.

RAO (1970) reported that patients who had suffered a recent myocardial infarction had a significantly lower androsterone/etiocholanone ratio that did normals.

Androsterone (41), an endogenous hypocholesterolemic hormone, also decreases plasma fibrinogen levels and stimulates fibrinolysis. Etiocholanone (42) significantly increases plasma fibrinogen levels. Therefore, a low androsterone/etiocholanone ratio might favor the progress of atherogenesis. Determination of the urinary excretion ratio of the steroid metabolites 41 and 42 is useful for obtaining information about

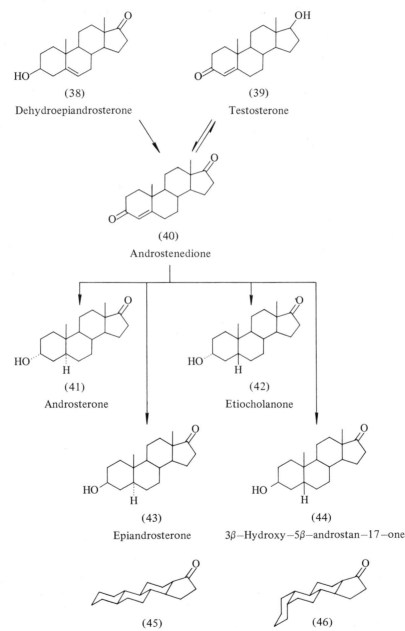

(38)
Dehydroepiandrosterone

(39)
Testosterone

(40)
Androstenedione

(41)
Androsterone

(42)
Etiocholanone

(43)
Epiandrosterone

(44)
3β−Hydroxy−5β−androstan−17−one

(45)
5−alpha H (A : B trans)

(46)
5−beta H (A : B cis)

the relative activities of the 5-α and 5-β reductases. According to a review by So-LYOM (1972), decrease in this ratio was found in patients with hyperlipemia or myx-edema, and also after myocardial infarction or prolonged corticosteroid therapy. KAPPAS et al. (1972) found that administration of thyroid hormone appeared to stimulate hepatic 5-α steroid reductase and could restore the 5-α/5-β steroid urinary excretion ratio to normal.

The effect of estrogen and thyroid hormones on the ratio of metabolites 41 to 44 has been discussed by BENCZE et al. (1969). Epiandrosterone (43) has been found to be a more abundant metabolite than androsterone (41) in patients with ischemic heart disease. Estrogen therapy appears to stimulate the enzyme producing the 3-α-hydroxy metabolite 41. BENES et al. (1970) found that epiandrosterone (43) caused maximal inhibition of placental glucose-6-phosphate dehydrogenase (G-6-PD). De-hydroepiandrosterone (38) has also been reported by BENES et al. (1970a) to be the strongest inhibitor of human red blood cell G-6-PD. It has been postulated that increased G-6-PD activity produces a high level of NADPH concentration which in turn enhances the biosynthesis of fatty acids. Consequently, an increase in the availa-bility of the ketosteroids 38 and 43 acting as inhibitors of G-6-PD, would result in a dimished rate of lipid biosynthesis.

The prospects of the utilization of certain androgen derivatives to afford selective shifts among plasma proteins, such as a reduction of apolipoprotein A concentra-tion, has been discussed by SOLYOM (1972). Selective regulation of apolipoprotein A and fragments thereof may influence lipoprotein lipase enzyme systems, cholesterol biosynthesis and distribution. In contrast, impairment of the biogenesis of apolipo-protein B does not appear to be a desirable goal, because it is associated with a massive fatty infiltration of the liver. WINDMUELLER and LEVY (1967) found that administering a diet containing 1% orotic acid resulted in a decrease of the plasma β-lipoprotein concentration to less than 1% of the normal level, while the lipid content of the liver increased.

XII. Substituted Phenyl- and Phenyloxy-acetic Acids

The first observation that phenylacetic acid derivatives cause a reduction in plasma cholesterol levels both in the rat and man was made by REDEL and COTTET (1953). The historical aspects and structure activity relationships of 48 representative phenyl-, biphenylyl-, naphthyl-, and phenoxy-acetic acids have been thoroughly dis-cussed by BENCZE et al. (1969). The purpose of this chapter is to present the main features of the hypolipidemic profile of clofibrate (48) and the ensuing efforts of medicinal chemists and pharmacologists in their search for an improved clofibrate type drug. Although p-chlorophenoxyisobutyric acid (CPIB) (47) had been prepared by GALIMBERTI and DEFRANCESCHI (1948) and the ethyl ester of this acid, clofibrate (48) had been reported by JULIA et al. (1956), it was THORP and WARING (1962) who discovered that this acid and its aethyl ester possessed a novel type of hypolipidemic activity in experimental animals. In the past decade clofibrate has become by all odds the most widely used hypolipidemic drug. During the same time four new derivatives of phenoxy-acetic acid, compounds 49 to 52 have been developed. Each of these four substances possess more potent hypolipidemic activity than clofibrate.

Early in their studies of the structure-activity relationships of aryloxyisobutyrate derivatives, THORP and WARING (1962) observed the strange dependence of the hypolipidemic response of the experimental animals to clofibrate treatment on their hormonal state. Particularly marked was the influence of the thyroid hormone. It has been found that both clofibrate (48) and methyl clofenapate (49) are rapidly hydrolyzed to the corresponding free acids in the organism, and that these acids are adsorbed to and transported by albumin. A crucial physiological role of albumin is the transport of the plasma free fatty acids, a portion of thyroxine, the acid sulfate conjugates of steroid hormones and probably many more acids possessing important metabolic functions. The competitive binding of aryloxyisobutyric acids and thyroxine to albumin was found to be very intense and selective. Consequently, the I.C.I. team developed an *in vitro* test system based on the competitive affinity of thyroxine and phenoxyisobutyric acids to occupy the same binding sites on albumin. Based on such screening procedures, THORP (1970) selected the free acid of compound 49, clofenapic acid, that was adsorbed to albumin very extensively more than 99% and was found to reduce by 50% the primary association constant of the binding of L-T_4 to human albumin. Due to the great affinity of clofenapic acid to the "albumin space" and its extremely long serum half-life of 30 to 40 days, it was found that in man an initial period of treatment at 20 mg per day for 6 weeks, followed by the maintenance dose of 10 mg (0.13 mg/kg/day), was sufficient to afford a persistent hypolipidemic activity.

The thyroxine hypothesis has been supported by RUEGAMER et al. (1969) who found that a single dose of clofibrate (48) caused a displacement of ^{131}I-labeled thyroxine from the plasma into the liver. Hence, clofibrate rendered the liver hyper-

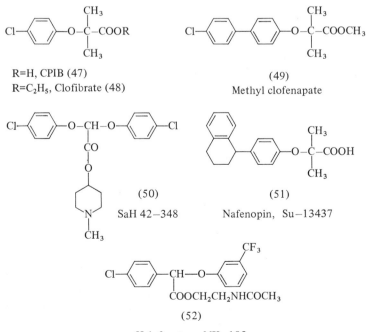

thyroid, while the rest of the organism remained euthyroid as evidenced by the lack of change in the basic metabolic rate. WESTERFELD et al. (1968) included clofibrate 0.3% in the diet of rats and observed a fourfold rise of the hepatic mitochondrial alpha-glycerol phosphate dehydrogenase level. Liver and adipose tissue malic enzyme levels were also increased. These enzymes are also stimulated by thyroxine. The authors listed the following hepatic effects of clofibrate which may be thryroxine-mediated: increase in hepatic protein synthesis, depletion of liver glycogen, increase in liver mitochondria, and increase in prothrombin time.

Nevertheless, there are other responses of clofibrate administration which are not thyroxine-like effects. Thus, STEINBERG (1970) pointed out that clofibrate reduces the levels of the S_f 20-400 lipoproteins and often causes in increase in the S_f 0-20 lipoprotein fraction. Conversely, thyroxine reduces primarily the S_f 0-20 lipoprotein fraction. Another effect of the phenoxyisobutyric acids which is not thyroxine-mediated was described by WESTERFELD et al. (1972). These authors fed orotic acid to thyroidectomized rats producing fatty livers and a diminished intensity of the β-lipoprotein band in the electrophoretic pattern. Addition of clofibrate (48) or Su-13437 (51) to the diet restored the β-lipoprotein band and prevented the development of the fatty liver. These effects being manifested in thyroidectomized animals cannot be thyroxine-mediated.

STEINBERG (1970) reasoned that the shunting of thyroid hormone into the liver is probably not the mechanism through which clofibrate exerts its hypocholesterolemic activity. Thyroid hormones are known to increase the rate of hepatic biosynthesis of cholesterol and also the oxidative elimination of cholesterol, while administration of clofibrate has been found to reduce hepatic cholesterol synthesis. SODHI et al. (1971) administered ^{14}C-acetate and ^{3}H-mevalonate to normal subjects and patients with hyperlipemia. Their data supported the hypothesis, based on animal studies, that the site of the inhibitory action of clofibrate in the hepatic synthesis of cholesterol in man is between acetate and mevalonate. GRUNDY et al. (1972) studied the influence of clofibrate administration on cholesterol emtabolism in all categories of hyperlipidemia. The bulk of the obtained data suggested that in all forms of hyperlipidemia, except fat-induced hypertriglyceridemia, the drug causes an increased output of cholesterol while simultaneously inhibiting any compensatory increase in cholesterol synthesis. As a consequence, cholesterol stores in tissues appeared to be depleted. Previous clinical reports on the resolution of xanthomata as a result of clofibrate administration are in agreement with this study. WITIAK and WHITEHOUSE (1969) noted that rat plasma albumin reacted differently from that of 10 other species in regard to the binding of acids. No relationship was discovered between albumin binding and hypocholesterolemic activity in vivo in a series of phenoxyacetic acids related to clofibrate.

The hypotriglyceridemic effect of all five hypolipidemic agents 48 to 52 is even more marked than their hypocholesterolemic property. Conflicting results have been reported about the mechanism of the reduction of serum triglycerides. GOULD et al. (1966) have shown that in the clofibrate treated rat the rate of liver triglyceride synthesis was increased. In a similar fashion, DUNCAN and BEST (1969) demonstrated that administration of compounds 48 or 51 to the rat resulted in a higher rate of incorporation of radioactive carbon from ^{14}C-acetate into liver total fatty acids. Using the same technique, SODHI et al. (1971a) found that clofibrate administration to man also increased the rate of acetate incorporation into fatty acids by the liver. Contrary to these reports, AZARNOFF et al. (1965) noted that the concentration, as well as the total quantity of cholesterol and triglyceride, decreased in the liver of male and female rats that were fed clofibrate. FALLON et al. (1972) provided evidence that clofibrate lowers hepatic triglyceride levels. MARAGOUDAKIS et al. (1972) showed that the livers of rats treated with substance 51 exhibited significantly lower levels of acetyl coenzyme-A carboxylase activity than those of control animals. Inhibition of acetyl coenzyme-A carboxylase, the key enzyme of fatty acid synthesis may be responsible for at least a part of the hypotriglyceridemic action of the phenoxyisobutyrate type hypolipidemic agents.

The role of the skin, an organ actively participating in the biosynthesis of cholesterol and other lipids, has been studied by FULTON and HSIA (1969). Specimens of epidermis from patients treated with clofibrate were incubated with $1\text{-}^{14}C$-acetate. Incorporation of radioactive carbon into all lipid fractions was suppressed by 50 to 70%.

In consideration of the complex nature of the lipoprotein lipase enzyme systems it is not surprising to find seemingly contradictory reports about the effect of clofibrate upon these enzymes. NESTEL et al. (1970) did not find any influence of clofibrate on rat adipose tissue lipoprotein lipase activity, whereas TOLMAN et al. (1970) observed that lipoprotein lipase activity of homogenates of adipose tissue from rats fed clofibrate was consistently higher than that from animals fed the same diet without the drug. Large doses of clofibrate (400 mg/kg/day) administered to rats inhibited heart lipoprotein lipase activity *in vitro* in the hands of CRATNETTER and GEIZEROVA (1971). Some light might be shed on these controversial reports by the study of BORENSZTAJN et al. (1972), who came to the conclusion that the lipoprotein lipase enzyme system of the rat is regulated differently in the heart and adipose tissues. In fed rats, adipose tissue lipoprotein lipase activity is high while that in the heart is low. The converse situation exists in fasted animals.

In human subcutaneous adipose tissue specimens obtained by needle biopsy from patients who responded to clofibrate treatment PERSSON et al. (1972) found no drug-induced alteration of the lipoprotein lipase activity.

A somewhat clearer picture emerged from the observations about the effect of clofibrate treatment on the plasma lipoproteins. The general consensus is that clofibrate therapy may bring about a reciprocal shift in the concentration of very low and low density lipoproteins in man. WILSON and LEES (1972) observed that clofibrate administration to normal subjects and patients with hyperlipidemia resulted in a decrease in very low-density lipoprotein cholesterol content and a compensatory increase in low density lipoprotein cholesterol levels. The reciprocal increase in LDL concentration as a response to clofibrate therapy does not appear to occur in type III hyperlipoproteinemia. However, many patients with type II hyperlipoproteinemia and increased VLDL concentrations (type II b) will show an increase in plasma LDL concentrations following clofibrate administration. It should be mentioned here that the classical typing of the states of hyperlipoproteinemia by FREDRICKSON et al. (1967) has been adopted and slightly modified by the World Health Organization. The modification included the division of type II into II a and II b subgroups (see BEAUMONT et al., 1970).

A different response of type II and IV patients was recorded by HORLICK et al. (1971). These authors demonstrated that administration of clofibrate resulted in a consistent increase of fecal neutral and acidic sterols during the treatment period in type II patients only. Type IV subjects showed no changes in fecal neutral or acidic sterols. The response to clofibrate treatment among patients with type II or III may also be different. SCOTT and HURLEY (1969) found four patients among a larger group of type II and III patients whose LDL levels did not show the compensatory increase, but have been lowered instead. It could then be construed as a substantial gain in the treatment of hyperlipidemia when the newer and more potent analog of clofibrate, methyl clofenapate (49) was found to lower LDL levels in both type IIa and IIb patients in the clinical trials conducted by CRAIG and WALTON (1972). Alas, this very potent hypolipidemic agent had to be withdrawn from clinical trials because of hepatotoxic effects in mice and rats (see CRAIG, 1972).

A potent hypolipidemic agent, SaH-42-348 (50) has been developed by TIMMS et al. (1969). The active hypolipidemic moiety is again the free parent acid of the basic ester 50, i.e. bis-p-chlorophenoxyacetic acid. Compound 50 has been found to be several times more active than clofibrate and to lower the levels of all major classes of serum lipids in the rat. It was not possible to demonstrate that SaH-42-348 (50) inhibited cholesterol biosynthesis in vivo from radioactive acetate, while the inhibitory activity of clofibrate was readily demonstrated. In addition, propylthiouracil inhibited the hypocholesterolemic activity of clofibrate in the rat, whereas the activity of substance 50 was unaffected under the same conditions. BERKOWITZ (1969) reported that SaH-42-348 (50), as well as compound 51, were effective in producing significant decreases in plasma cholesterol levels in type II patients, the majority of whom had previously been unresponsive to clofibrate.

Another potent hypolipidemic agent, nafenopin, Su-13437 (51) has been announced by HESS and BENCZE (1968). Structurally, substance 51 is related to a group of naturally occurring lignans. Nafenopin is a derivative of 1-phenyl tetraline; consequently it can be resolved. BENCZE et al. (1970) determined the absolute configuration of the component enantiomers. SCHACHT et al. (1972) showed that the two antipodes of nafenopin (51) possess the same degree of hypolipidemic activity. Several hepatic enzymes regulating lipid and sugar metabolism were altered by both enantiomers in a similar fashion as by the racemate 51. HESS et al. (1969) reported that nafenopin inhibited serum cholesterol levels in male rats at a dose of 10 mg/kg/day, while the rise in triglyceride in fructose-induced hypertriglyceridemia was inhibited at doses of 1 to 30 mg/kg.

The first extensive clinical evaluation of nafenopin (51) has been carried out by HARTMANN and FORSTER (1969). Even type II patients consistently responded to the drug, though to a lesser degree than those of types III, IV, and V. No escape or tachyphylaxis has been observed during the treatment periods of up to 2 years. DUNCAN and BEST (1970) reported that compound 51 caused a reduction in serum total cholesterol levels of 22%, and triglycerides of 51%. BOBERG et al. (1970) concluded that administration of nafenopin (51) to patients with hyperlipidemia resulted in a decrease of plasma triglyceride levels due to an increase in the peripheral clearance of triglycerides. Intravenous fat tolerance had been low in 8 patients and had improved by 100% during treatment. The VLDL class was reduced by 50%, and the LDL by 15%, while the HDL had a tendency to rise.

The fifth hypolipidemic agent in this series is halofenate, MK-185 (52). Halofenate is rapidly hydrolyzed after oral administration to rats, dogs, monkey, and man to the corresponding free acid. The acid is extremely bound to plasma protein. The plasma half-life time is 24 hrs in man (HUCKER et al., 1971). MORGAN et al. (1971) and SIRTORI et al. (1972) found that administration of compound 52 to patients with hyperlipidemia caused significant reduction in serum triglyceride levels. It had minimal effects on cholesterol, but decreased serum uric acid concentration. It has been noted in an EDITORIAL review (1969) that hyperuricemia can be taken to be an attribute associated with coronary heart disease. JEPSON et al. (1972) observed that halofenate (52) was more effective in mixed hyperlipoproteinemias and in reduction of serum uric acid levels than clofibrate.

XIII. Hepatic Action of Clofibrate and Its Analogs

A great wealth of knowledge about lipid metabolism emerged from the study of the effects of clofibrate and its analogs upon the liver. All five drugs 48 to 52 cause pronounced hepatomegaly in the rat and several other species after oral administration for a week or longer. The liver enlargement consists of hypertrophy of the hepatocytes rather than hyperplasia. Several intracellular organelles, among them mitochondria, microsomes, and most typically the peroxisomes or microbodies are altered upon administration of compounds 48 to 52 to the rat.

A. Mitochondria

KORUP et al. (1970) found that the liver content of mitochondria was doubled on feeding clofibrate to rats or mice. In the Wistar rat even a single oral dose of clofibrate increased the volume of the hepatic mitochondrion threefold, while in the desert rat the volume of the mitochondrion remained the same but the number of them increased, as reported by RIEDE et al. (1972). PEREIRA and HOLLAND (1970) showed that there was an increase in the rate of incorporation of labeled leucine into hepatic mitochondrial protein following clofibrate administration to the rat. The authors speculate that the hypolipidemic action of clofibrate may be due, in part, to the induction of mitochondrial protein synthesis, in particular that of α-glycerophosphate dehydrogenase. A sixfold increase in the activity of this enzyme in the liver of rats treated with clofibrate had been demonstrated by HESS et al. (1965).

An *in vitro* assay for the relative potencies of hypolipidemic drugs has been developed in the laboratory of KRITCHEVSKY. Mitochondrial preparations from the livers of rats fed the hypolipidemic agent showed an increased capacity to oxidize cholesterol-26-^{14}C to labeled CO_2. However, the stimulation of the mitochondrial enzyme system performing this oxidation functioned only in the absence of a boiled supernatant factor. New and valuable information about this sterol redox enzyme system may be gained by isolation and characterization of the heat stable factor. The degree of the enhancement of cholesterol side-chain oxidation by rat liver mitochondrial preparations has been studied by prefeeding the rat with clofibrate (48), KRITCHEVSKY et al. (1969a); nafenopin (51), KRITCHEVSKY and TEPPER (1969); and halofenate (52), KRITCHEVSKY and TEPPER (1972).

B. Microsomes

The hepatic microsomes consist of fragments of the endoplasmic reticulum. They are eminently known to be involved in the performance of a variety of specific chemical reactions, like N- and O-demethylations, aromatic hydroxylations, etc. The activation of the microsomes can be induced or inhibited by a variety of drugs, e.g., phenobarbital (53) is an inducer, SKF-525A (54), or metyrapone (55) are inhibitors. The pharmacological implications of microsomal enzyme induction has been reviewed by CONNEY (1967).

The administration of phenobarbital (53) inhibited the increase in serum concentration of cholesterol and phospholipids, as well as the development of atheromata in the aorta of the cholesterol-fed rabbit (SALVADOR et al., 1970). Stimulation of the activity of the microsomal enzymes that hydroxylate testosterone in the 6-β, 7-α, and 16-α positions has been reported by the same authors. The microsomal enzyme induction by phenobarbital may be very selective and species- or even subspecies-specific. Thus, SHEFER et al. (1972) found that Wistar rats pretreated with phenobarbital showed a sixfold enhancement in the activity of hepatic microsomal cholesterol-7-α hydroxylase. In Charles River rats there was no increase in the activity of this enzyme, though liver weights and microsomal protein contents were increased by phenobarbital treatment in both strains. ARIYOSHI and TAKABATAKE (1971) reported that the total phospholipid content of hepatic microsomes was increased in female rats pretreated with phenobarbital.

In general, the clofibrate type hypolipidemic agents are also inducers of hepatic microsomal enzymes. SALVADOR et al. (1970b) demonstrated that clofibrate (48) and SaH 42-348 (50) induced in the liver microsomes the formation of the enzyme system that metabolizes testosterone to more potent metabolites, whereas the enzymes which metabolize pentobarbital and 3,4-benzopyrene were not affected. SCHACHT and GRANZER (1970) found that administration of nafenopin (51) to rats substantially increased the microsomal NADPH oxidase activity.

Another type of microsomal enzyme system has been investigated by SCHWEPPE and JUNGMAN (1971). These authors showed that clofibrate treatment enhanced the formation of cholesteryl oleate and linoleate, SaH 42-348 (50) affected the rate of formation of cholesteryl oleate and palmitate, while nafenopin (51) stimulated the synthesis of all cholesterol esters.

Inhibitors of hepatic microsomal enzyme systems may also be capable of eliciting hypolipidemic activity. A few pertinent properties of two representative inhibitors, SKF-525A (54) and metyrapone (55) are discussed here.

The history and the hypolipidemic activity of SKF-525A (54) has been reviewed by HOLMES (1964). Compound 54 has been shown to inhibit the metabolism of most

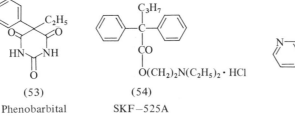

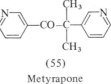

| (53) | (54) | (55) |
| Phenobarbital | SKF—525A | Metyrapone |

substrates that are amenable to the action of hepatic microsomal mixed-function oxidase systems. A metabolite of SKF-525A has been shown to form a stable complex of ferrous cytochrome P-450 to furnish a new species of cytochrome P-455. It has been suggested by SCHENKMAN et al. (1972) that this new complex may be responsible for the noncompetitive inhibition of microsomal oxidation of several substrates by SKF-525A. An obscure observation was recorded by JENNER and NETTER (1972). These authors found that the non-competitive inhibition of liver microsomal activity elicited by SKF-525A, was converted to an apparent competitive type inhibition by recrystallization of the drug SKF-525A from benzene.

Metyrapone (55) is being employed as a clinical diagnostic agent for the semiquantitative assessment of pituitary reserve capacity. The chemistry and structure-activity relationships of metyrapone analogs as selective inhibitors of steroid hydroxylase enzymes has been discussed by BENCZE and DESTEVENS (1967). Recently, DINGMAN (1972) reported that metyrapone (55) administration to four patients with type II b hyperlipidemia elicited a marked hypocholesterolemic and hypotriglyceridemic effect. Metyrapone administration causes a selective inhibition of steroidal 11-β-hydroxylase and results in a reduction of plasma hydrocortisone levels, which in turn elicits a compensatory rise in endogeneous ACTH output. The stimulation of ACTH secretion, however, is not the only cause of the hypolipidemic action of metyrapone. A hypotriglyceridemic but no hypocholesterolemic response to administration of a synthetic ACTH fragment has been reported by MATSUZAKI et al. (1971). The fact that metyrapone (55) is an effective inhibitor of liver microsomal hydroxylases both *in vivo* and *in vitro* has been emphasized by NETTER et al. (1967).

C. Peroxisomes (Microbodies)

PAGET (1963) observed that in the liver cells of rats treated with clofibrate there was a proliferation of "dense bodies" and he provisionally identified them as lysosomes. HESS et al. (1965) noted that these dense bodies are modified microbodies, or peroxisomes, as they were then named by DEDUVE and BAUDHUIN (1966). These subcellular organelles have been found only in two mammalian tissues, the liver and kidney. The role of the peroxisomes in lipid metabolism is obscure. RIEDE et al. (1972) hinted that the participation of the peroxisomes in the oxidative elimination of extramitochondrial NADPH may be anticipated.

The enzyme catalase accounts for about 16% of the total protein content of the peroxisomes. A several-fold increase in hepatic catalase was found by HESS et al. (1965) upon administration of clofibrate (48) to rats. Several oxidases as well as catalase are coupled to the pyridine nucleotide redox system. Therefore catalase may be capable of influencing the NADP/NADPH ratio.

There appears to be a correlation between the inhibitory activity of several chemical agents on hepatic catalase and the increased excretion of porphyrins caused by these agents. GOLDFISCHER et al. (1972) demonstrated that experimental porphyria induced in the rat by a single injection of allylisopropylacetamide could be inhibited by clofibrate treatment. This protective action of clofibrate is probably due to its stimulatory action on hepatic peroxisomal catalase.

D. Cytoplasm

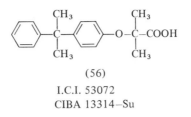

(56)
I.C.I. 53072
CIBA 13314–Su

Several enzymes in the cytoplasmic space of liver cells exert a regulatory action in lipid and sugar metabolism. PLATT and COCKRILL (1967) examined the influence of clofibrate (48), I.C.I. 53072 (CIBA 13314-Su) (56), phenobarbital (53), and the hepato-toxic agents DDT, thioacetamide, and carbon tetrachloride on the activity of four liver dehydrogenase enzymes. Two of the four enzymes studied, Glucose-6-phos-phate dehydrogenase (G6PDH) and lactate dehydrogenase (LDH), have been stimu-lated by oral administration of clofibrate (48) and compound 56 to rats for 14 days. The activities of two other hepatic dehydrogenases have been diminished. The pat-tern of stimulation or inhibition caused by phenobarbital and the hepatotoxic agents varied and was different from that caused by the two hypolipidemic agents 48 and 56. Quantitatively, compound 56 exerted the same degree of stimulatory activity on LDH as clofibrate, but the activity of G6PDH appeared to be ten times more enhanced by substance 56 than by clofibrate. SCHACHT and GRANZER (1970) found that administration of nafenopin (51) to rats did not influence hepatic G6PDH activity. Assuming that substantial differences in the activation of G6PDH elicited by various analogs of substituted phenoxyacetic acids ware real and reproducible, the influence of these agents on intermediary lipid and sugar metabolism must also differ correspondingly. It has been thought that increased activity of G6PDH results in stimulation of lipogenesis by the production of an abundance of the reducing units NADPH$_2$.

The effect of nafenopin (51) on another enzyme system regulating lipogenesis has been intensively studied by MARAGOUDAKIS et al. (1972a). The authors reported that a genetically obese strain of mice exhibits hepatic acetylcoenzyme A carboxylase activity levels at least sixfold higher than their lean siblings. On treatment with nafenopin (51) the obese mice showed about 50% depression of lipogenesis from labeled glucose as compared to controls. Tissue lipids were lowered too. In contrast, CENEDELLA (1970) treated normal male mice with the same drug (51) and observed a large increase in the incorporation of radioactive acetate into the total fatty acids of both the whole liver and per gram tissue of liver. LENZ and FLEISCHMAN (1971) fed nafenopin (51) to rats with congenital hypertriglyceridemia. Total and relative lipid, cholesterol, and FFA levels in the liver were lowered by the drug.

Lactate dehydrogenase (LDH) also plays a prominent regulatory role in sugar and lipid metabolism. McINTOSH and TOPHAM (1972) reported that LDH activity was stimulated in rat but not in mouse liver on addition of clofibrate to the diet.

XIV. Extrahepatic Enzymes Influenced by Clofibrate

It would be especially valuable to know to what extent administration of clofibrate alters lipid and sugar utilization in the heart. Information in this respect is yet scarce. MRHOVA et al. (1971) studied the effect of clofibrate on the activity of lactate dehydrogenase and a few other enzymes in rat aorta and myocardium. The turnover of lactate in human myocardium has been studied intensively in the past decade. It appears that the normally oxygenated human myocardium extracts lactate from the blood, whereas inadequate oxygen or blood supply to the myocardium leads to anaerobic glycolysis with resultant lactate production. Temporal relationships of myocardial lactate metabolism at rest and during angina precipitated by exercise have been quantitatively assessed by PARKER et al. (1969).

The undesirable stimulation of an extrahepatic enzyme system in a few patients due to clofibrate treatment has been reported by LANGNER and LEVY (1968). The authors found that in about 15% of their patients receiving clofibrate serum creatine phosphokinase levels were elevated. In two of these patients severe myalgia and muscle stiffness developed. Cessation of therapy resulted in prompt resolution of symptoms. Creatine phosphokinase is absent from the liver and may originate from muscle. This problem has been reexamined by SMITH et al. (1970). Serum creatine phosphokinase was not raised in 195 men receiving clofibrate, and there was no instance of myalgia recorded in 452 men who received clofibrate for one year. BRIDGMAN et al. (1972) correlated the muscular pain following clofibrate treatment of patients with nephrotic syndrome. In all of these patients hyperlipemia was associated with nephrotic syndrome and the plasma half-life of clofibrate increased from the normal 12 hrs to 36 hrs. The diminished capacity of the serum albumin in these patients to bind clofibrate was thought to be the cause of the undesirable side effects.

XV. Potential Antiatherosclerotic Effect of Clofibrate

In a short-term experiment, KRITCHEVSKY et al. (1968a) induced atheromata in rabbits by an atherogenic diet. When 0.3% clofibrate was added to the regimen, atheromata in the aortic arch were significantly less frequent, but thoracic atheromata were not affected.

Secondary prevention trials in ischemic heart disease using clofibrate were conducted in Scotland and Newcastle, in which physicians watched 1214 patients for 4 or 5 years. In a joint commentary, DEWAR and OLIVER (1971) came to the following conclusions: Administration of clofibrate to patients who had angina resulted in a significant reduction in mortality. The drug seemed to offer protection particularly against sudden death. The beneficial effect bore no apparent relation to the initial serum cholesterol levels, nor to the hypolipidemic effect of clofibrate. The overall mortality or morbidity rates in patients admitted to the Scottish trials, with a history of infarct without preceding angina, were not altered. In one subgroup of patients there was an adverse effect in the clofibrate-treated group. The authors cautioned that the ethics in the design of further clinical trials will have to be appraised carefully.

Another prevention trial in coronary heart disease was conducted in the United States by KRASNO and KIDERA (1972) among 3286 male employees of the United

Airlines over periods of two to five years. In this study, it has been shown that clofibrate exerted a favorable effect on morbidity in coronary heart disease by causing a reduction in the rate of nonfatal myocardial infarction from 6.6 or 5.0/1000 year, as observed in untreated men, to 1.89 or 0.64/1000 year in the treated group. As in the British study, this protection was found to be unrelated to the hypolipidemic effect of clofibrate. There was no significant difference in the mortality rates between the treated and untreated groups. The authors speculate that the protection offered by the drug, as evidenced by the reduction of the nonfatal myocardial infarction rate, may be due to its ameliorating effect on platalet aggregation, fibrinolysis, permeability of endothelial cells, or other yet unknown atherogenic processes.

A controlled, small trial of clofibrate in cerebral vascular disease was conducted by ACHESON and HUTCHINSON (1972). The study lasted for seven years. In the treated group 66% of the patients experienced further episodes of cerebral ischemia, in the placebo group 60%. No protective effect was offered by the drug in this trial.

HEADY (1973) described the design, methods, and progress of a large, cooperative trial on the primary prevention of ischemic heart disease using the hypolipidemic agent clofibrate. This project is coordinated and controlled by a committee of investigators assembled by the World Health Organization. The required 15000 subjects have been admitted to the trial as of 1973. The fate of clofibrate may well be determined by the results of this large investigation.

The long-awaited analysis of the effect of clofibrate on the mortality rate of survivors of heart attacks has been presented in an initial report of the CORONARY DRUG PROJECT RESEARCH GROUP (1975). The five-year total mortality rate was 20.0% for the clofibrate group and 20.9% for placebo. Even this small, statistically insignificant difference vanished when the total follow-up experience, up to 8.5 years, was taken into consideration.

In search of more promising prospects for the demonstration of possible beneficial effects of the administration of clofibrate in the treatment of patients with ischemic heart disease, Imperial Chemical Industries of Great Britain announced the introduction of clofibrate and the cardioselective β-adrenergic blocking agent practolol (25). It appears that the introduction of this particular combination may be a stillborn effort. RAFTERY (1974) noted that practolol seems to be unique among the β-blocking agents in producing the syndrome of disseminated lupus erythematosus in patients. In addition, sclerosing peritonitis appears to be another undesired complication in some patients caused by the administration of practolol, as reported by BROWN et al. (1974) and others.

XVI. Derivatives of Dialkylaminoethanol

2-Dimethylamino-, or 2-diethylaminoethanol do not exhibit hypocholesterolemic activity even when administered at high-dose levels. However, a number of ester, e.g. SKF-525A (54), or ether derivatives of dialkylaminoethanol possess marked hypocholesterolemic properties. Thousands of such basic ether derivatives of natural and synthetic estrogens have been evaluated as hypolipidemic agents during the past two decades. Structure-activity relationships of about 20 basic ether derivatives have been discussed by BENCZE et al. (1969). Only five representative compounds 57 to 61 will be discussed in this section.

A substantial amount of clinical and pharmacological data has been recorded on the hypolipidemic action of triparanol (MER-29) (57). HOLMES (1964) reviewed the mechanism of the hypolipidemic action of triparanol. It has been reported in several studies that triparanol reduced plasma cholesterol levels in man and in experimental animals, mostly at the expense of a compensatory increase in the blood level of 24-dehydrocholesterol (desmosterol). The rate of deposition of cholesterol or desmosterol into atheromatous plaques has been found to be approximately the same. Therefore, the therapeutic value of compond 57 became questionable. Due to toxic side effects, substance 57 is no longer clinically available.

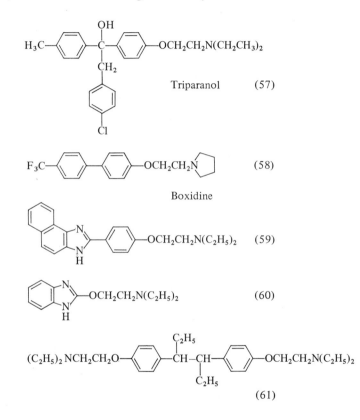

The extremely potent hypocholesterolemic agent boxidine (58) has been developed by BACH et al. (1968). Oral administration of boxidine at 0.0003% of diet to rats caused a 20% decrease in serum cholesterol concentration. GORDON and CEKLENIAK (1968) reported that the fall in plasma cholesterol levels was partially compensated by the appearance of 7-dehydrocholesterol in the blood. GAILANI et al. (1972) gave boxidine to 13 terminal cancer patients. A definite decrease in serum cholesterol was observed in 9 out of the 13 patients. 7-Dehydrocholesterol appeared in the serum of all the patients tested. Objective tumor regression was observed only in one patient with adrenal carcinoma.

It appears that the inhibition of hepatic cholesterol synthesis at the last steps is frequently encountered among dialkylaminoethyl derivatives. A study by BLACK et al. (1968) of the mode of action of the two analogs 59 and 60, closely related in structure, illustrates that caution is required in presuming that like structures exert their hypocholesterolemic activity by the same mechanism. The authors found that compound 59 inhibited sterol $\triangle$-24-reductase, while substance 60 blocked sterol $\triangle$-7-reductase.

Species differences in the hypolipidemic response elicited by drugs of this series are often observed. Thus ADACHI et al. (1972) reported that the basic ether derivative of hexestrol (61) exerted a cholesterol-lowering effect in the rat. The same drug elicited a marked elevation of blood cholesterol levels in humans. Compound 61 also caused the appearance of desmosterol in the liver and spleen of the treated rats.

XVII. Unsaturated Fatty Acids

Twenty years have passed since it was found that addition of unsaturated fat to the diet brings about a reduction of serum cholesterol levels. However, not all the unsaturated acids may qualify as useful adjuncts of dietary antiatherogenic treatment. KRITCHEVSKY et al. (1971) supported the concept that two saturated acids that are components of peanut oil may be responsible in part for the unexpected atherogenic effect of peanut oil. Often the same unsaturated fats will produce different responses in metabolically different individuals. Thus CONNOR (1971) indicated that in normal men, polyunsaturated fat in the diet increased fecal bile excretion as serum cholesterol levels were decreased. This was, however, not the case in type II hypercholesterolemic patients. Moreover, the same unsaturated fatty acid may furnish different prostaglandins, which in turn will elicit various hormonal and metabolic responses in the same organism.

The usefulness of unsaturated fats as hypocholesterolemic agents was questioned by GRUNDY and AHRENS JR. (1970), who observed that in the majority of patients with various hyperlipoproteinemia, unsaturated dietary fats changed neither the rate of cholesterol synthesis nor the conversion of sterols to bile acids. Consequently the hypocholesterolemic effect must be interpreted as a result of redistribution of cholesterol into tissue pools.

$$CH_3CH_2CH_2CH_2-(CH_2CH=CH)_2(CH_2)_6CH_2CO-R$$

R = OH , linoleic acid (62)

R = NH$-C_6H_{11}$ (cyclohexyl) (63)

R = NH$-CH(CH_3)C_6H_5$ (64)

R = NH$-CH(C_6H_5)H_2C$—⟨ ⟩—CH$_3$ (65)

$C_6H_5-CH=C(CH_3)-CH_2COOH$ (66)

$CH_2=CHCH_2CH_2COOH$ (67)

$CH_3CH_2CH_2CH_2CH(C_2H_5)COOH$ (68)

A disturbing note about the potential toxicity of unsaturated fat was recorded by Dayton et al. (1969) and Pearce and Dayton (1971). These authors claimed that in their clinical trial of a diet high in unsaturated fat, the incidence of cerebral fatal atherosclerotic events was lower, but that of fatal carcinomas was higher in the experimental group. Ederer et al. (1971) analyzed the combined results of five studies and noted that cholesterol-lowering diets do not influence cancer risk. In a similar fashion, Miettinen et al. (1972) found that during a twelve-year crossover trial, cholesterol-lowering diet reduced the mortality rate of the male participants to one half or less of that of the control group. However, differences in the mortality from malignant neoplasms were small and showed no consistent pattern. Mead (1972) discussed the potential toxicity of dietary polyunsaturated fatty acids and suggested that they be accompanied by adequate amounts of dietary antioxidants. Reproducible pharmacological and clinical results can only be obtained by the study of the effects of chemically well-defined hypolipidemic agents. Dietary unsaturated fats are complex mixtures of triglycerides. Hence progress in this field was ensured when a group of Japanese investigators initiated a long-term study of the potential hypocholesterolemic and antiatherogenic effects of a series of amides 63 to 65 of the essential fatty acid, linoleic acid (62). Nakatani et al. (1966) observed that the metabolic fate and the hypocholesterolemic effect of N-substituted amides of linoleic acid was different from that of linoleic acid (62). Kritchevsky and Tepper (1967) noted that N-cyclohexyl linoleamide (63) significantly reduced liver and serum cholesterol levels in cholesterol-fed rabbits at a dosage of 300 mg/day but had no effect upon atheromata. Antiatherogenic response was observed, however, at a dose of 600 mg/day. Kritchevsky et al. (1968 b) also found that the synthesis of cholesterol from acetate or mevalonate by liver slices from rats fed 0.6% dietary N-cyclohexyl linoleamide (63) was diminished. There was no effect, however, at a dietary level of 0.3%.

The potency of the hypocholesterolemic and antiatherogenic activity of substance 63 could be progressively increased by the development of compounds 64 and 65. Thus, Fukushima et al. (1969) reported that N-(α-methylbenzyl) linoleamide (64) lowered serum cholesterol levels and exhibited antiatherogenic activity at a dose level of 25 mg/day (10 mg/kg/day) in the cholesterol-fed rabbit. The third amide in this series (-)N-α-phenyl-β(p-tolyl)ethyl linoleamide (65) exhibited the same activity as did compound 64, even at doses of 2 mg/kg/day, as indicated by Nakatani et al. (1970). The synthetic substance β-benzal-butyric acid (66) has been reported by Giorgini and Porcellati (1969) to inhibit the incorporation of labeled acetate into cholesterol. Speranza et al. (1970) suggested that compound 66 may act via inhibition of oxidative phosphorylation.

The small unsaturated fatty acid, 4-pentenoic acid (67) has been found to inhibit coenzyme A-linked oxidation of fatty acids by isolated rat liver mitochondria. Fukami and Williamson (1971) interpreted the sequence of events elicited by compound 67 as follows: inhibition of β-oxidation of fatty acids, depletion of coenzyme A levels, decreased gluconeogenesis, and hypoglycemia.

Although the branched-chain acid, 2-ethyl-n-caproic acid (68) is a saturated acid, it has been included in this section. Chung et al. (1969) reported that aortic involvement in the development of atherosclerotic lesions in the cholesterol-fed rabbit was reduced from 46.5 to 12.9% by the administration of acid 68. Serum lipid was not affected, but glyceride synthesis in rats was inhibited by compound 68.

XVIII. Compounds Containing Sulfur

Probucol, DH-581, 4,4'-(isopropylidenedithio)bis-(2,6-di-t-butylphenol), (69) has been prepared by NEUWORTH et al. (1970) and found to be the most potent hypolipidemic agent among 37 analogs. KRITCHEVSKY et al. (1971a) observed that compound 69 decreased the severity of atheromata in the cholesterol-fed rabbit at a dose level of 1%. At this dose, serum and liver cholesterol concentration was also decreased. Serum triglyceride levels were variable. MIETTINEN (1972) studied the mode of action of stubstance 69 in patients with familial hypercholesterolemia in a metabolic ward. Serum free- and total cholesterol was reduced in all patients by 27% on average. However, after administration of the drug for 6 to 7 months, the patients tended to show their mean initial high serum cholesterol level. Conformation of this "escape" phenomen in a larger number of patients would detract from the value of this novel hypolipidemic agent.

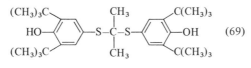

$$(69)$$

Probucol

$$HO-CH_2CH_2-S(CH_2)_{10}-S-CH_2CH_2-OH \quad (70)$$

$$CH_3-SO-CH_2-CH(NH_2)COOH \quad (71)$$

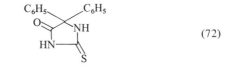

$$(72)$$

A French research group presented another sulfur-containing hypolipidemic agent, bis(hydroxy-ethyl-thio) 1-10-decane, (70). ASSOUS et al. (1972) claimed that compound 70 possessed the same type and degree of hypolipidemic activity as clofibrate (48), but with a lesser degree of toxicity. ROUFFY and LOEPER (1972) gave oral doses of 1.2 to 3.6 g of compound 70 to 77 patients with essential hyperlipoproteinemia. Total serum cholesterol was reduced 15.8% in type II hyperlipoproteinemia, triglyceride 26% in mixed hyperlipemia and 65% in endogeneous hypertriglyceridemia. There were no side effects.

A sulfur-containing amino acid, S-methyl-L-cysteine sulfoxide (71) has been isolated from cabbage. FUJIWARA et al. (1972) reported that substance 71 is a potent anti-hypercholesterolemic agent in the rat when administered at the high doses of 182.2 and 364.4 mg/kg/day for two weeks.

The hypolipidemic effects of diphenylhydantoin and its 2-thio-analog were compared by DALTON and VEREBELY (1972). Oral administration of 5,5-diphenyl-2-thiohydantoin (72) to rats caused a 60 to 80% decrease in serum triglyceride levels, accompanied by an increase in liver and thyroid weight, as well as liver total lipid and phospholipid content. There was a smaller decrease in serum cholesterol and phospholipid levels at lower doses, and elevated serum cholesterol and phospholipid levels when high doses of compound 72 were administered to rats. A hypotriglyceridemic effect was not observed with equivalent doses of 5,5-diphenylhydantoin. The authors suggested that substance 72 lowers serum triglycerides by a mechanism unrelated to its antithyroid properties and differing from that of known antihyperlipidemic agents. Administration of thioamides or thiolactams to rats may often give rise to fatty infiltration of the liver.

XIX. Indole-2-Carboxylic Acids

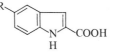

| | Activity: | | |
	hypocholesterolemic,	hypoglycemic	
R = Cl	+	−	(73)
R = H	+	+	(74)
R = Br	+	+	(75)
R = CH$_3$	+	+	(76)
R = OCH$_3$	−	+	(77)

The chlorosubstituted indolecarboxylic acid (73) was found to be the most potent hypocholesterolemic compound in a series of substituted indole-2-carboxylic acids tested by KARIYA et al. (1972). This substance was twice as active as clofibrate (48), and it did not cause hepatomegaly. A single large dose was inactive. The activity was demonstrable upon feeding the substance to rats for 10 days. Triton induced hyperlipemia was not reversed and there was no effect on plasma triglycerides. Thus, the mode of action of substance 73 differs from that of clofibrate. The mode of action of compound 73 was also different from that of nicotinic acid, because norepinephrine-induced lipolysis in isolated fat cells was not inhibited by acid 73. Finally, this acid did not elicit hypoglycemic activity in the rat. In contrast, the methoxy-substituted acid (77) has been reported to reduce plasma glucose levels in fasted rats (see BAUMAN and PEASE, 1969). The authors proposed that the hypoglycemic effect was due to inhibition of gluconeogenesis. Compound 77 did not possess hypocholesterolemic activity. The other three acids, compounds 74 to 76 exhibited both hypocholesterolemic and hypoglycemic activities in the rat.

XX. Hydroxylamine Derivatives

LUDWIG et al. (1967) reported the synthesis and hypocholesterolemic, as well as the antiatherogenic activity of a large number of hydroxylamine derivatives. Only one compound of this series is discussed here, namely N-γ-phenyl-propyl-N-benzyloxy-acetamide, beloxamide, (W-1372, Wallace), (78).

$$C_6H_5-(CH_2)_3-N-OCH_2C_6H_5$$
$$\vert$$
$$COCH_3 \qquad \text{beloxamide} \quad (78)$$

BERGER et al. (1969) compared the activity of compound (78) and clofibrate (48) in rats. The hypocholesterolemic effect of substance 78, unlike that of clofibrate, was found to be greater in rats on a high fat diet. Effects on liver cholesterol and triglycerides, the rapid exchange cholesterol pool, and liver protein also differed. KRITCHEVSKY et al. (1969) reported that administration of substance 78 at a level of 2% in the diet to cholesterol-fed rabbits: inhibited weight gain, did not alter serum cholesterol, raised serum triglycerides, lowered liver cholesterol, inhibited the development of atheromata, and reduced exacerbation of preestablished atheromatous lesions. Upon feeding compound 78 to the rat at a level of 0.3% of diet for 3 weeks, KRITCHEVSKY and TEPPER observed hepatomegaly and a hypotriglyceridemic effect. Serum cholesterol levels were not influenced. Mitochondrial fractions from the livers of the treated rats oxidized more cholesterol-26-^{14}C to radioactive carbon dioxide than did control preparations. However, when equivalent levels of mitochondrial protein were taken, no difference was observed.

A direct antiatherogenic property of compound 78 has been described by BERGER et al. (1970). The authors observed that administration of beloxamide (78) produced regression of the lipid deposits in the heart of rats fed an atherogenic diet.

The drug may not be free of potential hepatotoxic effects. KHANDEKAR et al. (1971) noted that rats receiving oral doses of 5 to 10 mg of beloxamide per day for 3 days developed lipid and liposome accumulation and altered rough-surfaced endoplasmic reticulum in the liver.

XXI. Pyridinolcarbamate

The story of pyridinolcarbamate began more than a decade ago when SHIMAMOTO et al. (1961) announced the antiatherogenic activity of nialamide (79), a monoamine-oxidase inhibitor. The authors thought that this effect of compound 79 may be due to its weak activity as a bradykinin antagonist. Subsequently, SHIMAMOTO et al. (1966) developed their own bradykinin antagonist, pyridinolcarbamate (80) and reported that this new compound prevented the atheromatous changes and deposition of cholesterol in the aortic wall of rabbits fed a high cholesterol diet.

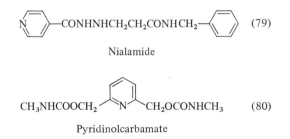

$$N\langle\rangle-CONHNHCH_2CH_2CONHCH_2-\langle\rangle \quad (79)$$

Nialamide

$$CH_3NHCOOCH_2-N-CH_2OCONHCH_3 \quad (80)$$

Pyridinolcarbamate

KRITCHEVSKY and TEPPER (1971) observed that pyridinolcarbamate (80) caused a slight increase in liver size, markedly reduced plasma and liver triglycerides, but did not affect plasma free fatty acid and cholesterol levels in the rat.

The proceedings of an international symposium on Atherogenesis, Thrombogenesis, and Pyridinolcarbamate Treatment was edited by SHIMAMOTO and NUMANO

(1969). This report contains 24 clinical papers on the effect of substance 80 in angina pectoris, coronary heart disease, atherosclerosis obliterans, diabetic retinopathy, and cerebrovascular disease.

Western research groups, in general, were not always able to demonstrate the antiatherogenic effects of pyridinolcarbamate. MALINOW et al. (1972) reported that addition of compound 80 to an atherogenic diet fed to cynomolgous monkeys at a level of 400 to 1000 mg/kg in the food has been found ineffective in preventing the development of cholesterol-induced aortic and coronary atherosclerosis. The same authors, MALINOW et al. (1968), noted that the drug was also found ineffective in preventing atherosclerotic lesions in the squirrel monkey.

Among the dehydrogenase enzymes, increased lactate dehydrogenase activity and decreased ATP-ase activity has been observed in the aortic intima of cholesterol-fed rabbits. MOETTOENEN et al. (1972) showed that pyridinolcarbamate had no effect on the activity of these two enzymes.

HESS et al. (1972) treated 42 patients having atherosclerosis obliterans with pyridinolcarbamate for 3 months. The arterial lesions remained constant in 75% and showed deterioration in 15% of the patients. The authors concluded that pyridinolcarbamate is not an effective antiatherosclerotic agent.

XXII. Eritadenine

A natural compound has been isolated from the edible mushroom Lentinus edodes. The active principle eritadenine (81) was chemically identified as 2(R),3(R)-dihydroxy-4-(9-adenyl)-butyric acid by two independent groups of investigators, CHIBATA et al. (1969) and KAMYA et al. (1969). Eritadenine (81) was formerly called lentinacin or lentysine. TAKASHIMA et al. (1973) reported that compound 81 lowered the plasma levels of cholesterol, triglycerides, and phospholipids in the rat. The substance was found to be more than ten times as active as clofibrate when administered in the diet.

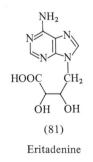

(81)

Eritadenine

DOLE (1961) demonstrated that adenosine inhibited lipolysis in tissues of experimental animals *in vitro*. Adenosine is rapidly deaminated *in vivo*. Therefore, high doses are needed to detect the antilipolytic activity *in vivo*. Phenylisopropyl adenosine (27) resists metabolic deamination and exhibits high potency as an inhibitor of lipid mobilization. Although eritadenine (81) and substance 27 are both derivatives of adenine, their antilipolytic effects may be elicited by totally different mechanisms.

Rokujo et al. (1970) noted that compound 81 reduces serum cholesterol, phospholipids, and triglycerides both in intact rats and in animals fed a high fat diet. Hepatomegaly and changes in liver lipid levels have not been observed.

There has been a flurry of reports of elegant syntheses of eritadenine and analogs. A convenient method of synthesis has been described by Okomura et al. (1971). A few years later Okomura et al. (1974) reported the synthesis of more than 100 analogs of eritadenine. Some compounds were found to be 50 times more active than eritadenine in lowering the serum cholesterol concentration in the rat at a dose of 0.0001% in the diet.

XXIII. Miscellaneous Compounds

Blohm (1972) discussed the hypolipidemic activity of the experimental drug treloxinate, a dibenzo-dioxacin derivative (82). The compound is a ring-closed homolog of the parent acid of SaH-42-348 (50). In rats treloxinate is 8 times as potent as clofibrate in reducing plasma cholesterol levels, and 30 times as potent in lowering plasma triglyceride concentration. The chemistry of treloxinate (82) and related dibenzodioxocin derivatives, as well as their hypocholesterolemic and hypotriglyceridemic activities in Wistar rats were explored by Grisar et al. (1972).

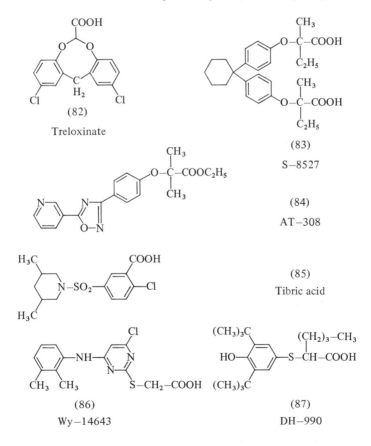

(82) Treloxinate

(83) S–8527

(84) AT–308

(85) Tibric acid

(86) Wy–14643

(87) DH–990

A compound containing two phenoxyacid moieties, S-8527 (83) was introduced by Toki et al. (1973). This dicarboxylic acid elicited a more pronounced reduction of serum cholesterol and triglyceride levels than clofibrate (48) in rats. The hepatomegalic effect was slight. Kritchevsky and Tepper (1973) studied the effect of substance 83 on cholesterol metabolism and liver lipids in rats. The data obtained were consistent with the hypothesis that the mechanism of the hypolipidemic action of S-8527 involves both inhibition of cholesterol synthesis and reduction of lipoprotein release from the liver. However, oxidation of labeled cholesterol to $^{14}CO_2$ by rat liver mitochondria from rats fed clofibrate was significantly higher than that observed in rats fed compound 83.

In the laboratories of Takeda Chemical Industries a new series of substituted 1,2,4-oxadiazoles has been evaluated as hypolipidemic agents by Imai et al. (1973). One compound in this series, possessing the phenoxyisobutyrate as well as the 3-pyridyl groups, has been found to reduce plasma cholesterol levels in the rat. In contrast to clofibrate, substance 84 had little or no effect on plasma triglycerides and phospholipids.

An extensive search for structurally novel hypolipidemic agents in the Pfizer laboratories has led to the potent hypolipidemic sulfamylbenzoic acids. Holland and Pereira (1974) announced that tibric acid (85) was about ten times more potent than clofibrate in the rat. Ryan et al. (1974) treated 40 hyperlipemic (type IV) patients with tibric acid for a period of up to 12 months. Serum triglyceride levels decreased from 262 to 170 mg per 100 ml. There was no effect on serum cholesterol concentration. However, there was an increase in serum creatine phosphokinase levels. Another small clinical trial with tibric acid was conducted by Sirtori et al. (1974) who administered the drug to patients with hyperlipoproteinemia. The new hypolipidemic agent (85) was found to be well tolerated and effective in the patients with type IV hyperlipoproteinemia. The type IIb subjects proved to be rather resistant to treatment with tibric acid.

A potent antihypercholesterolemic agent, in the form of a thioacetic acid derivative has been found in the Wyeth Laboratories. Santilli et al. (1974) reported that the pyrimidinylthio-acetic derivative, Wy-14643 (86) reduced serum cholesterol levels of hypercholesterolemic male rats by 50% at a dosage of 1 mg/rat/day.

Another sulfur-containing acid is the subject of a report that is just as preliminary as the preceding one. During the study of potential metabolites of probucol (69) Wagner (1975) prepared a number of hydroxy-mercaptophenol derivatives. Among them, the tert. butyl-substituted phenylthio-hexanoic acid, DH-990 (87) was found to lower serum cholesterol concentration by 29% in the rat and by 45% in the Rhesus monkey. Rat serum triglyceride levels were diminished by 70% from the control values. Compound 87 also prevented cholesterol deposition in the livers of cholesterol-fed rabbits and prevented the formation of atherosclerotic plaques in their aortas. Clinical studies of this new hypolipidemic agent (87) have been initiated.

XXIV. Cholestyramine

Hepatic biosynthesis of cholesterol in man amounts to approximately 1 to 2 g/day, whereas only about one tenth of this amount is absorbed from the diet. More than 90% of cholesterol leaves the body in the feces in the form of bile acids, predominantly as cholic acid. Bile acids recirculate several times during a day via the entero-hepatic circulation. Removal of bile acids from the intestinal tract with adsorbants affords an effective measure to deplete cholesterol from the rapid exchange pool in those species which cannot synthesize cholesterol fast enough to compensate for the artificial drainage of bile acids. TENNENT et al. (1959) developed for this purpose a high-molecular-weight nonabsorbable, quaternary ammonium-exchange resin known as cholestyramine. The rat and pig are able to compensate fast enough for the loss of bile acid caused by cholestyramine so that reduction of plasma concentration of cholesterol cannot be achieved by the resin. In the rabbit, dog, chicken, and man cholestyramin administration will result in effective depletion of cholesterol from the hepatic and plasma compartments.

That cholestyramine actually increases fecal bile acid excretion in man was first shown by CAREY and WILLIAMSON (1961). These authors recorded an eightfold increase of fecal desoxycholic acid output in a normal man. MIETTINEN (1970) estimates that administration of the resin increased threefold the biosynthesis of cholesterol in the liver and intestines. Type II hypercholesterolemic patients also respond with increased bile acid secretion and cholesterol biosynthesis, but to a lesser degree than normal subjects. NAZIR et al. (1972) performed short-term sterol balance studies in a few patients with familial hypercholesterolemia during treatment with cholestyramine. The observed increment in the acidic fraction of excreted endogenous fecal steroids was greater than that of the neutral sterol fraction.

In the rat the stimulation of the oxidative conversion of cholesterol to bile acids as elicited by cholestyramine coincides with an increased activity of hepatic microsomal cholesterol 7-α-hydroxylase (see BOYD and LAWSON, 1970, and JOHANSSON, 1970).

XXV. Neomycin

Neomycin is an antibiotic mixture from which three components, closely related in their chemistry, neomycin A, B, and C have been separated. Neomycin B, for example, is composed of the units: D-ribose, neamine, and neosamine (see the Merck Index for the structural formula). This antibiotic mixture is readily soluble in water, both in the free base and salt forms.

Neomycin effectively reduces serum cholesterol levels in man and in the chicken. MIETTINEN (1970) reports that this antibiotic is ineffective, or even hypercholesterolemic in the rat. Observations made by FALOON et al. (1969) suggest that the cholesterol lowering effect of oral neomycin in man is due to bile acid binding and removal. The antibiotic action of neomycin is probably not involved, because VAN DEN BOSCH and CLAES (1967) found that the N-methylated derivative, which is devoid of antibacterial activity, equally reduced serum cholesterol levels and markedly increased fecal excretion of neutral sterols and bile acids in man. Both neomycin and its N-methyl analog are unabsorbable, polybasic substances. They precipitate bile acids *in vitro*. Therefore, it has been suggested that they exert their hypocholesterolemic activity in a way similar to that of the insoluble anion exchange resin cholestyramine.

Cholestyramine and neomycin provided suitable tools for the analysis of the turnover curve of radioactive plasma cholesterol. Such studies revealed the presence of rapid and slow turnover-rate compartments of cholesterol in man. The rapid turnover pool contains about 25 g of cholesterol. GOODMAN and NOBLE (1968) administered cholestyramine at a dose of 12 g/day and observed an average decrease of 13% in the plasma cholesterol levels. They also found that the resin produced an increase in the production rate and an even greater increment in the elimination of cholesterol from the rapid turnover pool without a significant alteration of the size of this pool. In contrast, SAMUEL et al. (1968) showed that oral administration of neomycin, 2 g/day, led to a reduction of up to 44% in the rapid-turnover cholesterol pool in man, which was even greater than the decrease in serum cholesterol levels. Later, SAMUEL et al. (1970) observed an impressive average decrease of 38% in serum cholesterol levels in the typical drug-resistant type II patients during treatment with the combined regimen of neomycin and clofibrate.

XXVI. Rifampin

When rifampin was undergoing chronic toxicity studies, WARNER and STEPHENSON (1971) noted that single daily oral doses of 40, 80, and 120 mg/kg of this semisynthetic antibiotic elicited a marked lowering of serum cholesterol levels in the cynomulgus monkey. In contrast to neomycin, rifampin is readily absorbed from the intestinal tract and was shown to be transported in the enterohepatic circulation. Chemically, rifampin is the 3-(4-methylpiperazinyl iminomethyl) derivative of rifamycin, a natural macrolide antibiotic.

XXVII. Concluding Remarks

DEWAR (1972) noted that among patients treated with clofibrate there were fewer sudden deaths and fewer new infarcts. Protection was particularly marked in heavy smokers.

Recent literature on biochemical and enzymic alterations induced by smoking, discloses some correlations that may be relevant to the protective effect of clofibrate.

Epidemiological studies generally will list smoking as a risk factor of atherosclerosis. Nicotine has been assumed to be the offending constituent of the cigarette. Indeed, ARONOW and SWANSON (1969) reported that nicotine is capable of lowering the exercise threshold in angina. GOLDSMITH (1969) however, blamed enhanced atherosclerosis on the carbon monoxide present in cigarette smoke. In the presence of carboxyhemoglobin, oxygen is more strongly bound to hemoglobin. Consequently, there will be less dissociation of oxygen from hemoglobin at a given oxygen tension when carboxyhemoglobin is present in the blood. ASTRUP (1967) and KJELDSEN et al. (1968 and 1969) demonstrated in a series of experiments that carbon monoxide or reduced oxygen tension accelerated, and hyperoxia reversed atheromata in cholesterol-fed rabbits. WHEREAT (1970) interpreted the role of carbon monoxide and other environmental respiratory inhibitors in atherosclerosis by postulating a biochemical mechanism. He proposed that inhibition of cytochrome oxidase will result in a high NADH/NAD ratio. Normally, this ratio is less than 0.1 in the mitochondria of the heart and aorta. Thus, lipid synthesis, which is a reductive process, is negligible in these tissues, because the source of hydrogen, i.e. the level of NADH, is low. When, however, the oxidation of the NADH to NAD in the mitochondrial respiratory chain is impaired, the increased reducing-power of NADH will find an outlet in the increase of fatty acid synthesis and a decrease of fatty acid oxidation. The current concensus is that lipid synthesis in the heart and aortic wall takes place mainly inside the mitochondrion, and the hydrogen donor is NADH. In the adipose tissue and liver, not NADH but NADPH is the source of hydrogen for lipid synthesis, which is carried out in the cytoplasmic space by an extramitochondrial enzyme system.

ASTRUP (1972) reviewed the experimental data on the effects of carbon monoxide, e.g. in tobacco smoke, on the vascular system. Carbon monoxide, at a level of 0.018% in the air, and hypoxia produced identical lesions in the vascular wall of rabbits, indistinguishable from those of spontaneous atherosclerosis.

The hypothesis put forward by WHEREAT (1970) was that carbon monoxide, as well as hypoxia, brings about a high NADH/NAD ratio, which in turn favors lipogenesis and diminishes lipid oxidation. Treatment with clofibrate may counteract these enzymic alterations. PLATT and COCKRILL (1966) reported that the administration of clofibrate to rats resulted in a shift in the hepatic NADH/NAD ratio; in particular, the NAD concentration was raised. It is possible that the same alteration of the NADH/NAD ratio could be induced in the human vascular system by long-term clofibrate treatment.

Inhibition or stimulation of glucose-6-phosphate dehydrogenase (G-6-PD) by chemical agents is another way to modulate the stores of NADH and NADPH. Among the phenoxyisobutyrate-type hypolipidemic agents, compound 56 seemed to stimulate G-6-PD activity; clofibrate also did so to a lesser extent, and nafenopin (51) appeared to exert no influence on G-6-PD activity. Consequently, the selection of a hypolipidemic agent that would stimulate G-6-PD activity less than clofibrate, or even inhibit it, might furnish a potentially more efficacious antiatherosclerotic drug.

The usefulness of clofibrate in the treatment of coronary heart disease associated with atherosclerosis became questionable. Upon the completion of the secondary prevention trials conducted in Scotland and Newcastle DEWAR and OLIVER (1971) commented that the drug seemed to offer protection particularly against sudden death. However, the surprisingly strange observation has been made that the beneficial effect bore no apparent relation to the initial cholesterol levels, nor to the hypolipidemic effect of clofibrate.

The findings of the CORONARY DRUG PROJECT RESEARCH GROUP (1975) about the effectiveness of clofibrate and nicotinic acid in the primary prevention of mortality were scarcely encouraging. Indeed, the poor results will be agonizingly remembered by the avid advocators of hypolipidemic therapy in coronary heart disease for many years to come.

A third and even larger trial of clofibrate has been launched under the auspices of the World Health Organization. The design of this international, cooperative study has been described by HEADY (1973). Before the still outstanding results of this acid test make a shambles of our endeavour, we have to grope for the light at the end of the tunnel. In the meantime, all of the investigators engaged in basic research on lipid metabolism, as well as the medicinal chemist, biochemist, and pharmacologist, should also be prepared to face the justified nagging petulance of the clinicians. Many of them may be inclined to hector us about our aberrations in submitting totally useless, if not outright harmful drugs to be used in painstaking and astronomically expensive clinical trials.

All of us have to ponder the facts. Hyperlipidemia has never been irrefutably identified as a causative factor of atherosclerosis. There is merely a reasonably secure association between the two. The relative ease with which the development of a seemingly good model of atherosclerosis can be induced in experimental animals by cholesterol feeding is a fact. On the human scale the dramatic stages of fatal atherosclerotic heart disease: Hypercholesterolemia, xanthomata, angina pectoris, myocardial infarctions in the youthful Lebanese patients with familial type II hyperlipidemia, as described by KHACHADURIAN (1968) will also remain facts. The interpretation of these findings has been duly generalized, extrapolated, and grossly oversimplified. The resulting plausible conclusion was that hypolipidemic treatment of atherosclerotic heart disease would be a sound and reasonable approach. The more cautious and timid investigators may have simply contended that the lowering of plasma lipid levels in man would allay the atherogenic processes. This hypothesis still may be true and realistic if restricted to the very initial stages of atherogenesis.

The sinuous complexity of lipid metabolism is no excuse for dismissal of the further exploration of already known chemical agents as regulators of lipid metabolism. In the rapid expansion of knowledge we must search for improved agents as well as interpretations that fit the facts better than those previously. To date most of our hypolipidemic agents have been selected by their effects elicited in the liver. In the heart, however, the transport, absorption, storage, and utilization of both lipid and sugar substantially differ from that in the liver. The wealth of knowledge accumulated about the activity of clofibrate in the liver is in sharp contrast to the scarceness of data about its effects in the heart. It is concievable that during the initial stages of atherogenesis the beneficial hepatic effects of a drug such as clofibrate may alleviate the still budding processes of atherogenesis. However, when atherosclerotic heart disease becomes clinically manifest it may be risky, if not fallacious, to resort to the use of a drug that has been explored only for its hepatic effects.

A more careful consideration of the metabolism of the ischemic myocardium may become a cornerstone in the routine management of myocardial infarction. It is known that high concentrations of circulating FFA can themselves induce arrhythmias. High plasma FFA levels also diminish glucose extraction by the ischemic heart. Consequently, reduction of plasma FFA levels will also improve glucose uptake.

The myocardial protective effects of the β-adrenergic blocking agents have been discussed in this review. Recently, the effect of a lipolytic agent from the nicotinic acid series on the human myocardium has been explored by ROWE et al. (1975). This controlled trial revealed that antilipolytic treatment of patients admitted to a coronary-care unit with 5-fluoro-3-hydroxymethyl-pyridine (14) afforded a reduction of elevated plasma FFA to normal levels. When treatment with the lipolysis inhibitor (14) was started within 5 hrs of the onset on the symptoms of myocardial infarction, the number of patients developing ventricular tachycardia was significantly reduced, provided that plasma FFA levels were rapidly lowered and maintained at normal levels for 24 hrs.

In conclusion, both the medicinal chemist and the pharmacologist are now faced with the fresh challenge of finding ways and means to restore the normal responsiveness of the myocardium to catecholamines and to correct deranged insulin-mediated lipid and sugar storage and utilization.

Considering the progress—both negative and positive—made in the course of the past decade, the decision to study the action of chemical agents on lipid metabolism, in the hope that this might lead to the still elusive antiatherosclerotic drugs, appears to have been a sound one. The dedication of the determined students of lipid metabolism will not merely endure, it will prevail.

References

ACHESON, J., HUTCHINSON, E. C.: Controlled trial of clofibrate in cerebral vascular disease. Atherosclerosis **15**, 177—183 (1972).

ADACHI, S., MATSUZAWA, Y., YOKOMURA, T., ISHIKAWA, K., UHARA, S., YAMAMOTO, A., NISHIKAWA, M.: Drug-induced lipidosis (V). Changes in the lipid composition of rat liver and spleen following the administration of hexestrol bi(2-diethylaminoethoxy) ether. Lipids **7**, 1—7 (1972).

AHLQUIST, R. P.: A study of the adrenotropic receptors. Amer. J. Physiol. **153**, 586—600 (1948).

ALFIN-SLATER, R. B., AFTERGOOD, L.: Lipids and the pill. Lipids, **6**, 693—705 (1971).

ALTSCHUL,, R., HOFFER, A., STEPHEN, J. D.: Influence of nicotinic acid on serum cholesterol in man. Arch. Biochem. Biophys. **54**, 558—559 (1955).

ANDERSSON, R., HOLMBERG, S., SVEDMYR, N., ABERG, G.: Adrenergic α and β receptors in coronary vessels in man. Acta med. scand. **191**, 241—244 (1972).

ARESKOG, N. H., ADOLFSSON, L.: Effects of a cardio-selective β adrenergic blocker (I.C.I. 50172) at exercise in angina pectoris. Brit. med. J. **1969** II, 601—603.

ARIYOSHI, T., TAKABATAKE, E.: Effects of phenobarbital, ethanol and ethionine on the content and fatty acid composition of hepatic microsomal phospholipids. Chem. Pharm. Bull. **20**, 170—174 (1971).

ARNOLD, A.: Differentiation of receptors activated by catecholamines. Farmaco. Sci. **29**, 79—100 (1972).

ARONOW, W. S., SWANSON, A. J.: The effect of low-nicotine cigarettes on angina pectoris. Ann. intern. Med. **71**, 599—601 (1969).

ASSOUS, E., POUGET, M., NADAUD, J., TARTARY, G., HENRY, M., DUTEIL, J.: Etude d'un nouvel hypolipidémiant, le bis(hydroxy-éthyl-thio) 1-10 décane: LL 1558. I. Etude toxicologique et pharmacologique. Thérapie **27**, 395—411 (1972).

ASTRUP, P., KJELDSEN, K., WANSTRUP, J.: Enhancing influence of carbon monoxide on the development of atheromatosis in cholesterol-fed rabbits. J. Atheroscler. Res. **7**, 343—354 (1967).

ASTRUP, P.: Pathological effects of moderate carbon monoxide exposure. Staub-Reinhalt. Luft. **32**, 146—150 (1972), Chem. Abs. **77**, 70941 w (1972).

AVOGARO, P., CAPRI, C., CAZZOLATO, G., PAIS, M., TRABUIO, G. F.: Effects of the combination of nicotinic acid and propranolol in very low doses on blood lipids in man. Atherosclerosis **10**, 395—400 (1974).

AZARNOFF, D. L., TUCKER, D. R., BARR, G. A.: Studies with ethyl chlorophenoxyisobutyrate (clofibrate). Metab. Clin. Exp. **14**, 959—965 (1965).

BACH, F. L., BARCLAY, J. C., KENDE, F., COHEN, E.: Nonsteroidal hypocholesterolemic agents. II. The synthesis and serum cholesterol lowering properties of 4-(2'-dialkylaminoalkoxy)-4'-substituted biphenyls. J. med. Chem. **11**, 987—993 (1968).

BAILEY, D. M., WOOD, D., JOHNSON, R. E., McAULIFF, J. P., BRADFORD, J. C., ARNOLD, A.: Lowering of serum lipid levels by "masked" nicotinic acid derivatives. J. med. Chem. **15**, 344—348 (1972).

BARBORIAK, J. J., FRIEDBERG, H. D.: Propranolol and hypertriglyceridemia. Atherosclerosis **17**, 31—35 (1973).

BARNES, B. O.: The coronary drug project. J. Amer. med. Ass. **221**, 918 (1972).

BAUMAN, N., PEASE, B. S.: Effects of 5-methoxyindol-2-carboxylic acid on carbohydrate metabolism. Biochem. Pharmacol. **18**, 1093—1101 (1969).

BEAUMONT, J. L., CARLSON, L. A., COOPER, G. R., FEJFAR, Z., FREDRICKSON, D. S., STRASSER, T.: Classification of hyperlipidemias and hyperlipoproteinemias. Bull. Wld Hlth Org. **43**, 891—908 (1970).

BECHTOL, L. D., WARNER, W. L.: Dextrothyroxine for lowering serum cholesterol. Analysis of data on 6066 patients. Angiology **20**, 565—579 (1969).

BENCZE, W. L., DESTEVENS, G.: Chemical control of hormone action and fertility. Ann. N.Y. Acad. Sci. **136**, 487—522 (1967).

BENCZE, W. L., HESS, R., DESTEVENS, G.: Hypolipidemic agents. In: JUCKER, E. (Ed.): Progress Drug Res., Vol. 13, pp. 217—292. Basel: Birkhaeuser 1969.

BENCZE, W. L., KISIS, B., PUCKETT, R. T., FINCH, N.: The absolute configuration of a hypolipidemic 1-aryl tetralin, nafenopin. Tetrahedron **26**, 5407—5414 (1970).

BENES, P., MENZEL, P., OERTEL, G. W.: Inhibition of glucose-6-phosphate dehydrogenase by steroids. II. Effects of 17-oxo-C 19-steroids upon human placental glucose-6-phosphate dehydrogenase. J. Steroid Biochem. **1**, 291—293 (1970).

BENES, P., FREUND, R., MENZEL, P., STARKA, L., OERTEL, G. W.: Inhibition of glucose-6-phosphate dehydrogenase by steroids. I. Effects of 3-hydroxy-Δ^5-steroids of the C 19 and C 21-series upon human red blood cell glucose-6-phosphate dehydrogenase. J. Steroid Biochem. **1**, 287—290 (1970 a).

BERGER, F. M., DOUGLAS, J. F., LU, G. G., LUDWIG, B. J.: Effect of N-γ-phenylpropyl-N-benzyloxy acetamide (W-1372) and of clofibrate on the lipids of normal and hypercholesterolemic rats. Proc. Soc. exp. Biol. (N.Y.) **132**, 293—297 (1969).

BERGER, F. M., DOUGLAS, J. F., LU, G. G., LUDWIG, B. J.: The effect of N-γ-phenylpropyl-N-benzyloxy acetamide (W-1372) and clofibrate on lipid deposits induced in rats by a high fat diet. Fed. Proc. **29**, 385 abs. 790 (1970).

BERKOWITZ, D.: Clinical experiences with two new lipid lowering agents. Circulation **40** (Suppl. III), 44 (1969).

BERKSON, D. M., STAMLER, J., LINDBERG, H. A., MILLER, W. A., STEVENS, E. L., SOYUGENC, R., TOKICH, T. J., STAMLER, R.: Heart rate: An important risk factor for coronary mortality.—Ten-year experience of the Peoples Gas Co. In: JONES, R. J. (Ed.): Atherosclerosis, Proc. 2nd Internat. Symp., pp. 382—389. Berlin-Heidelberg-New York: Springer 1970.

BIECK, P., FINGERHUT, M., WESTERMANN, E.: Adenosinderivate als Hemmstoffe der Lipolyse *in vivo*. Naunyn-Schmiederbergs Arch. Pharm. **264**, 217—218 (1969).

BIZZI, L., GROSSI, E.: The evaluation of 3-pyridineacetic acid as a hypocholesterolemic substance. Arzneimittel-Forsch. **11**, 265—266 (1961).

BLACK, J. W.: The predictive value of animal tests in relation to drugs affecting the cardiovascular system in man. In: WOLSTENHOLME, G., PORTER, R. (Eds.): Drug responses in man. Symposium at the CIBA Foundation, pp. 111—124. London: Churchill 1967.

BLACK, M. L., RODNEY, G., CAPPS, D. B.: Simultaneous inhibition of alternative pathways of cholesterol biosynthesis by two related hypocholesterolemic agents. Biochem. Pharmacol. **17**, 1803—1814 (1968).

BLOHM, T. R.: Atherosclerosis. Chapter 16. In: HEINZELMAN, R. V. (Ed.): Annual Reports in Medicinal Chemistry, Vol. 7, pp. 169—181. New York: Academic Press 1972.

BOBERG, J., CARLSON, L. A., FROEBERG, S. O., OROE, L.: Effect of a hypolipidemic drug (CH 13437) on plasma and tissue lipids, and on the intravenous fat tolerance in man. Atherosclerosis **11**, 353—360 (1970).

BORENSZTAJN, J., WISSLER, R. W., RUBENSTEIN, A. H.: Regulation of rat heart and adipose tissue lipoprotein lipase activity. Diabetes **21** (Suppl. I), 344 (1972).

BOYD, G. S., LAWSON, M. E.: Studies on the catabolism of cholesterol to bile acids in liver: cholesterol-7α-hydroxylase. In: JONES, R. J. (Ed.): Atherosclerosis. Proc. 2nd Internat. Symp., pp. 286—289. Berlin-New York-Heidelberg: Springer 1970.

BRATTGARD, S. O., BRATTSAND, R., HARTHON, J. G. L.: Resorption, Blutspiegel und Ausscheidung von Meso-inositol-^{14}C-hexanikotinat nach peroraler Gabe an Katzen. Arzeimittel-Forsch. **16**, 145—146 (1966).

BRATTSAND, R., LUNDHOLM, L.: The effect of nicotinic acid and pentaerythritol tetranicotinate upon experimental atherosclerosis in the rabbit. Atherosclerosis **14**, 91—105 (1971).

BRAUN, T., HECHTER, O.: Comparative study of hormonal regulation of adenyl cyclase activity in rat and rabbit fat cell membranes. In: JEANRENAUD, B., HEPP, D. (Eds.): Adipose tissue, regulation and metabolic functions, pp. 11—19. Stuttgart: Thieme 1970.

BRENNER, G., BRENNER, H.: Die Einwirkung von Xanthinolnikotinat auf den Stoffwechsel des Gehirns. Arzneimittel-Forsch. **22**, 754—759 (1972).

BRIDGMAN, J. F., ROSEN, S. M., THORP, J. M.: Complications during clofibrate treatment of nephrotic syndrome hyperlipoproteinemia. Lancet **1972 II**, 506—509.

BROWN, P., BADDELEY, H., READ, A. E., DAVIES, J. D., McGARRY, J.: Sclerosing peritonitis, an unsusual reaction to a β adrenergic blocking drug (practolol). Lancet **1974 II**, 1477—1481.

BRUCE, R. A., COBB, L. A., WILLIAMS, R. H.: Effects of exercise and isoproterenol on free fatty acids and carbohydrates in cardiac patients. Amer. J. Med. Sci. **241**, 59—67 (1961).

BRUNNER, H., HEDWALL, P. R., MEIER, M.: General concepts in the use of β-blockers: The relative roles of specific and nonspecific effects. Naunyn-Schmiedebergs Arch. Pharm. **269**, 219—231 (1971).

BUTCHER, R. W.: The second messenger concept and lipid metabolism. Naunyn Schmiedebergs Arch. Pharm. **269**, 358—372 (1971).

CAREY, J. B., WILLIAMS, G.: Relief of the pruritus of jaundice with a bile-acid sequestering resin. J. Amer. med. Ass. **176**, 432—435 (1961).

CARLSON, L. A.: Inhibition of the mobilization of free fatty acids from adipose tissue. Ann. N.Y. Acad. Sci. **131**, 119—142 (1965).

CARLSON, L. A., EKELUN, L. G., OROE, L.: Clinical and metabolic effects of different doses of prostaglandin E_1 in man. Acta med. scand. **183**, 423—430 (1968).

CARLSON, L. A., HEDBOM, C., HELGSTRAND, E., SJOEBERG, B., STJERNSTROM, N. E.: Pyridines affecting FFA (free fatty acid) mobilization *in vivo*. In: HOLMES, W. L. (Ed.): Advan. Exp. Med. Biol., Vol. 4, pp. 85—92. New York: Plenum Press 1969.

CARLSON, L. A., BUTCHER, R. W., MICHELI, H.: Fat moblilizing lipolysis and levels of cyclic AMP in human and dog adipose tissue. Acta med. scand. **187**, 525—528 (1970).

CARLSON, L. A., HEDBOM, C., HELGSTRAND, E., MISIORNY, A., SJOEBERG, B., STJERNSTROM, N. E., WESTIN, G.: Potential hypolipidemic agents. 1. Synthesis of esters realated to 5-fluoro- and 5-chloronicotinic acid and the corresponding alcohols. Effects on noradrenaline-stimulated free fatty acid mobilization. Acta Pharm. Suec. **9**, 221—228 (1972).

CENEDELLA, R. J.: Effects of Su-13437, a new hypolipidemic drug upon lipogenesis *in vivo*. Pharmacologist **12**, 238 abs. 217 (1970).

CHARMAN, R. C., MATTHEWS, L. B., BRAEULER, C.: Nicotinic acid in the treatment of hypercholesterolemia. A long-term study. Angiology **23**, 29—35 (1972).

CHIBATA, E., OKUMURA, K., TAKEYAMA, S., KOTERA, K.: Lentinacin: a new hypocholesterolemic substance in Lentinus edodes. Experientia (Basel) **25**, 1237—1238 (1969).

CHUNG, T. H., VAHOUNY, G. V., TREADWELL, C. R.: Dietary inhibition of experimental atherosclerosis in rabbits by 2-ethyl-n-caproic acid. J. Atheroscler. Res. **10**, 217—227 (1969).

CONNEY, A. H.: Pharmacological implications of microsomal enzyme induction. Pharm. Rev. **19**, 317—366 (1967).

CONNOR, W. E.: The effects of dietary lipid and sterols on the sterol balance. In: JONES, R. J. (Ed.): Atherosclerosis, Proc. 2nd Internat., Symp., pp. 253—261. Berlin-Heidelberg-New York: Springer 1970.

CORBIN, J. D., KREBS, G.: A cyclic AMP-stimulated protein kinase in adipose tissue. Biochem. biophys. Res. Commun. **36**, 328—336 (1969).

CORBIN, J. D., REIMANN, E. M., WALSH, D. A., KREBS, E. G.: Activation of adipose tissue lipase by skeletal muscle cyclic adenosine 3′,5′-monophosphate-stimulated protein kinase. J. biol. Chem. **245**, 4849—4851 (1970).

CORONARY DRUG PROJECT RESEARCH GROUP: The Coronary Drug Project. Initial findings leading to modifications of its research protocol. J. Amer. med. Ass. **214**, 1303—1313 (1970).

CORONARY DRUG PROJECT RESEARCH GROUP: The Coronary Drug Project. Findings leading to further modifications of its protocol with respect to dextrothyroxine. J. Amer. med. Ass. **220**, 996—1008 (1972).

CORONARY DRUG PROJECT RESEARCH GROUP: The Coronary Drug Project. Findings leading to discontinuation of the 2.5 mg/day estrogen group. J. Amer. med. Ass. **226**, 652—657 (1973).

CORONARY DRUG PROJECT RESEARCH GROUP: Clofibrate and niacin in coronary heart disease. J. Amer. med. Ass. **231**, 360—381 (1975).

COUNCIL ON DRUGS of the American Medical Association: Evaluation of a hypocholesterolemic drug. Dextrothyroxine sodium (Choloxin). J. Amer. med. Ass. **208**, 1014—1015 (1969).

CRAIG, G. M.: A comparison of clofibrate and its derivative methyl clofenapate. Atherosclerosis **15**, 265—271 (1972).

CRAIG, G. M., WALTON, K. W.: Clinical trial of methyl clofenapate (a derivative of clofibrate) in patients with essential hyperlipidemias. Atherosclerosis **15**, 189—198 (1972).

CRATNETTER, D., GEIZEROVA, H.: Effect of clofibrate on lipoprotein lipase. Arch. int. Pharmacodyn. **193**, 73—79 (1971).

DALTON, C., VAN TRABERT, T. C., DWYER, J. X.: Relationship of nicotinamide and nicotinic acid to hypolipidemia. Biochem. Pharmacol. **19**, 2609—2619 (1970).

DALTON, C., VEREBELY, K.: Hypotriglyceridemic activity of 5,5-diphenyl-2-thiohydantoin (DPTH). J. Pharmacol. exp. Ther. **180**, 484—491 (1972).

DAYTON, S., PEARCE, M. L., HASHIMOTO, S., DIXON, W. J., TOMIYASU, U.: A controlled clinical trial of a diet high in unsaturated fat. Circulation **40** (Suppl. 2), 1—63 (1969).

DEDUVE, C., BAUDHUIN, P.: Peroxisomes (microbodies and related particles). Physiol. Rev. **46**, 323—357 (1966).

DEWAR, H. A., OLIVER, M. F.: Secondary prevention trials using clofibrate: A joint commentary on the Newcastle and Scottish trials. Brit. med. J. **1971 I**, 784—786.

DEWAR, H. A.: Long-term therapy of ischemic heart disease. Arzneimittel-Forsch. **22**, 1835—1840 (1972).

DINGMAN, J. F.: Treatment of familial hypercholesterolemia with metyrapone. New Engl. J. Med. **286**, 1214—1215 (1972).

DOLE, V. P.: Effect of nucleic acid metabolites on lipolysis adipose tissue. J. biol. Chem. **236**, 3125—3130 (1961).

DUNCAN, C. H., BEST, M. M.: Stimulation of hepatic synthesis of fatty acids by clofibrate and by a tetralin phenoxyisobutyric acid. Circulation **40** (Suppl. 3), 6 (1969).

DUNCAN, C. H., BEST, M. M.: Effects of a phenolic ether, Su-13437, on serum cholesterol, triglyceride, and transaminase levels of human subjects. Circulation **42**, 859—856 (1970).

EDERER, F., LEREN, P., TURPEINEN, O., FRANTZ, I. D.: Cancer among men on cholesterol-lowering diets. Lancet **1971 II**, 203—206.

EDGREN, R. A., JONES, R. C., PETERSON, D. L.: Biological classification of progestational agents. Fertil. and Steril. **18**, 238—256 (1967).

EDITORIAL: Serum uric acid and coronary heart disease. Lancet **1969 I**, 358.

EFENDIC, S.: Influence of prostaglandin E_1 on lipolysis induced by noradrenaline, isopropyladrenaline, theophylline, and dibutyryl c-AMP in human omental adipose tissue *in vitro*. Acta med. scand. **187**, 503—507 (1970).

FABIAN, H. E. M., CHEMERINSKY, E., MERLO, A. B., IZQUIERDO, J. A.: Effect of propranolol on free fatty acids of mice plasma during passive avoidance test. Psychopharmacologia (Berl.) **30**, 369—374 (1973).

FALLON, H. J., ADAMS, L. L., LAMB, R. G.: A review of studies on the mode of action of clofibrate and β-benzalbutyrate. Lipids **7**, 106—109 (1972).

FALOON, W. W., RUBULIS, A., RUBERT, M.: Cholesterol lowering and fecal bile acid and neutral sterol alteration during oral neomycin. Clin. Res. **17**, 158 (1969).

FITZGERALD, J. D.: Experimental approaches to prophylaxis and treatment of ischemic heart disease. Postgrad. med. J. **47**, 36—43 (1971).

FORREST, W. A.: A total of 254 cases of angina pectoris treated with oxprenolol in hospital practice—a monitored release study. Brit. J. clin. Pract. **26**, 217—222 (1972).

FREDRICKSON, D. S., LEVY, R. I., LEES, R. S.: Fat transport. An integrated approach to mechanisms and disorders. New Engl. J. Med. **276**, 32—44, 94—103, 148—156, 215—226, 273—281 (1967).

FREYSS-BEGUIN, M., VAN RUSSEL, E., LECHAT, P.: Comparative effect of pyridinecarboxylic and piperidinecarboxylic acids on the serum fatty acid content of rats treated with triton WR-1-339. Therapie **25**, 857—862 (1970).

FUJIWARA, M., ITOKAVA, Y., UCHINO, H., INOUE, K.: Anti-hypercholesterolemic effect of a sulfur-containing amino acid, S-methyl-L-cysteine sulfoxide, isolated from cabbage. Experientia (Basel) **28**, 254—255 (1972).

FUKAMI, M., WILLIAMSON, J. R.: On the mechanism of inhibition of fatty acid oxidation by 4-pentenoic acid in rat liver mitochondria. J. biol. Chem. **246**, 1206—1212 (1971).

FUKUSHIMA, H., TOKI, K., NAKATANI, H.: The effect of N-(α-methylbenzyl) linoleamide on experimental atherosclerosis in rabbits. J. Atheroscler. Res. **9**, 57—64 (1969).

FULTON JR., J. E., HSIA, S. L.: Lipid synthesis in human skin and its suppression by ethyl 2-(p-chlorophenoxy)-2-methyl-propionate (clofibrate). Circulation (Suppl. 3) 9 (1969).

FURMAN, R. H.: Endocrine factors in atherogenesis. In: SCHETTLER, F. G., BOYD, G. S. (Eds.): Atherosclerosis, pp. 375—454. Amsterdam: Elsevier 1969.

DE GAGLIARDINO, E. P., DE YASHAN, A. M. G., MONTUORI, E., GAGLIARDINO, J. J.: Effect of a potent hypolipemic agent on glycogen metabolism. Experientia (Basel) **28**, 579—580 (1972).

GAILANI, S., HOLLAND, J. F., GLICK, A.: Effects of boxidine on human sterols and neoplasms. Clin. Pharmacol. Therap. **13**, 91—96 (1972).

GALIMBERTI, P., DEFRANCESCHI, A.: Synthesis of some α-derivatives of isobutyric acid. Gazz. Chim. Ital. **77**, 431—438 (1947); Chem. Abs. **42**, 336 li (1948).

GAUT, Z. N., POCELINKO, R., SOLOMON, H. M., THOMAS, G. B.: Oral glucose tolerance, plasma insulin, and uric acid excretion in man during chronic administration of nicotinic acid. Metabolism **20**, 1031—1035 (1971).

GERRITSEN, G. C., DULIN, W. E.: Development of tachyphylaxis to the antilipolytic, hypoglycemic agent 5-methyl-pyrazol-3-carboxylic acid, U-19425. Proc. Soc. exp. Biol. (N.Y.) **126**, 524—527 (1967).

GILLIS, R. A., MELVILLE, K. I.: Cardiac adrenergic mechanisms in rabbits with experimentally produced coronary atherosclerosis. Atherosclerosis **15**, 71—76 (1972).

GIORGINI, D., PORCELLATI, G.: Inhibition of liver cholesterol biosynthesis by butyric acid derivatives. Farmaco (Pavia) Ed. Sci. **24**, 392—401 (1969).

GLUECK, C. J., SWANSON, F., STEINER, P.: Estrogens and progestins: opposite effects in patients with hyperlipidemia. Clin. Res. **18**, 624 (1970).

GLUECK, C. J.: Effects of oxandrolone on plasma triglycerides and postheparin lipolytic activity in patients with types III, IV and V familial hyperlipoproteinemia. Metab. clin. Exp. **20**, 691—702 (1971).

GLUECK, C. J., SCHEEL, D., FISHBACK, J., STEINER, P.: Progestagens, anabolic-androgenic compounds, estrogens: Effects on triglycerides and postheparin lipolytic enzymes. Lipids **7**, 110—113 (1972).

GLUECK, C. J., SCHEEL, D., FISCHBACK, J., STEINER, P.: Estrogen-induced pancreatitis in patients with previously covert familial type V hyperlipoproteinemia. Metabolism clin. Exp. **21**, 657—666 (1972a).

GOLDFISCHER, S., BIEMPICA, L., KOSOWER, N.: Inhibition by ethyl α-chlorophenoxyisobutyrate (atromid S) of experimental porphyria induced by a single injection of allylisopropylacetamide. Lab. Invest. **26**, 476 (1972).

GOLDSMITH, J. R.: Carbon monoxide and coronary heart disease. Ann. intern. Med. **71**, 199—201 (1969).

GOODMAN, DE WITT, S., NOBLE, R. P.: Turnover of plasma cholesterol in man. J. clin. Invest. **47**, 231—241 (1968).

GORDON, S., CEKLENIAK, W. P.: 1-(2-[4'(trifluoromethyl)-4-biphenyloxy]ethyl)pyrrolidine. A potent hypocholesterolemic agent. J. med. Chem. **11**, 993—996 (1968).

GOULD, R. G., SWYRYD, E. A., COAN, B. J., AVOY, D. R.: Effect of chlorophenoxyisobutyrate (CPIB) on liver composition and triglyceride synthesis in rats. J. Atheroscler. Res. **6**, 555—564 (1966).

GRISAR, J. M., PARKER, R. A., KARYA, T., BLOHM, T. R., FLEMING, R. W.; PETROW, V., WENSTRUP, D. L., JOHNSON, R. G.: Treloxinate and related hypolipidemic 12H-Dibenzo[d,g][1,3]dioxocin-6-carboxylate derivatives. J. med. Chem. **15**, 1273—1278 (1972).

GRUNDY, S. M., AHRENS, JR., E. H.: The effects of unsaturated dietary fats on absorption, excretion, synthesis and distribution of cholesterol in man. J. clin. Invest. **49**, 1135—1152 (1970).

GRUNDY, S. M., AHRENS, JR., E. H., SALEN, G., SCHREIBMAN, P. H., NESTEL, P. J.: Mechanism of action of clofibrate on cholesterol metabolism in patients with hyperlipidemia. J. Lipid Res. **13**, 531—551 (1972).

HAMILTON, J. G., SULLIVAN, A. C., GUTIERREZ, M., MILLER, O. N.: The effect of some analogs of nicotinic acid on the biosynthesis of cholesterol and fatty acids in rat liver. Fed. Proc. **30**, 519 (Abstr. 1810) (1971).

Hartmann, G., Forster, G.: Clinical evaluation of a new hypolipidemic drug, CIBA 13437-SU. J. Atheroscler. Res. **10**, 235—246 (1969).

Havel, R. J.: Catecholamines. In: Paoletti, R., Destevens, G. (Eds.): Lipid pharmacology, Vol. 2 of: Medicinal Chemistry. New York: Academic Press 1964.

Hazzard, W. R., Spiger, M. J., Bagdade, J. D., Bierman, E. L.: Studies on the mechanism of increased plasma triglyceride levels induced by oral contraceptives. New Engl. J. Med. **280**, 471—474 (1969).

Heady, J. A.: A cooperative trial on the primary prevention of ischemic heart disease using clofibrate: design, methods, and progress. Bull. Wld Hlth Org. **48**, 243—256 (1973).

Hess, H., Goossens, N., Keil-Kuri, E., Zollner, R., Meyer, A.: Über die Wirkung von Pyridinolcarbamat auf Blutgerinnung und Thrombolyse bei Patienten mit obliterierender Arteriopathie. Vasa **1**, 206—211 (1972).

Hess, R., Bencze, W. L.: Hypolipidemic properties of a new tetralin derivative (CIBA 13437-SU). Experientia (Basel) **24**, 418—419 (1968).

Hess, R., Maier, R., Staeubli, W.: Evaluation of phenolic ethers as hypolipidemic agents. Effects of CIBA 13437-SU. In: Holmes, W. L. (Ed.): Drugs affecting lipid metabolism. Advanc. Exp. Med. Biol., Vol. 4, pp. 483—489. New York: Plenum Press 1969.

Hess, R., Staeubli, W., Riess, W.: Nature of the hepatomegalic effect produced by ethyl chlorophenoxyisobutyrate in the rat. Nature (Lond.) **208**, 856—858 (1965).

Holcomb, G. N.: Antidiabetics. In: Cain, C. K. (Ed.): Annual reports in medicinal chemistry, 1968, pp. 164—177. New York: Academic Press 1969.

Holland, G. F., Pereira, J. N.: Heterocyclic tetrazoles, a new class of lipolysis inhibitors. J. med. Chem. **10**, 149—154 (1967).

Holland, G. F., Pereira, J. N.: Tibric acid: A new, structurally distinct, hypolipidemic agent. Abs. Papers, Am. Chem. Soc. 168th Meet. MEDI 30 (1974).

Hollobaugh, S. L., Kruger, F. A., Hamwi, G. J.: The effect of a pyrazole derivative on plasma free fatty acids in man. Metab. clin. Exp. **16**, 996—1000 (1967).

Holmes, W. L.: Drugs affecting lipid synthesis. In: Paoletti, R. (Ed.): Lipid Pharmacology, Vol. 2 of Medicinal Chemistry. Destevens, G. (Ed.), pp. 131—184. New York: Academic Press 1964.

Horlick, L., Kudchodkar, B. J., Sodhi, H. S.: Mode of action of chlorophenoxyisobutyric acid on cholesterol metabolism in man. Circulation **43**, 299—309 (1971).

Hucker, H. B., Grady, L. T., Michniewicz, B. M., Stauffer, S. C., White, S. E., Maha, G. E., McMahon, F. G.: Metabolism of a new hypolipidemic agent, 2-acetamidoethyl alpha-(p-chlorophenyl)- alpha-(m-trifluoromethylphenoxy)acetate (halofenate) in the rat, dog, rhesus monkey and man. J. Pharmacol. exp. Ther. **179**, 359—371 (1971).

Huttunen, J. K., Steinberg, D., Mayer, S. E.: Protein kinase activation and phosphorylation of a purified hormone sensitive lipase. Biochem. biophys. Res. Commun. **41**, 1350—1356 (1970).

Illiano, G., Cuatrecasas, P.: Endogenous prostaglandins modulate lipolytic processes in adipose tissue. Nature (Lond.) New Biol. **234**, 72—74 (1971).

Imai, Y., Matsumura, H., Tamura, S., Shimamoto, K.: Biological studies of AT-308. Part 2. Hypocholesterolemic effect of At-308, a new derivative of 1,2,4-oxadiazole, in rats. Atherosclerosis **17**, 131—137 (1973).

Jenner, S., Netter, K. J.: On the inhibition of microsomal drug metabolism by SKF 525A. Biochem. Pharmacol. **21**, 1921—1927 (1972).

Jepson, E. M., Small, E., Grayson, M. F., Bance, G., Billimoria, J. D.: A comparative study of a new drug MK 185 with clofibrate in the treatment of hyperlipidemias. Atherosclerosis **16**, 9—14 (1972).

Johansson, G.: Effect of cholestyramine and diet on hydroxylations in the biosynthesis and metabolism of bile acids. Europ. J. Biochem. **17**, 292—295 (1970).

Julia, M., Baillarge, M., Tchernoff, G.: Sur quelque nouveaux derives aryloxyisobutyriques et apparentes. Bull. Soc. chim. France, **1956**, 776—783.

Kamya, T., Saiton, Y., Hashimoto, M., Seki, H.: Structure and synthesis of lentysine, a new hypocholesterolemic substance. Tetrahadron Letters **1969**, 4729—4732.

Kappas, A., Bradlow, H. L., Gillette, P. N., Levere, R. C., Gallagher, T. F.: A defect of steroid hormone metabolism in acute intermittent porphyria. Fed. Proc. **31**, 1293—1297 (1972).

Karia, T., Grisar, J. M., Wiech, N. L., Blohm, T. R.: Hypocholesterolemic indole-2-carboxylic acids. J. med. Chem. **15**, 659—662 (1972).

KEKKI, M., NIKKILAE, E. A.: Plasma triglyceride turnover during use of oral contraceptives. Metab. Clin. Exp. **20**, 878—889 (1971).

KHACHADURIAN, A. K.: The effect of clofibrate (Atromid S) on the plasma lipids and lipoproteins in various types of hyperlipidemias. Abstracts 3rd International symposium on drugs affecting lipid metabolism, p. 136, Milan, (1968).

KHANDEKAR, J. D., GARG, B. D., KOVACS, K.: Beloxamide effects on the liver ultrastructure in rats. Arch. Path. **92**, 221—230 (1970).

KJELDSEN, K., ASTRUP, P., WANSTRUP, J.: Reversal of rabbit atheromatosis by hyperoxia. J. Atheroscler. Res. **10**, 173—178 (1969).

KJELDSEN, K., WANSTRUP, J., ASTRUP, P.: Enhancing influence of arterial hypoxia on the development of atheromatosis in cholesterol-fed rabbits. J. Atheroscler. Res. **8**, 835—845 (1968).

KLAINER, L. M., CHI, YM., FREIDBERG, S. L., RALL, T. W., SUTHERLAND, E. W.: Adenylcyclase. IV. The effects of neurohormones on the formation of adenosine-3',5'-phosphate by preparations form brain and other tissues. J. biol. Chem. **237**, 1239—1243 (1962).

KOBAYASI, T.: Fine structure of arteriosclerosis induced in rabbit aorta by epinephrine and thyroxine. Acta. path. microbiol. scand. **76**, 193—202 (1969).

KRASNO, L. R., KIDERA, G. J.: Clofibrate in coronary heart disease. Effect of morbidity and mortality. J. Amer. med. Ass. **219**, 845—851 (1972).

KRITCHEVSKY, D., TEPPER, S. A.: Linolexamide (N-cyclohexyl linoleamide) in experimental atherosclerosis in rabbits. J. Atheroscler. Res. **7**, 527—530 (1967).

KRITCHEVSKY, D.: The use of pharmalogic agents in atherosclerosis therapy. Ann. N. Y. Acad. Sci. **149**, 1058—1068 (1968).

KRITCHEVSKY, D., SALLATA, P., TEPPER, S. A.: Effect of D-thyroxine on experimental atherosclerosis in rabbits. Comparison of two preparations. G. Arterioscler. **6**, 267—269 (1968).

KRITCHEVSKY, D., SALLATA, P., TEPPER, S. A.: Influence of ethyl p-chlorophenoxyisobutyrate (CPIB) on establishment and progression of experimental atherosclerosis in rabbits. J. Atheroscler. Res. **8**, 755—761 (1968a).

KRITCHEVSKY, D., SALLATA, P., TEPPER, S. A.: Effect of N-cyclohexyl linoleamide on cholesterol metabolism in rats. Proc. Soc. exp. Biol. (N.Y.) **127**, 132—135 (1968b).

KRITCHEVSKY, D., SALLATA, P., TEPPER, S. A.: Effect of N-gamma-phenylpropyl-N-benzyloxy-acetamide (W-1372) on experimental atherosclerosis in rabbits. Proc. Soc. exp. Biol. (N.Y.) **132**, 303—306 (1969).

KRITCHEVSKY, D., TEPPER, S. A.: Influence of 2-methyl-2- [(p-l, 2,3,4-tetrahydro-l-naphthyl)phenoxy] propionic acid on the oxidation of cholesterol by rat liver mitochondria. Experientia (Basel) **25**, 699—700 (1969).

KRITCHEVSKY, D., TEPPER, S. A., SALLATA, P., KABAKJIAN, J. R., CHRISTOFALO, V. J.: Effect of the ethyl ester and sodium salt of alpha-p-chlorophenoxyisobutyric acid on cholesterol oxidation by rat liver mitochondria. Proc. Soc. exp. Biol. (N.Y.) **132**, 76—82 (1969a).

KRITCHEVSKY, D., TEPPER, S. A.: Oxidation of cholesterol by rat liver mitochondria: Effect of N-gamma-phenylpropyl-N-benzyloxy-acetamide (W-1372, Wallace). Arzneimittel-Forsch. **20**, 584—585 (1970).

KRITCHEVSKY, D., Tepper, S. A.: Influence of pyridinolcarbamate on oxidation of cholesterol by rat liver mitochondria. Arzneimittel-Forsch. **21**, 146—147 (1971).

KRITCHEVSKY, D., TEPPER, S. A., VESSELINOVITCH, D., WISSLER, R. W.: Cholesterol vehicle in experimental atherosclerosis. Part II. Peanut oil. Atherosclerosis **14**, 53—64 (1971).

KRITCHEVSKY, D., KIM, H. K., TEPPER, S. A.: Influence of 4,4'-(isopropylidenedithio) bis (2,6-di-tert.-butylphenol) (DH-581) on experimental atherosclerosis in rabbit. Proc. Soc. exp. Biol. (N.Y.) **136**, 1216—1221 (1971a).

KRITCHEVSKY, D., TEPPER, S. A.: Effect of 2-acetamidoethyl-(p-chlorophenyl), (m-trifluoromethylphenoxy)acetate (halofenate) on cholesterol oxidation by rat liver mitochondria. Proc. Soc. exp. Bid. (N.Y.) **139**, 1284—1287 (1972).

KRITCHEVSKY, D., TEPPER, S. A.: The influence of 1,1- bis [4'-(1''-carboxy-l''-methylpropoxy)-phenyl] cyclohexane (a new aryloxy compound, S-8527) on cholesterol metabolism in rats. Atherosclerosis **18**, 93—99 (1973).

KUPIECKI, F. P.: Stimulation of lipolysis by inhibition of lipid mobilization. Fed. Proc. **29**, 879 abs. 3704 (1970).

KURUP, C. K. R., AITHAL, H. N., RAMASARMA, T.: Increase in hepatic mitochondria on administration of ethyl alpha-p-chlorophenoxyisobutyrate to the rat. Biochem. J. **116**, 773—779 (1970).

LAMBERT, D. M. D.: Beta blockers and life expectancy in ischemic heart disease. Lancet **1972 I**, 793—794.

LANGNER, T., LEVY, R. I.: Accute muscular syndrome associated with administration of clofibrate. New Engl. J. Med. **279**, 856—858 (1968).

LASSERS, B. W., WAHLQVIST, M. L., KAIJSER, L., CARLSON, L. A.: Relationship in man between free fatty acids and myocardial metabolism of carbohydrate substrates. Lancet **1971 II**, 448—452.

LEFKOWITZ, R. J., LEVEY, G. S.: Norepinephrine: Dissociation of beta receptor binding from adenylate cyclase activation in solubilized myocardium. Life Sci. **11**, part II, 821—828 (1972).

LENGSFELD, H., GEY, K. F.: Mechanism of the plasma cholesterol depression in fasted rats by beta-pyridylcarbinol. In: BERG, G. (Ed.): Hyperlipidaemien, Symposium 1970. p. 82—90. Stuttgart: Georg Thieme 1971.

LENZ, P. H., FLEISCHMAN, A. I.: Hypolipidemic effect of 2-methyl-2 p-(1,2,3,4-tetrahydro-1-naphthyl)phenoxy propionic acid (Su-13437) in rats with natural endogenous hypertriglyceridemia. Lipids **6**, 783—785 (1971).

LEON, A. S., WHITE, F. C., BLOOR, C. M., SAVIANO, M. A.: Reduced myocardial fibrosis after dimethylsulfoxide (DMSO) treatment of isoproterenol-induced myocardial necrosis in rats. Amer. J. med. Sci. **261**, 41—45 (1971).

LEVEY, G. S., EPSTEIN, S. E.: Myocardial adenyl cyclase. Activation by thyroid hormones and evidence for two adenyl cyclase systems. J. clin. Invest. **48**, 1663—1669 (1969).

LINDGREN, I.: Angina pectoris. A clinical study with special reference to neurosurgical treatment. Acta med. scand. Suppl. **243**, 11—203 (1950).

LIPSON, M. J., NAIMI, S., PROGER, S.: Synergistic effect of propranolol and nicotinic acid on the inhibition of plasma free fatty acid release in the dog. Circulation Res. **28**, 270—276 (1971).

LLOYD-MOSTYN, R. H., LEFEVRE, D., LORD, P. S., DOIG, E., KRIKLER, D. M.: The effects of beta adrenergic blocking agents on serum lipids. Atherosclerosis **14**, 283—287 (1971).

LOTTI, B., VEZZOSI, O.: Derivati pirazolici ad attivita ipoglicemizzante. Farmaco (Pavia) Ed. Sci. **27**, 313—316 (1972).

LOVRIEN, F. C., STEELE, A. A., BROWN, J. D., STONE, D. B.: Effect of amitriptyline on lipolyis and cyclic AMP concentration in isolated fat cell. Metab. clin. Exp. **21**, 223—229 (1972).

LUDWIG, B. J., DUERSCH, F., AUERBACH, M., TOMECZEK, K., BERGER, T. M.: The synthesis of hydroxylamine derivatives possessing hypocholesterolemic activity. J. med. Chem. **10**, 556—564 (1967).

MALINOW, M. R., MCLAUGHLIN, P., PERLEY, A.: The effects of pyridinolcarbamate on induced atherosclerosis in cynomulgus monkeys (Macaca ira). Atherosclerosis **15**, 31—36 (1972).

MALINOW, M. R., PERLEY, A., MCLAUGHLIN, P.: The effects of pyridinolcarbamate on aortic and coronary atherosclerosis in squirrel monkeys (Saimiri sciurea). J. Atheroscler. Res. **8**, 455—461 (1968).

MANCHESTER, J. R., SHELBURNE, J. C.: Propranolol-induced decrease in the oxygen affinity of hemoglobin. Science **175**, 1372—1373 (1972).

MARAGOUDAKIS, M. E., HANKIN, H., WASVARY, J. M.: On the mode of action of lipid lowering agents. VII. In vivo inhibition and reversible binding of hepatic acetyl coenzyme A carboxylase by hypolipidemic drugs. J. biol. Chem. **247**, 342—347 (1972).

MARAGOUDAKIS, M. E., HANKIN, H., WASVARY, J. M.: Acetyl coenzyme A carboxylase inhibition in genetically obese mice. Fed. Proc. **31**, 475 abs. 1468 (1972a).

MARMO, E., IMPERATORE, A., CAPUTI, A., CATALDI, S.: Sugli effetti ipocolesterolemizzanti ed ipolipidemizzanti del p-clorofenossi-alpha-isobutirrato di 3-idrossimetilpiridina cloridato. Farmaco (Pavia) Ed. Prat. **26**, 557—584 (1971).

MARMORSTON, J., MOORE, F. J., HOPKINS, C. E., KUZMA, O. T., WEINER, J.: Clinical studies of long term estrogen therapy in men with myocardial infarction. Proc. Soc. exp. Biol. (N.Y.) **110**, 400—408 (1962).

MAROKO, P. R., KJEKSHUS, J. K., SOBEL, B. E., WATANABE, T., COWELL, J. W., ROSS, J. JR., BRAUNWALD, E.: Factors influencing infarct size following experimental coronary artery occlusion. Circulation **43**, 67—82 (1971).

MATSUZAKI, F., KOMIYAMA, M., SHIZUME, K.: Hypotriglyceridemic action of synthetic ACTH. Endocr. Jap. **18**, 511—516 (1971).

MATTSON, F. H., VOLPENHEIM, R. A.: Hydrolysis of fully esterified alcohols containing from one to eight hydroxyl groups by the lipolytic enzymes of rat pancreatic juice. J. Lipid Res. **13**, 325—328 (1972).

MAY, B., LEINWEBER, W.: Antilipolytic action of phenylisopropyl adenosine in man. Naunyn-Schmiedebergs Arch. Pharmak. **269**, 467—468 (1971).

MAYER, S., MORAN, N.C., FAIN, J.: The effect of adrenergic blocking agents on some metabolic actions of catecholamines. J. Pharmacol. exp. Ther. **134**, 18—27 (1961).

MCDEWITT, D. G., SHANKS, R. G., HADDEN, D. R., MONTGOMERY, D. A. D., WEAVER, J. A.: The role of the thyroid in the control of heart rate. Lancet **1968 I**, 998—1000.

MCINTOSH, D. A. D., TOPHAM, J. C.: A comparison of mouse and rat liver enzymes and their response to treatment with various compounds. Biochem. Pharmacol. **21**, 1025—1029 (1972).

MEAD, J. F.: Dietary polyunsaturated fatty acids as potential toxic factors. Chem. Technol. **1972**, 70—71 (1972).

MIETTINEN, T. A.: Drugs affecting bile acid and cholesterol excretion. In: JONES, R. J. (Ed.): Atherosclerosis, Proc. 2nd Internat. Symp., pp. 508—515, Berlin-Heidelberg-New York: Springer 1970.

MIETTINEN, T. A.: Mode of action of a new hypocholesterolemic drug (DH-581) in familial hypercholesterolemia Atherosclerosis **15**, 163—176 (1972).

MIETTINEN, M., KARVONEN, M. J., TURPEINEN, O., ELOSNO, R., PAAVILAINEN, E.: Effect of cholesterol lowering diet on mortality from coronary heart-disease and other causes. Lancet **1972 II**, 835—838.

MOETTOENEN, M., PANTIO, M., NIEMINEN, L.: Enzyme histochemical observations on the effect of pyridinolcarbamate on cholesterol-induced atherosclerosis. Atherosclerosis **15**, 77—82 (1972).

MORGAN, J. P., BIANCHINE, J. R., HSU, T. H., MARGOLIS, S.: Hypolipidemic, uricosuric and thyroxine-displacing effects of MK-185 (Halofenate). Clin. Pharmacol. Ther. **12**, 517—524 (1971).

MOSHER, L. R.: Nicotinic acid side effects and toxicity. A review. Amer. J. Psychiat. **126**, 1290—1296 (1970).

MRHOVA, O., GRAFENETTER, D., JANDA, J., LINHART, J.: Effect of atromid-S on the activity of vascular enzymes in rats. Biochem. Pharmacol. **20**, 3069—3076 (1971).

MUELLER, H., AYRES, S. M., GIANELLI, S. Jr., CONKLIN, E. F., MAZZARA, J. T., GRACE, W. J.: Cardiac performance and metabolism in shock due to acute myocardial infarction in man: Response to catecholamines and mechanical cardiac assist. Transactions N. Y. Acad. Sci. Ser. II, **34**, 309—333 (1972).

MUELLER, H. S., AYRES, S. M., RELIGA, A., EVANS, R. G.: Propranolol in the treatment of acute myocardial infarction. Effect on myocardial oxygenation. Circulation **49**, 1078—1087 (1974).

NAKATANI, H., AONO, S., SUZUKI, Y., FUKUSHIMA, H., NAKAMURA, Y., TOKI, K.: The effect of (-)N-α [Phenyl-β-(p-tolyl)ethyl] linoleamide on experimental atherosclerosis in rabbits. Atherosclerosis **12**, 307—311 (1970).

NAKATANI, H., FUKUSHIMA, H., WAKIMURA, A., ENDO, M.: N-cyclohexyl linoleamide: Metabolism and cholesterol-lowering effects in rats. Science **153**, 1267—1269 (1966).

NAZIR, D. J., HORLICK, L., KUDCHODKAR, B. J., SODHI, H. S.: Mechanism of action of cholestyramine in the treatment of hypercholesterolemia. Circulation **46**, 95—102 (1972).

NESTEL, P. J.: Practolol in the treatment of ischemic heart pain: results of a controlled trial. Med. J. Aust. **59 I**, 1033—1035 (1972).

NESTEL, P. J., AUSTIN, W.: The effect of ethyl p-chlorophenoxyisobutyrate (CPIB) on the uptake of triglyceride fatty acids, activity of lipoprotein lipase and lipogenesis from glucose in fat tissue of rats. J. Atheroscler. Res. **8**, 827—833 (1968).

NETTER, K. J., JENNER, J., KAJUSCHKE, K.: Über die Wirkung von Metyrapon auf den mikrosomalen Arzneimittelabbau. Naunyn-Schmiedebergs Arch. Pharmakol. **259**, 1—16 (1967).

NEUWORTH, M. B., LAUFER, R. J., BARNHART, J. W., SEFRANKA, J. A., MCINTOSH, D. D.: Synthesis and hypocholesterolemic activity of alkylidenedithio bisphenols. J. med. Chem. **13**, 722—725 (1970).

Nordoey, A., Roedset, J. M.: Platelet function and platelet phospholipids in patients with hyper-betalipoproteinemia. Acta med. scand. **189**, 385—389 (1971).

Okumura, K., Oine, T., Yamada, Y., Tomie, M., Adachi, T., Nagura, T., Kawazu, M., Mizogu-chi, T., Inoue, I.: Synthetic studies on eritadenine. I. Reactions of some purines with the 2,3-0-protected dihydroxybutyrolactone. J. Org. Chem. **36**, 1573—1579 (1971).

Okomura, K., Matsumoto, K., Fukamizu, M., Yasuo, H., Taguchi, Y., Sugimara, Y, Inoue, I., Seto, M., Sato, Y., Takamura, N., Kanno, T., Kawazu, M., Mizoguchi, T., Saito, S., Tak-ashima, K., Takayema, S.: Synthesis and hypocholesterolemic activities of eritadenine deriva-tives. J. med. Chem. **17**, 846—855 (1974).

Oliver, M. F.: Hormones. In: Schettler, F. G., Boyd, G. S. (Eds.): Atherosclerosis, pp. 865—881. Amsterdam: Elsevier 1969.

Oliver, M. F.: Oral contraceptives and myocardial infarction. Brit. med. J. **1970 II**, 210—213.

Oliver, M. F., Boyd, G. S.: Influence of reduction of serum lipids on prognosis of coronary heart disease. A five-year study using estrogens. Lancet **1961 II**, 499—505.

Olsson, A. G., Oroe, L., Roessner, S.: Clinical and metabolic effects of pentaerythritol tetranico-tinate (perycit) and a comparison with plain nicotinic acid. Atherosclerosis **19**, 61—73 (1974).

Osman, M. M., Toppozada, H. K., Ghanem, M. H., Guergis, F. K.: The effect of an oral contra-ceptive on serum lipids. Contraception **5**, 105—118 (1972).

Paget, G. A.: Experimental studies of the toxicity of atromid with particular reference to fine structural changes in livers of rodents. J. Atheroscler. Res. **3**, 729—736 (1963).

Palonkangas, R., Vihko, V.: Effects of noradrenaline, propranolol, and corticosterone on the concentration of free fatty acids in the plasma of the titmouse (Parus major). Comp. Biochem. Physiol. B. **40**, 813—818 (1971).

Parker, J. O., West, R. O., Case, R. B., Chiong, M. A.: Temporal relationships of myocardial lac-tate metabolism, left ventricular function, and S-T segment depression during angina precipi-tated by exercise. Circulation **40**, 97—111 (1969).

Parsons, Jr. W. B.: Studies of nicotinic acid use in hypercholesterolemia. Arch. intern. Med. **107**, 653—667 (1961).

Parsons, Jr. W. B.: Chemotherapy of hyperlipidemia. Mayo clin. Proc. **40**, 822—829 (1965).

Pearce, M. L., Dayton, S.: Incidence of cancer in men on a diet high in polyunsaturated fat. Lancet **1971 I**, 464—467.

Pereira, J. N., Holland, G. F.: The development of resistance to a potent lipolysis inhibitor, 3-methylisoxazole-5-carboxylic acid. J. Pharmacol. exp. Ther. **157**, 381—387 (1967).

Pereira, J. N., Holland, G. F.: Studies of the mechanism of action of p-chlorophenoxyisobutyrate (CPIB). In: Jones, R. J. (Ed.): Atherosclerosis, Proc. Int. Symp. 2nd 1969. 549—554, New York: Springer 1970.

Pereira, J. N., Holland, G. F., Hochstein, F. A., Gilgore, S., Defelice, S., Pinson, R.: The phar-macology of 5-(3-pyridyl)-tetrazole, a hypocholesterolemic lipolysis inhibitor. J. Pharm. exp. Ther. **162**, 148 (1968).

Pereira, J. N., Mears, G. A.: Biphasic effect of nicotinic acid on plasma FFA (free fatty acid) levels. Life Sci. **10**, 1—8 (1971).

Persson, B., Schroeder, G., Hood, B.: Lipoprotein lipase activity in human adipose tissue. Assay methods. Atherosclerosis **16**, 37—49 (1972).

Platt, D. S., Cockrill, B. L.: Changes in the liver concentrations of the nicotinamide adenosine dinucleotide coenzymes and in the activities of oxido-reductase enzymes following treatment of the rat with ethyl chlorophenoxy isobutyrate (Atromid S). Biochem. Pharmacol. **15**, 927—935 (1966).

Platt, D. S., Cockrill, B. L.: Liver enlargement and hapatotoxicity: An investigation into the effects of several agents on rat liver enzyme activities. Biochem. Pharmacol. **16**, 2257—2270 (1967).

Ponari, O., Civardi, E., Poti, R.: Action of some beta blockers on plasma fibrinolysis *in vitro* and *in vivo* in man. Arneimittel-Forsch. **22**, 629—631 (1972).

Preziosi, P., Loscalzo, B., Marmo, E., Miele, E.: Decrease of blood cholesterol and lipids by components with a pyridine core: Relations between structure and activity and between dos-age and effectiveness. Arch. ital. Sci. Farmacol. **11**, 386—389 (1961).

PRICHARD, B. N. C., GILLAM, P. M. S.: Assessment of propranolol in angina pectoris. Clinical dose response curve and effect on electrocardiogram at rest and on exercise. Brit. Heart J. **33**, 473—480 (1971).

RAAFLAUB, J.: Zur Umwandlung von β-pyridylcarbinol in Nikotinsäure im tierischen Organismus. Experientia (Basel) **22**, 258—259 (1966).

RAFTERY, E. B.: Cutaneous and ocular rections to Practolol. Brit. med. J. **1974 IV**, 653.

RAO, L. G. S.: Urinary steroid excretion patterns after acute myocardial infarction. Lancet **1970 II**, 390—391.

RATTI, G., DEFINA, E.: Effect of 3-pyridineacetic acid on serum lipids. Lancet **1959 II**, 917.

REDEL, J., COTTET, J.: Action hypocholesterolemiante de quelques acides acetiques disubstitues. C. R. Acad. Sci. (Paris) **236**, 2553—2555 (1953).

RIEDE, U. N., ETTLIN, CH., VON ALLMEN, R., ROHR, H. P.: Vergleichende ultrastrukturell-morphologische Untersuchung zwischen der Leberparenchymzelle der Wistarratte (Rattus norvegicus) und der Wüstenratte (Meriones crassus). Naunyn-Schmiedebergs Arch. Pharmakol. **272**, 336—350 (1972).

RIEGEL, E. R., ZWILGMEYER, F.: Chelidonic acid. Org. Synth. coll. **2**, 126—128 (1943).

RODBELL, M.: The fat cell in mid-term: Its past and future. In: JEANRENAUD, R., NEPP, D. (Eds.): Adipose tissue, regulation and metabolic function, pp. 1—4. Stuttgart: G. Thieme 1970.

ROESSNER, S., LARSSON-COHN, U., CARLSON, L. A., BOBERG, J.: Effects of an oral contraceptive agent on plasma lipids, plasma lipoproteins, the intravenous fat tolerance and the postheparin lipoprotein lipase activity. Acta med. scand. **190**, 301—305 (1971).

ROKUJO, T., KIKUCHI, H., TENSHO, A., TSUKITANI, Y., TAKENAWA, T., YOSHIDA, K., KAMIYA, T.: Lentysine. A new hypolipidemic agent from a mushroom. Life Sci. **9**, II. 379—385 (1970).

ROUFFY, J., LOEPPER, J.: Effets hypolipidémiants du bis (hydroxy-2-éthylthio) 1,10-décane (LL1558). A partir de 77 observations d'hyperlipidémie essentielle. Thérapie **27**, 433—444 (1972).

ROWE, M. J., DOLDER, M. A., KIRBY, B. J., OLIVER, M. F.: Effect of a nicotine acid analogue on raised plasma free-fatty-acids after acute myocardial infarction. Lancet **1973 II**, 814—817.

ROWE, M. J., NEILSON, J. M. M., OLIVER, M. F.: Control of ventricular arrhythmias during myocardial infarction by antilipolytic treatment using a nicotinic acid analogue. Lancet **1975 I**, 295—300.

RUEGAMER, W. R., RYAN, N. T., RICHERT, D. A., WESTERFELD, W. W.: The effects of p-chlorophenoxyisobutyrate on the turnover rate and distribution of thyroid hormone in the rat. Biochem. Pharmacol. **19**, 613—624 (1969).

RYAN, J. R., JAIN, A. K., MCMAHON, F. G.: Tibric acid treatment of hyperlipemia. Clin. Pharmacol. Ther. **15**, 218 (1974).

SACHS, B. A., WOLFMAN, L.: Effect of oxandrolone on plasma lipids and lipoproteins in patients with disorders of lipid metabolism. Metab. clin. Expt. **17**, 400—410 (1968).

SALVADOR, R. A., ATKINS, G., HABER, S., KOZMA, C., CONNEY, A. H.: Effect of phenobarbital and chlorcyclizine on the development of atherosclerosis in the cholesterol-fed rabbit. Biochem. Pharmacol. **19**, 1975—1981 (1970).

SALVADOR, R. A., HABER, S., ATKINS, C., GOMMI, B. W., WELCH, R. M.: Effect of clofibrate and 1-methyl-4-piperidyl bis (p-chlorophenoxy)acetate (Sandoz 42—348) on steroid and drug metabolism by rat liver microsomes. Life Sci. **9**, part II. 397—407 (1970 b).

SAMUEL, P., HOLTZMAN, C. M., MEILMAN, E., PERL, W.: Effect of neomycin on exchangeable pools of cholesterol in the steady state. J. clin. Invest. **47**, 1806—1818 (1968).

SAMUEL, P., HOLTZMAN, C. M., MEILMAN, E., SEKOWSKI, I.: Reduction of serum cholesterol and triglyceride levels by the combined administration of neomycin and clofibrate. Circulation **41**, 109—114 (1970).

SANTILLI, A. A., SCOTESE, A. C., TOMARELLI, R. M.: A potent antihypercholesterolemic agent: [4-chloro-6-(2,3 xylidino)-2-pyrimidinylthio] acetic acid (Wy-14643). Experientia (Basel) **30**, 1110 (1974).

SCHACHT, U., GRANZER, E.: On the effect of the hypolipidemic phenyl ether CH 13437 on the liver metabolism of the rat. Biochem. Pharmacol. **19**, 2963—2971 (1970).

SCHACHT, U., SCHMITT, K., GRANZER, E.: Comparative studies on the action of the optical antipodes of the hypolipidemic aryloxyalkanoic acid CH-13437, on liver enzymes of the rat. Experientia (Basel) **28**, 788—790 (1972).

SCHENKMAN, J. B., WILSON, B. J., CINTI, D. L.: Diethylaminoethyl 2,2-diphenylvalerate HCl (SKF-525 A) *in vivo* and *in vitro* effects of metabolism by rat liver microsomes—formation of an oxygenated complex. Biochem. Pharmacol. **21**, 2373—2383 (1972).

SCHRAVEN, E., NITZ, R. E., TROTTNOW, D.: Beeinflussung der Resorption von Magnesium-28 durch Dehydrocholsäure und Nikotinsäure. Arzneimittel-Forsch. **22**, 511—513 (1972).

SCHWABE, U., EBERT, R.: The effect of heterocyclic inhibiting agents of lipolysis on the activity of 3',5'-AMP-phosphodiesterase. Naunyn Schmiedebergs Arch. Pharmak. **263**, 251—252 (1969).

SCHWEPPE, J. S., JUNGMANN, R. A.: The effects of hypocholesterolemic agents on cholesterol esterification *in vitro*. Proc. Soc. exp. Biol. (N. Y.) **136**, 449—451 (1971).

SCOTT, P. J., HURLEY, P. J.: Effect of clofibrate on low density lipoprotein turnover in essential hypercholesterolemia. J. Atheroscler. Res. **9**, 25—34 (1969).

SHARMA, B., MEERAN, M. K., GALVIN, M. C., TULPULE, A. T., WHITAKER, W., TAYLOR, S. H.: Comparison of adrenergic β blocking drugs in angina pectoris. Brit. med. J. **1971 III**, 152—155.

SHEFER, S., HAUSER, S., MOSBACH, E. H.: Stimulation of cholesterol 7-α-hydroxylase by phenobarbital in two strains of rats. J. Lipid Res. **13**, 69—70 (1972).

SHIMAMOTO, T., NUMANO, F., FUJITA, T.: Atherosclerosis-inhibiting effect of an antibradykinin agent pyridinolcarbamate. Amer. Heart J. **71**, 216—227 (1966).

SHIMAMOTO, T., NUMANO, F. Editors. "Atherogenesis." Proceedings of the first international symposium on atherogenesis, thrombogenesis and pyridinolcarbamate treatment. Amsterdam: Excerpta Medica Found 1969.

SHIMAMOTO, T., YAMAZAKI, H., INOUE, M., FUJITA, T., SAGAWA, N., SUNAGA, T., ISHIOKA, T.: Discovery of antithromboembolic effect of nialamide-protection of siliconlike property of blood vessels by nialamide. Proc. Japan Acad. **36**, 240—245 (1960). Chem. Abstr. **55**, 799d (1961).

SHIO, H., SHAW, J., RAMWELL, P.: Relation of cyclic AMP to the release and actions of prostaglandins. Ann. N. Y. Acad. Sci. **185**, 327—335 (1971).

SIMONS, L. A., MYANT, N. B.: The effect of D-thyroxine on the metabolism of cholesterol in familial hyperbetalipoproteinemia. Atherosclerosis **19**, 103—117 (1974).

SIRTORI, C., HURWITZ, A., SABIH, K., AZARNOFF, D. L.: Clinical evaluation of **MK-185**: A new hypolipidemic drug. Lipids **7**, 96—99 (1972).

SIRTORI, C. R., ZOPPI, S., QUARISA, D., AGRADI, E.: Clinical evaluation of tibric acid, a new hypolipidemic agent. Pharmacol. Res. Commun. **6**, 445—456 (1974).

SKIDMORE, I. F., SCHOENHOEFER, P. S., KRITCHEVSKY, D.: Effects of nicotinic acid and some of its homologs on lipolysis, adenylcyclase, phosphodiesterase and cyclic AMP accumulation in isolated fat cells. Pharmacology **6**, 330—338 (1971).

SMITH, A. F., MACFIE, W. G., OLIVER, M. F.: Clofibrate, serum enzymes, and muscle pain. Brit. med. J. **1970 II**, 86—88.

SNEYD, J. G. T., CORBIN, J. D., PARK, C. R.: The role of cyclic AMP in the action of insulin. In: BACK, N., MARTINI, L., PAOLETTI, R. (Eds.): pp. 367—376. Pharmacology of hormonal polypeptides and proteins, New York: Plenum Press 1968.

SODHI, H. S., KUDSCHODKAR, B. J., HORLICK, L., WEDER, C. H.: Effects of chlorophenoxyisobutyrate on the synthesis and metabolism of cholesterol in man. Metab. clin. Exp. **20**, 348—359 (1971).

SODHI, H. S., KUDCHODKAR, B. J., HORLICK, L.: Effect of chlorophenoxyisobutyrate on the metabolism of endogenous glycerides in man. Metab. clin. Exp. **20**, 309—318 (1971 a).

SOLYOM, A.: Effect of androgens on serum lipids and lipoproteins. Lipids **7**, 100—105 (1972).

SPERANZA, M. L., GAITI, A., DE MEDIO, G. E., MONTANINI, I., PORCELLATI, G.: The inhibition of mitochondrial respiration by beta benzal butyric acid and the possible relationship to cholesterol biosynthesis. Biochem. Pharmacol. **19**, 2737—2743 (1970).

SRIKANTIA, S. G., RAO, K. S. J., PRASAD, P. S. K.: Effect of C-17 alkylated steroid methandrostenolone on plasma lipids of normal subjects. Amer. J. med. Sci. **254**, 201—204 (1967).

STAMLER, J., PICK, R., KATZ, L. N., PICK, A., KAPLAN, B. M., BERKSON, D. M., CENTURY, D.: Effectiveness of estrogens for therapy of myocardial infarction in middle-aged men. J. Amer. med. Ass. **183**, 632—638 (1963).

STEINBERG, D.: Drugs inhibiting cholesterol biosynthesis, with special reference to clofibrate. In: JONES, R. J. (Ed.): Atherosclerosis, Proceedings second internat. symp. pp. 500—508. Berlin-Heidelberg-New York: Springer 1970.

STOKES, T. WYNN, Y.: Serum lipids in women on oral contraceptives. Lancet. **1971 II**, 677—680.

SUTHERLAND, E. W.: Studies on the mechanism of hormone action. Science **177**, 401—408 (1972).

TAGGART, P., CARRUTHERS, M.: Suppression by oxprenolol of adrenergic response to stress. Lancet. **1972 II**, 256—258.

TAGGART, P., CARRUTHERS, M., SOMERVILLE, W.: Electrocardiogram, plasma catecholamines and lipids, and their modification by oxprenolol when speaking before an audience. Lancet **1973 II**, 341—346.

TAKASHIMA, K., IZUMI, K., IWAI, H., TAKEYAMA, S.: The hypocholesterolemic action of eritadenine in the rat. Atherosclerosis **17**, 491—502 (1973).

TAMASI, G., BORSY, J., PATTHY, A.: Comparison of the antilipemic effect of nicotinic acid and 3-methylpyrazol-5-carboxylic acid in rats. Biochem. Pharmacol. **17**, 1789—1794 (1968).

TENNENT, D. M., SIEGEL, H., ZANETTI, M. E., KURON, G. W., OTT, W. H., WOLF, F. J.: Reduction of plasma cholesterol in animals with bile acid sequestrants. Circulation **20**, 969—970 (1959).

THORP, J. M., WARING, W. S.: Modification of metabolism and distribution of lipids by ethyl chlorophenoxyisobutyrate. Nature (Lond.) **194**, 948—949 (1962).

THORP, J. M.: Hypocholesterolemic and other effects of methyl clofenapate, a novel derivative of clofibrate. In: JONES, R. J. (Ed.): Atherosclerosis, Proceedings second internat. symp. pp. 541—544. Berlin-Heidelberg-New York: Springer 1970.

TIMMS, A. R., KELLY, L. A., HO, R. S., TRAPOLD, J. H.: Laboratory studies of l-methyl-4-piperidyl bis(p-chlorophenoxy)acetate, SaH 42—348, a new hypolipidemic agent. Biochem. Pharmacol. **18**, 1861—1871 (1969).

TOKI, K., NAKAMURA, Y., AGATSUMA, K., NAKATANI, H., AONO, S.: Hypolipidemic action of a new aryloxy compound (S-8527) in rats. Atherosclerosis **18**, 101—108 (1973).

TOLMAN, E. L., TEPPERMAN, H. M. TEPPERMAN, J.: Effect of ethyl p-chlorophenoxyisobutyrate on rat adipose tissue lipoprotein lipase activity. Amer. J. Physiol. **218**, 1313—1318 (1970).

TRACY, R. E.: That estrogens may have nothing to do with coronary heart deaths. Fed. Proc. **25**, 665 (Abstr. 2690) (1966).

VAN DEN BOSCH, J. F., CLAES, P. J.: Correlation between the bile-salt precipitating capacity of derivatives of basic antibiotics and their cholesterol lowering effect in vivo. Progr. biochem. Pharmacol. **2**, 97—104 (1967).

VAUGHAN, M.: An in vitro effect of triiodothyronine on rat adipose tissue. J. clin. Invest. **46**, 1482—1491 (1967).

VAUGHAN, M., MURAD, F.: Adenyl cyclase activity in particles from fat cells. Biochemistry **8**, 3092—3099 (1968).

WAGNER, E. R.: The hypolipidemic properties of 3,5-di-t-butyl-4-hydroxymercaptophenol derivatives. Abs. Papers 169th Meeting Am. Chem. Soc. MEDI 33 (1975).

WARNER, S. D., STEPHENSON, M. F.: Hypocholesterolemic effect of rifampin in the monkey (M. fasicularis). Proc. Soc. exp. Biol. (N.Y.) **137**, 194—195 (1971).

WEEKS, J. R.: Biological significance of prostaglandins with special reference to their effects on metabolism. Naunyn-Schmiedebergs Arch. Parmak. **269**, 347—357 (1971).

WEGENER, M., GEBHARDT, W., CLOTTEN, R.: Blutfette nach medikamentöser beta-Rezeptoren-Blockade. Dtsch. med. Wschr. **94**, 904—908 (1969).

WENKE, M.: Adrenotropic drugs in lipid mobilization. In: JEANRENAUD, B., HEPP, D. (Eds.): Adipose tissue, regulation and metabolic function, pp. 55—62. Stuttgart: Thieme 1970.

WESTERFELD, W. W., ELWOOD, J. C., RICHERT, D. A.: Effect of clofibrate on the handling of dietary and liver fat. Biochem. Pharmacol. **21**, 1117—1125 (1972).

WESTERFELD, W. W., RICHERT, D. A., RUEGAMER, W. R.: The role of the thyroid hormone in the effect of p-chlorophenoxyisobutyrate in rats. Biochem. Pharmacol. **17**, 1003—1016 (1968).

WESTERMANN, E., STOCK, K.: Inhibitors of lipolysis. Potency and mode of action of alpha and beta adrenolytics, methoxamine derivatives, prostaglandin E, and phenylisopropyl adenosine. In: JEANRENAUD, B., HEPP, D. (Eds.): Adipose tissue, regulation and metabolic functions, p. 47—54. Stuttgart: G. Thieme 1970.

WEXLER, B. C.: Protective effects of propranolol on isoproterenol-induced myocardial infarction in arteriosclerotic and nonarteriosclerotic rats. Atheriosclerosis **18**, 11—42 (1973).

WHEREAT, A. F.: Is atherosclerosis a disorder of intramitochondrial respiration? Ann. intern. Med. **73**, 125—127 (1970).

WHITTINGTON-COLEMANN, P. J., CARRIER, O. JR., DOUGLAS, B. H.: The effects of propranolol on cholesterol-induced atheromatous lesions. Atherosclerosis **18**, 337—345 (1973).

Wilhelm, M., Hedwall, P., Meier, M.: o-Allyloxy-pheonoxy-propanolamine, eine neue Gruppe adrenergischer beta-Receptoren-Blocker. Experientia (Basel) **23**, 651—652 (1967).

Wilson, D. E., Lees, R. S.: Metabolic relationships among plasma lipoproteins. Reciprocal changes in the concentrations of very low and low density lipoproteins in man. J. clin. Invest. **51**, 1051—1057 (1972).

Wilson, D. F., Watson, O. F., Peel, J. S., Turner, A. S.: Trasicor in angina pectoris: a double blind trial. Brit. med. J. **2**, 155—157 **1969 II**.

Windmueller, H. G., Levy, R. I.: Total inhibition of hepatic beta-lipoprotein production in the rat by orotic acid. J. biol. Chem. **242**, 2246—2254 (1967).

Witiak, D. T., Whitehouse, M. W.: Species differences in the albumin binding of 2,4,6-trinitrobenzaldehyde, chlorophenoxyacetic acids, 2(4′-hydroxybenzeneazo)benzoic acid and some other acidic drugs — the unique behavior of rat plasma albumin. Biochem. Pharmacol. **18**, 971—977 (1969).

Zampaglione, N. G., Lech, J. J., Calvert, D. N.: Diethyl chelidonate, a specific inhibitor of hormone-stimulated lipolysis. Biochem. Pharmacol. **19**, 2157—2164 (1970).

Zoellner, N., Wolfram, G.: Die Behandlung der Xanthome bei Hypercholesterinaemie. Hautarzt **21**, 443—445 (1970).

CHAPTER 10

The Rationale for Hypolipemic Therapy

I. D. FRANTZ

A satisfactory discussion of this topic is impossible at the present time. Only opinions based on incomplete evidence can be expressed. The field has been in this unhappy state for many years. It is not likely to change until additional clinical trials of primary and secondary prevention have been completed. How can one weigh the benefits of treatment against its dangers if one is not sure that reduction in blood lipids causes any reduction at all in the risk of heart attack and stroke? The best that can be done is to put together the evidence from all the trials that have been completed, include a factor based on data from animal experimentation, and arrive at a not very well educated guess.

Some workers do not feel this absolute requirement for experimental proof. They find the epidemiological evidence convincing in itself. According to this point of view, no cause and effect relationship can be logically postulated between the low prevalence of coronary heart disease in certain populations and the other characteristics of these populations, except for the low blood cholesterol concentrations and reduced dietary intake of animal fat. It is probably true that these circumstances favor the diet-lipid hypothesis as the most likely explanation of the observed facts. Nevertheless, the chain of logic is incomplete. Other as yet unidentified environmental factors may play the major role. Definitive clinical trials are necessary. Probably no single trial can be sufficient. Bias in the design, unknown to the investigator and undetectable in his reports, can lead to false conclusions from almost any scientific experiment.

In the paragraphs to follow, an evaluation of some of the more important clinical trials completed to date will be attempted. A point of view towards hypolipidemic therapy will be presented, based on the degree of certainty that now exists as to the value of such therapy, the risks associated with omitting treatment, and the potential dangers of the treatments themselves.

Cholesterol Lowering by Diet

References could be given to a few comparatively small clinical trials of cholesterol lowering diets completed several years ago for which statistically significant beneficial results were reported. The design of these trials was condemned by the statisticians, and it is better that they be disregarded. More recently, several more reliable dietary trials demand serious consideration. Without examining an exhaustive list or suggesting that trials not mentioned did not add valuable information, let us consider those trials which have most strongly influenced my own attitudes.

Leren carried out a randomized 5-year secondary prevention trial in 412 men aged 30 through 67. The serum cholesterol fell an average of 17.6% in the experimental group, and 3.7% in the controls. The combined incidence of myocardial reinfarction, acquired angina pectoris, and sudden death was reduced in the experimental group by 29%, a result which was statistically significant. The incidence of the comparatively soft end-point, acquired angina pectoris, was reduced by 66%, while myocardial reinfarction was reduced by only 33%, and sudden death was not affected. Despite this circumstance, the Oslo trial creates a prima facie case for the beneficial effect of a diet low in cholesterol and saturated fats in male survivors of a myocardial infarction.

Another important dietary trial is that of Dayton et al. They divided 846 male residents of a Veterans Administration domiciliary, aged 50 through 89, randomly into a control group and a group maintained on a cholesterol lowering diet. The mean fall in serum cholesterol of the experimental group below the controls was 12.7%. After more than 8 years, 119 "hard" events attributable to atherosclerosis had occurred in the control group, and 85 in the treated group. Although a wider variety of events was included in this analysis than in the original definition of the end-point, the observed difference was statistically significant.

Miettinen et al. have presented preliminary results from a 12 year dietary trial in two mental hospitals in Finland. In this trial, the experimental diet was fed in one hospital for 6 years, and the control diet in the other. The diets in the two hospitals were then reversed. Although full details are not yet available, the trends in this trial also seem to have been favorable.

Two British trials of secondary prevention were less encouraging. Rose et al. randomized 80 male survivors of myocardial infarction into 3 groups. One group served as controls. The other two groups were given a dietary supplement of 80 g/day of either olive oil or corn oil, on a double-blind basis. The serum cholesterol levels in the corn oil group fell, averaging about 26 mg/100 ml below the pre-trial values. Serum cholesterol levels did not change significantly in the two other groups. After 2 years, 75% of subjects in the control group remained free of major cardiac events, but only 57% of the olive oil group and 52% of the corn oil group. Although the numbers are too small to establish an unfavorable effect of the oils, the probability that the observed results would have occurred in the presence of a substantial true difference in the opposite direction is very slight.

The other London trial, conducted by a Research Committee to the Medical Research Council, involved 393 male survivors of a single myocardial infarct, aged 60 or under at the time of the infarct. 199 of these men, allocated randomly to the experimental group, were given a diet low in saturated fats and containing 85 g of soy bean oil daily. The diet of the 194 control subjects was unchanged. Time of the trial for the different subjects varied from 2 to $6^3/_4$ years. The results were mildly suggestive of a favorable effect of the diet, but much less so than in the OSLO trial. For example, 74 "first relapses" occurred in the control group and 62 in the experimental, but the number of major relapses was 39 and 40, respectively. The number of fatal reinfarctions was 25 in each group. The average fall in serum cholesterol after 6 months was 22% for the experimental group and 6% for the control group, so that the disappointing outcome can scarcely be attributed to inadequate lipid response.

Conclusions from the Dietary Trials

If one considers all of the trials that have been conducted, the weight of evidence definitely favors the conclusion that dietary treatment is beneficial. DAYTON has reviewed several more of the smaller trials, not discussed above, and most of these were ostensibly highly successful. They achieved statistical significance because of apparent reductions in event rates far exceeding those reported for the larger trials which we have considered in more detail. This circumstance is disquieting. Although it is often difficult to suggest a reasonable hypothesis to account for totally incorrect results, one is left in a state of mind favoring the attitude of many statisticians, that results are to be disregarded unless all of the niceties of experimental design to avoid bias were meticulously followed. An extension of this pessimism is to wonder if in the larger, more tightly designed studies, the mildly favorable results obtained might have been due to the effects of similar bias, largely but not completely eliminated in the design.

Cholesterol Lowering with Clofibrate

One primary prevention trial and two secondary prevention trials have been reported with clofibrate.

KRASNO and KIDERA pair-matched 1001 men free of coronary heart disease for risk factors. One group was treated with clofibrate for 39 months, and the other group was untreated. An additional 67 men with known coronary heart disease were also included. Among this latter group, there were 20 events in the controls and only 8 in the treated group. In the men previously free of coronary heart disease, 19 events occurred in the controls, and 5 in the group receiving clofibrate. If the groups are combined, the difference is significant at the 0.001 level. A surprising feature of this trial was that there seemed to be no relation between the protective effect of clofibrate and its lipid lowering action. Although 37% of men with hypercholesteremia and 29% of men with hypertriglyceridemia failed to show a lipid response to clofibrate, none of the events occurred in this group.

Two comparatively large secondary prevention trials with clofibrate have been reported. In the first of these, by a group of physicians of the Newcastle upon Tyne region, 497 patients with ischemic heart disease were assigned randomly to clofibrate and placebo groups. The trial was double-blind, and the patients were observed for 5 years. Sixty new infarcts occurred in the placebo group, and only 37 in the clofibrate group. Forty-eight cardiac deaths occurred in the placebo group, and 27 in the clofibrate group. As in the Krasno trial, protection by clofibrate could not be related to the cholesterol response. Protection was greatest in patients with angina. It was greater against sudden death than against non-fatal infarct, in sharp contrast to the results of the Oslo dietary trial. It was greater for smokers than for non-smokers. To quote the authors, "It would seem likely, therefore, that clofibrate has its most striking, though not its only, effect in ischaemic heart disease by protecting patients who suffer from angina from succumbing to dysrhythmic sudden deaths, and this effect is mediated through some other mechanism than its cholesterol- and triglyceride-reducing properties".

The other secondary prevention trial was reported by a research committee of the Scottish Society of Physicians. 350 patients were assigned to clofibrate and 367 to placebo. The trial lasted for 6 years, but some patients were observed for no longer than about 18 months. There were 34 deaths and 25 non-fatal infarcts in the clofibrate group. The numbers for the placebo group were 38 and 41, respectively. When calculated as a rate per 1200 patient-months, the only statistically significant difference was in the group of patients who presented initially with both angina and a previous infarct (clofibrate, 3.84; placebo, 8.82). In most other sub-groups, the trend was favorable.

DEWAR and OLIVER presented a joint commentary on the Newcastle and Scottish trials. Their conclusions: "Clofibrate is a beneficial drug in the treatment of ischaemic heart disease in patients who first present with angina and in those who continue to have angina after mycardial infarction". "The effect of the drug in reducing serum lipids was maintained up to five years, but in neither trial has it been possible to prove that this effect and the improved prognosis are causally related".

FRIEDEWALD and HALPERIN have written a commentary on the Newcastle and Scottish trials. They have pointed out some of the imperfections in design, discrepancies between the results, and possible pitfalls in interpretation, "without denying that, in some respects, clofibrate treatment appears to be beneficial".

A series of letters appeared in the correspondence section of the British Medical Journal, critical of various aspects of the Newcastle and Scottish trials. These culminated in a more conservative interpretation of the results by Dr. OLIVER:

"These trials were not specifically designed to study the effects of the drug in patients with angina. They have shown an unexpected result, which was derived from relatively small numbers when one considers the sample size usually required for secondary prevention trials."

"The main conclusion of both trials was that clofibrate had a beneficial effect in reducing mortality and, to a lesser extent, morbidity in patients with angina. This may well prove to be accurate, but it is my view that further appraisal is necessary and confirmation should be sought."

Extrapolations between Different Lipid Lowering Techniques

Suppose that a given hypolipidemic drug is ultimately shown beyond doubt to lower the incidence of cardiovascular events attributable to atherosclerosis. Do we have a right to conclude that other drugs or diets which produce similar effects on the blood lipids will be similarly beneficial? One would be inclined to believe that a conclusion based on such an extrapolation would be more likely to be right than wrong. And yet the results of both the United Air Lines (Krasno) and Newcastle trials suggest that properties of clofibrate other than its lipid lowering action produced the benefits. Such a result is a priori extremely unlikely. It is no more likely than that one of the millions of known organic compounds should have been chosen at random and been found effective. And yet the facts at present point to the conclusion that this unlikely but happy accident has occurred. In this particular instance, we have no right to extrapolate to other lipid lowering regimes.

What about extrapolations from primary to secondary prevention, and vice versa? Most observers would be inclined to doubt that a regimen found capable of preventing first infarcts would necessarily be beneficial in the face of disease which had already progressed to the point of serious complications. The opposite extrapolation seems more permissible, with the reservation that antiarrhythmic effects would probably be less important in the absence of a previous infarct.

Summary of Opinions

The rationale for hypolipemic therapy is a highly controversial topic. It is not surprising that it should have generated expressions of opinion ranging all the way from complete rejection of any form of hypolipemic therapy to insistence that elevated blood lipids should always be treated. Without claiming that bias did not enter into the selection, I would like to present some recent quotations from scientists whose contributions to and long association with the field entitle them to be heard.

We begin with two quotations from J. C. LA ROSA:

"While experts disagree as to when the cholesterol level becomes dangerous in terms of atherogenesis, a prudent policy is to prescribe dietary therapy in all patients who have cholesterol levels between 240 and 300 mg per 100 ml or triglyceride levels over 250 mg per 100 ml. If diet is not sufficient to lower cholesterol below 280 mg and triglycerides below 250 mg, drug therapy should be seriously considered."

"With adequate attention to diagnosis, the majority of patients can be successfully treated. Whether treatment will ultimately prevent or reverse atherosclerosis remains to be seen. However, because the risks are so high and the therapy is relatively benign, it seems prudent to make every effort to seek out and identify patients with hyperlipoproteinemia and to give them adequate treatment."

The following quotation from RICHARD HAVEL is representative of the skepticism still widespread among responsible investigators, despite the apparently successful clinical trials cited above:

"The effort involved in these studies implies provisional acceptance by many investigators of a causal relationship between the level of certain serum lipids and the development of the atherosclerotic lesion and its ischemic complications. Although such a relationship is supported by studies of the pathogenesis of the atherosclerotic plaque in experimental animals, by epidemiological studies among and within population groups, and by the association of ischemic arterial disease with hereditary hyperlipidemic disorders, proof that either prevention or amelioration of coronary heart or peripheral atherosclerotic vascular disease follows successful lipid-lowering remains to be obtained."

The current edition of GOODMAN and GILMAN's textbook contains a chapter entitled, "Drugs used in the Prevention and Treatment of Atherosclerosis". The title seems to imply acceptance of the value of treatment, but the author, HOWARD A. EDER, while obviously inclined towards that position, recognizes the limitations of our current knowledge: "While there is as yet no definitive proof that the lowering of plasma lipoprotein concentrations by either drugs or diet is effective in the prevention of atherosclerosis, either in the total population or in high risk patients, there is strong indirect evidence to suggest that such therapeutic efforts are reasonable."

The Inter-Society Commission for Heart Disease Resources recommended, among many other things, "that adequate resources be committed to accomplish changes in diet to prevent or control hyperlipidemia ..." It also recommended "coordinated plans for large-scale, long-term trials to determine the effect of various interventions particularly diet modification on the rates of premature atherosclerotic diseases in the United States". The first of these recommendations would seem to prejudge the outcome of the trials called for in the second. Nevertheless, my own conclusions are not greatly different.

Conclusions

In dealing with patients and disease, one cannot wait for the evidence to become conclusive, but must adopt a position on the basis of facts available at a given moment. The following conclusions are subject to continuous modification, as knowledge grows.

1. The evidence in favor of hypolipidemic therapy is insufficient to preclude the conduct of additional randomized, double-blind clinical trials. Current public attitudes and dietary patterns remain compatible with such trials. The medical profession has a strong obligation to obtain the additional evidence needed to settle this matter conclusively.

2. If circumstances do not permit entry of a given patient with hyperlipoproteinemia into a randomized trial, the physician is justified in prescribing dietary treatment, supplemented with drugs if needed to obtain an adequate blood lipid response.

3. Persons with blood lipid concentrations average for the western world are well advised to adopt a diet lower in saturated fats and cholesterol, pending the outcome of ongoing research.

References

Controlled trial of soya-bean oil in myocardial infarction: Report of a research committee to the Medical Research Council. Lancet **1968 II**, 693—700.

Dayton, S., Pearce, M. L., Hashimoto, S., Dixon, W. J., Tomiyasu, U.: A controlled clinical trial of a diet high in unsaturated fat. Circulation **39** and **40**, Suppl. 2, II-1-63 (1969).

Dewar, H. A., Oliver, M. F.: Secondary prevention trials using clofibrate: a joint commentary on the Newcastle and Scottish trials. Brit. med. J. **1971 IV**, 784—786.

Eder, H. A.: Drugs used in the prevention and treatment of atherosclerosis, in Goodman, L. S., Gilman, A. (Eds.): The pharmacological basis of therapeutics, pp. 764—772, 4th Ed. New York: Macmillan 1970.

Friedewald, W. T., Halperin, M.: Clofibrate in ischemic heart disease. Ann. intern. Med. **76**, 821—823 (1972).

Group of Physicians of the Newcastle upon Tyne Region: Trial of clofibrate in the treatment of ischaemic heart disease. Brit. med. J. **1971 IV**, 767—775.

Havel, R. J., Kane, J. P.: Drugs and lipid metabolism. Ann. Rev. Pharm. **13**, 287—308 (1973).

Inter-Society Commission for Heart Disease Resources: Primary prevention of the atherosclerotic diseases. Circulation **42**, A-55—A-95 (1970).

KRASNO, L. R., KIDERA, G. J.: Clofibrate in coronary heart disease. Effect on morbidity and mortality. J. Amer. med. Ass. **219**, 845—851 (1972).

LA ROSA, J. C.: Hyperlipoproteinemia. 3. Drug Therapy. Postgrad. Med. **52**, 128—132 (1972).

LEREN, P.: Effect of plasma cholesterol lowering diet in male survivors of myocardial infarction. Acta med. scand. Suppl. 466 (1966).

MIETTINEN, M., TURPEINEN, O., KARVONEN, M. J., ELOSUR, R., PAAVILAINEN, E.: Effect of cholesterol-lowering diet on mortality from coronary heart-disease and other causes. A twelve-year clinical trial in men and women. Lancet **1972 II**, 835—838.

OLIVER, M. F.: Trial of clofibrate. Brit. med. J. **1972 II**, 227.

Research Committee of the Scottish Socity of Physicians: Ischaemic heart disease: a secondary prevention trial using clofibrate. Brit. med. J. **1971 IV**, 775—784 (1971).

ROSE, G. A., THOMAS, W. B., WILLIAMS, R. T.: Corn oil in treatment of ischaemic heart disease. Brit. med. J. **1965 I**, 1531—1533.

TURPEINEN, O., MIETTINEN, M., KARVONEN, M. J., ROINE, P., PEKKARINEN, M., LEHTOSUO, E. J., ALIVIRTA, P.: Dietary prevention of coronary heart disease: Long-term experiment. Amer. J. clin. Nutr. **21**, 255—276 (1968).

Author Index

Page numbers in *italics* refer to bibliography.

Numbers shown in square brackets are the numbers in the bibliography

Subject Index

Handbuch der experimentellen Pharmakologie/
Handbook of Experimental Pharmacology
Heffter—Heubner, New Series